VIOLENCE AND CRIME

This book examines the critical connections between criminal justice and public health perspectives on violence and crime. Violent crime involves not only criminal justice agencies, but social agencies, community groups, and public and private healthcare organizations. The authors provide a broad overview of prevalent forms of violence, focusing on how criminal justice and public health perspectives converge in the examination of and response to these issues.

The book looks at the nexus of public health with problems as varied as assaultive violence, child abuse, rape and sexual abuse, interpersonal violence, elder abuse, suicide, police violence, teenage bullying, workplace violence, firearm injuries, and opioid addiction. The authors lay out a structure for an epidemiological approach to studying violent crime and offer policy recommendations for using both criminal justice and public health approaches to prevent violence.

This volume spotlights the connections between violent crime and public health and urges a consideration of public health in efforts to prevent and control violent crime. It is ideal for courses on violence in criminology, criminal justice, sociology, and social work, and an invaluable tool for practitioners, policymakers, researchers, advocates, and community volunteers in criminal justice, public health, and social service.

James F. Anderson received a Ph.D. in criminal justice from Sam Houston State University and an M.S. in criminology from Alabama State University. He has taught criminal justice and criminology courses for over 30 years to undergraduate, graduate, and doctoral students. He is currently Professor in the Department of Criminal Justice and Criminology at East Carolina University. His areas of research include crime and public health, epidemiological approaches to crime, alternatives to incarceration, elderly and child abuse, intimate personal violence, and criminological theory. He is the author of several books, book chapters, and journal articles on criminal justice-related issues.

Kelley Reinsmith-Jones received a Ph.D. in leadership from Gonzaga University and an M.S. in social work from Eastern Washington University. She is Associate Professor and Graduate Program Director in the School of Social Work at East Carolina University.

While there, she created and taught a series of leadership development courses with funds awarded by the BB&T Leadership Center. Prior to teaching in North Carolina, she taught as an adjunct for Eastern Washington University in the social work and substance abuse departments. She also held an administrative position in public mental health working closely with social workers, psychiatrists, and care teams while specializing in managed care, residential care, and state/community psychiatric care. She was director of a HUD SPINS grant that provided housing and other services to migrant workers with HIV or AIDS, working closely with public health providers. In Alaska, she worked primarily in creating and providing substance abuse prevention, intervention, treatment, and aftercare services to youth, ages 14–24 years, and their families. She worked for the Juneau Recovery Hospital and was an affiliate staff of Bartlett Regional Hospital.

Tazinski P. Lee received a Ph.D. in public policy and administration from Jackson State University and an M.S. in criminal justice from Grambling State University. Professor Lee has taught criminal justice, criminology, and public administration courses for over 30 years. She is currently Professor and Head of Criminal Justice at Grambling State University. Her research focuses on race, crime, and gender, female sex offenders, and public policy. She has published in several journals in the areas of public health, race and ethnicity, alternatives to incarceration, and others.

VIOLENCE AND CRIME

A Public Health Perspective

James F. Anderson, Kelley Reinsmith-Jones and Tazinski P. Lee

Routledge
Taylor & Francis Group

NEW YORK AND LONDON

Designed cover image: Getty Images

First published 2026
by Routledge
605 Third Avenue, New York, NY 10158

and by Routledge
4 Park Square, Milton Park, Abingdon, Oxon, OX14 4RN

Routledge is an imprint of the Taylor & Francis Group, an informa business

ISBN: 9781032446066 (hbk)
ISBN: 9781032446059 (pbk)
ISBN: 9781003373001 (ebk)

DOI: 10.4324/9781003373001

Typeset in Sabon
by Newgen Publishing UK

The use of any figure or data taken from NIH does not represent an endorsement from NIH.

CONTENTS

1 Introduction   1

2 Epidemiology and Criminology of Violence   26

3 Data Sources for Victimization   73

4 Assaultive Violence and Public Health   99

5 Child Abuse and Public Health   135

6 Rape and Sexual Assault and Public Health   187

7 Intimate Partner Violence and Public Health   224

8 Elderly Abuse and Public Health   264

9 Suicide and Public Health   295

10 Police Violence and Public Health   332

11 Teenage Bullying and Public Health   375

12 Workplace Violence and Public Health   402

13 Firearm Injuries and Public Health   436

14 Opioid Addiction and Public Health   485

15 Toward an Epidemiological Approach to Study Violence and Crime   524

Index   *564*

1
INTRODUCTION

Introduction

After agreeing to visit a sorority sister, Michelle booked a flight to Chicago. Three weeks after exiting the *O'Hare International Airport*, she took a shuttle to the rental car center to take possession of the vehicle she reserved to drive to her friend's suburban apartment. However, in the car rental garage, Michelle was accosted, robbed, and sexually assaulted at gun point by two men. Because of the surveillance at the airport and rental car center, police were able to quickly apprehend her attackers who were arrested and charged with robbery and sexual assault. At trial, Michelle was able to identify and give eyewitness testimony about the circumstances surrounding the crime which helped the district attorney build a strong case against the defendants. Subsequently, the jury found the accused men guilty, and they were given a 25-year sentence. While this example may satisfy the requirements for criminal justice, the event did not end there for Michelle, since she was hospitalized after the initial victimization, not to mention she experienced several negative health consequences from the encounter that included being tested for STIs, depression, trauma, and counseling to cope in the aftermath. To some experts, violence and crime do not always end with criminal justice responses, since some acts of violence spill over into the healthcare systems (Anderson et al., 2017).

Available statistics from the *Uniform Crime Reports* (UCR) reveal that violent crime continued to increase into 2022 (Berk, 2023) including mass shootings where four or more deaths occurred in a single criminal episode. While the number of violent crimes is increasing, experts contend that the crime rate is modest compared to statistics from several decades ago. For example, violent crime from the 1990s through 2020s was at an all-time high in the 1990s but began a downward trend in 2000. At that time, it showed signs of stabilizing, but declined in 2005 only to increase in 2006, and declined until 2014 and increased until 2017 when it declined until 2020. Research experts argue that violent crime increased during the COVID-19 pandemic (Grawert & Kim, 2022; Berk, 2023). Correspondingly, homicides, which represent the smallest category of violent crime rates, mirrored the trends in violent crimes that occurred from 1990 to 2020, but increased by nearly 30% nationwide in the

DOI: 10.4324/9781003373001-1

inner cities, suburbs, and rural areas (Grawert & Kim, 2022). Moreover, the number of assaults increased by more than 10%. Evidence suggests that 75% of the murders in 2020 were perpetrated with a firearm. Impoverished communities experienced the most violent crimes since it rose in 2020. It was disproportionately committed by younger Americans. In fact, arrest data provide that 40% of people arrested for murder in 2020 were between the ages of 20 and 29. Its victim's ages ranged between the ages of 20 and 40. Some experts also observe divergence between property and violent crime in 2020. That is, violent crimes continued to rise into 2021, while property crime either stabilized or declined. The same experts contend that in the absence of completed national data from the FBI's UCR, divergence continues (Grawert & Kim, 2022).

What Is Violence and Crime?

Since violence and crime continues to rise in America, a working definition is necessary to better understand their magnitude, scope, and pervasiveness. Perhaps the definition used by the *World Health Organization* (WHO) provides a global and more encompassing framework. It defines violence as:

> The intentional use of physical force or power, threatened, or actual against oneself, another person, or against a group or community, that either assault in or has a high likelihood of resulting in injury, death, psychological, harm, maldevelopment or deprivation.
>
> *(p. 5)*

This definition encompasses a broad range of outcomes that include physical as well as psychological harm. Therefore, one can easily understand that murder, rape, assault, robbery, child abuse, intimate personal violence, suicide, elderly abuse, bullying, firearms injuries, and the harm left in the aftermath of these actions come under the auspices of violence. Public health researchers and crime experts recognize that an understanding of violence must include behavior that does not always result in death but, rather, has an adverse or negative effect on people, families, communities, and healthcare systems globally (Krug et al., 2002), since these types of victimizations happen to men, women, children, and the elderly often resulting in physical, psychological, and emotional problems that could last for decades (Rauf, 2022; Wolke & Lereya, 2015).

Crime is defined as any action that is committed or omitted in violation of a law forbidding or commanding it (Anderson, 2015). This definition covers commissions as well as omissions and it brings a broad range of behaviors under the rule of law (i.e., criminal, civil, regulatory). For example, it governs behavior such as street crime, political crime, organized crime, medical crime, white collar crime, governmental crime, cybercrime, and others. While these crimes are harmful to the victims and others, some of them cause more serious harm compared with others. Fortunately, when a street crime such as a murder or homicide is committed, most people in society quickly recognize and identify it as being prohibited by law and wait for the criminal justice system to mete out punishment and dispense justice. They may also understand that the death of a loved one will have a negative impact on surviving family members. Unfortunately, when political crimes or governmental crimes are committed which arguably take a greater toll on society, many people fail to recognize them or understand their impact on society owing to having a limited social reality of such crime, victimization, and negative health consequences. They affect large numbers of people in the population.

Consider the following examples. First, it is well-established in the literature that when certain segments of the population experience violence and terror from police or state repression, they along with others suffer negative health consequences in the aftermath that may include acute stress, chronic fear, trauma, stroke, ulcers, diabetes, heart disease, depression, autoimmune disorders, accelerated aging and death (Alang et al., 2017). Second, in 2014, Flint, Michigan experienced water contamination that devastated several Black communities. The incident made national news after the story reported that lead and legionnaire bacteria infected the tap water of nearly 100,000 residents from 2014 to 2015. Ray (2022) reported that in 2014, the city of Flint switched its water supply from the *Detroit Water and Sewage Department* to the Flint River after deciding it would be more cost-effective. Residents immediately reported a change in the quality of water but were told to boil the water because of the presence of dangerous levels of bacteria. By 2015, residents were informed that elevated levels of carcinogenic trihalomethanes were detected in Flint's water but were told, it was safe to drink. Public health experts in Flint also reported that levels of lead were also detected but Flint's emergency manager refused to go public. It was later revealed that city officials' decisions were based on cost-effectiveness. Consequently, 12 people were killed from a type of pneumonia-causing bacteria found in Legionella, and many others who were exposed to lead poisoning continued to suffer severe negative health consequences such as miscarriages and increased risk of fetal death, while children have been diagnosed with high blood count levels and intellectual disabilities (Lee et al., 2023). Public health officials declared the matter a public health crisis that endangered the health of nearly all residents in Flint. A civil court agreed, and the residents of Flint were awarded $626 million in a class action lawsuit in 2021 against the state of Michigan, the city of Flint, an engineering company, and hospital (Lee et al., 2023). Despite the financial award, the health problems continue to plague many residents.

What Is Public Health?

Schneider (2021) argues that public health is defined as the science of protecting, improving the public's health by preventing disease, prolonging life, and promoting physical and psychological health through community efforts designed to ensure conditions in which people can be healthy. Perhaps Acheson (1988) captured public health best when he explained it is concerned with improving the overall health of the population through collective actions that are coordinated to promote health, prevent, mitigate, and treat diseases and use public policy to act on social and ecological factors that challenge the health of the community. Public health focuses on protecting and improving the well-being of a community or the health of the population. Consequently, those in public health focus on preventing incidents that threaten the physical and psychological health of residents or large groups of people such as violence, crime, disease, contaminated water, drugs, police violence, and other actions that negatively affect the public's health.

Public health efforts are broad measures that span from neighborhoods to cities, regions of the country, and even to different nations in the global community. To accomplish their goals, public health experts rely on education to promote healthy lifestyles. More specifically, they conduct extensive research on preventing diseases and injuries that contribute to human suffering and result in a diminished quality of life before they reach epidemic proportions. Unlike other professionals who respond to crises, public health officials must be proactive in their efforts to address and prevent problems from happening, spreading, and recurring. Consequently, they engage in aggressive educational outreach programs that are designed to educate the public about the dangers of disease, violence, crime, and other behaviors that threaten the public, where to seek health care and services, and they also recommend appropriate policies to adopt as measures toward prevention.

Major U.S. Inequalities and How They Correlate with Crime and Public Health

While studies show that no one in society is exempted from exposure to violence and crime, the research literature is replete with evidence that reveals an established relationship between the disproportionality of access to health care, and violence and crime experienced by inequities based on race, socioeconomic status, gender, and one's neighborhood (Centers for Disease Control and Prevention [CDC], 2016; Armstead et al., 2021). As previously stated, the national homicide rate is higher among younger Americans. Neighborhoods characterized as low-income experience more violent and property crime compared with high-income areas. This also includes child abuse, elderly abuse, intimate personal violence, firearm violence, and injuries. Health experts contend that many people who experience crime also suffer from mental distress and a diminished quality of life. Their situation is exacerbated by the fact that they also suffer health disparities owing to a lack of access to health services that are typically measured by differences in incidence, prevalence, mortality, diseases, and other negative health conditions (National Institutes of Health [NIH], 2014). Gramham (2004) explains it by stating that health disparities stem from health inequities of groups and communities that occupy unequal positions in society (Phelan et al., 2010). To some, this may suggest that inequities in the structure of society may have a lot to do with or is a root cause of the amount of violence people experience owing to social and structural determinants of health. Health experts argue that whether people are healthy is determined by their circumstances and physical environment.

NIH suggests that social and structural factors play a twofold purpose in health disparities. First, social determinants that affect one's health are beyond individual control, since they are in the social environment where one is born, lives, and reared. Social determinants of health are shaped by the distribution of money, power, and resources in the local community, nation, and global community (NIH, 2014). For example, one could be exposed to what is found in an impoverished environment, namely racism and discrimination and a lack of access to material and symbolic resources compared with a life of affluence and having access to the best health and treatment services. Some experts refer to them as the intermediate determinants of health. Second, structural determinants are the social, political, and economic factors that shape and influence the quality of social determinants of health that people in certain economic class positions experience in their neighborhood. One's socioeconomic status also affects access to the resources that are necessary for health services. Typically, structural position determines the degree of access or at least to the extent access is equitably distributed. The structure in stratified societies such as the U.S. is based on race, gender, social class, and other social constructions.

Violence and Crime Are Public Health Problems

Experts report that the three leading causes of death in the U.S. for people between the ages of 15 and 34 are unintentional injuries, homicide, and suicide. The same experts also report that violent deaths are typically linked to the use of a firearm (Freire-Vargas, 2018). The U.S. also has the dubious distinction of being the homicide leader in the world when compared with other advanced and high-income nations. Homicides are committed by firearms at a rate of 25 times higher than other nations (Grinshteyn & Hemenway, 2016). In the U.S., the homicide rate is more pronounced for impoverished Black males between the ages of 10 and 25, a rate that is 25 times higher than their White counterparts in the same age group (CDC, 2014). Despite homicides, each year, the U.S. also experiences high numbers of random shootings and injuries related to intimate personal violence, sexual assaults of adults as well as children, and gunshot wounds (intentional and unintentional) that may not result in death but may manifest in the form of paralysis or other physical disabilities. In fact, there is so much violence and crime committed each year that health experts agree that they should be considered as epidemics and treated using the healthcare approach (Marquez et al., 2015).

Public health officials argue that violence and crime take on many forms that include interpersonal, self-directed, and collective. When either type occurs, the consequence can manifest in physical or psychological injuries, disabilities, or premature deaths. When this occurs, the matter transcends the need for a criminal justice response and enters the area of public health because of the treatment needed for victims and others in the aftermath. Other experts contend that exposure to violence increases the likelihood of medical illnesses such as hypertension, heart disease, strokes, asthma, and cancer. Despite these physical ailments, violence also has a psychological effect on victims and others. For example, research finds that violence contributes to depression and PTSD. Some health experts also report that the victims of violence tend to smoke more, sleep less, and self-isolate which could lead to a premature death (Moffitt and The Klaus-Grave 2012 Think Tank, 2013; Krug et al., 2002; World Health Organization [WHO], 2014a). Because of the health outcomes associated with violence and crime, public health officials argue that it is a public health issue that requires epidemiological approaches as well as assessment to effectively combat the problem since public health approaches are aimed at proactively preventing violence and crime instead of responding to the devastation they cause.

Prevention and Intervention

Prevention and intervention are separate objectives that are often confusing and tend to overlap (Roberts, 2016). In fact, they are sometimes referred to as preventive interventions (Krug et al., 2002). On one hand, prevention in public health is designed to improve a person's or community's well-being by addressing factors that negatively impact one's behavior or health. Prevention can take place either before, immediately after, or as a disease or injury occurs. Some public health officials argue that prevention can also occur during the long term of either. Most conventional researchers who study violence prevention subscribe to the definition that targets the group that is the focus of the investigation. As such, the definition often has broad range encompassing universal interventions, selected interventions, and indicated interventions. According to experts, universal interventions are strategies that focus on groups or a general population without concerns of individual risk for violence or disease, and indicated interventions are strategies used on people who have already engaged in violence or who have contracted a disease. In this case, the intervention could be treatment (Krug et al., 2002). On the other hand, intervention is action taken with the goal of improving human health by preventing disease or violence by either curing or reducing the severity of either and restoring function to what was lost from either the disease or violence (Smith, 2015). Moreover, intervention involves the process of identifying those who are at risk, clarifying if they are at risk, and taking steps to make sure that safety measures are taken. Therefore, intervention requires deliberate steps or a protocol to increase safety for people or communities (Roberts, 2016). Some health experts argue that there are two categories of intervention. Those that are referred to as prevention interventions that are designed to prevent diseases and violence from occurring thereby reducing the number of incidence or new cases, and those interventions that are therapeutic and designed to treat, mitigate, or postpone violence or a disease to reduce either fatality or grave injury caused by either. Public health officials also point out that some interventions can accomplish both (Smith, 2015).

Criminal Justice Reactive Approaches to Solving Violence and Crime

Apprehending, Prosecuting, and Punishing Offenders

The criminal justice system is designed to dispense justice in the areas of policing, courts, and corrections. While it primarily works toward doing justice to the offenders that are processed through the system, it also desires to reduce the number of crimes that are committed, the number of offenders who committed them, and ultimately, the number of victims that are impacted by violence and crime. The justice system is sworn to serve and protect the community it serves (Siegel, 2011). However, the system is reactionary and not proactive. It responds to crime and does not spend a great deal of time or resources on actively trying to prevent crimes from occurring nor was it made to treat crime victims. For example, police, the gate keepers of the justice system, rarely happen on crime in progress, but rather, officers are typically dispatched when a citizen calls police for assistance in the aftermath of violence and crime. In their reactionary role, police are tasked with quickly apprehending suspects to hold them criminally responsible if they commit the prohibited behavior. Sometimes the process is very slow given that offenders often remain at large until they are eventually apprehended. When they are found, police will affect an arrest, read them their rights, take them into custody, interrogate them, and book them for the criminal offense. This is followed by an arraignment (Siegel, 2011).

When suspects are indicted, a grand jury or prosecutor has determined that enough probable cause exists to hold them criminally responsible to stand trial and account for the alleged criminal wrongdoing. After this occurs, a trial date is set, and the defendant is provided an attorney to represent their legal interest. During this prosecutorial phase of the justice process, a district attorney will use evidence (material and testimonial) collected by police to win a criminal conviction. At the same time, the accused lawyer will attempt to refute or rebut the evidence to establish the client's innocence. In the end, either a judge or jury will determine the defendant's guilt. If the defendant is found not guilty, he will be released from custody and set free. However, if the defendant is found guilty of the criminal changes, he will be remanded to the department of corrections that has jurisdiction over the case and crime which is determined by the gravity of the criminality committed (Siegel, 2011). This brief example of the reactive nature of the criminal justice system is instructive in several regards. First, it demonstrates the role of the police in removing dangerous and violent offenders from society. The role of policing does not extend to providing services to crime victims, especially those who suffer negative health outcomes of crime. Second, it reveals the procedures that occur when cases go to trial.

A reality about justice in the U.S. is that about 90–95% of all criminal cases (state and federal) are resolved through negotiated plea bargaining where suspects agree to a lesser charge and a reduced sentence rather than take their chances in a criminal proceeding (Johnson, 2023). When a plea agreement is made, victims are not included in the process and should consider themselves fortunate if police officers provide them with a follow-up regarding the status of their case. In other words, the court proceeding often leaves victims out of the process unless the prosecutor intends to call them as material or eyewitnesses to the crime in those few cases that make it to trial. Despite this, some public health officials contend that the use of victim impact statements before sentencing can be therapeutic to surviving family members since it offers them an opportunity to express how the crime has affected their physical and emotional well-being. Third, corrections are focused on the level of custody that the accused will receive after a determination of guilt. As stated earlier, the accused is remanded over to the penal institution or correctional setting that has jurisdiction over the case to serve the pronounced sentence that has been imposed by the state. In essence, the accused is removed from society to ensure safety and that he will no longer pose a threat to the community. In doing so, the presumption is this form of social control sends a twofold message. The first is deterrence and the second is community safety. The justice system functions from a deterrence perspective or philosophy in that it is hoped that when punishment is meted out, others will not commit crime out of fear that they will face similar consequences for their behavior. In doing so, the justice system believed that this promotes community safety since the offender is no longer free to victimize others (Siegel, 2011).

Community Policing

A progressive strategy that some law enforcement agencies use to fight violence and crime is community policing. It is designed to promote better police community relationships that build trust between police and the community it serves. Police experts report it requires an effort from both police and the community. They contend that the philosophy behind this strategy is to make community residents more aware of police activities, educate them on self-protection efforts, and improve attitudes toward policing (Gaines & Miller, 2010). Community policing is premised on creating partnerships with the public since successfully combating crime and keeping the community safe is contingent on the community's involvement. This approach to policing is grounded in the idea that who better than the residents of their own community to understand the dynamics and elements in their own neighborhood. Experts argue that this is implemented when officers engage in foot patrol to get to know the people they serve instead of being anonymous in a patrol vehicle (Trojanowicz & Bucqueroux, 1990).

Problem-Solving Policing (PSP) -Hot Spots

Another policing strategy that holds promise because it is also proactive rather than reactive is referred to as problem-solving policing (PSP), or problem-oriented policing. PSP is implemented after police agencies identify long-term community problems such as drug dealing, prostitution, and gang activity. PSP is a prevention strategy with the goal of eliminating the community problem (Goldstein, 1979). Similarly, to community policing efforts, to be effective, police must rely on community residents to solve problems. More specifically, police managers are tasked with developing community resources, designing cost-effective solutions to problems and advocating for the communities they serve. To address specific problems in certain communities, some police departments use available intelligence to address urban crime found in a few "hot spots" or urban areas (Sherman et al., 1989). The logic of the strategy is to concentrate law enforcement efforts in those few areas that are saturated with crime such as certain apartment complexes, malls, bars, and hotels (Renauer, 2007). This proactive effort is believed to have an appreciable impact on crime reduction and community safety.

Effective Crime Prevention Strategies

Effective crime prevention is referred to as any action that causes a reduction in the amount of crime, victims, and criminal offenders. These efforts tend to focus on what causes crime as well as what reduces or eliminates factors that lead to crime. Crime experts contend that prevention can be categorized into three phases that include *primary, secondary,* and *tertiary prevention. Primary crime prevention* strategies are focused on stopping the problems before they start. This suggests that prevention efforts should target reducing criminal opportunities from occurring. This can be accomplished by strengthening the community and social structures where people reside by improving both the physical and social environment. Therefore, *primary prevention* strategies often focus on social and structural factors. Experts postulate that social factors such as low educational attainment, unemployment, poverty, and poor health contribute to the decision to commit crime. Therefore, to offset these factors, prevention measures such as community-based programs (e.g., local resident action groups that offer guardianship is needed) and school-based programs (e.g., truancy initiatives) should be implemented. Where structural prevention is concerned, it addresses the environment and matters such as how buildings are designed and land scapes, and the products that people use (Hsu et al., 2022). *Secondary crime prevention* is a strategy that is used to change people, especially those who are at a higher risk of engaging in crime. Some experts refer to this process as preemptively targeting the activities of potential offenders. These efforts should offer early and effective interventions such as youth programs. Experts contend that high-risk neighborhoods are prime locations to target these interventions. They also postulate that primary crime prevention requires active support based on offenders' commitment to not reengage in crime.

Tertiary crime prevention examines how the criminal justice system addresses the aftermath of violence and crime. For example, how does the justice system intervene in the lives of offenders or prevent recidivism or keep them from reoffending. This approach often varies from offender to offender since the type of *tertiary prevention* strategy can be different contingent on the type of sentence or punishment an offender received for their crime. For example, those placed or returned to the community under probation supervision will require a different strategy compared with offenders who are paroled after serving part of a prison sentence. The same is true for offenders who were sentenced to a year or less in a county jail. Nevertheless, some *tertiary crime prevention* strategies could include community-based sanctions and treatment programs designed to reintegrate the offender back into society on conditions of release that require contact with either a probation or patrol officer (Pease, 2002).

Public Health Approaches to Preventing Violence and Crime

Those working to prevent violence must view it as a societal problem that requires input from multiple agencies to effectively address it. That is, violence and the consequences it brings demand more than a criminal justice response. Therefore, no one agency can adequately address it since it requires a range of agencies to partner with officials as well as community organizations to meet the needs of offenders and victims in general, and to primarily keep the community safe. Violence prevention is vast and requires the help of community and civic leaders since they play key roles in efforts to reduce and prevent violence. Some contend that partnerships must emerge from strategic planning by justice agencies and community efforts to implement early intervention, treatment given to offenders and victims, as well as support services to assist crime victims (Local Government Association, n.d.).

Public health officials argue that unlike criminal justice responses to violence and crime that are made after the fact, public health approaches are proactive and have been successfully implemented in the past when used to prevent the transmission of diseases, motor vehicle deaths, the adverse health consequences, and premature deaths linked to cigarette smoking, and other behaviors (Schneider, 2021). They contend that the same success can be achieved to improve community safety (e.g., from intimate personal violence, mental illness, substance abuse, suicides and violent injuries and death linked to firearms), if efforts are made to follow the data. These experts contend that the use of available data allows for the creation of layered approaches to prevent violence, especially premature deaths and nonfatal injuries owing to the use of firearms. Public health experts argue that their approaches to preventing crime and violence are anchored in the use of evidence-based methodologies to keep communities safe (Schneider, 2021).

Surveillance

Surveillance is used to closely monitor disease, violence, and other adverse public health issues. Surveillance in public health is concerned about the ongoing and systematic collection, analysis, and interpretation of health-related data that are used to plan, implement, and evaluate the practice of public health (Thacker & Birkhead, 2008). Some health experts contend that surveillance provides information about "who" and "where" health problems are occurring along with who is affected most by the problems (Caves, 2004). Data used in public health are taken from a variety of sources that include the following: surveys, medical records, electronic health records, public health investigations, and others (Rojanaworarit, 2015). After these data are collected, they are disseminated to public health authorities charged with preventing the devastation that comes with violence and crime. More specifically, surveillance data are given to public health personnel, government leaders, and those in the general public to help shape and influence public health policies and programs (Smith et al., 2013). Experts contend that the purpose of surveillance is to collect and provide information to be used to promote public health by tracking emerging health related issues and providing a solution before they escalate.

While surveillance is conducted for several reasons by public health officials, experts suggest the reasons are sevenfold. First, to identify patients or victims and their contacts for intervention and treatment. Second, to detect epidemics (e.g., large amounts of violence), health problems, and changes in behavior. Third, to estimate the magnitude and scope of health problems. Fourth, to measure trends and characterize violence and disease. Fifth, to monitor changes in violence, or infectious and environmental agents. Sixth, to assess the effectiveness of programs designed to prevent and control violence and diseases. Seventh, to develop hypotheses and stimulate research (Thacker & Birkhead, 2008).

Public health surveillance is not singular, but rather, there are several types that include *passive surveillance, active surveillance, sentinel surveillance, and syndromic surveillance. Passive surveillance* occurs when diseases and infections are reported by health providers. The process is less time consuming. For example, if a doctor encounters a case or disease listed by Centers for Disease Control and Prevention (CDC) surveillance and sends it to the local and state health departments, she must report the matter to the appropriate local or state health agency (Aker et al., 2013). However, it tends to underreport some injuries and diseases owing to reporting practices and the quality of reporting. *Active surveillance* occurs when health agencies are visited, and health providers are asked to present medical records for review and to determine health status. Unlike the *passive* type, active surveillance ensures that reports are more complete. The method is used in combination with certain types of epidemiological investigations. Experts argue that it is highly appropriate when addressing epidemics, or when diseases have been targeted for elimination. *Sentinel surveillance* occurs when a select number of health professionals provide a report in a certain geographical area. Health experts contend that sentinel surveillance can be interpreted as active or passive. *Syndromic surveillance* targets one or more symptoms instead of a physician's diagnosed or laboratory confirmed disease (WHO, 2014b).

What is the problem?

Health experts contend that defining the problem is essential to the public health approach. For example, in the case of violence, they argue that while the problem will be determined based on what is derived from the continuous and systematic collection, analysis, and interpretation of health data, one must also engage in a robust need assessment concerning violence. This must include a focus on which type of violence is concerning. To be effective requires having a clear understanding of risk and protective factors that can be targeted among individuals, families, communities as well as populations to effectively reduce and prevent violence (CDC, 2020).

Risk Factors

In the prevention of violence and crime, understanding risk factors and or protective factors is important and must be ascertained by an evidence-led approach (Armstead et al., 2018). Health experts contend that prevention requires an understanding of causality. As such, those using the public health approach must be able to recognize risks and protective factors and understand the interplay between both. When this occurs, interventions targeted at the individual, family, community, and population are more likely to meet with success. For example, if it is determined that alcohol and drug use lead to more crime and violence, these issues can be targeted with intervention groups. On the other hand, interventions should also target strengthening protective factors that mediate the use of violence. These could be the influence of parents, teachers, and role models. If it is determined that the latter are protective factors, efforts must be made to get them involved in helping to prevent violence (Armstead et al., 2018).

Intervention Evaluation

To address the problem of violence, one must develop and identify effective interventions. Local areas are encouraged (when resources are available) to defray the cost for evidence-based intervention that have been proven successful at reducing violence. For example, an anti-violence crime policy should emerge to address a need in a neighborhood, community, or population. Specifically, what causes violence. Experts suggest that the intervention or strategy that is created should receive agreement from all stakeholders involved in the process. They also recommend that strategies are designed to be measurable, relevant, achievable, and have goals that specify a timeline. The strategy should not be used alone, but rather, it should be part of a broader approach that includes partnerships with the local community, health personnel, and others to ensure local ownership of the strategy or intervention. Experts believe this will allow for the strategy to be implemented as it was designed or intended (Armstead et al., 2018).

Implementation

When prevention strategies are implemented, experts advise that they should reflect the agreed upon design model. This requires consideration of the context in which the intervention will be placed. When the risk factors in a community are determined to be the excessive use of alcohol and drugs, changing the social and cultural context may be difficult and time consuming. Therefore, the community where the intervention is targeted must understand and accept that immediate impact might be unrealistic, but rather, interventions and programs often take time to meet a desired outcome. According to Rosenberg and Fenley (1991), implementing a strategy to prevent assaultive violence must rely on broad social changes in its overall approach to violence and specific interventions in cases of potential and actual violence and different forms of abuse. Interventions must be far reaching and able to reach people before a pattern of victimization is established. They may also attempt to minimize the consequences of violence by providing victims with support and offenders with the help to change. Public health researchers suggest that community resources should be used to educate residents that violence is a problem that can be addressed. Specific attention should be placed on violence and acted out in the neighborhood.

What Is Public Health Surveillance?

Effective violence and disease prevention programs rely on effective surveillance and response systems that are influenced by data that have been systematically collected, analysed, and interpreted to prevent disease and injuries (Massetti et al., 2016). For example, WHO, CDC,

NIH, and other institutions use databases and automated electronic reporting systems to track and monitor outbreaks of diseases and high levels of violence (Nsubuga et al., 2006). Health experts argue that better surveillance increases the likelihood that communities will be able to effectively identify violence and disease prevention priorities, plan to give the population better health options, inform and educate stakeholders, and implement evidence-based interventions that are proven to be successful. Interventions will be monitored to determine if they have issues that need to be addressed. Moreover, surveillance should be seen as a common or routine public service that relies on similar structures, processes, and resources that recognize that there are different types of violence and diseases that threaten the safety of a community and therefore, they often require specialized types of surveillance needs (Massetti et al., 2016). Consequently, this may require blending core functions (e.g., detection, confirmation, analysis, response) and support functions (e.g., training, supervision, communication, resource management) (WHO, 2023). The public health approach relies on institutions and experts from many disciplines to apply a four-step process to prevent violence and other health problems. The approach is designed to define and monitor the problem; identify protective and risk factors; develop and test prevention strategies; and assure widespread adoption (Schneider, 2021).

Define and Monitor the Problem

To effectively prevent violence and other health problems, one has to define and monitor the problem. As such, one must use the systematic data collection to understand the "who," "what," "when," "where," and "how" associated with the behavior. This requires knowing what behavior is detrimental to individuals, communities, and populations. It also requires an understanding of the magnitude of or how pervasive the problem is. Health experts argue that it requires knowing where the problem is located within the population. It also requires understanding how the problem works. Researchers contend that to answer these questions, it is necessary to collect and analyse reliable data (e.g., police records, medical examiners files, vital statistics, surveys, registries, and others) that provide the number of violence incidents and related behavior, injuries, and deaths. Data must detail the scope and complexity of the problem. To determine if the problem constitutes a public health issue, data should reveal the frequency of the problem, its patterns, and trends, who the perpetrators are as well as the victims (WHO, 2023). Public health data help health officials identify trends, guide priorities, understand risk factors, and develop and evaluate targeted prevention strategies (Dalberg & Krug, 2002).

Identifying Risk and Protective Factors

While understanding the nature and extent of the problem is important, those who are engaged in violence prevention must do research to understand those factors that place people at risk of violence and other health problems. To that end, the public health approach addresses population level risk factors that lead to violence and protective factors that reduce violence. Health researchers contend that some factors can protect or shield people from engaging in violence, other factors can place people at risk of experiencing violence. Stated differently, certain factors protect people from perpetrating violence and other factors place people at risk of becoming crime victims. Public health officials are tasked with understanding risk and protective factors to identify where prevention efforts should be placed. Research reveals that risk factors exist on the individual, community, and societal levels that increases the likelihood that violence will occur. While addressing these, public health experts do not believe that risk factors cause violence since the presence of risk factors does not mean that everyone exposed to them will be victimized or injured; however, their presence means that the likelihood is greater compared with them not being present. Therefore, risk factors are defined as characteristics that increase the likelihood that a person will either become a victim or perpetrator of violence. Protector factors are elements that decrease the likelihood that a person will become a victim or perpetrator of violence. In the end, data analysis and research should identify factors that increase or decrease the risk of violence and other health problems (Dahlberg & Krug, 2002).

Develop and Test Prevention Strategies

Policymakers and practitioners use the public health approach to create and test prevention strategies that are supported by findings from the research literature, community surveys, collaborative interviews, needs assessment data, and focus groups (Schneider, 2021). According to experts, these data and findings should be properly vetted and recognized as evidence-based approaches to planning effective programs. The interventions or strategies must address the risk factors that have been identified as those that increase the likelihood that violence will occur (Schweig, 2014). Researchers advise that interventions should be tested on a regular basis to determine if they are effective as well as equitable. In fact, they argue that testing methods should be rigorous given that interventions have the potential of being adopted and modeled either locally, regionally, or nationally depending on need and effectiveness. When programs are created, policymakers can advocate that more interventions are developed and designed to target behavioral risk factors for violence. They can also advocate that interventions are created to target community risk factors that promote violence (Schweig, 2014).

Ensure Widespread Adoption of Strategies

After the strategy or intervention is determined to be effective, it should be implemented and adopted on a broadscale. Health experts warn that prevention policies are only effective to the extent that they are properly implemented and enforced. Stated differently, when an intervention has been observed to reduce violence, its measures should be shared and widely disseminated to others. Therefore, public health officials encourage communities to be receptive toward implementing proven strategies that are based on the best available evidence. However, they are also encouraged to continue assessing the intervention to determine if it meets the community needs, whether it addresses the community context and ultimately, whether it prevents violence and other health related issues. Experts also suggest that communities should not be hesitant about implementation since workshops are offered on best practices to assist in training, networking, and providing technical assistance as well as evaluation (Dahlberg & Krug, 2002). Policymakers, practitioners, and public health officials contend that the public health approach is also focused on allocating monies for implementing and evaluating violence prevention strategies at the local, state, and federal levels. They also state that these funds should be allocated to train stakeholders to ensure that new policies and programs are adopted properly and have measurable outcomes (WHO, n.d.).

Goal of Public Health Surveillance

Public health surveillance is what anchors the practice of public health since it is regarded as critical to improving the population health (Holland, 2002). Surveillance provides information about when and where health problems are occurring along with who is affected most by the problem (Caves, 2004). According to health experts, it provides current and updated data and information that presents the distribution of negative health events, prioritizes public health action, monitors the impact of control measures, and identifies emerging conditions that may adversely affect the health of the population (Groseclose & Buckeridge, 2017, p. 58). Public health surveillance is viewed as the most potent weapon in the health arsenal to fight epidemics since it serves five essential functions: population health assessment; health surveillance; health promotion; disease and injury prevention; and health protection (Choi, 2012).

Some public health researchers contend that surveillance is contingent on the use of systems or collectives of processes and components to measure the health of the population. More specifically, they provide that surveillance is about data collection, data quality, monitoring, data management, data analysis, interpretation of analytical results, information dissemination, and applying the information to programs designed to promote a healthy community and population (Groseclose & Buckeridge, 2017). Others argue that public health surveillance systems are created to increase the efficiency and effectiveness of public health system's ability to determine and address those factors that are detrimental to the public's health. As a result of the systems' efforts, all information is given to public health practitioners, public health officials, and stakeholders to inform the decisions they make and the actions they take to improve public health (Burris et al., 2016). Similarly, Bernstein and colleagues (2015) contend that surveillance systems produce information that drives action which requires that these systems generate quality data in a timely fashion to match public health objectives. The major goals of public health surveillance are sixfold. First, identify diseases of public health importance. Second, quickly identify any outbreaks, epidemics, or usual events. Third, identify risk factors. Fourth, identify high-risk populations. Fifth, monitor disease trends. Sixth, access current disease control activities.

Surveillance Process

The public health approach requires several integrative steps to use to carry out surveillance on a targeted health problem. It also relies on the help of many people in the process. The steps entail a fivefold process that include the following: (1) identifying, defining, and measuring the health problem; (2) collecting and compiling data about the problem and factors that influence it; (3) analysing and interpreting data; (4) providing data and their interpretation to those responsible for controlling the health problem; and (5) monitoring and making periodic evaluations of the usefulness and quality of surveillance to improve it for future use (Thacker & Stroup, 1998). The surveillance process requires that people such as healthcare providers (e.g., doctors, nurses, and social workers, and others) report information about patients that they have examined during routine medical practices. Someone typically associated with health authorities must also be responsible for collecting data from healthcare providers and gathering it together for epidemiologists and others who are trained to analyse health surveillance. These analyses usually focus on revealing the magnitude, pattern, and trends of specific health problems. These reports often calculate rates of diseases and violence and the changes in prevalence of diseases and violence (Thacker & Stroup, 1998).

Researchers often focus on incidences (including persons at risk, place at risk, time at risk). Health experts contend that the analysis often relies on descriptive epidemiological methods to reveal the magnitude and patterns of health problems. Moreover, they can also use longitudinal data collection that reveal trends overtime (Rojanaworarit, 2015). After data are analysed, public health authorities at the local, state, and federal levels are tasked with determining what must be done based on the results of the data analysis. Data interpretation is critical since it leads to consideration about what public health action is needed. For example, if there are observed increases in a disease, public health action should be immediate. Public health researchers argue that if any step in the process is not carried out, the information derived from the process will be viewed as unusable regarding taking appropriate public health action (Rojanaworarit, 2015).

Data Dissemination and Link to Public Health Action

Surveillance information should be disseminated to health officials who need the information to make informed decisions about public health issues. These officials must be provided with an accurate response in cases that require immediate action such as an outbreak or epidemic. Therefore, the information should be linked to public health action in cases where quick actions are needed or in cases regarding planning. Policy should be implemented based on judgment and application important to the context and setting by health officials (Rojanaworarit, 2015).

Logic of Viewing Violence and Crime as Epidemics

When infectious diseases (e.g., Influenza, AIDS, COVID-19, and other viruses) emerge and threaten the health of the population because large numbers of people are adversely impacted, the situation requires a national response from public health surveillance systems such as the CDC, NIH, and others to quickly mount a response using the best available data that inform strategies and interventions developed by public health officials to reduce and prevent the spread or the continuation of the disease to ensure the overall health and safety of the population (Schneider, 2021).

Because crime and violence are often pervasive and threaten many people in the U.S., it is concerning to all Americans from every segment of the population. For example, homicide, suicide (self-harm), and interpersonal violence are among the top 15 leading causes of death in the U.S. (CDC, 2009). However, crime surveillance statistics (e.g., *UCR, NCVS,* and *SRS*) reveal that while no one in society is completely immune from being a crime victim, violence and crime is more pronounced in certain socioeconomic areas of the country and tend to disproportionately impact specific racial and ethnic minorities. In fact, some experts contend that they can easily be viewed as constituting an epidemic with adverse health consequences, including a diminished quality of life for the community as well as the society at large (Williams et al., 2016).

The idea of violence and crime as epidemics in need of a public health response is nothing new, but rather, it emerged in the 1980s and early 1990s, when the homicide and suicide rates reached epidemic proportions in certain segments of the population, mainly among young minority males during the crack cocaine epidemic and the violence that followed in its wake and aftermath. More specifically, from 1985 to 1991, the homicide rate for males between the ages of 15 and 19 increased by 154%, while the suicide rate for young adults between the ages of 15 and 24 almost tripled between 1950 and 1990 (CDC, 2008). Researchers contend there are other reasons why violence and crime are public health issues. For example, for decades, the public health community has accepted behavioral factors in the etiology and prevention of violence that has led health officials to believe that the same behavioral modifications used to prevent some of the leading causes of death in the U.S. (e.g., heart disease, cancer, and strokes) can be used to prevent violence and crime. Put differently, because the public health approach has been highly effective at reducing the threat of infectious diseases, epidemiologists believe that it can be just as successful at reducing violence and crime.

These same experts contend that when violence and crime reach epidemic proportions, it requires not only a criminal justice response, but also a public health response since some of the consequences of violence and crime are that they are contagious and cause a vicious cycle that is perpetuated from generation to generation. They also require medical and psychological treatment of victims after certain crimes (e.g., gun violence, physical and sexual assaults) have been committed. In fact, after hospitalization is received, many surviving victims may require decades of physical therapy, counseling, medication, and other forms of treatment protocols post-victimization. Sometimes, communities with high incidence of violence will need to develop effective interventions to reduce and prevent the continuation of violence (Rosenburg & Finley, 1991).

Success of Public Health Approaches in Addressing Problems Such as Smoking, STIs, and Auto-Accidents

The history of success using the public health approach is well documented in the areas of preventing smoking, STIs, and automobile accidents. In fact, the literature indicates that the health and life expectancy of Americans improved dramatically during the 20th century given that public health responses included help from the medical profession, epidemiology, public health organizations, intervention and prevention programs, consumer advocates, public education and training, and others (Sleet et al., 2007). Health experts contend that the public health prevention model introduced tools, methods, applications, and systems combined with its infrastructure to identify, track, and monitor targeted issues that were not used to solve problems prior to this time (Sleet & Gielen, 1998). Researchers attribute the increase in life expectancy to new advances and discoveries made in public health and implemented throughout the nation (Morbidity and Morality Weekly Report [MMWR], 1999; Bunker et al., 1994). While there have been many accomplishments and success stories in public health, some that bare mentioning includes the eradication of smallpox, the elimination of poliomyelitis in the Americas, control of measles, rubella, tetanus, diphtheria, and others. It is undeniable that the public health approach has proven successful when used to safeguard and protect the overall health and wellness in the U.S.

Pierce and colleagues (2016) provide that as early as the 1960s, public health approaches were used to reduce the negative health consequences of cigarette smoking, namely because it was viewed as the primary cause of the global lung cancer epidemic. More specifically, the U.S. *Department of Health and Human Services* targeted high-risk populations such as women, Black adults, and people with a high school education or less for smoking cessation programs. Healthcare providers discovered that to achieve long-term health and economic benefits of reducing the nation's overall level of smoking, efforts needed to be made to develop intensive smoking prevention programs. Researchers discovered that each year, one million young persons started to smoke which cost the healthcare system an estimated $10 billion during their lifetime for treatment in the U.S. After 50 years, the results reveal a 70% decline from its peak consumption in the U.S. Moreover, researchers report that public health efforts that targeted smoking brought about a reduction in the number of coronary heart diseases and strokes owing to risk-factor modification that include smoking cessation and blood pressure control, along with access to early detection and more effective treatment. Consequently, the prevalence of smoking among adults has decreased and millions of smoking-related deaths have been prevented. Some physicians estimate that the number of coronary heart disease has declined by 51% (Public Health Services, 1994).

STIs including AIDS are a public health issue that threatens the health and economy of the U.S. CDC researchers posit that STIs have a huge impact on the health and well-being of the country. In fact, epidemiologists report that since 2014, the rate of STIs has continued to increase and access to reliable data to use in their prevention has never been more important to inform policy and decision-making of public health officials. This growing concern has been sparked by the prevalence of infections along with new emerging incidences within a specific timeframe. For example, statistics reveal that in 2018, there was an estimated 67.6 million prevalent STIs in the U.S. There were also additional 26.2 million incidents of STIs in the U.S. in 2018. Surveillance data indicate that 45% of all 2018 incidents of STIs were acquired by persons 15–24 years old. Experts contend that STIs in the U.S. are common and costly and pose a threat to the healthcare system costing billions each year. In fact, *CDC* data estimate that new infections in 2018 cost a total of $16 billion in direct medical costs. However, society is also adversely impacted by STIs to the extent that they contribute to loss of productivity, psychological effects, sick days taken from work, and others. This has led some public health officials to contend that the nonmedical costs of STIs may exceed the medical costs associated with this public health threat (CDC, n.d.). Other healthcare experts report that the discovery of antimicrobial therapy has been critical to the success of the public health system's ability to control infections such as tuberculosis and STIs. For example, advocating the use of contraceptives has prevented the transmission of human immunodeficiency virus and other STIs.

Health officials also view motor vehicle injuries and deaths as a public health threat that is preventable. As such, they frame the problem as a predictable and preventable public health issue that is amendable to change contingent on convincing the public and policymakers that something can be done to save lives (Sleet et al., 2007). Research shows that prior to the U.S. viewing automobile accidents as a public health problem with devastating consequences for many Americans, the number of injuries and fatalities was concerning.

In fact, statistics from the Department of Health and Human Services (1992) reveal that in the past 100 years, there have been over 2.8 million deaths and nearly 100 million injuries on U.S. roads and highways. Moreover, traffic injuries were the leading cause of death for children, adolescents, and young adults and accounted for the deaths of adults in every age group. Officials with the National Highway Traffic Safety Administration (NHTSA) (2006) reported that in 2005, automobile accidents were responsible for 43,443 deaths and an estimated 2.7 million nonfatal injuries. However, after traffic safety was accepted as a public health concern, there were drastic improvements in motor vehicle safety. For example, public health approaches were used to advocate making highway construction safer, and changing the behaviors of drivers, pedestrians, and cyclists by convincing them that auto-accidents and their injuries (fatal and nonfatal) are preventable. These efforts led to a substantial decrease in the number of accidents and fatalities (Sleet et al., 2007). Despite that motor vehicle injuries accounted for an estimated $89 billion of the total lifetime costs for injuries in 2000, economists contend that motor vehicle-related injuries also cost 2.3% of the gross national product and employee accidents (that occur at and away from work) cost employers almost $60 billion annually (Network of Employers for Traffic Safety, 2006). For these reasons, public health officials contend that traffic crashes have an adverse effect on the transportation system, economic system, health system, jobs, families, and the culture of safety in the U.S. (Sleet et al., 2007).

Use of Educational Campaigns to Effect Massive Behavioral Changes

In response to the danger of smoking, public health professionals have relied on multilayered intervention designs used to prevent young people from obtaining access to tobacco products. The interventions have targeted school-based tobacco-use prevention programs that include mass media campaigns that target high-risk groups, increase excise taxes on tobacco products, increase the minimum age on those who can purchase tobacco products, prohibit manufacturers from marketing tobacco products to minors, eliminate the sale of tobacco products through vending machines, and enforce tobacco access laws for minors (Public Health Services, 2000). Pierce and colleagues (2016) contend that other interventions that can be effectively used to prevent the dangers of smoking include increasing the price of tobacco products, mass media anti-smoking advertising, smoke free policies, creating anti-smoking curricula in schools, restricting opportunities the tobacco industry from marketing to adolescents, and creating a comprehensive tobacco control campaign designed to de-normalize smoking.

Public health officials report that STIs can be prevented and controlled by relying on three strategies that include the following: reducing the risk of transmission via any sexual encounter by using a condom, reducing the number of sex partners, and reducing the period of infectiousness in individuals (Catchpole, 2001). Therefore, the challenge for the public health system is to counsel and educate the public by increasing its level of awareness and having an openness about sexual health discussions within the broader context of health. Epidemiologists and health providers report that having a comprehensive sexuality education program, condom promotion, STI and HIV pretest information and posttest counseling, safer sex/risk reduction counseling, along with interventions that focus on key populations are successful in preventing and protecting the public's health from STIs. Other health experts recommend community engagement methods and partnerships to create local STD prevention and control capacity or community approaches to reduce sexually transmitted disease (CARS) that are designed to support planning, implementation, and evaluation of interventions that enhance STD and personal health services for certain at-risk groups, namely adolescents and sex workers, men who have sex with men, transgender people, prisoners, and those who inject drugs.

Similarly, when it comes to preventing injuries and untimely deaths related to automobile accidents owing to speeding, alcohol, lack of using a safety belt, and pedestrian and bicycle safety, public health officials have relied on several groups to educate the U.S. population about the culture of safety. According to Sleet and colleagues (2007), these groups include the private sector, voluntary organizations, and nonprofit groups such as *SafeKids Worldwide*, and the *Association for Safe International Road Travel* (ASIRT). They also rely on advocacy groups such as *Mothers against Drunk Drivers* (MADD), *Physicians for Auto Safety*, the *Insurance Institute for Highway Safety*, and the *AAA Foundation for Traffic Safety*. Through the combined effort of these groups and organizations, public health officials have been able to influence state and federal public health agencies' efforts that have led to the passage of legislation and public policy that supports victims' rights, and sponsored research in traffic safety and public health (Sleet et al., 2007). The public health approach has called for drivers to use safety belts, motorcycle helmets, abstain from drinking and driving, and to use child safety seats and other devices (Bolen et al., 1997).

Need for Criminal Justice and Epidemiological Approaches to Combat Violence and Crime

As early as 1985, Surgeon General, C. Everett Koop, recognized the need and called for the incorporation of public health strategies to be used with law enforcement efforts to prevent violence (Koop, 1985). Because violence is a public health, as well as a criminal justice problem, that threatens the health of the community, scholars argue that efforts to prevent and address this issue should include both approaches, but for different reasons. First, offenders who engage in crime should be arrested and punished before they victimize others. This allows the community to feel safe, and it reduces the number of crime victims. Second, the criminal justice system is case-focused, reactive, and punitive, but justice experts tend to disagree contending that what most people see as reactive is preventative since the system strives to achieve specific and general deterrence. Despite this goal, there is little evidence that supports that criminal justice approaches alone are effective at preventing crime and violence. Notwithstanding, the justice system intervenes after the fact, when crimes have been committed, while the public health approach is proactive. That is, it takes effect before crimes are committed by reducing risk factors to decrease the number of potential offenders as well as victims. Moore (1995) argues that both public health and criminal justice approaches should be used to address violence since they are complementary. Some observers report that law enforcement and public health have similar models for addressing problems (Markovic, 2012). Their combined efforts can address primary, second, and tertiary levels of intervention. More specifically, health researchers point out that the public health system focuses on primary prevention, while the criminal justice system addresses preventing violence at the secondary and tertiary levels.

Since violence is pervasive in the U.S., coordinating the public health approach with the law enforcement sector will expand the level of observation and intervention, along with medical expertise and needed resources to develop more effective strategies and interventions based on best practices and updated surveillance data from the justice department as well as the public health system. Some experts believe that coordination will balance prevention and reactivity. While both systems can be used to address crime and violence, there are different views regarding this matter. For example, criminal justice experts view interpersonal violent (e.g., homicide, rape, robbery, assault, and others) attacks as "crime," while public health experts see interpersonal violent attacks as "intentional and unintentional" injuries that threaten the health of the community. As such, criminal justice experts see crime, especially violence, as threating to the social fabric of society. Consequently, they make efforts to prosecute and incarcerate offenders to safeguard the well-being of the community. As a result, the justice system seeks the cause of crime and violence from within the offender by focusing on intent or motivation. Public health experts view unintentional and intentional injuries as part of a category of health problems that include disease, crime, violence, and injuries. Unlike their counterparts, they are not concerned with intent, but rather, they see the cause of violence as more complex stemming from factors that will either increase the likelihood that one will commit an offense or become a victim of violence. Stated differently, public health experts seek to identify the commonalities shared by offenders and victims through risk and protective factors (Swensen et al., 2020). Public health professionals argue that small risk factors (e.g., structural and cultural) in the environment often shape the decision to engage in violence, but they can be used to target where intervention is needed.

The commonality that both the criminal justice and public health systems share is that they aim to improve the health and safety of community residents. They also impact morbidity and mortality of U.S. citizens (Moore, 1995). While both systems are concerned about violence, the public health system emphasizes prevention programs, social support, and case management as the most effective strategy to assess problems and protect the public (Wolfe, 2012). Public health also brings a highly effective and successful model to prevent violence that surpasses what is currently found in criminal justice strategies. Perhaps the most compelling reason for the need to partner criminal justice and public health approaches lies in the fact that by partnering in the prevention of violence, it allows both systems the opportunity to share methodologies, information, data analysis, and best practices that are selected from evidence-based research that has found success at increasing coordination and community cohesion that leads to community safety through violence prevention interventions that enable stakeholders to track high crime areas, social network, and address societal, socioeconomic, and environmental causes that are more effective at preventing violence and its increasing numbers of offenders as well as victims (Markovic, 2012; Joyce & Schweig, 2014).

Summary

Violence and crime are pervasive in the U.S. and while criminal justice responses are often used to prevent such actions, some experts believe that violence and crime are also a public health problem. Some experts contend that the inequities in the U.S. may also account for rates of violence and healthcare disparities found throughout the social structure. Since crime and violence are viewed as a public health issue, health officials contend that efforts to address them should be based on prevention and interventions, rather than, reactive approaches that are used by the criminal justice system that focuses on arresting and prosecuting offenders. Public health officials view such methods as reactive and punitive.

However, there may be common ground since police agencies often engage in cooperative efforts such as community policing and problem-solving policing, which closely align with proactive approaches used in public health. The public health approach to preventing violence and crime relies on surveillance data that are collected from several agencies such as the CDC, NIH, WHO, and the department of health. It is concerned about risk factors, intervention evaluations, and implementation. Public health surveillance data are used to help define and monitor health problems including violence, identify risk factors, develop and test prevention strategies, and ensure widespread adoption of strategies. While the role of public health surveillance varies, there are several types that include passive and active surveillance. The steps in the surveillance process include data collection, data analysis, data interpretation, data dissemination, and link to action. Public health surveillance is action-based and is used to describe potential violence, monitor trends and patterns of violence, risk factors, detect sudden changes in violence occurrences, provide data for programs, policies, and priorities, and evaluate prevention and control efforts. The logic of viewing crime and violence as epidemics is to treat them as a threat to the health of the community and population like those in public health view diseases and use the public health's epidemiological approach to address them given that the approach has a proven record of success when treating and preventing tobacco smoking, STIs, and auto accidents. The public health approach uses massive educational campaigns to reach large populations to inform them about the negative health consequences of matters that threaten the nation's health. Experts argue that since many of the techniques used in criminal justice and public health often parallel, efforts should be made to use both approaches to prevent violence.

Discussion Questions

1 What is the relationship between crime and public health?
2 What is the public health approach to violence prevention?
3 How can surveillance data help to inform prevention interventions?
4 What is the logic of viewing violence and crime as epidemics?
5 Discuss several benefits of using both criminal justice and public health approaches to prevent violence.
6 What approaches does the criminal justice system rely on to prevent violence?

References

Acheson, E.D. (1988). On the state of public health (the Fourth Duncan lecture). *Public Health*, 102(5), 431–437.

Akers, T.A., Potter, R.H., & Hill, C.V. (2013). *Epidemiological criminology: A public health approach to crime and violence*. Jossey-Bass.

Alang, S., McAlpine, D., McGrcedy, E., & Harderran, R. (2017). Police brutality and black health: Setting the agenda for public health scholars. *American Journal of Public Health*, 107(5), 662–665.

Anderson, J.F. (2015). *Criminological theories: Understanding crime in America* (2nd ed.). Jones and Bartlett.

Anderson, J.F., Reinsmith-Jones, K., & Reddington, F.P. (2017). *Criminological theories: Understanding crime in America* (2nd ed.). Jones and Bartlett.

Armstead, T.L., Wilkins, N., & Amanda, D. (2018). Indicators for evaluating community and societal level risk and protective factors for violence prevention: Finding from a review of literature. *Journal of Public Health Management and Practice*, 24(1), S42–S50.

Armstead, T.L., Wilkins, N., & Nation, M. (2021). Structural and social determinants of inequities in violence risk: A review of indicators. *Journal of Community Psychology*, 49(4), 878–906.

Berk, R. (2023). Is violent crime increasing? https//crim.sas.upenn.edu/fact-check/violent-crime-inc reasing

Bernsteins, J.A., Friedman, C., Jacobson, P., & Rubin, J.C. (2015). Ensuring public health's future in a national-scale learning health system. *American Journal of Preventive Medicine*, 48, 480–487.

Bolen, J.R., Sleet, D.A., Chorba, T. et al. (1997). Overview of efforts to prevent motor vehicle-related injury. In Prevention of motor vehicle-related injuries: A compendium of articles from the Morbidity and Mortality Weekly Report, 1985–1996. Atlanta, Georgia: US Department of Health and Human Services, Centers for Disease Control and Prevention, National Center for Injury Prevention and Control.

Braveman, P. (2014). What are health disparities and health equity? We need to be clear. *Public Health Reports*, 129(1), 5–9.

Bunker, J.P., & Frazier, H.S. (1994). Improving health: Measuring effects of medical care. *Milbank Quarterly*, 72, 225–258.

Burns, S., Hitchock, L., Ibrahim, J., Penn, M., & Ramanathan, T. (2016). Policy surveillance: A vital public health practice come of age. *Journal of Health Politics, Policy and Law*, 41(6), 1151–1183. https://doi.org/10.215/03616878-3665931

Catchpole, M. (2001). Sexually transmitted infections: Control strategies. BMJ, 322:1135–1136.

Caves, R.W. (2004). *Encyclopedia of the city* (p. 548). Routledge. ISBN97804152256.

Centers for Disease Control and Prevention (CDC). (2008). *National Center for Health Statistics. Leading causes of death 1900–1998.* www.cdc.gov/nchs/data/dvs/lead1900-98. pdf. Accessed November 18, 2008.

Centers for Disease Control and Prevention (CDC). (2009). *National Center for Injury Prevention and Control.* Web-based injury Statistics Query and Reporting System (WISQAS). https://wisqars. cdc.gov. Accessed November 18, 2008.

Centers for Disease Control and Prevention (CDC). (2014). *National Center for Injury Prevention and Control.* Web-based injury Statistics Query and Reporting System (WISQARS) (online). Retrieved from: https://wisqars.cdc.gov/

Centers for Disease Control and Prevention (CDC). (2016). *Preventing multiple forms of violence: A strategic vision for connecting the dots.* Atlanta, GA: National Centers for Injury Prevention and Control, Centers for Disease Control and Prevention. Retrieved from www.cdcgov/violenceprevent ion/pdf/strategic-visions

Centers for Disease Control and Prevention (CDC). (2020). *The public health approach to violence prevention.* National Center for Injury Prevention and Control, Division of Violence Prevention.

Centers for Disease Control and Prevention (CDC). (n.d.). *Calculating the burden of sexually transmitted infections in the United States: New CDC research streamlines data analysis.* Centers for Disease Control and Prevention. National Centers for HIV/AIDS, Viral Hepatitis, STD, an TB Prevention. www.cdc.gov

Choi, B.C. (2012). The past, present, and future of public health surveillance. *Scientifica*, https://pmc. ncbi.nlm.nih.gov/articles/PMC9384415/

Dahlberg, L.L., & Krug, E.G. (2002). Violence a global public health problem. In E. Krug, L.L. Dahlberg, J.A. Mercy, A.B. Zwi, & R. Lozano (Eds.), *World report on violence and health* (pp. 1–21). World Health Organization.

Department of Health and Human Services (1992). Public health service. Position papers from the Third national injury control conference: Setting the national agenda for injury control in the 1990s. Washington, DC: Government Printing Office, DHHS Pub. No. 1992-634-66.

Freire-Vargo, L. (2018). Violence as a public health issue. *Journal of Ethics, American Medical Association*, 20(1), 25–28.

Gaines, L.K., & Miller, R.L. (2010). *Criminal justice in action: The core* (5th ed.). Wadsworth Cengage Learning.

Gebo, E. (2022). Intersectional violence prevention: The potential of public health-criminal justice partnership. *Health Promotion International*, 37(3), daccCO62. https://doi.org/10.1093/heapro/daac062

Goldstein, H. (1979). Improving policing: A problem-oriented approach. *Crime and Delinquency*, 25, 236–258.

Graham, H. (2004). Social determinants and their unequal distribution: Clarifying policy misunderstanding. *The Milbank Quarterly*, 82(1), 101–124.

Grawert, A., & Kim, N. (2022). Myths and realities: Understanding recent trends in violent crime. *Brennen Center for Justice*. https://www.brennancenter.org

Grinshteyn, E., & Hemenway, D. (2016). Violent death rates: The US compared with other high-income OECD countries. *The American Journal of Medicine*, 129(3), 266–273.

Groseclose, S.L., & Buckeridge, D.L. (2017). Public health surveillance systems. Recent advances in their use and evaluation. *Annual Review of Public Health*, 38, 57–79.

Holland, W.W. (2002). A dubious future for public health. *Journal of the Royal Society of Medicine*, 95(4), 182–188.

Hsu, S.C., Chen, K.Y., Lin, C.P., & Su, W.H. (2022). Knowledge development trajectories of crime prevention domain: An academic study based on citation and main path analysis. *International Journal of Environmental Research and Public Health*, 19(17), 1–20. https://doi.org/10.3390/ijerph191710616

Johnson, C. (2023). The vast majority of criminal cases end in plea bargains, a new report finds. www.npr.org/2023/02/23/1158356619

Joyce, N., & Schweig, S. (2014). Preventing victimization: Public health approaches to fight crime. *The Police Chief Magazine*, 38–41.

Koop, C. (1985). Welcome and "change" to the participants. Surgeon Generals' Workshop on violence and public health. Health Resources and Services Administration; US Public Health Service; US Department of Health and in Human Services (DHHS Publication No. HRS-D-MC 86-1).

Krug, E.G., Dahlberg, L.L., Mercy, J.A., Zwi, A.B., & Lozano, R. (2002). *World report on violence and health*. World Health Organization.

Krug, E.G., Mercy, J.A., Dahlberg, L.L., & Zwi, A.B. (2002). The world report on violence and health. *The Lancet*, 360(9339), 1083–1088.

Lee, J., Negussie, T., & Zaru, D. (2023). Flint residents grapple with water crisis 9 years latter: No justice. https://abcnews.go.com. April 21, 2023

Local Government Association (n.d.). Public health approaches to reducing violence. www.local.gov.uk/sites/default/files/documents/15.32%20-%20Reducing%20family%20violence_03.pdf

Markovic, J. (2012). Criminal justice and public health approaches to violent crime: Complementary perspectives. *Geography and Public Safety*, 3(2), 1–18.

Marques, A.H., Oliveira, P.A., Scomparini, L.B., Silva, U., Silva, A., Doretto, V. Filho, M.,& Scivoletto, S. (2015). Community-based global health program for maltreated children and adolescents in Brazil: The equilibrium program. *Frontiers in Psychiatry*, 6(102), 1–8.

Massetti, G.M., Holland, K.M., & Gorman-Smith, D., (2016). Implementation measurement for evidence-based violence prevention programs in communities. *Journal of Community Health*, 41, 881–894.

Moffitt, T.E., & The Klaus-Grave 2012 Think Tank (2013). Childhood exposure to violence and lifelong health: Clinical intervention science and stress biology research join forces. *Development and Psychology*, 25, 1619–1634.

Moore, M.H. (1995). Public health and criminal justice approaches to prevention. *Crime and Justice*, 19, 237–262.

Morbidity and Mortality Weekly Report (MMWR). (1999). Ten great public health achievements – United States, 1990–1999. US Department of Health and Human Services, Centers for Disease Control and Prevention.

National Highway Traffic Safety Administration (NHTSA). (2006). Motor vehicle traffic crash fatality events and estimates of people injured for 2005. DOT HS 810 639, August 2006.

Network of Employers for Traffic Safety. (2006). Advancing Safety. ww.trafficsafety.org. Accessed October 1, 2006.

Nsubuga, P., White, M.E., Thackers, S.B., et al. (2006). Public health surveillance: A tool for targeting and monitoring interventions. In D.T. Jamison, J.G., Brennan, & A.R. Measham, et al. (Eds.), *Disease Control Priorities in Developing Countries* (2nd ed.). World Bank, Chapter 53.

Pease, K. (2002). Crime reduction. In M. Maguire & Reiner, R. (Eds.), *The Oxford handbook of criminology* (pp. 947–979). Oxford University Press.

Peirson, L., Mu, A., Kenny, M., Raina, P., & Sherifali, D. (2016). Interventions for prevention and treatment of tobacco smoking in school-aged children and adolescents: A systematic review and meta-analysis. *Prevention Medicine*, 85, 20–31.

Phelan, J.C., Link, B.G., & Tehranifer, P. (2010). Social conditions as fundamental causes of health inequalities: theory evidence and policy implications. *Journal of Health and Social Behavior*, 51, S28–S40.

Public Health Services. (1994). For a healthy nation: Returns on investment in public health. Atlanta, Georgia: US Department of Health and Human Services, Public health Service, Office of Disease Prevention and Health Promotion an CDC.

Rauf, D. (2022). Childhood abuse can lead to physical and mental problems decades later: Counseling may help reduce negative health outcomes. www.everydayhealth.com/emotional-health/childhood-abuse-can-lead-to-physical-and-mental-problems-decades-later

Ray, M. (2022). *Flint water crisis: Public health crisis*, Flint, Michigan, United States. www.britannica.com/event/Flint-water-crisis

Renauer, B. (2007). Reducing fear of crime. *Police Quarterly*, 10, 41–62.

Roberts, S. (2016). What's the difference between prevention and intervention when dealing with suicide? www.linkedin.com/pulse/whats-difference-between-prevention-intervention

Rojanaworarit, C. (2015). Principles of public health surveillance: A revisit to fundamental concepts. *Journal of Public Health and Development*, 13(1), 13–46.

Rosenberg, M.L., & Fenley, M.A. (1991). *Violence in America: A public health approach*. Oxford University Press.

Schneider, M.J. (2021). *Introduction to public health* (6th ed.). Jones and Bartlett Learning.

Schweig, S. (2014). Healthy communities may make safe communities: Public health approaches to violence prevention. *NIJ Journal*, 273. www.OJP.gov/pdffilesNo.1/nij/244150.pdf

Sherman, L., Gartin, P., & Buerger, M. (1989). Hot spots of predatory crime: Routine activities and the criminology of place. *Criminology*, 27, 27–55.

Siegel, L.J. (2011). *Essentials of criminal justice* (7th ed.). Wadsworth Cengage Learning.

Sleet, D.A., & Gielen, A. (1998). *Injury prevention*. In J. Arnold and S. Gorin (Eds.), *Health promotion handbook* (pp. 247–275). Mosby.

Sleet, D.A., Dinh-Zarr, B., & Dellinger, A.M. (2007). Traffic safety in the context of public health and medicine (pp. 41–58). Foundation for Traffic Safety. Washington, DC. https://aaafoundation.org/wp-content/uploads/2018/02/ImprovingTrafficSafetyCultureinUSReport.pdf

Smith, P.F., Hadler, J.L., Stanbury, M., Rolfs, R.T., & Hopkins, R.S. (2013). "Blueprint Version 2.0": Updating public health surveillance for the 21st century. *Journal of Public Health Management and Practice*, 19(3), 231–239. www.jstor.org/stable/48566839

Smith, P.G. (2015). Types of intervention and their development. In P.G. Smith, R.H. Marrow, and D.A. Ross (Eds.), *Field trials of health intervention: A toolbox* (3rd ed.). Oxford University Press. www.ncbi.nlm.nih.gov

Swensen, K., Murza, G., Sulzer, S., & Voss, M. (2020). Public health violence prevention: Supporting law enforcement. Can public health efforts reduce crime and resolve inequities? https://extension.usu.edu/heart/research/violence-prevention-supports-law-enforcement

Teutsch, S.M., & Churchill, R.E. (2000). *Principles and practice of public health surveillance*. Oxford University Press.

Thacker, S.B., & Birkhead, G.S. (2008). *Field epidemiology.* Oxford University Press.

Thacker, S.B., & Stroup, D.S. (1998). *Public health surveillance in applied epidemiology: Theory to practice* (pp. 105–135), edited by R.C. Brownson & D.B. Petitti. Oxford University Press.

Trojanowicz, R., & Bucqueoux, B. (1990). *Community policing: A contemporary perspective.* Anderson.

WHO Global Consultation on Violence and Health. (1996). Violence: A public health priority. Geneva, World Health Organization (document WHO/EHA/SPI. POA.2).

Williams, D.R., Priest, N., & Anderson, N.B. (2016). Understanding associations among race, socio-economic status and health: Patterns and prospects. *Health Psychology*, 35(4), 407–4011.

Wolf, R.V. (2012). The overlap between public health and law enforcement: Sharing tools and data to foster healthier community. *International Review of Law, Computer & Technology*, 26(1), 97–107.

Wolke, D., & Lereya, S.T. (2015). Long-term effects of bullying. *Archives of Disease in Childhood*, 100(9), 879–885.

World Health Organization (WHO). (2014a). Global status report on violence prevention 2014. United Nations Office on Drugs and Crime. United Nations Development Programme.

World Health Organization (WHO). (2014b). Surveillance for vaccine preventable diseases. World Health Organization: Immunization, Vaccines and Biologicals. Archived from the original on April 1, 2014. Retrieved October 19, 2016.

World Health Organization (WHO). (2023). Public health surveillance. www.emro.who.int/health-topics/public-health-surveillance/index.html

2

EPIDEMIOLOGY AND CRIMINOLOGY OF VIOLENCE

Introduction

John, a Black resident of a marginalized community, works at a neighborhood grocery store and is fatally struck by bullets to his chest as he enters the grocery store to start his morning shift. The assailant is Angela, a known substance abuser who stopped John the day before the shooting, asking for money. On this day, she holds John at gunpoint in an effort to rob him. Subsequently, she shoots him twice. As Angela is retrieving money from John's wallet, Michael, the security guard at the store, hits Angela over the head with his gun and knocks her out. Michael retrieves her gun, and bystanders hold her until the police arrive. Angela is arrested, convicted of John's murder, and confined in a women's prison serving a life sentence, but offered no treatment for her substance abuse. A study conducted in the aftermath of this murder revealed several residents of the community who were eyewitnesses to the murder as well as others who were not, experienced health issues such as increased blood pressure rates, anxiety, depression, and substance abuse. Acts of violence such as the above scenario can occur among all classes of people and in any neighborhood, often posing detriments to individuals' health status. Among health studies that have been conducted regarding individuals in disadvantaged neighborhoods, Akers and Lanier (2009) suggested that marginalized populations are often at risk of violent crimes which also places them at risk of developing health-related issues. This is most concerning due to the rising impact of violent acts and the unintended health consequences that result from the violence on persons residing in marginalized neighborhoods who may be the perpetrators of the violence, firsthand victim(s) of the violence, or witnesses to the violence.

Etiological, Theoretical, and Epidemiological Causes of Violent Crime

According to the World Health Organization (WHO), violence is defined as:

> the intentional use of physical force or power, threatened or actual, against oneself, another person, or against a group or community, that either results in, or has a high likelihood of resulting in injury, death, psychological harm, maldevelopment or deprivation.

DOI: 10.4324/9781003373001-2

In 2002, the WHO regarded violent crime as a global health epidemic in its first *World Report on Violence and Health*. What emerged from the report was the need to better understand the causes of violent crime and the manner(s) in which it could be reduced (Krug et al., 2002). When examining the etiology of violent crime, it is unpredictable and can be explained by various theoretical explanations, which include poverty, genetic predisposition, personality characteristics, and substance abuse, to name a few. However, understanding the etiology of violent crime has eluded criminologists, political scientists, economists, social and behavioral scientists, and public health experts for years. Perhaps this is due to there being so many theoretical causes of violence, but no solution. While several fields of study, such as the social behavioral sciences, including criminology, have made attempts to explain the etiology of violence, epidemiologists have studied violence as a public health issue. As such, epidemiologists study the disease of violence and its distribution in populations. Epidemiology combines research methodology with theoretical concepts to determine the causes of violence and those impacted by it. For example, epidemiologists study the effectiveness of firearm laws to determine if violence will result. Epidemiologists determined that young people between the ages of 15 and 34 are disproportionately affected by injuries from firearms and deaths in their communities and suffer from short-term chronic mental and physical health conditions as well as behavioral issues (Centers for Disease Control and Prevention [CDC], 2024). In the following section, we examine health disparities and how epidemiology works.

Impact of Health Disparities

Defining Health Disparity

To begin understanding health disparities, it is best to start with an understanding of health equity. *Health equity* has been defined by the CDC (2022) as "The state in which everyone has a fair and just opportunity to attain their highest level of health" (p. 1). In other words, according to Braveman (2014a), equity is justice. The movement toward health equity requires the reduction of health disparities by improving the health of those considered most underprivileged such as persons of color, members of the LGBTQ community, battered women and children, those who have a socially stigmatizing disability, those most economically poor such as the homeless, and others who have been marginalized from the mainstream of society. *Health disparities* are "preventable differences in the burden of disease, injury, violence, or opportunities to achieve optimal health" (CDC, 2022) as experienced by the aforementioned groups and numerous others. Health disparities may also affect persons based on where they are located geographically, their age, their citizenship status, and the language they speak (Ndugga & Artiga, 2023).

Disparities are measured by the differences in which populations of persons experience life expectancy, mortality, mental health disorders, including post-traumatic stress disorder, and conditions such as asthma, malnutrition, cancer, and diabetes (University of Southern California, 2023). Life-threatening disparity also exists in people's access to medical and behavioral health care and their ability to have medical insurance. For example, in 2022, multiracial adults demonstrated more mental illness than any other racial group (Substance Abuse and Mental Health Services Administration, 2022). In this case, adult multiracial persons experienced a disparity in mental illness as a group due to the high numbers of persons reporting mental illness when compared to other racial/ethnic groups.

Notable Health Disparities

For many years, the definitions of health disparity and minority health were intertwined because of the undue burden that health disparities have placed upon minority populations. Adding to the definitions of health equity and health disparity provided above. *Minority health* is defined as, "The distinctive health characteristics and attributes of racial and/or ethnic minority groups, as defined by the U.S. Office of Management and Budget (OMB), that can be socially disadvantaged due in part to being subject to potential discriminatory acts" (National Institute on Minority Health and Health Disparities, 2024). Groups included definitionally are American Indian or Alaska Native, Asian, Black, Native Hawaiian or Pacific Islander, and Latino or Hispanic. While other racial or ethnic groups are certainly affected by health disparities, these populations are statistically impacted by disparities to a greater degree. Factors other than race or ethnicity compound the weight of disparities: lower socioeconomic status (SES), residing in rural communities, membership of sexual and gender minority (SGM) groups, and living with one or more disability. Major health disparities in the U.S. include, but are not limited to, infant mortality, heart disease and stroke, cancer, mental health, and Type 2 Diabetes (National Institutes of Health, n.d.). These disparities are more prevalent in the groups mentioned above compared with other groups in the U.S.

Infant Mortality

When a child dies before 12 months of age, it is referred to as *infant mortality* (National Institute of Child Health and Human Development, 2021). While U.S. infant mortality has decreased 10% overall, the rate for Black babies is 1.9 times the national rate per 1,000 births (March of Dimes, 2023). For the period 2019–2021, infant mortality was at 10.5% for Blacks and 7.7% for American Indians and Alaskan Natives (AI/AN) compared with 4.8% for Hispanics, and 4.4% for Whites.

Cardiovascular Disease (CVD) and Stroke

Between the years 2017 and 2020, 59.0% of Black females and 58.9% of Black males were diagnosed with a type of cardiovascular disease (CVD), the largest percentage for any U.S. racial population (Tsao et al., 2023). CVD has been linked to risk factors such as smoking, low physical activity, obesity, and problems with cholesterol, blood pressure, and glucose control. These factors are prevalent in populations bearing the burden of health disparities. It has also been reported that the rate of stroke is two times greater for Blacks of any gender compared with Whites, although rates have varied by U.S. region (Saller et al., 2010).

Cancer

Cancer prevalence and deaths vary by gender, race, ethnicity, geographic location, and socioeconomics. For example, males (undivided by race) in the U.S. Appalachia area experience lung cancer rates 26% higher than in any other U.S. region, which is likely attributed to occupation and environmental circumstances (DeBolt et al., 2021). The rate of risk for triple-negative breast cancer for Black women is three times that of other female U.S. groups (McCarthy et al., 2021). Black women are also likely to have poorer treatment outcomes compared with their White counterparts who are diagnosed with this cancer type (Cho et al., 2021). Black males have twice the rate of colon cancer deaths of any other male U.S. racial group. Socioeconomics and insurance play a role in cancer treatment disparities. For example, Noel and colleagues (2023) found that bladder cancer patients from a higher SES with private insurance received the proper standard of care, while those from a lower socioeconomic group received a lower standard of care.

Mental Health

Mental illness disorders continue to be a leading cause of disability in the U.S. They are among the costliest conditions for those between 18 and 64 years old (National Institute of Mental Health [NIMH], 2023). In 2017, persons identifying as bi-racial reported the highest rate (24.9%) of mental illness, followed by AI/AN (22.7%), followed by Whites (19%), and Blacks (16.8%), respectively. While the rate of mental illness for Blacks is not the highest, Blacks and Hispanics have reported more persistent symptoms (Budhwani et al., 2015). Not only do AI/AN experience higher rates of post-traumatic stress disorder and alcohol use disorders (NIMH, 2023), but they also carry the burden of the highest suicide rates for adults between the ages of 35–46 years old: 41.3 suicides per 100,000 for AI/AN men compared with 35.7 per 100,000 for White men as well as 12.8 per 100,000 for AI/NA women compared with 10.7 per 100,000 White women (CDC, 2023a). Another disparity is gender orientation: lesbian, gay, and bisexual high school students attempting suicide had a rate five times higher than non-LGB high schoolers (Jones et al., 2021).

Type 2 Diabetes

Type 2 diabetes is a leading cause of death in the U.S., affecting approximately 38.4 million or 11.6% of the population, and it is estimated that at least 8.7% more persons have diabetes diagnosed, but have not been diagnosed (CDC, 2023c). Of the adult U.S. population, from 2019 to 2021, Type 2 Diabetes was highest among AI/AN at 14.5%, followed by Blacks (12.1%), Hispanics (11.7%), Asians (9.1%), and Whites (6.9%) (CDC, 2023c).

Some Consequences of Health Disparity

The impacts of health disparities are many and often include high death and uninsured rates, physical and mental disability, the economic burden of illness, and increased homicide rates. Below, we take a closer look at two of these impacts.

High Death Rates and Lack of Insurance

Health disparities have different forms, such as the absence of care alone or in conjunction with the lack of health insurance to acquire care. Of all wealthy nations, the U.S. is the only country that does not provide universal government-funded health insurance and has the lowest life expectancy rate (Gunja et al., 2023). In 2022, approximately 26 million people in the U.S. were without health insurance, a slight drop from pre-pandemic numbers (Tolbert et al., 2023). According to Tolbert and colleagues (2023), data on the uninsured show that nearly 73.3% had one or more full-time workers in the family, with only 15.8% showing no workers in the household. Additionally, 80.8% of nonelderly uninsured people were in families with incomes below 400% of the federal poverty level. Racially, of those nonelderly uninsured for 2022, 40% were Hispanic, 37.7% White, and 12.8% Black. Though the number of nonelderly Whites is the highest among racial groups, "people of color made up 45.7% of the nonelderly U.S. population but accounted for 62.3% of the total nonelderly uninsured population" (p. 12). Among the top six reasons for being uninsured, affordability was number one.

Accordingly, death rates are highest for minority, underserved, and uninsured U.S. populations. Woolhandler and Himmelstein (2017) found studies demonstrating how uninsured persons have a lower chance of survival since a lack of insurance typically leads to a lower rate of preventive services use. A 2022 U.S. White House briefing stated that "lack of health insurance coverage was associated with higher excess mortality rates during the pandemic, even after controlling for differences in vaccination rates" (p. 2) and other factors such as age, pre-existing conditions, and state restrictions during the pandemic. Again, the connection between COVID deaths and race is undeniable: it is estimated that 97.9 of every 100,000 Blacks died from COVID-19—a death rate one-third higher than for Latinos and double that for Whites (Reyes, 2020).

Economic Burden

Economic burden can be viewed as the direct costs of having an illness (e.g., treatment and related care) as well as indirect costs (e.g., lost wages, lost costs due to early death, and nonmedical expenses) (Weintraub, 2023). According to a 2018 study funded by the National Institute on Minority Health and Health Disparities (NIMHD), "racial and ethnic health disparities cost the U.S. economy $451 billion annually, a 41% increase from the previous estimate of $320 billion in 2014" and that the " burden of education-related health disparities for persons with less than a college degree in 2018 reached $978 billion" (LaVeist et al., 2023).

Nationally, in 2018, the Black U.S. population carried the weight of the economic burden because of premature mortality, or rather, years of life lost before the age of 70. Per person, however, Native Hawaiian/Pacific Islander and Alaskan Native and Native American populations had the highest burden. State data confirmed that Black and African-American populations had the greatest burden. Persons not completing a GED or receiving a high school diploma bore the most economic burden when considering education (LaVeist et al., 2023).

Conceptualizing Criminogenic Health Disparities

Criminogenic health disparities can be thought of as those disparities correlated with criminal behavior over time. Listed below are two of the many health disparities that research has shown to shape a person's behavior and potentially lead to criminal justice involvement.

Lead Poisoning

According to Housing and Urban Development lead paint surveys from 1990 to 2019, the number of homes with lead paint has decreased (Jacobs & Brown, 2023). However, old home stock, most affordable for low-income populations and with deteriorated lead paint, increased. Racial occupancy in these homes has varied over the years. However, research has demonstrated that the continued presence of lead paint is linked to poor environmental regulations and "residential segregation, concentrated poverty, discrimination in housing markets, and neighborhood disinvestment" related to "racial and class inequalities in exposure to lead" (Winter, 2020, 2). Muller et al. (2018) found that from 1995 to 2013, in Chicago black neighborhoods, inhabitants reliably demonstrated the highest prevalence of lead in tested blood levels, with lower levels found in Hispanic communities, and the lowest levels found in White neighborhoods.

Several studies have supported the link between elevated lead blood levels in persons and problem behaviors, poor health outcomes, and low educational achievement. Even at low levels, lead has been found to cause irreversible effects such as attention span problems, learning disabilities, hyperactivity, and other "health, intellectual, and behavioral problems" (p. 4), and at high levels may cause "mental retardation, coma, convulsions, and even death" (p. 5) (National Center for Healthy Housing, 2023). Sampson and Winter (2018) reported that lead exposure could harm younger children's brain and nervous system development, leading to academic and behavioral problems. Talayero and colleagues (2023) reported that in-utero and childhood lead exposure might be correlated with criminal justice involvement for adults. After conducting a systematic review of 17 manuscripts and 13 studies about childhood exposure to lead and subsequent criminal involvement, they found an association between exposure to lead and the later development of "delinquent, antisocial, and criminal behavior" (p. 19).

Exposure to Firearm Violence

Firearm violence is recognized as a public health issue. As of 2023, firearm violence was the leading cause of death for children and teenagers between the ages of 1–17, and reports demonstrate that the U.S. child firearm mortality rate doubled from 2013 to 2021 (McGough et al., 2023). Firearm deaths can be viewed in three categories: accidental, suicide, and assault. U.S. teen firearm assault mortality rates peaked in 2021 at a rate of 3.9 per 100,000, and the child/teen firearm suicide mortality rate increased by 21% from 2019 to 2021. For Black male youth, there was a 39.2% increase in firearm mortality from 1999 to 2020, resulting in a 47.1% rate for Black male youth ages 1–19 years old, with White male youth at 31.6%, and Hispanic male youth at 18.1% (Mariño-Ramírez et al., 2022). Firearm suicide rates among Black children and teens have, for the first time recorded, surpassed that of their White counterparts (Johns Hopkins Bloomberg School of Public Health, 2023).

Whether exposure to firearm violence is direct or indirect (e.g., witnessing firearm violence, knowing someone who was lost to firearm violence, or even living in a neighborhood where firearm violence occurs), adverse personal short and long-term consequences can occur. Children are exposed to violence in many ways, including through domestic violence, all forms of bullying, child abuse, and neighborhood violence (National

Institute of Justice [NIJ], 2016). Exposure to violence, and the possible consequential trauma, has been linked to the onset of academic problems (Crouch et al., 2019), drug or alcohol use (Halpern, 2018), aggression, depression (Humphreys et al., 2020), and/ or other mental health problems, and further victimization (Ports et al., 2016), physical conditions (Gilbert et al., 2015), as well as juvenile delinquency and adult criminal behavior (Lo et al., 2020).

How Epidemiology Works

Epidemiology is an approach that many fields use, public health particularly, to study the occurrence of a disease or other harmful agents in populations of persons, rather than within individuals: it could be described as *societal* rather than *clinical* (Farmer & McDonald, 1988). Epidemiology goes beyond describing and studying singular or small group accounts of an occurrence to searching for patterns of occurrence across larger numbers of people. Therefore, this approach is used by many health departments, government divisions, the military, hospitals, clinics, and other entities concerned with public or population health.

Data required for epidemiology involves "evidence-informed risk and protective factors, and service outcomes" (Government of South Australia, n.d., 2). For example, well-studied *risk factors* of a specific population that make it *vulnerable to* a defined occurrence or *protective factors* that buffer that population from a defined occurrence. For our purposes here, that occurrence is violence. Paramount to epidemiology is prevention and the outcomes of services used for addressing a disease or event. Epidemiology uses two types of frequency measures: incidence and prevalence rates, which are useful in identifying the causes of a disease or injury. *Prevalence* rates indicate the number of persons affected by a determined occurrence or injury over a specific period (CDC, 2023b). *Incidence* rates demonstrate the number of occurrences or injuries occurring in a given sample over a defined period (CDC, 2023b).

The epidemiological approach to addressing and preventing injury or disease involves following patterns of onset and occurrence rates in the population being studied, identifying risk and protective factors, developing intervention and prevention measures, evaluating those measures, and disseminating successful prevention methods to the public (Government of South Australia, Human Services, n.d., 3). Based on data collected and analyzed during research activities, conclusions can be made based on comparative studies, high and highest-risk subsets of populations can be identified, and long-term surveillance can occur to monitor the efficacy of interventions over time (BMJ, 2024).

Violence is a multidisciplinary problem, and therefore, the epidemiological approach utilizes resources from varied disciplines to address it. Schneider (2000) references four of these specialties: (1) biomedical sciences (a combination of biology and medicine); (2) environmental health sciences (includes chemical exposure, noise, and elements of the physical environment); (3) social sciences (the study of society and the interpersonal relationships between people and their environment); and (4) the behavioral sciences (studies of mental health and behavior) (Schneider, 2000). Therefore, the work of identifying causative factors of violence and constructing intervening or preventive measures is done collaboratively.

The Epidemiological Triangle

The epidemiological triangle is a tool used by public health when examining how a disease moves throughout a population and how to intervene with and prevent it. The epidemiologic triangle has three parts: agent, host, and environment (River University, 2024). The *agent* is considered the cause of what is being studied, the *host* is considered the carrier or transmitter of what is being studied, and the *environment* refers to all the outside factors that play some part in how the disease or other circumstance is being carried throughout a population. Consider smoking as an example. A carcinogen in the smoke of a cigarette is considered the agent, people who smoke or inhale second-hand smoke become the hosts, and the environment contains the many reasons that people smoke tobacco, as well as the frequency they use cigarettes and how long a period that they have been a smoker (River University, 2024).

For this discussion, the disease is violence or violent crime. Using the triangle to examine violence, the agent would be the violent crime itself; persons who commit the violence, or even who are affected by the violence, are the hosts; and the environment consists of causal and/or determinate factors that assist in the prevalence and occurrence of violent crime among a subset of people. Using the epidemiological triangle, success in intervening with or preventing violence would be considered as breaking one of the triangle's sides, disrupting the continuation of the violent crime that the triangle represents.

While the triangle can be a simple epidemiological representation of violent crime, each point of the triangle (i.e., the agent, the host, and the environment) is complex. This model could be used to look at several types of violent crime simultaneously and even be used in comparative studies, such as violent crime against women and violent crime against members of the LGBTQ community (Figure 2.1).

By examining one type of violence, prevention or intervention methods found to have efficacy with one population may work with another, even in a modified form, or by placing the prevention on a different side of the triangle, as with the Against Women diagram.

Major Theoretical Explanations for Violence from Criminal Justice and Public Health

Bartol and Bartol (2002) suggest that the theoretical causes of violence include biological, socialization, cognitive, and situational factors. Biological factors include physiological,

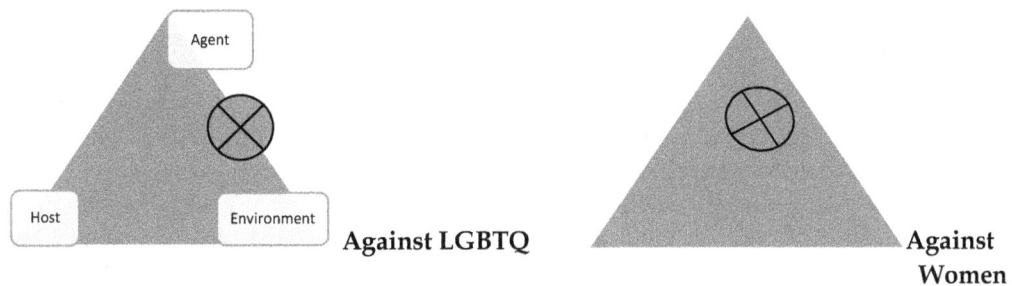

Against LGBTQ   **Against Women**

FIGURE 2.1   The Epidemiological Triangle.

chemical, and neurological influences on an individual's aggression and violence. Interactions between the social environment and biological factors can influence the development of children. Linkages have been found between brain damage and aggressive behavior in children, which has resulted from head injuries, lead paint, deficiencies in children's diet, the mother's using alcohol and drugs prior to birth, and trauma caused during birth. This aggressive behavior is often treated with medication.

In describing socialization factors, Bartol and Bartol (2002) assert that children learn attitudes and norms of how to interact with others from observing social behavior; they also learn in what situations to use this behavior. Therefore, children learn violence from those they hold in high esteem as well as fictional characters. Bartol and Bartol (2002) describe cognitive factors as the patterns of thinking that emerge from interactions with the world over one's lifetime, but state violent individuals have different ways of processing this information and will resolve disagreements and conflicts in a violent manner. Situational factors refer to environmental characteristics such as stress or aggression that bring violent behavior. For example, any adverse situation such as an unfavorable living condition can trigger violence and the presence of a weapon can increase the likelihood of violence. Bartol and Bartol argue that childhood aggression can be a predictor of adult violence. However, Cavanaugh (2012) postulates that psychodynamic and/or social factors have historically been used to reduce the occurrence of violent behavior, but provide little information regarding the theoretical causes of violence. She states, "psychology highlights intra-psychic attributes and behaviors; sociology features the influence of social factors and structures; and anthropology points to socio-cultural influences and traditions," but there is no one theory or paradigm that can be used to fully explain the etiological causes of violence (Cavanaugh, 2012, p. 608). Therefore, there is a need to intertwine the various theories to perhaps develop an answer to the question, "What causes violent crime?"

When examining violence from a public health approach, Perry (2009) suggests that public health is atheoretical, and since the 20th century, it has been based on theories of biomedical science, behavioral psychology, and public administration, but has relied on theoretical orientations in the fields of criminology, sociology, and psychology to guide it. Kleinman (2010, p. 1518) adds to this argument by stating that the field of medicine has not been rich in theory, but the health field is "evidence-based and theory oriented." As such, Gilligan (2001) proposed a useful public health theory of violence, The Germ Theory of Disease, which views violence as a disease, and as an emotion that brings shame and humiliation. Shame and humiliation are described as violating one's self-respect and dignity and possibly leading to childhood cruelty/neglect; inequalities in status in society, and it is controlled by punishment and humiliation in the criminal justice system. The theory would view the act of murder as the ultimate defense mechanism against the shame of such acts once committed against the murderer, such as child molestation, racial discrimination, or other social injustices. Here, the commission of the murder restores a sense of power to the murderer over the victim, a sense of "getting even" approach.

Gilligan views violence as a health problem that can be prevented and his theory not only explains the causes of violence, but its prevention. To eliminate the shame, Lawson and King (2012, p. 518) suggest that for Gilligan, violence produces suffering for the victim as well as the predator, and it is not a legal issue that can be resolved by inflicting more punishment on the predator through the justice system. The criminal justice system serves as a continuation of the shame from arrest to imprisonment and, therefore, a continuation of the violence.

Gilligan rejects the classical school of thought's notion of punishment fitting the crime, in this view, severe punishment imposed by the criminal justice system only manifests the shame of crime and produces more crime among members of oppressed communities. Members of these communities have been victimized by such social inequalities as unemployment, dilapidated housing, crime, and the lack of education, which lead to poor health issues. For members of deprived communities, violence can be an everyday occurrence that produces such health issues such as hypertension, suicide/suicidal attempts, strokes, and psychological illnesses. Gilligan's theory suggests treatment and education are needed in communities and prisons to prevent the spread of violence.

Briceno-Leon and colleagues (2008) proposed a sociological model of violence that examined the relationship between individuals and various factors and suggested that violence is a product of multiple levels of influence on behavior. Exposure to violence can be influenced by the individual, relational, community, and society levels. At the individual level, such biological factors as one's beliefs and attitudes, and personal history can determine if one becomes a perpetrator or victim. At the relationship level, close social relationships determine violence. One's workplace, neighborhood, school, and environmental characteristics can contribute to violence or protect against it. Societal factors include conditions of society that either encourage violence or prevent it. Briceno-Leon and colleagues concluded that influences on violence were unemployment opportunities, social inequalities, urban segregation, widespread use of alcohol, drug markets, and the availability of guns. There also needs to be the understanding that when oppressed individuals, particularly persons of color, are forced to live in substandard conditions, they "fight" for daily survival; therefore, violence ensues and becomes a public health problem in marginalized communities. Gilligan's theory and Briceno-Leon and colleagues' sociological model of violence resonate with McDonald's (2000) notion of the public health approach to violence which focuses on the health of the population by seeing the predator as a victim of society who in most cases should not be punished for his/her violent behavior. Rather, there needs to be an understanding of the causes and risk factors of violence.

Mercy and others (1993) suggest that the public health approach views violence as a social problem. As such, public health analyzes violence based on the theory of causation and intervention. It defines the problem and collects data on it; identifies the causes, risks, and protective factors of the problem; develops and tests interventions to find out what works under what circumstances; and shares what works and its impact on the population at large.

Bucerius and others (2022) suggest that violence is no longer just a social, criminal justice, or economic problem; it is also a global public health issue. As such, public health is grounded in the science of epidemiology and benefits from an approach that embraces various disciplines (Donnelly et al., 2014). In essence, what is warranted is the need to view violence as not only a criminal justice issue, but also as a public health issue. Just as there are several public health explanations about the etiology of violence, there are also criminological theories.

Criminological Explanations

Several criminological explanations have been used to explain the etiology of violence. The etiology of violence is explained from the perspectives of the following theoretical conceptions: choice, social structure, social processing, and social conflict theories.

Choice Theories

The premise of choice theory is that people choose all behavior, including criminal behavior. However, an individual's choice can be controlled by the fear of punishment. Some of the various types of choice theory in criminology are *general deterrence* (e.g., the offenders' punishment serves as an example to others who have not engaged in criminal activity to deter their behavior), *specific deterrence* (e.g., the punishment is enough to prevent the criminal from engaging in criminal/violent behavior again; for example, shock sentencing or corporal punishment), and *rational choice* (e.g., assumes individuals rely on reason and logic when making choices) (Siegel, 2013). Of particular concern is rational choice theory (RCT) and its explanation of violence. RCT is concerned with the importance that satisfying one's self-interest plays in understanding human behavior. During the 1960s, Becker (1968) brought more attention to RCT by suggesting that criminal behavior was similar to economic behavior, in that both were guided by rational decisions of costs and benefits. In essence, RCT can be approached from an economic standpoint in that criminals conduct a cost–benefit analysis prior to engaging in crime (Piquero & Hickman 2002).

Social scientists have used RCT to explain human behavior. RCT has also been used to explain any array of violent crimes, ranging from robbery to murder. Muro-Ruiz (2002) contends that violence, according to RCT, can be a cold and calculated action that is carried out deliberately to achieve a purpose other than injuring the victim, or it can also be an emotional reaction governed primarily by the desire to hurt someone.

McCartney and Chaudharry (2014) suggest that RCT refers to a set of notions as to the relationship between an individual's preference and the choices they make. Individuals make rational choices based on their goals, and it is those choices that govern behavior. Therefore, Walters (2015) contends that the difference between criminals and non-criminals according to RCT is found in the choices they make. Criminals examine the relationship between what one likes and the risk (e.g., the fear of criminal penalties associated with being caught and convicted for law violations) associated with the choices they make to acquire it. Paternoster and colleagues (2017) suggest that RCT implies "offending is based upon a self-interested appraisal of the costs and benefits of alternative courses of action, with the action taken being the one with the greatest perceived utility." According to Clarke and Cornish (2001), RCT assumes that criminals make purposive decisions to offend. Criminals perform deliberate acts with the sole purpose of benefiting themselves. McCartney and Chaudharry (2014) further contend that the cost of crime for a criminal may include the legitimate loss of wages, incarceration, and rejection by a significant other. These authors characterize the benefits of crime as an increase in money, the thrill of committing the crime, or the notion of achieving a new status resulting from the crime.

Beaudry-Cyr (2015) and Turner (1997) make the following suppositions regarding RCT in criminology:

1 Humans possess the power to freely choose their conduct.
2 Humans are goal-oriented and purposive.
3 Humans have hierarchically ordered utilities or preferences.
4 Humans act based on rational judgments pertaining to:

The utility of alternatives based on their hierarchically ordered preferences.
The cost of each alternative.
The best opportunity to maximize utility.

There are various critics of RCT. Simpson and colleagues (2002) argue that individuals' decisions are usually made without accurate information or careful consideration of evidence, out of habit, or under pressure from others. Crime involves knowing the risks and facts of a particular behavior, and criminals may not know everything associated with a crime. O'Grady (2011) contends that not all individuals are capable of making rational decisions because some individuals are mentally incapable of doing such; he reasons that some individuals are not criminally responsible due to having a mental disorder. For example, an individual with dementia who has access to a gun and kills her family members.

Gul (2009) suggests the advantage of RCT is its usefulness in the field of criminal justice because it provides a framework for understanding all types of crime and is useful in suggesting new avenues of prevention. Clarke and Cornish (1987) argue that RCT is useful for understanding policies that try to control crime. These authors argue that a distinction should be made between one's criminal involvement, which includes the factors that lead to an individual's "readiness" to commit a crime, and the criminal events, which are the factors that influence the commission of specific offenses. Here there is more focus on individual and situational factors surrounding crime which are similar to the Neoclassical School of Criminology. Tibbetts and Hemmens (2014) suggest that rational choice theorists' basic argument is that individuals are not purely rational when making decisions, but consider the costs and benefits of their decisions. Likewise, Lilly and colleagues (2019, p. 359) argue that:

> rational choice theory represents an important advance in criminological thought because it shows the need to study offenders not as "empty vessels" propelled to commit crime by background factors but, rather as conscious decision makers who weigh options and act with a purpose.

The schools and theories to be examined here are the Neoclassical School of Criminology and the Routine Activity Theory (RAT).

Neoclassical School of Criminology

The Neoclassical School of Criminology became the new Classical School due to the Classical School dismissing the intent or *mens rea* of an offender and only focusing on the act or *actus reus* the offender caused to society. When determining the charges to be brought against an offender, the Neoclassical School examines the intent or circumstantial factors as well as individual factors that may have given rise to the commission of a crime and may increase or decrease punishment. For instance, a 7-year-old who suffers from severe schizophrenia and violently murders his neighbor would probably not receive the same punishment as a 40-year-old who commits the same offense.

Gabriel Tarde, René Garraud, and Henri Joly are credited with modifying the classical school with the development of the neoclassical school which viewed children, the elderly, and the mentally challenged as being less capable of exercising free will and, thus less responsible for their actions (Burke, 2009). The Neoclassical School continued to contain elements of the classical school which include the ability to make choices, decisions, and have free will. However, the neoclassical school addressed the flaws of the classical school by evaluating its assumptions. Neoclassical criminology utilizes scientific evidence to determine the just punishment for crimes. Neoclassical criminology takes into consideration that crime can result from psychological, emotional, environmental, and other factors that may lead an individual to commit crime or violence. As Amarasinghe (2020) suggests, there may be external or mental factors that prohibit one from acting on his free will. For example, individuals residing in poverty-stricken communities with little or no education or employment may be prone to criminal behavior in order to survive in society. The view of this school is that all individuals who commit illegal acts cannot be punished equally.

Criticisms of the Neoclassical School include Cornish and Clarke's (1986) suggestion that several offenders commit crimes on impulse without weighing the cost and benefits of the crime. As Lilly and colleagues (2019) argue, the brains of humans are not designed to weigh all decisions in a rational manner, and as a result, individuals rely on rules of thumb and impulse decisions, which are often irrational. Such decisions may lead to confinement in prison. The Neoclassical School is flawed by the notion that punishment is not always applied based on the circumstances or situation of the offense. There have been various persons of color who have committed the act of murder under the same circumstances/ situation as Whites, but the punishment received has been more severe for the persons of color. An additional criticism is that the theory argues that offenders can make the decision to commit a crime without the influence of others. For example, the neoclassical school provides no account for juveniles who are influenced to commit delinquent acts by their peers nor for adults who may be influenced by others to commit a criminal act.

The Neoclassical School of Criminology expands Rational Choice Theory so that it includes an understanding of individual behavior. Crime is influenced by the criminal opportunity to commit it. Amarasinghe suggests the Neoclassical School is premised on the idea of "just deserts" as a method of deterrence which is the notion that an individual who commits a crime must be punished for her wrongdoings. In essence, due process must exist, and punishment should be meted out in proportion to the crime, but must also weigh the physical and psychological condition of the perpetrator. Therefore, judges and other court personnel must consider such characteristics as the mental status and age of offenders. Likewise, Thilakarathna (2019) argues that the insane and minors should receive lenient punishment due to their inability to distinguish between right and wrong. The Neoclassical School of Criminology was the groundbreaker for establishing due process, legal rights, and alternative sentencing.

Routine Activity Theory

RAT was derived from the Neoclassical School of Criminology and was proposed by Lawrence Cohen and Marcus Felson (1979). Bruinsma and Johnson (2018) and Wilcox and Cullen (2018) suggest that RAT is labeled as Environmental Criminology or as an opportunity theory due to it examining how aspects of the physical and social environment can produce opportunities for criminal behavior. For opportunity theorists, the way to prevent crime is to reduce the opportunities for criminal behavior to occur. RAT views crime as occurring during the functions of one's daily activities. For a crime to occur, three elements must be present: a *motivated offender*, a *suitable target*, and *no capable guardian present* (Cohen & Felson, 1979). According to RAT, committing a crime involves a motivated offender and the opportunity to act on those motivations. There must exist a suitable target such as a person or object that the offender would like to have or control. RAT also involves the absence of a capable guardian who can prevent crime such as a police officer, security guard, parent, teacher, dog, or alarm.

To prevent crime, RAT suggests that individuals reduce contact with those who are motivated to commit crime and when individuals remove one of the elements needed for the crime to occur. This might include removing a suitable target such as a diamond necklace or staying near security when attending a party. RAT requires that all three elements must converge in time and place (Cohen & Felson, 1979). Similarly, Miro' (2014) suggests, "routine activity is the study of crime as an event, highlighting its relation to space and time and emphasizing its ecological nature and the implications thereof."

There are several criticisms of RAT. First, it argues that criminal activity can be prevented without a major cultural or social revolution (Lilly et al., 2019, p. 348). Does this mean that all burglaries can be prevented by merely installing an alarm system, or all aggravated rapes can be prevented by purchasing a guard dog? Second, Akers (1997) argues that RAT does not define the characteristics of motivated offenders or why one offender may be more motivated than another to commit a crime. Finally, Garland (1999) argues that RAT aligns with social and economic policies that ignore groups of people, and with "zero tolerance" police policies that repress minor crimes.

Felson (1998) contends that RAT ignores how poverty and inequality could generate crime or produce the motivation to commit crime. He argued that "poverty areas" can increase "temptations" and "decrease" controls. Individuals living in poverty usually live in areas where there are shopping malls, hospitals, and bars; areas in which the temptation to commit crime can be present due to money, drugs, and liquor being readily available; moreover, these areas have little security at night. For the criminal justice system, RAT serves as an indicator of why some locations have more criminal behavior than others. RAT has become a modern approach to predict and reduce criminal behavior. For example, geographical mapping and the Global Positioning System (GPS) are modern approaches developed based on the premises of RAT to predict and prevent crime.

Social Structure Theories

Social Structure Theories are premised on social disorganization, strain, and cultural deviance theories. "Social Structure Theories suggest that crime is caused by the way societies are structurally organized" (Tibbetts & Hemmens, 2014, p. 229). These theories argue that there are certain groups in society who are more likely to commit criminal behavior due to disadvantages or cultural differences that result from the way society is structured. In essence, there are certain racial and ethnic groups in society who are prone to crime as well as members of lower-class groups who are overrepresented in criminal behavior. Unlike previous theories, social structure theories are concerned with the criminal behavior of groups and not individuals.

Social Disorganization Theory

The proponents of social disorganization theory were Clifford Shaw and Henry McKay, who examined juvenile court statistics to map the spatial distribution of delinquency in

Chicago. Relying on maps created by Parks and Burgess, Shaw and McKay theorized that certain neighborhoods in the "zone of transition," located near factories and railroads, and characterized as slum areas, had more delinquent and criminal behavior because of their location. The further the neighborhood was away from these factors, the more affluent the neighborhood was, with little to no crime. Data analysis confirmed Shaw and McKay's theory that delinquency was more present in the zone of transition. This led to the notion that neighborhoods with high delinquency or crime rates tend to suffer from social illnesses such as poverty, physical dilapidation, infant mortality, disease, heterogeneity, and low birth rate which overlap with delinquency and crime. Here, the conditions of the neighborhood lead to social disorganization, which causes crime and delinquency. However, Shaw and McKay's findings indicated that the further one moved away from the zone, the less criminal or delinquent behavior was present. Moreover, Shaw and McKay's findings reveal that regardless of which ethnic group one belonged to, all groups living in such conditions were prone to delinquent or criminal behavior. Tibbetts and Hemmens (2014) argue that delinquent behavior is often learned in children from older youth. This theory's notion is that it is not one's culture that influences crime and delinquency, but the criminogenic nature of one's environment.

Kubrin and Wo (2016) suggest that issues such as poverty, unemployment, racial composition, and family disruption are ecological characteristics of great importance to social disorganization researchers. These researchers argue that while such community characteristics as poverty or residential instability are related to crime, they are not the initial causes of crime. These characteristics are indirectly related to crime by such neighborhood processes as informal social control which is the scope of collective intervention that the community directs toward local problems, including crime (Kornhauser, 1978).

It is the informal, non-official actions taken by residents that combat crime in their communities, for example, elderly neighbors who inform parents about their children's misbehavior may keep the child from engaging in delinquency. Kubrin and Wo describe this as informal surveillance when neighbors act as the "eyes and ears" of the community. According to the theory, socially disorganized neighborhoods have lower levels of informal social control and thus experience higher crime rates when compared to more socially organized neighborhoods (Kubrin & Wo, 2016). Lilly and colleagues (2019) argue that, according to social disorganization theory, the best method for reducing crime is to reorganize society.

Social disorganization theory has also been criticized. The theory ignores the fact that crime occurs in affluent communities. In addition, all neighborhoods do not practice or have methods of informal social control. For example, in most neighborhoods, it may be a rarity for neighbors to hold casual conversations with each other and even more to inform a neighbor as to the wrongdoings of their child. Bursik (1988) suggests that social disorganization theory has been criticized for its assumption of stable ecological structures that have not been justified by long-term historical evidence. Moreover, Burski also suggests that Shaw and McKay did not make a clear distinction between the anticipated outcome of social disorganization and the disorganization itself, and confusion exists as to the conceptualization of social disorganization.

Strain Theories

Strain theorists view strain as the major cause of criminal behavior. Robert Merton's article, "Social Structure and Anomie," is primarily responsible for the origination of strain theory. Merton's article was written in 1938 during the Great Depression when the economic structure led to once affluent individuals becoming poor and committing crimes to survive (Tibbetts & Hemmens, 2014). Merton surmised that everyone, despite social class position, was socialized to believe in the American Dream which meant if one worked hard for what they wanted or needed, they could achieve material wealth or have economic prosperity, also known as the "American Dream." However, Merton did caution that only a small percentage of individuals would be able to achieve wealth. For some juveniles and adults, impoverished communities that lacked access to structural and institutionalized means such as having a lack of or limited education, as well as being underemployed or having no employment. As a result, strain is produced because of the inability to achieve the culturally induced goal of the American Dream through conventional means. Jang and Agnew (2015) suggest that this culturally induced goal can produce criminal activity, frustration which causes one to strike another, or drug use. "Merton thought the United States epitomized the type of society that overemphasized the goal of economic disparity far more than the means. This disequilibrium is emphasized between the goals and means of society" (Tibbets & Hemmens, 2014, p. 237). Anomie, which comes from the French means "normlessness" and was used by Emile Durkheim to explain, how a breakdown of predictable social conditions can lead to feelings of personal loss and dissolution. In Durkheim's writings, anomie was a feeling of strain that resulted from not being personally embedded in society. However, Merton used anomie to refer to the contradiction between society's cultural aspirations and society's legitimate means to obtain them.

Merton saw Americans as being too focused on material wealth and developed five typologies that individuals use to respond to the strains associated with the inability to attain wealth. These typologies are also referred to as modes of adaptation. The first adaptation is *conformity*, in which an individual accepts both the cultural goals and the institutional means of obtaining success. Here, individuals work to achieve legally what they desire. Most members of the middle and upper class in society fit into this mold. The second adaptation, *innovation*, occurs when the cultural goals are accepted, but the legitimate means of obtaining them are rejected. Many lower-class individuals become innovative. An example of the adaptation of innovation is a lower-class female who has accepted the traditional goal of success and desires an expensive purse, but resorts to committing the crime of theft to achieve it. The third adaptation, in contrast to *innovation*, is *ritualism*. Ritualists are individuals who do not take risks. The fourth adaptation is *retreatism*. Retreatists reject the cultural goals of society as well as the means for achieving them. These individuals turn away from society and live by their own rules. Such individuals may suffer from mental illnesses, they may be homeless, and they may be addicted to drugs. The final adaptation is *rebellion*. Individuals who often fit into this adaptation want to change the cultural goals and structural means of society. Such people are revolutionaries and radicals who wish to create alternative lifestyles or activists who wish to promote equality; they can also be terrorists.

Additional theorists presented variations of Merton's strain theory. In the 1950s, Albert Cohen (1955), a former student of Merton examined Merton's theory of strain and expanded his assumptions of the lower class, male gangs, and adolescents. Cohen developed the theory of Lower-Class Status Frustration and Gang Formation. Cohen's assumption was that lower-class youth internalize middle-class goals of success, but develop strain or status frustration due to their inability to attain them. To cope with strain, they join delinquent gangs or engage in malicious acts (Bartollas & Schmalleger, 2014). Jang and Agnew (2015) assert that the lower class's hostility toward what those in the middle-class value leads the lower-class to reject middle-class values. For example, those in the middle class may value legal behavior, while those in the lower class may value illegal behavior. Cohen also concluded that the rejection of middle-class values by those in the lower class is what causes gang activity (Tibbetts & Hemmens, 2014). Another variation of Merton's Strain Theory was presented after Cohen by Richard Cloward and Lloyd Ohlin. Like Cohen's theory, Cloward and Ohlin's theory was a structural strain theory of gang formation and behavior (Tibbetts & Hemmens, 2014).

Cloward and Ohlin's theory developed the perspective of differential opportunity. Although Cloward and Ohlin also held the assumption that all individuals are socialized to be successful and follow the American Dream, but become frustrated and strained when they cannot, their theory differed from Merton and Cohen's in that it identified three types of gangs that could emerge from the lower-class culture. Cloward and Ohlin proposed the characteristics of gangs varied due to the illegal opportunities present in the social structure of the neighborhood (Tibbetts & Hemmens, 2014). The three types of delinquent subcultures they identified are: (1) criminal subcultures/gangs which developed in lower-class communities where criminal role models are prominent. For example, older gang members recruit youth and teach them criminal behavior; (2) conflict subcultures/gangs, in which disorganized gangs are formed without the skills and knowledge to profit from crime, therefore, they use violence to gain respect in their communities; and (3) retreatists subcultures/gangs that withdraw from society and engage in drug use. Tibbetts and Hemmens (2014) assert that Cloward and Ohlin's typologies of gangs helped to lead to the Juvenile Delinquency Prevention and Control Act of 1961. Jang and Agnew (2015) suggest that although Merton, Cohen, and Cloward and Ohlin's theories of strain differ, they all share the assumption that strain involves the inability of all groups in society to acquire the goal of success through legitimate structural means.

Robert Agnew (1992) developed a theory of general strain that did not restrict criminal behavior to members of the lower class exclusively. Agnew's theory explained crime from an individual perspective as opposed to Merton's social class notions. According to Agnew, adverse emotions such as frustration and anger that result from negative social relationships with others may cause individuals to engage in crime. Agnew argued that there are other types of situations that may produce strain and cause individuals to commit crimes. According to Lilly and colleagues (2019), Agnew identified the sources of strain that can result in criminal behavior as: (1) *Failure to achieve positively valued goals* (e.g., the loss of a loved one may lead to drug addiction to manage the stress); and (2) *Removal of positive stimuli* (e.g., an individual responds to the adversity by removing the source; for example, a wife who murders her husband for sexually abusing their child). A critique of Agnew's theory is that while there is evidence that the combination of strain and anger can increase the risk of crime,

what remains to be clarified, however, is whether strain creates anger, which then leads to crime, or whether people who are angry are more likely to create strain in their lives, which then leads to crime. Of course, both causal links to crime are possible.

(Mazerolle et al., 2000)

Additional criticisms of strain theories have also been made. According to Brym and Lie (2007), strain theory suggests that one's social class plays a major role in whether an individual will engage in crime. The theory assumes that crime only occurs among the lower class in society and ignores that both the middle class and upper class can experience strain and engage in criminal behavior, beyond white-collar crime. Several studies (Tittle & Villemez, 1977; Hindelang, 1980; Thornberry & Farnsworth, 1982) that examined self-reported delinquent behavior found little or no relationship between social class and criminal behavior. According to Lilly and colleagues (2019), Cohen portrayed delinquents as embracing "nonutilitarian, malicious, and negativistic" values, but some youths' criminality is consumption-oriented and ostensibly utilitarian. Lilly and colleagues also recognized Cloward and Ohlin's three distinctions of delinquent subculture types: criminal, conflict, and retreatist, but observed that delinquents often mix these activities and rarely engage in only one. For example, delinquents may not limit themselves to smoking marijuana; they may also drink alcohol or engage in gang activity. Despite their differences, the classical strain theories of Merton, Cohen, and Cloward and Ohlin share the idea that strain involves the inability to achieve conventional culturally induced success goals through legitimate structural means.

Cultural Deviance Theories

The assertion of Cultural Deviance Theory is that crime is influenced by one's community, the individuals they are surrounded with, and the socioeconomic conditions of one's environment. The theory places a great deal of concern with the values found in some lower-class cultures. Bartollas and Schmalleger (2014, p. 84) suggest "central to cultural deviance theory is the belief that delinquent and criminal behavior are expressions of conformity to cultural values and norms that are in opposition to those of the larger society." Essentially, the assumption is that due to the frustrations of everyday life, members of the lower class develop their own subculture with rules and values unique to them.

Walter Miller's (1958) theory of focal concerns identified values unique to members of the lower-class culture. Miller regarded these focal concerns as trouble, toughness, excitement, smartness, fate, and autonomy. Miller's assumption was that *trouble* was seen as a symbol of status and prestige to stay in trouble. Physical strength and endurance are seen as signs of *toughness* and fearlessness of nothing, including law enforcement in the lower class. *Smartness* is seen as the ability to outwit another, to be cunning or manipulative; for example, hiding from the police when being chased. Lower-class individuals are thrill-seekers who enjoy *excitement* which may lead to gang activity or using drugs. Individuals in the lower-class place value on *fate or luck* when feeling disempowered; according to Miller, this is an enabler of delinquency. Finally, lower-class individuals often feel controlled by institutions or those in authority; therefore, they value *autonomy*, which can result in petty crimes. The premise of Miller's theory is that lower-class individuals have their own subculture, and adhering to the values of that subculture leads to delinquency/crime.

Cultural deviance theory has received various criticisms. Kornhauser (1978) suggests that individuals are so surrounded by criminal culture that it is normal for them to commit crimes. The theory fails to realize that a person's culture does not control them and leads them into criminal behavior. Cultural deviance stereotypes members of the lower class by regarding them as deviant, criminal, cunning, tough, and always in trouble for violating the law without realizing that both the middle and upper class may also engage in such behavior.

Social Process Theories

Social process theories are concerned with the interactions that individuals have with other individuals, their environment, and organizations. Its notion is that criminal and delinquent behavior is learned through a process of interaction with others and the socialization process that occurs through membership in the group. For example, these groups may comprise one's family, peers, colleagues, or gangs who instill their views and values in their members (Schmalleger, 2009). Social process theories view violence as a product of socialization and interactions with influential others that determine what one learns, one's level of control, and formal as well as informal labeling. The social process theories are learning, containment, social control, and labeling.

Learning Theories

Learning theories assume that all individuals are born with a blank slate and believe what they are told to believe and act as they are told to act by those they socialize with. Learning theories suggest that criminal behavior is influenced by cultural norms and the social environment. Bandura (1973) suggests that violence is not a trait one is born with, but rather one learns aggressive behavior through life experiences. Learning theories are differential association theory, differential identification theory, differential reinforcement theory, and neutralization theory/techniques of neutralization.

Differential association theory was introduced by Edwin Sutherland in 1939 in his text *Principles of Criminology* (Schmalleger, 2009). Sutherland viewed criminal behavior as being learned through differential association, a process through which criminal and delinquent behavior is learned from exposure to an excessive number of antisocial values and attitudes (Siegel, 2009). Sutherland disputed the notion that criminal behavior was caused by biological or psychological reasons, but instead it was learned from others. Sutherland presented the seven propositions of differential association:

1 Criminal behavior can be learned; it is an acquired trait.
2 Criminal behavior can be learned through the process of verbal and nonverbal communication with others.
3 Criminal behavior is learned through intimate primary groups.
4 Learning criminal behavior includes learning the techniques of committing a crime which includes the attitudes, motives, and drives.
5 One must learn the motives and drives of criminal behavior from perceptions of favorable or unfavorable definitions of the legal code. According to Sutherland, this causes cultural conflict due to the opposing views of what is right and what is wrong.
6 One becomes a criminal or delinquent because of an excess of definitions favorable to violating the law as opposed to those that are unfavorable.
7 Whether one learns to obey the law or commit a crime is influenced by the frequency, duration, intensity, and priority of one's social interaction. For example, if a child is

exposed to criminal behavior early in life, the criminal behavior will have a further-reaching effect.

8 One learns criminal or delinquent behavior just as one learns the processes and mechanisms involved in learning anything else.

9 Criminal and delinquent behavior could be an expression of needs and values but so is non-criminal behavior. In essence, both behaviors have needs, therefore, for example, motives to accumulate money are just as likely to produce non-criminal behavior and be acquired by working to achieve the money.

Bartollas and Schmalleger (2014) suggest that according to Sutherland, people become criminals or delinquents because they accept more reasons favorable to engaging in criminal behavior than conformity. While differential association theory has had an impact on the way we view crime and delinquency, evaluations of the theory have yielded several criticisms. Bartollas and Schmalleger (2014) contend that the terminology used by the theory is vague and makes it difficult to empirically test the theory. For example, *frequency*, *duration*, and *priority* cannot be studied. They also suggest that the theory fails to explain the effects that punishment has on delinquent or criminal behavior. Siegel (2009) acknowledges that research testing its assumptions has been limited. Differential association theory fails to explain why one individual who is exposed to criminal or delinquent behavior submits to it and others in the same condition do not. The theory fails to explain how the first individual who taught the criminal/delinquent behavior was taught; how did the behavior get passed down. The theory also does not explain why people who act spontaneously and commit crimes do so, such as serial killers (Siegel, 2009). However, differential association theory can account for criminal and delinquent behavior occurring in all social classes. According to Tibbetts and Hemmens (2014), Jeffrey (1965) argued that differential association theory did not take into consideration that individuals can also be conditioned to act or behave in a certain manner such as being rewarded for conforming to the behavior.

Differential reinforcement theory is another learning theory that attempts to explain crime and delinquency. This theory was popularized in 1966 by Robert Burgess and Ronald Akers who criticized Jeffrey's argument and incorporated some of Sutherland's principles to obtain a better understanding of criminal behavior. Akers and Burgess combined Sutherland's principles with B.F. Skinner's theory of operant conditioning in which learning is a form of association that is created through positive and negative reinforcements such as punishments and rewards. However, Akers and Burgess's modifications to differential association theory were based on the notions of reinforcement and punishment (Lilly et al., 2019). Akers suggests that it is through interactions with significant others and groups in their lives that individuals learn to evaluate their own behavior. These groups control sources and patterns of reinforcement, define behavior as right or wrong, and provide behaviors that can be modeled through observational learning. The more individuals learn to define their behavior as good or at least as justified, rather than as undesirable, the more likely they are to engage in it (Siegel, 2009). Rowan and McGuire (2023) contend there are four types of reinforcement or punishments:

1 **Positive reinforcement**: reinforcements, such as money, and social status with friends that reward behavior and increase the likelihood that an action is taken.

2 **Positive punishment**: the presentation of a negative consequence, such as being arrested or injured after a behavior is displayed to decrease the likelihood it will happen again.
3 **Negative reinforcement**: reinforcements that help avoid the negative consequences of a behavior, such as avoiding getting arrested, or facing disappointment from others, that increase the likelihood that an action is taken.
4 **Negative punishment**: the removal of positive reinforcement after displaying an undesirable behavior to decrease the likelihood of a person engaging in that behavior again. For example, the removal of access to the internet if a child is disruptive at school.

Differential reinforcement theory is concerned with what occurs after a criminal or delinquent act and whether that behavior is rewarded or punished by one's family, friends, or institutions in society (Tibbetts & Hemmens, 2014). Borrowing from principles of operant conditioning, Burgess and Akers (1966) argued that differential reinforcements are the driver of whether individuals engage in crime. The essence of differential reinforcement theory is that individuals usually repeat the behavior that they are rewarded for. For example, an individual receives money for murdering someone and thus makes this her career; here, the act of murder is reinforced through the funds received for so doing. Therefore, criminal behavior is explained by one's rewards and punishments for present, past, and future actions.

Gresham Sykes and David Matza are primarily noted for the development of the techniques of neutralization theory. Neutralization theory is a learning theory that contends that youth can vacillate between conforming behavior and non-conforming behavior. In other words, youth know the difference between right and wrong (Bartollas & Schmalleger, 2014). Sykes and Matza's neutralization theory examines how juveniles justify their responsibility for delinquent behavior. As such, Sykes and Matza developed five techniques delinquents use to justify their behavior and make it acceptable. These techniques of neutralization are as follows:

1 Denial of responsibility ("I didn't mean it.")
2 Denial of injury ("I didn't really hurt anyone.")
3 Denial of the victim ("They had it coming to them.")
4 Condemnation of the condemners ("Everyone is picking on me.")
5 Appeal to higher loyalties ("I didn't do it for myself.")

Tibbetts and Hemmens (2014) argue that neutralization theory received its name due to individuals justifying their behavior by neutralizing it or making it appear not so serious. Individuals make excuses for behavior they know is delinquent/criminal so they will not feel guilty; it is a defense mechanism. Siegel (2009, p. 208), suggests that neutralization theory with delinquents

> can account for the aging-out process: youths can forgo criminal behavior as adults because they never really rejected the morality of normative society. It helps explain the behavior of the occasional or non-chronic delinquent, who can successfully age out of crime.

Learning theories have been criticized due to the failure to define how the first person who committed a crime learned the definition of a crime and the techniques involved in committing a crime. According to Siegel (2009), there is little evidence to suggest that individuals who are deviant seek out other individuals with the same lifestyle. Learning theories add to the study of criminal and delinquent behavior across all classes of society.

These theories also demonstrate the importance of learning the proper techniques and criminal attitudes to commit a criminal or delinquent act.

Control Theories

Control theory's assumption is that all individuals would naturally commit crimes if it were not for the restraints on their selfish tendencies (Tibbetts & Hemmens, 2014). In essence, there is an internal mechanism that represses the urge to commit delinquency and criminal behavior. Since control theory assumes that humans have selfish tendencies, it questions why more individuals do not commit crimes.

Control theorists view crime and delinquency as resulting from a deficiency and can only be controlled by some absent force (Bartollas and Schmalleger, 2014). As suggested by Bryjak and Soroka (1997, p. 262), control theories "focus on the class between deviant motivation and the extent to which this motivation is held in check by an individual's commitment to societal values and norms and integration into various nondeviant groups." Albert Reiss (1951 as cited in Tibbetts & Hemmens) had an early version of control theory in which he found that delinquency occurred because there were no restraints against it. Reiss assumed if parents and the community imposed adequate discipline, then delinquency would not occur. He was also of the view that if juveniles denied self-gratification, delinquency would not occur. Yet, there was no empirical evidence to support his claims. However, Walter Reckless's containment theory and Travis Hirschi's social bonding theory are the most developed examples of this theory.

Containment theory was developed by sociologist Walter Reckless during the 1950s to explain criminal and delinquent behavior. Reckless contends that one's social environment as well as individual disorders can push them into delinquent or criminal behavior (Tibbetts & Hemmens, 2014). For example, such entities as the lack of employment, associating with gangs, having a mental disorder, or having a risk-taking personality can push an individual toward criminal or delinquent behavior. Reckless also suggested that there are factors that might pull an individual into criminal or delinquent behavior such as associating with delinquents or criminals or watching violent television productions; one might add listening to music in which individuals are degraded in a violent manner. According to Lilly and others (2019, p. 94), Reckless' argument was, "that to commit crime or delinquency requires the individual to break through a combination of outer and inner containment that together tend to insulate the person from both the internal pushes and external pulls." However, when the outer and inner containments were weak, criminal or delinquent behavior can occur.

According to Tibbetts and Hemmens (2014), internal containment refers to strengthening one's sense of self so that the urge to engage in criminal/delinquent behavior is repressed. External containment includes social institutions such as the church, schools, or clubs that build positive bonds that prevent individuals from being pushed or pulled into criminal/delinquent behavior. A replica of Lilly and colleagues' (2019, p. 96) chart summarizing Reckless' Containment Theory is provided below. This chart describes the Sources of Criminal Motivation, the Types of Containment, and the Components of Inner Containment (Figure 2.2).

Sources of Criminal Motivation

Pushes refer to factors that propel or motivate offenders toward crime, including biophysical forces, psychological pressures, and social conditions such as poverty.

Pulls refer to factors for crime that entice individuals to offend, such as the presence of illegitimate opportunities or peers who offend. Differential association and subculture theories are "pull" explanations.

Types of Containment

Outer containment refers to factors within an organized group that serve to reinforce conventional behavior, encourage internalization of rules, and offer supportive relationships that are not found in socially disorganized neighborhoods.

Inner containment refers to internal factors that insulate, or allow individuals to resist, the pushes and pulls toward crime that they encounter.

Components of Inner Containment

Self-concept refers to positive views of self as a law-abiding citizen. Anticipated the concept of "resilience."

Goal orientation refers to realistic views of aspirations that success goals are attainable.

Frustration tolerance refers to self-control to cope with failures and problems in life.

Norm retention and erosion refers to acceptance or belief in conventional values, laws, customs, and ways of behaving. Weakening or erosion of normative commitment can lead to crime.

FIGURE 2.2 Summary of Reckless' Containment Theory.

Criticisms have been led against containment theory. The first criticism is that the theory is complex and has too many constructs, per the chart, to be measured (Lilly et al., 2019). Second, according to Tibbetts and Hemmens (2014), there is less support for the theory from minorities and females because they may be influenced by peers or other influences; therefore, the theory may hold more validity for White males. Another criticism by Tibbetts and Hemmens is that the theory does not thoroughly explore the factors that predict crime among specific groups. Various factors, as noted by Tibbetts and Hemmens could be described as either a pull or push toward criminal/delinquent behavior as well as an inner or outer containment of criminal/delinquent behavior.

The theorist most closely identified with social control theory is Travis Hirschi who argued that delinquency results when a juvenile's bond to society is weak or broken. According to Bartollas and Schmalleger (2014), Hirschi viewed all humans as having the motivation to commit criminal or delinquent behavior unless there is a reason for them to refrain from so doing. Hirschi was a proponent of Social Control Theory which questioned, "Why do individuals break the law." To address this question, Hirshi argued that most individuals have a close bond with family, church, school, and their peers, and the stronger the commitment to the bond, the less likely they are to engage in delinquent or criminal behavior. They develop a commitment to these bonds which prevent them from engaging in criminal/delinquent behavior because they fear jeopardizing the relationship over poor choices they might make. For example, being caught with drugs in a car could jeopardize a college student's future career and her relationship with her family.

According to Bartollas and Schmalleger (2014), Hirschi identified four elements of having strong social bonds. These elements are attachment, commitment, involvement, and beliefs. The first element, attachment, includes the affection one has for parents, and peers, as well as the respect for elders and authority figures such as the police and teachers. Attachment concerns the care one gives to another. If the attachment is strong, especially to parents, the individual will consider the ties that he has with the sources of attachment when tempted to commit a criminal/delinquent act. Siegel (2009) states that psychologists view an individual with no attachments as someone who could become a psychopath and not be able to relate coherently to others.

The second element, commitment, is the activity for which an individual is willing to invest the time and energy to achieve with no desire to engage in any activity (i.e., criminal behavior) that poses a risk to the activity. For example, an individual invests time and energy in obtaining an education or having a good reputation. Conversely, if an individual has no commitment to conventional values, criminal/delinquent behavior may occur since he has nothing to lose (Siegel, 2009).

According to Bartollas and Schmalleger (2014), Hirschi viewed the third element, involvement, as shielding one from criminal/delinquent behavior. In essence, if one is busy working, meeting deadlines, and planning, there is little room for engagement in illegal behavior. The fourth element, belief, refers to individuals who reside in similar social settings and share the same morals, beliefs, and uphold behavior that is socially acceptable. These individuals are law-abiding and believe in upholding the social norms of society. If these beliefs are not present, there is a likelihood that illegal behavior will occur since belief creates an obligation to follow societal rules.

Hirschi's social control theory does have its limitations. Hirschi viewed all people as having the potential to engage in delinquency and crime if they have a weak or broken social bond. He did not consider the role that racial disparities could have on persons of color. Moreover, social control theory does not consider the impact that changing gender roles, or deteriorating communities have on one committing crimes (Lilly et al., 2019). Social control theory assumes that a strong commitment to one's family will prevent one from engaging in criminal or delinquent behavior because the individual does not want to disappoint or bring shame to the family; however, the theory provides little if any consideration to individuals who have strong bonds to an unconventional family, do these individuals engage in criminal/delinquent behavior so as not to disappoint their family?

Labeling Theories

The labeling theory is concerned with how one's personal characteristics and identity can be tagged or stigmatized as deviant, delinquent, or criminal. As the frequency and duration of the labeling take place, the person who is labeled conforms to the label and engages in delinquent or criminal behavior. Once the individual is processed through the criminal justice system, the labeling continues by both society and law enforcement. Bartollas and Schmalleger (2014, p. 131) describe labeling theory as, "the view that society creates the delinquent by labeling those who are apprehended as different from other youths when in reality they are different primarily because they have been tagged with a deviant label." Bryjak and Soroka (1997, p. 533) defines labeling theory in a similar manner, but argued that "society is responsible for creating deviance by imposing laws with infractions that constitute deviance, but only applying those laws to certain individuals." An example is the act of racial profiling of persons of color by law enforcement officers. The premise of labeling theorists is how and why some people are labeled as delinquent/criminal and how the label affects their future (Orcutt, 1973).

Early proponents of the labeling theory were Frank Tannenbaum and Edwin Lemert. Tannenbaum wrote the book *Crime and the Community* in 1938. He observed juveniles once they came to the attention of the justice system and were processed through the system. Tannenbaum's observation revealed that as the juvenile was processed, society treated the juvenile differently and tagged the juvenile as a delinquent. As a result of the tagging, the juvenile begins to associate with other delinquents to escape the society that labeled him as delinquent. Tannenbaum referred to this process as the "Dramatization of Evil." Tannenbaum theorized that the less society dramatizes evil, the less likely juveniles are to engage in deviant behavior (Bartollas & Schmalleger, 2014).

Edwin Lemert developed the concept of primary and secondary deviance. Primary deviance occurs when an offender commits her initial offenses, these are crimes that are not serious and that are easily forgotten by the offender. For example, an individual who steals a piece of candy from a local store when she is young, yet goes to college to become a physician and discovers the cure for cancer. The fact that the offender shoplifted as a juvenile did not prevent the offender from becoming successful. Secondary deviance occurs when the deviant act comes to the attention of others who apply a negative label to the offender (Siegel, 2009). Secondary deviance causes the labeled individual to internalize and assume the label. Evidence of internalizing the label can be found in the way the offender talks, dresses, and acts (Schmalleger, 2009). Lemert contends if a negative label is never applied to a first-time offender, then secondary deviance will not occur. Tibbetts and Hemmens (2014) suggest that "Lemert's model is highly consistent with the labeling approaches hands-off policies, such as diversion, decriminalization, and deinstitutionalization." However, there are unanticipated consequences of labeling individuals as criminal/delinquent because such labels may create the type of behavior one is trying to prevent (Lilly et al., 2019).

In the 1960s, Howard Becker published, *Outsiders: Studies in the Sociology of Deviance.* For Becker, society or social groups are responsible for creating "outsiders" or deviants/delinquents/criminals because social groups establish the rules of society and anyone who does not conform to the agreed-upon rules is labeled. Becker coined the term moral enterprise in his attempt to explain how some sanctions carry the full force of the law and others apply to marginal subcultures. A moral enterprise refers to "the efforts made by an interest group to have its sense of moral or ethical propriety enacted into law" (Schmalleger, 2009). A modern-day example of this is the "Three Strikes Laws" in which a group of community leaders can come together and engage in a discussion and formulate an objective to reduce crime, especially violent crime. As a result of their action, the *Violent Crime Control and Law Enforcement Act of 1994* was enacted and is now known as the "Three Strikes Law." This law requires a mandatory life sentence which targets habitual offenders who have a lengthy criminal history. One of the convictions must be a serious violent felony and the other offenses can be serious drug offenses. However, due to the nature of the "Three Strikes Law" people of color were disproportionately impacted.

According to Schmalleger (2009), Becker viewed labels as being applied to specific groups by society. This can also explain, in addition to racism, why persons of color are disproportionately represented in the criminal justice system, and why 87% of Blacks and 61% of Whites said the U.S. criminal justice system treats individuals of color less fairly than other individuals (Desilver et al., 2020).

The labeling theory assumes that individuals become delinquent, or criminal based on others' perception/treatment of them, individuals internalize the perceptions of others and act accordingly. However, the labeling theory has been criticized for its inability to identify why some individuals are labeled as criminal/delinquent and others are not. Title (1980) examined how labeling produces crime and discovered that many individuals do not engage in criminal careers after being labeled. Bartollas and Schmalleger (2014) contend that the labeling theory does not address the following key questions:

- Are the conceptions individuals hold of one another, correct?
- Does having a bad name indicate bad behavior?
- Why is it that some individuals who are labeled as delinquent age out of crime?

Social Conflict Theories

Social conflict theories suggest that those who are powerful and wealthy decide what is right and what is wrong in society. These people control the creation of the law and its enforcement (Petrocelli et al., 2003; Chamlin, 2009; Siegel, 2011). Social conflict theorists argue that crime in any society is caused by class conflict and that laws are created by those in power to protect their rights and interests (Schichor, 1980). Oberschall (1978, p. 291) argues that "social conflict refers to conflict in which the parties are an aggregate of individuals, such as groups, organizations, communities, and crowds, rather than, single individuals, as in role conflict." He further quotes Lewis Coser's definition of social conflict as, "a struggle over values or claims to status, power, and scarce resources, in which the aims of the conflict groups are not only to gain the desired values, but also to neutralize, injure, or eliminate rivals."

Conflict Theory

Conflict is present throughout society. There may be a conflict between races of people, conflict between countries, conflict between labor and management, and conflict between citizens and the police to name a few examples. Lilly and colleagues (2019) suggest that theories that focus attention on the struggles between individuals and/or groups regarding power differentials fall into the category of conflict theory.

Schmalleger (2009, p. 347) argues that the conflict perspective is "an analytical perspective on social organization that holds that conflict is a fundamental aspect of social life itself and can never be fully resolved." He further asserts that the conflict perspective views laws as a tool of the powerful that keeps others from taking control of social institutions. Bartollas and Schmalleger (2014) suggest that conflict theory argues that delinquency and crime are defined by socioeconomic class, power, and authority relationships, as well as group and cultural differences.

There are varying dimensions of conflict criminology. Conflict theorists focus on socioeconomic class, relationships between power and authority, and group and cultural conflict. Conflict theorists view crime, laws, and penalties for breaking laws as originating from the inequities of power and resources in society (Walsh & Hemmens, 2013). The leading conflict theories to be examined are Power Threat, Marxist, and Marxist feminist.

Power Threat Theory

During the 1950s through the 1960s, there was much unrest and demonstrations throughout the U.S. Most of this unrest stemmed from the Vietnam War and the Civil

Rights Movement. As a result of this unrest and oppression, the Power Threat Theory (PTT) emerged. The major proponent of the (PTT) is Hubert Blalock who presented this theory in 1967 to address how the dominant population imposes laws on members of the minority population whenever the minority population is seen as possibly threatening the existing social orders, political, or economic resources (Bodapati et al., 2008). An example of this occurred when the majority population feared the existing social order changing in southern states, prior to the passage of the Voting Rights Act in 1965, under Jim Crow Laws enforced by southern legislatures, Blacks were restricted from voting due to such practices as literacy test, poll taxes, all-White primaries, and grandfather clauses which were used to suppress the Black vote. More recently, in Galveston County, Texas, a redistricting plan was found to be in violation of the Voting Rights Act because it denied Black and Latino voters equal opportunity to participate in the political process. The U.S. District Court for the Southern District of Texas ruled that the Galveston County Commissioners Court must enact a redistricting plan in which at least one district provides Black and Latino voters with an equal opportunity to elect a candidate of their choice to the county government (U.S. Department of Justice, 2023).

PTT holds that when minority populations increase to the point where Whites have to compete instead of relying on White privilege, they will use punitive sanctions and other forms of social control to shift the balance of power back in their favor. Recently, these actions have become evident since demographers forecast that by the year 2042, Whites will no longer be the majority in the U.S. Consequently, this has manifested in an increase in hate crimes; hate group membership; as well as protests from domestic terrorists (Wilkerson, 2010). PTT postulates that in areas where minorities outnumber Whites, they immediately pose a threat to the White power base. For example, the majority views protests and demonstrations by minorities as threatening to the status quo. As such, law enforcement officers use violent militarized methods to subdue protesters. Officers often use excessive and deadly force on protesters exercising their right to peacefully demonstrate. Scholars, including critical race theorists, suggest Whites perceive minority protestors as threatening to their power base. Therefore, many Whites turn a blind eye to police brutality. PTT posits that large numbers of minority voters represent power that Whites fear will threaten their future dominance since a minority power base could demand equitable distributions of power and shift the balance of power. According to PTT, when the majority feels its power base is threatened, it will use punitive measures to incite fear. It may support racist politicians, ignore deadly force cases; uphold erroneous convictions; mete out capital punishment; and deny voting rights (Wilkinson, 2010).

Marxist Theory

Karl Marx is regarded as one of the best-known theorists of social conflict. During the Industrial Revolution of the mid-1800s, Marx examined the socioeconomic structures in society that control human relations. Marx's ideas were first published in the "Manifesto of the Communist Party," written in collaboration with Friedrich Engels in 1848 (Walsh & Hemmens, 2013).

Marx viewed society as being composed of two groups: the bourgeoisie and the proletariat. Marx referred to the owners of production in a capitalist society as the bourgeoisie, and those who worked to produce the production as the proletariat. As the bourgeoisie (i.e., the upper class) acquire more of society's wealth and the proletariat (i.e., the lower class) become more oppressed, their relationship becomes increasingly strained (Siegel, 2009). For Marx, it is the inequality caused by capitalism that produces this struggle between the classes. Therefore, in Marx's view, the way to eliminate class struggle in society is to eliminate capitalism. Although Marx wrote little regarding crime, he also viewed these class struggles resulting in crime. According to Wash and Hemmens (2013), Marx and Engels viewed crime as the reason for the social decline in society and referred to criminals as "social scum." Marx's views have been described as Marxist, critical, socialist, left-wing, new, or radical criminology (Bartollas & Schmalleger, 2014).

Willem Bonger was a follower of Marxist theory and is regarded as the first Marxist criminologist. Bonger suggested that society is divided between the haves and the have-nots. He acknowledged when he wrote, *Criminality and Economic Conditions* that some individuals are at a greater risk of engaging in criminal behavior than others due to their "innate social sentiments" which he regarded as *altruism*—a concern for the well-being of others and *egoism*—a concern for one's own selfish desires (Wash & Hemmens, 2013). Here, Bonger suggested that the economic system presented an unfavorable environment that encouraged individuals to seek pleasure and pitted one group against another which ultimately resulted in crime. Like Marx, Bonger viewed capitalism as the cause of societal conflict. According to Taylor (1971), Bonger is perhaps the only Marxist theorist to explore crime. Bonger suggested that poverty produced crime, and the effects of poverty could be traced to such factors as poor parental supervision of children, and the lack of education among the lower class and broken homes. However, Taylor does criticize Bonger for stating that poverty produced crime because it took away the Marxist view that capitalism was responsible for crime.

Marxist theorists Richard Quinney (2001) in his publication, *The Social Reality of Crime*, agreed with Marx when he wrote that in contemporary society, criminal law represented the interest of the dominant group in society. Quinney argues that laws are made by members of the upper class to control those in the lower class. Quinney suggested that conflicts between the upper and lower class determined the types of crimes each group would commit; the upper class committed crimes of domination and repression due to their desire to extract money from the lower class and to prevent the lower class from obtaining the upper class's position and power. The lower class commits crime due to their need for accommodation and resistance, their crimes are committed due to their frustration and rage with the upper class.

Bryjak and Soroka (1997) suggest that in a capitalist society, crime is the result of the struggle that exists between the upper class who controls the wealth and power in society to exploit those members of society who are less dominant, and members of the lower class. Here, the dominant class commits crimes due to their efforts to control the working class. Lower-class members of society resort to crime due to their treatment by the dominant class and due to their efforts to survive. Therefore, Bryjak and Soroka (1997) further argue that at the heart of Marxist theory are power, profit, and class struggle. They also suggest that Marxist capitalism is the real cause of crime. Moreover, Marxist theorists view laws as being created by the upper class and enforced by law enforcement officers, judges, and other criminal justice officers who work on behalf of the upper class. Tibbetts and Hemmens (2014) contend that Marx's writings suggest that those who are considered members of the upper class in society use the law to control the lower class which keeps them in a state of despair. This explains why members of the lower class (i.e., primarily persons of color) are disproportionately overrepresented in the criminal justice system in terms of arrest and charges.

The only solution Marxist theorists have for ending or perhaps reducing crime is to end capitalism. Bryjak and Soroka (1997, p. 262) suggests,

> Capitalism generates racism, sexism, and myriad social injustices, all of which directly or indirectly cause crime. The answer to the crime problem is a society established along socialist principles of criminal justice, a system that satisfies the needs of all members of society.

Marxist Theory has evolved over the years; however, the theory does not place enough emphasis on racism as a cause of social conflict. Marx is overly concerned with unequal power relations between the class structure instead of conflict due to race relations. The mere fact that most marginalized individuals are members of the lower class due to the color of their skin is evidence of a broader and more urgent example of social conflict that has resulted in global overt and covert racism. In addition, there is also the social conflict that exists due to issues of gender and sexuality.

Marxist Feminist Theory

MacKinnon (1989, p. 1) postulates that "sexuality is to feminism what work is to Marxism." In other words, relations between the sexes are similar to the Marxist conflict theory of the upper-class oppressing members of the lower class. It is a power and control relationship. Griffin (2017) argues that Marxist feminism derives from Marx's theory of capitalism and states that the oppression of women is tied to capitalism and private property. The oppression of women occurs due to men being paid for their labor and the inequality that occurs to women due to either being not paid or underpaid. Marxist feminists contend that gender and class divisions of labor determine male and female positions in society (Dekeseredy, 2011).

Daly and Chesney-Lind (1988) suggest that Marxist feminists hold the view that man's nature can be described as a product of history and culture, which is related to other systems of domination such as classism, racism, and imperialism. Likewise, Lilly and colleagues (2019) note Adler's argument, that both males and females are taught how to behave socially and culturally—males are taught to behave in the dominant role and females are taught to be passive and subordinate. Therefore, the oppression of women is natural to men because they have witnessed this display of domination throughout history and observed it in their culture, class, and race. Therefore, for men, it is second nature for them to treat women as inferior.

Barkan (2006) suggests that for Marxist feminists, women who are subordinated in a capitalist society may be victims of violence and rape. Marxist feminists argue that power differentials are also found among men employed in the justice system such as police, courts, judges, and corrections. They argue that vestiges of the past can be seen in the current social arrangement. These agencies and actors are not neutral, and therefore, women and other minorities are subject to abuse. Consequently, women who encounter the justice system experience intimidation, coercion, and violence from misogynists who symbolize social control and the interests of the powerful. Moreover, Marxist feminists argue that in capitalist societies, women are commodities like money for men to possess, especially where they are positioned in the social structure, class relations, and the mode of production (Schwendinger & Schwendinger, 1983).

"These class relations are used to control and subordinate women" (Einstadter & Henry, 1995, p. 264). Because of the structure in patriarchal societies, women experience sustained oppression in the home, public settings, as well as the workplace. Messerschmidt (1986) provides that capitalism permeates all aspects of social life by marginalizing women. Gender-variant women and women of color often experience double marginality. For example, because many are excluded from economic advancement in the labor force, they are denied status mobility. They are also marginalized from the family, in that many may be single, or divorced, and those who are gender variant are often disconnected from their biological families and discriminated against when they seek housing and employment opportunities. Some scholars argue that the powerlessness that women face makes them targets of violent crimes (Chapman, 1990). Marxist feminists believe that change can only occur when the existing social order becomes one that is based on the equal distribution of access to wealth and power, including decision-making within the justice system (Einstadter & Henry, 1995).

Public Health Perspectives

According to Dalberg and Mercy (2009), violence is considered a health issue because of its origins that include a multiplicity of stressors in the contextual, biological, environmental, systemic, and social domains, particularly those related to the growing number of homicides among young Black males and the increasing suicide rates for those between 15 and 24 years old. In other words, violence is not caused by people, but rather, it occurs because people are exposed to multiple risk and determinate factors (American Public Health Association [APHA], 2018, 3). Therefore, if specific risk factors are present, violence is likely to occur, and it becomes preventable when risk factors can be identified and addressed.

Stressors Leading to Violence

Contextual Stressors

The Institute of Medicine and National Research Council (IOM/NRC) (2013) consider the contextual influences on violence as the "systems and practices that contribute to the exacerbation, reduction, or prevention of violence, leveraging the classic epidemiologic model of infectious disease: spread, susceptibility, and immunity" (p. 28). There are several specific contextual factors highlighted by IOM/NRC such as place, poverty, culture and cultural context, historical oppression and trauma, race and racism, gender, mental illness and disabilities, and family. Several of these are discussed below:

Place

The effect or influence of *place* on violence can be explained as the proximity of persons to violence, the frequency of exposure to violence, if the violence is perceived as a normal reaction to violence being perpetrated, if persons have alternatives to violence, and whether there were non-violent response opportunities (IOM/NRC, 2013). Examples used to explain the effect of place on violence were juvenile detention facilities and prisons that, "exacerbate and spread violence" (p. 29). For example, Wolff and Shi (2009) reported on violence in prison related to gangs and gang structures, finding that being the victim of a gang crime increases the likelihood of becoming a gang member, and thus, the violence spreads and the gangs grow. When prisoners are released into communities, there is a strong potential for child abuse and intimate partner violence which can lead to intergenerational violence through children who experience and/or witness abuse (Oliver & Hairston, 2008; White et al., 2002).

Culture and Cultural Context

PrettyPaint, an internationally recognized expert in Native cultural resiliency and Indigenous evaluation methods, emphasized the importance of culture when discussing violence: "Culture confers certain worldviews and norms that need to be heeded" (IOM/ NRC, 2013). She explained that Native people believe that violence is something that someone can be healed from and that taking people out of their culture, or removing culture from people increases the chance of violence acting as an "infection" (p. 32). She spoke of the importance of culture for Native children: "Connection to culture and cultural practices helps create a place or meaningful connection of an individual to a greater whole," leading to an environment in which the spread of violence can be reduced (p. 32). PrettyPaint stresses the importance of people's ways of knowing and learning from watching, imitating, and noticing which behaviors are punished and which are rewarded.

Violence against women has a strong component of cultural norms (National Academies of Sciences, Engineering, and Medicine, 2018). Lori Heise of STRIVE Research Consortium states that behaviors, including violent behaviors, are "held in place by a matrix of norms, beliefs, and schemas" or rather, culture and cultural norms that lead to a condoning, tolerance, and normalization of violence against persons and animals. She explained that her work in gender violence and health confirms the existence of deeply embedded cognitive pathways that support the use of violence that is "often linked to norms of family [practice and] privacy," highlighting not only a cultural factor of violence, but also the impact of family structure. Heise believes that community-level interventions are best to reduce interpersonal violence and change norms.

Gender

Falk and colleagues (2014) reported that only 1% of the population was responsible for 63% of violent crime in the U.S. Risk factors for these individuals to engage in serious and persistent violent crime were found to be gender (i.e., male), mental illness, drug-related offenses, and substance use disorders (SUDs), in addition to being convicted of a violent crime before the age of 19 years. Among all risk factors for perpetrating violent crime, being a biological male is reported as the highest (Krug et al., 2002; Moffitt & Caspi, 2001). The 2020 female arrest rate for violent crime including murder, nonnegligent manslaughter, forcible rape, and aggravated assault was 5% for all ages (Office of Juvenile Justice and Delinquency Prevention, 2020).

Mental Illness

Among both males and females, mental illness, including psychopathy, is a common factor linked to committing violence (Brown et al., 2015; Olver & Wong, 2015). Persons diagnosed with psychopathy disorder may demonstrate "grandiosity, impulsivity, and possibly violent or aggressive behavior," yet little if any remorse or empathy (DeAngelis, 2022, 3). Psychopathology is believed to be one of the prominent factors for violent behavior in both men and women (Thomson, 2019) and persons diagnosed with psychopathology are reported to be responsible for over one-half of all violent crimes (Hare, 1993). Other psychiatric diagnoses associated with violent behavior include psychotic disorders, affective disorders, Cluster B personality disorders, conduct and oppositional defiant disorders, dissociative and post-traumatic stress disorders, intermittent explosive disorder, and sexual sadism (Petit, 2005).

However, mental illness alone is not a predictor of violence. Substance use and SUDs have been shown to play a major role in violence. Substance abuse, both among the general population (Pulay et al., 2008) and among violent offenders (Grann et al., 2008), increases the likelihood of violence occurring. A systematic review (Zhong et al., 2020) of crime and drug categories revealed that there are differences in the prevalence rates for crime dependent on the drug type being used by offenders. Yet, the use of any drug, even marijuana, increases the likelihood of violence occurring. Most significantly, Zong and colleagues (2020) found that persons with a SUD had a four to ten times greater chance of committing violence than someone without a SUD diagnosis. This is significant because SUDs are more prevalent than severe mental illness disorders, and therefore can have a greater impact on population health in terms of violence. Alcohol has been linked to various forms of crime, including aggression and acts of violence (Eisner & Malti, 2015), and is reported to be a key factor in homicide because of its effects on inhibitions and loss of emotional control (Karlsson, 1998).

Environmental

As with place, the environment in which people reside is a major factor in health, safety, and well-being. Many communities are plagued with violence, have unsafe drinking water, are built next to toxic industries such as factories and land waste dumps, and are classified as food deserts without places to acquire nutritious groceries (United States Department of Health and Human Services [USDHHS], n.d. a). As with many other factors involved with violence and health disparity, racial and ethnic minorities and those with lower incomes are the most affected by environmental factors. For example, persons who struggle economically are more likely to live in neighborhoods with more air pollution containing particulate matter from emissions such as from construction, highways, and diesel fuels, increasing their odds of developing chronic physical conditions (Tessum et al., 2021). Neighborhoods can also experience violence because of visible signs of disorder, such as run-down buildings, unkept lots, and yes, broken windows. As reported by Sampson and Raudensbush (2001),

> The broken windows metaphor is apt . . . as it asserts that physical signs of decay signal . . . unwillingness to . . . intervene when a crime is . . . committed or ask the police to respond.

(p. 1)

This constant disorder, or even a perceived state of disorder, can result in a cycle of decay (Office of Policy Development and Research, 2016, 1). Violent crime tends to reduce the value of a resident's property worse than even property crime (see Kirk & Laub, 2010). This is likely to leave those hit hardest economically without the means to move someplace safer and are, therefore, forced to live and raise children in very precarious circumstances. Even successful crime reduction acts in some of the most violent cities have not been able to reduce violent crime in the most violent communities (Friedson & Sharkey, 2015).

Systemic

Systemic factors of violence can also be considered systemic racism. For example, Braveman and colleagues (2022), define systemic and structural racism as "forms of racism that are pervasively and deeply embedded in systems, laws, written or unwritten policies, and entrenched practices and beliefs that produce, condone, and perpetuate widespread unfair treatment and oppression of people of color, with adverse health consequences" (p. 171). Looking at systemic causes of violence, this definition could be expanded to include other marginalized and disadvantaged populations. According to Braveman and colleagues (2022), examples of systemic racism include residential segregation, environmental injustice, inadequate education provided, and barriers to homeownership. It also includes income poverty and inequality.

Income Inequality

Income inequality is a systemic issue related to violence because of its effects on physical and behavioral health, housing, nutrition, education, and numerous environmental concerns such as the conditions of educational facilities and communities, and the location of housing developments. Income inequality is "the extent to which income is distributed unevenly in a group of people" (Equality Trust, n.d., 2). It is measured across an entire economic distribution. There are three primary kinds of economic inequality: income, unequal pay, and wealth inequality (the sum of resources of a person or household) (2–6).

According to the organization for Economic Co-operation and Development [OECD] (2022a), the U.S. ranked 35th out of 38 countries ranked low-to-high in income inequality, followed only by Turkey, Mexico, Chile, and Costa Rica. The U.S., also ranked very high (.180) in the global poverty rate (i.e., based on the ratio of the number of people in a given age group whose income falls below the poverty line) (OECD, 2022c) and ranked high again (.356) in global poverty gap, slightly below Romania (i.e., the ratio by which the mean income of the poor falls below the poverty line (OECD, 2022c). In fact, in 2020, the U.S. had the highest level of income inequality of all G7 nations (Schaeffer, 2020). As proof that income inequality is systemic, the Black–White income gap in the U.S. has persisted since 1970. Kent and Rickets (2024) report that during the third quarter of 2023, Black families owned 24 cents per one dollar of White wealth and Hispanic families owned 19 cents per 1 dollar of White wealth. According to Kent and Ricketts, the wealth gap can also be measured by household education: during the same third quarter of 2023, families headed by someone with a partial college education, but not a four-year degree, had 31 cents for each one dollar of wealth in families headed by someone with a college degree. In comparison, a family headed by someone with less than a high school diploma had 9 cents per 1 dollar of wealth in families where the head of household had a four-year college degree (7).

Children growing up in poverty are susceptible to living in areas with poor educational opportunities, lowering their likelihood of doing well in academics and graduating from high school or going to college. Braveman and colleagues (2022) stated, "Systemic racism is so embedded in systems that it often is assumed to reflect the natural, inevitable order of things" (p. 172). One example of systemic racism discussed by Braveman and colleagues was segregation. Segregation is persistent not only in communities but also in schools. A 2022 report from the U.S. Government Accountability Office showed that "During the 2020–21 school year, more than a third of students (about 18.5 million) attended schools where 75% or more students were of a single race or ethnicity" (p. 1) which leads to continued segregation because diversity in schools is related to its racial/ethnic makeup of the district and surrounding areas. The report demonstrated that the new school districts, most often more wealthy and better resourced, were predominantly attended by White students (73%). The remaining district students were 59% Black, 11% Hispanic, and 25% White. When looking at achievement scores and graduation rates, it can seem that minority children appear less capable than White children. However, it is the differences between experiences largely between Black and White children (the experience of more economic disadvantage, living in economically deprived neighborhoods, and attending underachieving schools) that can result in both lower academic achievement and later-life financial success (Condron et al., 2013).

Social Stressors

There are many social stressors related to violence. A person's relationships and interactions with family, friends, co-workers, significant others, and community are social factors that influence violence (USDHHS (n.d. b., *Social and Community Context*). The stress associated with these circumstances can be heightened because of their unpredictability and uncontrollability such as not being able to control the cost of food and rent, the safety of a neighborhood, or the security of income can be extremely stressful. For young children, parental incarceration, guardian substance abuse or mental illness, and being bullied are common social stressors. One of the greatest social stressors of late has been the COVID-19 pandemic and resulting periods of families being isolated in their homes, frequently small spaces not conducive to long-term confinement.

Unfortunately, stressors related to the pandemic resulted in increased child-to-parent violence, child witnessing violence between parents (Cano-Lozano et al., 2021), and parent-to-child violence (Elsayed, 2023). Confinement of multiple persons in one area for an extended time was not the only COVID-19 stressor. Families also faced lost income, food uncertainties, fear of eviction, online education for young persons, deaths of relatives, poor mental health, and others.

Family Violence: Child-to-Parent

Child-to-parent violence is defined as the aggression adolescents and young adults exert toward their parents or guardians, who may be elderly grandparents (Cano-Lozano et al., 2021). Although present before the pandemic, confinement stressors provided an environment that exacerbated incident rates. The Cano-Lozano and colleagues study examined the rate of violence in Hispanic homes among 2,245 young people (52.8% females) aged between 18 and 25 years. They found that 65.2% of the young participants demonstrated violence against their mother and 59.4% against their father. The behavior manifested in psychological violence (40.1%–61.3%), control and domination (36.5%–43%), economic violence (12%–16.6%), and physical violence (1.7%–3.3%) (p. 7). Social stressors reported by participants included worries about academic performance, employment, and overcrowding.

Family Violence: Parent-to-Child

Parent-to-child violence, or rather child abuse, was also studied during and after the pandemic to assess the impact of social stressors on the parent–child relationship. Elsayed (2023) found that parent-to-child aggression, for children whose parents stayed at home during the confinement periods, was at 79.84%. Approximately, 9,075 children of the United Arab Emirates were in the study population and there was a sample of 350 participants. For parental physical violence, there was a reported 81.67%, 74.12% for sexual violence, 84.98% for verbal violence, 74.47% for economic violence, and 83.97% for psychological violence. These percentages represent the weighted relative weight of the variable. Overall, girls were abused slightly more than boys, and children between the ages of 12–17 were abused more than younger children. Children from low-income families were at greater risk for abuse which is expected as income is a high-level social stressor, especially when adults cannot work as many experienced during the pandemic.

While these studies examined the impact of the pandemic within specific cultures, the study outcomes are similar to others examining child abuse during the pandemic mixture of cultures. A systematic review of pandemic child maltreatment and well-being found that the prevalence of child abuse reports increased internationally, citing social stress from parental work and financial issues as a primary factor (Or et al., 2023).

Potential Causes of Violence Using Theoretical and Conceptual Frameworks

Violence is a multidisciplinary issue. Although each discipline, be it social or behavioral sciences, criminology, psychology, public health, political, or other, has its own theoretical framework regarding the causes of violence, no discipline has the sole solution to preventing violence. However, each discipline informs and enhances our understanding of conceptualizing violence (Calhoun & Clarke-Jones, 1998).

Examinations of the multidisciplinary correlates of violence provide a view of its major theoretical perspectives. Biological theories contend that violent behavior depends on one's biological nature. Some individuals commit crimes due to genetic, hormonal, or neurological factors that are inherited or developed from an accident or illness; these theories focus on internal factors.

Social Learning Theories suggest that violence is learned just as one learns other actions from the family, school, and media. This theory rejects the notion of internal motivations and views violence resulting from child abuse in the home, discipline in the school, or being displayed through the media. Social Conflict Theories argue that violence results from an imbalance of power between the classes in which the dominant class imposes power on the weaker. The conflict may be religious, political, or ethnic and it can manifest into a cycle of violence.

Akers and Lanier (2009) suggest what is lacking is the methodological approaches in these disciplines that are needed to collect data and track the disease of violence. This approach can only be provided by merging these multiple theoretical disciplines with the discipline of epidemiology. This merger will provide a better understanding of not only the causes of violence, but its consequences, interventions, and preventions. Therefore, an integration of the theoretical disciplines with epidemiology will yield a new field of study; as Akers and Lanier (2009) have proposed the field of epidemiological criminology which will become the guiding framework for studying the causes of violent behavior.

Theories of Prevention and Solutions to Social Problems Caused by Violence

If we view violence as a public health problem, then theories of prevention and solutions to social problems caused by violence must also be viewed from a public health lens.

Social-Ecological Model

One promising public health prevention proposal is the *social-ecological model* that examines four levels of factors that protect people from or create susceptibilities to violence: individual, relationship, community, and societal (National Center for Injury Prevention and Control, 2022). This model highlights the influence of factors at one level upon the factors at the next level and suggests that prevention must simultaneously occur across many levels of the model (Figure 2.3).

The *individual level* in this model refers to the "biological and personal history factors that increase" one's susceptibility to becoming either victim or perpetrator of violence, such as "age, education, income, substance use, or history of abuse" (2). Effective violence prevention strategies at this level may be those promoting healthy attitudes and behaviors including skills in settling disputes, social-emotional learning curricula, and healthy-relationship practices. The second, or *relationship level*, highlights how close or intimate relationships affect a person's behavior. This typically includes peers, family, and significant others. Prevention efforts can include offering parenting classes and mentoring or peer programs that stress communication skills, healthy peer interactions, and supportive connections.

The third or *community level* considers one's larger, social environment. This can include schools, churches, recreational facilities, work settings, and communities. A goal is to understand which characteristics of these locations contribute to persons becoming

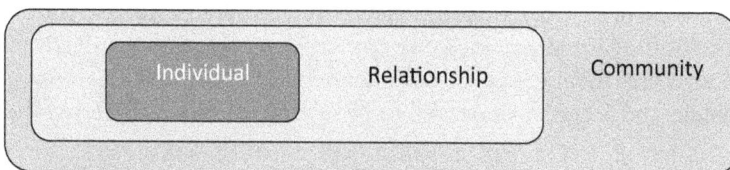

FIGURE 2.3   The Social-Ecological Model.

victims or perpetrators. Prevention efforts can seek improvements and safety in these areas by addressing functional aspects of crime such as neighborhood segregation and poverty, and/or by seeking overall advancements in well-being that include training in workplace harassment, more strategic planning in street lighting, and enhanced education for law enforcement about mental illness. The fourth or *societal level* pertains to the overall living or working environment and the extent to which violence is encouraged or dissuaded as a norm. Protective and preventive measures should include policy and educational goals that eliminate societal inequities and disparities that have been identified as risks and determinate factors that contribute to violent behavior.

This model exemplifies efforts that seek to prevent health inequalities, stemming from racial/ethnic and socioeconomic disparities associated with early delinquency. Jackson and Vaughn (2018) call for an integration of health disparity and life-course criminological frameworks. They incorporate an early developmental ecology concept with three health dimensions (health behaviors and lifestyles, health conditions, and access to health resources) as a basis for preventative model conceptualization. *Health behaviors* are a person's actions that either do or do not promote a healthy lifestyle. Some behaviors may be high-risk, while others may be protective. *Health conditions* refer to physical or mental expressions of poor health. *Health resources* are one's access to resources that assist in being healthy. Jackson and Vaughn propose that high-risk activities, poor health conditions, and limited health resources can lead to circumstances that predict the possibility of early onset of delinquency or aberrant behaviors. These behaviors, in turn, are associated with chronic offending and further criminal justice involvement, potentially leading to early morbidity and mortality (p. 92). In effect, they propose that health and criminal justice policies unite to assist one another in reaching an overarching goal of reducing or eliminating violence while supporting healthier communities and people. An example of this is explained by Vaugh and Jackson (p. 94): the reduction of food deserts is likely to result in improved child development and better long-term behavior while community crime reduction interventions may result in the creation of more businesses, such as grocery markets that offer varied and healthy foods (as compared to pre-packaged, highly refined foods). Prevention efforts such as this, recognize that violence is multidimensional and requires multi-systemic approaches in response.

Life-Course Approach

The life-course approach proposes that one's later life health reflects one's earlier life and that all economic and social factors (including health disparities) across the lifespan affecting well-being should be considered (Braveman, 2014b). It is also a framework for evaluating ethics and human rights. As humans, everyone has the right to health which Braveman (2014b) interprets as, "the right to achieve the health status experienced by the most economically and socially advantaged group in society" (p. 368). Using the life-course approach allows an examination of the disparities one has experienced from pre-birth to death and the policies and structures that created and/or maintained those disparities. Doing so allows for intervening where and when most needed to have the greatest effect across the lifespan.

Braveman (2014b) uses the example of a woman of color who is pregnant and delivers a child with an adverse birth outcome. By examining the woman's life, it is discovered that she experienced many challenges causing stress which could have, in turn, damaged her health and led to a high-risk adverse birth outcome (Lu & Halfon, 2003). This could be said for outcomes considered crime or criminal when looking at the same factors influencing an individual's health and behavior such as environmental toxins, inadequate schools, economically impoverished neighborhoods, and the consequences of psychosocial trauma.

Comparatively, a community-based program to address violence against women in India was designed using the social-ecological prevention model (Daruwalla et al., 2019). The program used three categories of intervention and prevention activities: "1) community mobilization, 2) crisis counseling, and 3) extended response for survivors of violence and work with police, medical, and legal, services" (p. 3). These activities included primary and secondary prevention strategies via neighborhood-led and hospital-based clinics, volunteers, and community resources.

Summary

Violence is one of the most tragic circumstances that impact the health of communities. Various efforts have been made to address the etiology of violence through theories of social science, criminology, and public health theories. It is only through awareness and understanding of these theories combined with knowledge from the field of epidemiology that effective and sustainable solutions can possibly be found to provide interventions and ultimately solutions to violence.

Discussion Questions

1 What is epidemiology?
2 What delineates an epidemiological factor of violence from a criminogenic factor?
3 What role does racism play in *Contextual, Biological, Environmental, Systemic, or Social stressors* related to violence? Choose one.
4 How does the epidemiological approach to violence intervention differ from the criminogenic approach?
5 Provide a discussion of the criminological explanations of violence.
6 What are some contextual stressors that lead to violence?

References

Agnew, R. (1992). Foundation for a general strain theory of crime and delinquency. *Criminology*, 30, 47–87.

Akers, R.L. (1997). *Criminological theories: Introduction and evaluation.* Roxbury Publishing Company.

Akers, T.A., & Lanier, M.M. (2009). "Epidemiological criminology": Coming full circle. *American Journal of Public Health*, 99(3), 397–402. https://doi.org/10.2105/AJPH.2008.139808

Albert, R. (1951). Delinquency as the failure of personal and social controls. *American Sociological Review*, 16, 196–207.

Amarasinghe, K. (2020, August). Pure-classical and neo-classical schools of criminology: Applicability into the present context of criminal law in Sri Lanka. *US-China Law Review*, 17(8), 348–355. https://doi.org/10.17265/1548-6605/2020.08.003

American Public Health Association (APHA). (2018). Violence is a public health issue: Public health is essential to understanding and treating violence in the U.S. https://apha.org/policies-and-advocacy/public-health-policy-statements/policy-database/2019/01/28/violence-is-a-public-health-issue

Bandura, A. (1973). *Aggression: A social learning analysis.* Prentice Hall.

Barkan, S.E. (2006). *Criminology: A sociological understanding* (3rd ed.). Pearson/Prentice-Hall.

Bartol, C.R., & Bartol, A.M. (2002). *Introduction to forensic psychology: Research and application* (6th ed.). SAGE Publications.

Bartollas, C., & Schmalleger, F. (2014). *Juvenile delinquency* (9th ed.). Pearson Education, Inc.

Beaudry-Cyr, M. (2015). Rational choice theory. In The encyclopedia of crime and punishment (pp. 1–3).https://doi.org/10.1002/9781118519639.wbecpx038

Becker, G.S. (1968) Crime and punishment: An economic approach. *Journal of Political Economy*, 76(2), 169–217.

BMJ. (2024). Epidemiology for the uninitiated, chapter 1: What is Epidemiology. British Medical Association. www.bmj.com/about-bmj/resources-readers/publications/epidemiology-uninitiated/1-what-epidemiology

Bodapati, M., Anderson, J.F., & Brinson, T.E. (2008). Revisiting Hubert Blalock's power threat theory to determine its effect on court workgroup behavior as it concerns structured sentencing. *Criminal Justice Studies: A Critical Journal of Crime, Law and Society*, 23(2), 109–134.

Bouffard, J., Bry, J., Smith, S., & Bry, R. (2008). Beyond the "science of sophomores" does the Rational Choice Explanation of crime generalize from university students to an actual offender sample? *International Journal of Offender Therapy and Comparative Criminology*, 52(6), 698–721.

Braveman, P. (2014a). What are health disparities and health equity? We need to be clear. *Public Health Reports*, 129(1_suppl2), 5–8. https://doi.org/10.1177/00333549141291S203

Braveman, P. (2014b). What is health equity: And how does a life-course approach take us further toward it? *Maternal and Child Health Journal*, 18(2), 366–372. https://doi.org/10.1007/s10995-013-1226-9

Braveman, P.A., Arkin, E., Proctor, D., Kauh, T., & Holm, N. (2022). Systemic and structural racism: Definitions, examples, health damages, and approaches to dismantling. *Health Affairs*, 41(2), 171–178. https://doi.org/10.1377/hlthaff.2021.01394

Briceno-Leon, R., Villaveces, A., & Concha-Eastman, A. (2008). Understanding the uneven distribution of the incidence of homicide in Latin America. *International Journal of Epidemiology*, 37, 751–757.

Brown, A.R., Dargis, M.A., Mattern, A.C., Tsonis, M.A., & Newman, J.P. (2015). Elevated psychopathy scores among mixed sexual offenders: Replication and extension. *Criminal Justice Behavior*, 42, 1032–1044. https://doi.org/10.1177/009385481557538

Bruinsma, G.J.N., & Johnson, S.D. (Eds.). (2018). *The Oxford handbook of environmental criminology*. Oxford University Press.

Bryjak, G., & Soroka, M. (1997) *Sociology: Cultural diversity in a changing world* (3rd ed.). Allyn and Bacon.

Bucerius, S.M., Oriola, T.B., & Jone, D.J. (2022). Policing with a public health lens – Moving towards an understanding of crime as a public health issue. *The Police Journal*, 95(3), 421–435. https://doi.org/10.1177/0032258X211009577

Budhwani, H., Hearld, K.R., & Chavez-Yenter, D. (2015). Depression in racial and ethnic minorities: The impact of nativity and discrimination. *Journal of Racial and Ethnic Health Disparities*, 2, 34–42. https://doi.org/10.1007/s40615-014-0045-z

Burgess, R. & Akers, R.L. (1966). A differential association-reinforcement theory of criminal behavior. *Social Problems*, 14(2), 128–147. https://doi.org/10.2307/798612

Burke, R.H. (2009). *An introduction to criminological theory* (3rd ed.). Willan Publishing.

Bursik, R. (1988). Social disorganization and theories of crime and delinquency: Problems and prospects. *Criminology* (26), 519–551.

Byym, R.J., & Lie, J. (2007). *Sociology your compass for a new world* (3rd ed., pp. 195–200, 13–19). Thomson Wadsworth.

Calhoun, A.D., & Clark-Jones, F. (1998). Theoretical frameworks: Developmental psychopathology, the public health approach to violence, and the cycle of violence. *Pediatric Clinics of North Amemrica*, 45(2), 281–291. https://doi.org/10.1016/S0031-3955(05)70005-5

Carmen Cano-Lozano, M., Navas-Martínez, M.J., & Contreras, L. (2021). Child-to-parent violence during confinement due to covid-19: Relationship with other forms of family violence and psychosocial stressors in Spanish youth. *Sustainability (Basel, Switzerland)*, 13(20), 11431. https://doi.org/10.3390/su132011431

Carmichael, S., & Piquero, A.R. (2004). Sanctions, perceived anger, and criminal offending. *Journal of Quantitative Criminology*. Special Issue: Offender Decision Making, 20(4), 371–393.

Cavanaugh, M. (2012). Theories of violence: Social science perspectives. *Journal of Human Behavior in the Social Environment*, 22, 607–618.

Centers for Disease Control and Prevention (CDC). (2004). *What is health equity?* What is Health Equity? | Health Equity | CDC. www.cdc.gov/health-equity/what-is/index.html

Centers for Disease Control and Prevention (CDC). (2023a). *About multiple cause of death, 2018–2021*. National Center for Health Statistics, National Vital Statistics System, CDC WONDER. http://wonder.cdc.gov/mcd-icd10-expanded.html

Centers for Disease Control and Prevention (CDC). (2023b). Health, United States, 2020–2021: Annual Perspective. https://dx.doi.org/10.15620/cdc:122044 .

Centers for Disease Control and Prevention (CDC). (2023c). *National diabetes statistics report*. www.cdc.gov/diabetes/php/data-research/

Centers for Disease Control and Prevention (CDC). (2024). Economics of injury and violence prevention. www.cdc.gov/injury-violence-prevention-economics.

Centers for Disease Control and Prevention (CDC). (2024). National diabetes statistics report. www.cdc.gov/diabetes/php/data-research/index.html

Chamlin, M.B. (2009). Threat to whom? Conflict, consensus, and social control. *Deviant Behavior*, 30, 539–559.

Chapman, J.R. (1990). Violence against women as a violation of human rights. *Social Justice*, 17, 54–71.

Cho, B., Han, Y., Lian, M., et al. (2021). Evaluation of racial/ethnic differences in treatment and mortality among women with triple-negative breast cancer. *JAMA Oncology*, 7(7), 1016–1023. https://doi.org/10.1001/jamaoncol.2021.1254

Cohen, A.K. (1955). *Delinquent boys: The culture of the gang*. Free Press.

Cohen, L., & Felson, M. (1979). Social change and crime rate trends: A routine activities approach. *American Sociological Review*, 44, 588–608.

Condron, D., Tope, D., Steidl, C., & Freeman, K. (2013). Racial segregation and the black/white achievement gap, 1992–2009. *Sociological Quarterly*, 54(1), 130–157. https://doi.org/10.1111/tsq.12010

Cornish, D., & Clarke, R. (1986). *The reasoning criminal: Rational choice perspectives on offending*. Springer-Verlag.

Cornish, D.B., & Clarke, R.V. (1987). Understanding crime displacement: An application of Rational Choice Theory. *Criminology*, 25(4), 933–948.

Cornish, D.B., & Clarke, R.V. (2001). Rational choice theory. In F.T. Cullen & P. Wilcox (Eds.), *Encyclopedia of criminology theory*. Volume 2, (pp. 216–220). Sage. https://doi.org/10.4135/9781412959193.n60

Crouch, E., Radcliff, E., Hung, P., & Bennett, K. (2019). Challenges to school success and the role of adverse childhood experiences. *Academic Pediatrics*, 19(8), 899–907. https://doi.org/10.1016/j.acap.2019.08.006

Dahlberg, L., & Mercy, J. (2009). History of violence as a public health problem. *AMA Journal of Ethics*, 11, 167–172. https://journalofethics.ama-assn.org/sites/joedb/files/2018-06/vm-0902.pdf

Daly, K., & Chesney-Lind, M. (1988). Feminism and criminology. *Justice Quarterly*, 5, 497–538.

Daruwalla, N., Jaswal, S., Fernandes, P., Pinto, P., Hate, K., Ambavkar, G., Kakad, B., Gram, L., & Osrin, D. (2019). A theory of change for community interventions to prevent domestic violence against women and girls in Mumbai, India. *Wellcome Open Research*, 4, 54–54. https://doi.org/10.12688/wellcomeopenres.15128.2

DeAngelis, T. (2022). A broader view of psychopathy: New findings show that people with psychopathy have varying degrees and types of the condition. *Monitor on Psychology*, 53(2). www.apa.org/monitor/2022/03/ce-corner-psychopathy

DeBolt, C.L., Brizendine, C., Tomann, M.M., & Harris, D.A. (2021). Lung disease in central Appalachia: It's more than coal dust that drives disparities. *Yale Journal of Biology and Medicine*, 94(3), 477–486. PMID: 34602885; PMCID: PMC8461577.

Dekeseredy, W. (2011). Feminist contributions to understanding women abuse, myths, controversies, and realities. *Aggression and Violent Behavior*, 16, 297–302.

Desilver, D., Lipka, M., & Fahmy, D. (2020, June). 10 things we know about race and policing in the U.S. Pew Research Center, www.pewresearch.org/short-reads/2020/06/03/10-things-we-know-about-race-and-policing-in-the-u-s/

Donnelly, Peter D., & Catherine L. Ward (eds). (2014). *Oxford textbook of violence prevention: Epidemiology, evidence, and policy*. Oxford Textbooks (Oxford, 2014; online edn). Oxford Academic. https://doi.org/10.1093/med/9780199678723.001.0001, accessed 16 July 2025.

Einstadter, W., & Henry, S. (1995). *Criminological theory: An analysis of its underlying assumptions*. Harcourt Brace & Company.

Eisner M.P., & Malti, T. (2015). Aggressive and violent behavior. In *Handbook of Child Psychology and Developmental Science* (pp. 794–841). https://doi.org/10.1002/9781118963418.childpsy319

Elsayed, W. (2023). Behind closed doors: Exploring the consequences of parents staying at home during the COVID-19 pandemic on the prevalence of parental violence against children. *RIMCIS: International and Multidisciplinary Journal of Social Sciences*, 12(3), 260–284. https://doi.org/10.17583/rimcis.12072

Equality Trust. (n.d.). *How is economic inequality defined?* https://equalitytrust.org.uk/how-economic-inequality-defined

Fagan, P.F. (1995) Real root causes of violent crime: The breakdown of marriage, family, and community. *The Heritage Foundation*, 1026, 1–36.

Falk, O., Wallinius, M., Lundström, S., Frisell, T., Anckarsäter, H., & Kerekes, N. (2014). The 1% of the population accountable for 63% of all violent crime convictions. *Social Psychiatry Psychiatry Epidemiology*, 49(4), 559–571. https://doi.org/10.1007/s00127-013-0783-y

Farmer, D., & McDonald, R. (1988). *Epidemiological model for crime control*. Virginia Commonwealth University. www.ojp.gov/ncjrs/virtual-library/abstracts/epidemiological-model-crime-control

Felson, M. (1998). *Crime and everyday life*. (2nd ed.). Pine Forge.

Friedson, M., & Sharkey, P. (2015). Violence and neighborhood disadvantage after the crime decline. *The Annals of the American Academy of Political and Social Science*, 660(1), 341–58. https://doi.org/10.1177/0002716215579825

Garland, D. (1999). Penal modernism and postmodernism. In R. Mathews (Eds.), *Imprisonment* (pp. 511–539). Dartmouth.

Gilbert, L., Breiding, M., Merrick, M., Thompson, W., Ford, D., Dhingra, S., & Parks, S. (2015). Childhood adversity and adult chronic disease. *American Journal of Preventive Medicine*, 48(3), 345–349. https://doi.org/10.1016/j.amepre.2014.09.006

Gilligan, J. (2001). *Violence: Reflections on our deadliest epidemic*. Jessica Kingsley.

Government of South Australia. (n.d.). *Epidemiological approach*. https://dhs.sa.gov.au/how-we-help/child-and-family-support-system-cfss/about-cfss/early-intervention-research-directorate/epidemiological-approach

Grann, M., Danesh, J., & Fazel, S. (2008). The association between psychiatric diagnosis and violent re-offending in adult offenders in the community. *BMC Psychiatry*, 8(1), 92–92. https://doi.org/10.1186/1471-244X-8-92

Griffin, G. (2017). *A dictionary of gender studies*. Oxford University Press.

Gul, S.K. (2009). An evaluation of the rational choice theory in criminology. *Journal of Social and Applied Science*, 4(8), 36–44.

Gunja, M., Gumas, E., & Williams, R. (2023, January 31). *U.S. health care from a global perspective, 2022: Accelerating spending, worsening outcomes.* Commonwealth Fund Issue Brief. https://doi.org/10.26099/8ejy-yc74

Halpern, S.C., Schuch, F.B., Scherer, J.N., Sordi, A.O., Pachado, M., Dalbosco, C., Fara, L., Pechansky, F., Kessler, F., & Von Diemen, L. (2018). Child maltreatment and illicit substance abuse: A systematic review and meta-analysis of longitudinal studies. *Child Abuse Review (Chichester, England: 1992),* 27(5), 344–360. https://doi.org/10.1002/car.2534

Hare, R.D. (1993). *Without conscience: The disturbing world of the psychopaths among us.* Guilford Press.

Hindelang, M.J. (1980). *Measuring delinquency.* Sage.

Humphreys, K.L., LeMoult, J., Wear, J.G., Piersiak, H.A., Lee, A., & Gotlib, I.H. (2020). Child maltreatment and depression: A meta-analysis of studies using the childhood trauma questionnaire. *Child Abuse & Neglect,* 102, 104361. https://doi.org/10.1016/j.chiabu.2020.104361

Institute of Medicine and National Research Council (IOM/NRC). (2013). Chapter 4/the role of contextual factors in the contagion of violence. In *Contagion of violence: Workshop summary.* The National Academies Press. https://doi.org/10.17226/13489

Jackson, D.B., & Vaughn, M.G. (2018). Promoting health equity to prevent crime. *Preventive Medicine,* 113, 91–94. https://doi.org/10.1016/j.ypmed.2018.05.009

Jacobs, D.E., & Brown, M.J. (2023). Childhood lead poisoning 1970–2022: Charting progress and needed reforms. *Journal of Public Health Management and Practice,* 29(2), 230–240. https://doi.org/10.1097/PHH.0000000000001664

Jang, S.J., & Agnew, R. (2015). Strain theories and crime. In D. James (Ed.), *Wright's international encyclopedia of the social and behavioral sciences* (2nd ed., Vol. 23, pp. 495–500). Elsevier.

Jeffery, C.R. (1965). Criminal behavior and learning theory. *Journal of Criminal Law, Criminology & Police Science,* 56(3), 294–300. https://doi.org/10.2307/1141238

Johns Hopkins Bloomberg School of Public Health. (2023). *CDC provisional data: Gun suicides reach all-time high in 2022, gun homicides down slightly from 2021.* https://publichealth.jhu.edu/2023/cdc-provisional-data-gun-suicides-reach-all-time-high-in-2022-gun-homicides-down-slightly-from-2021

Jones, S.E., Ethier, K.A., Hertz, M.S., DeGue, S., Le, V.D., Thornton, J., Lim, C., Dittus, P., & Geda, S. (2021). Mental health, suicidality, and connectedness among high school students during the COVID-19 pandemic—Adolescent behaviors and experiences survey, United States, January–June 2021. *CDC Morbidity and Mortality Weekly Report,* Suppl 2022, 71(Suppl-3), 16–21. http://dx.doi.org/10.15585/mmwr.su7103a3

Karlsson, T. (1998). Sharp force homicides in the Stockholm area, 1983–1992. *Forensic Science International,* 94, 129–139. https://doi.org/10.1016/S0379-0738(98)00067-X

Kent, H., & Ricketts, L. (2024). *The state of U.S. wealth inequality.* Federal Reserve Bank of St. Louis. www.stlouisfed.org/institute-for-economic-equity/the-state-of-us-wealth-inequality

Kent State University. (2025, April 10). Breaking down the epidemiological triangle: Key factors explained [Blog]. Kent State Online, Kent State University. The Epidemiological Triangle | Key Factors Explained

Kirk, D., & Laub, J. (2010). Neighborhood change and crime in the modern metropolis. *Crime and Justice,* 39(1), 441–502. https://doi.org/10.1086/652788

Kleinman, A. (May 1, 2010). Four social theories for global health. Volume 35, Issue 9+725. pp. 1518–1519. Perspectives www.thelancet.com/action/showpdf?pii=S0140-6736%2810%2960646-0]

Kornhauser, R.R. (1978). *Social sources of delinquency: An appraisal of analytical models.* University of Chicago Press.

Krug, E., Dahlberg, L., Mercy, J., Zwi, A., & Lozano, R. (2002). *World report on violence and health.* World Health Organization. https://iris.who.int/bitstream/handle/10665/42495/9241545615_eng.pdf?sequence=1

Kurbin, C. & Wo, J. (2016). Social disorganization theory's greatest challenge: Linking structural characteristics to crime in socially disorganized neighborhoods. In A.R. Piquero (Eds.), *Handbook of criminological theory* (pp.121–136). John Wiley & Sons

Lash, T.L., VanderWeele, T.J., Haneause, S., & Rothman, K. (2021). *Modern epidemiology* (4th ed.). Wolters Kluwer.

LaVeist, T., Pérez-Stable, E., Richard, P., Anderson, A., Isaac, L., Santiago, R., Okoh, C., Breen, N., Farhat, T., Assenov, A., & Gaskin, D. (2023). The economic burden of racial, ethnic, and educational health inequities in the US. *JAMA*, 329(19), 1682–1692. https://doi.org/10.1001/jama.2023.5965

Lawson, J., & King, B. (2012). Theories of violence: A review of textbooks on human behavior and the social environment. *Journal of Human Behavior in the Social Environment*, 22(5), 517–534. https://doi.org/10.1080/10911359.2011.598724

Lilly, R., Cullen, F.T., & Ball, R. (2019). *Criminological theory: Context and consequences* (7th ed.). Sage.

Lo, C.C., Ash-Houchen, W., Gerling, H.M., & Cheng, T.C. (2020). From childhood victim to adult criminal: Racial/Ethnic differences in patterns of victimization-offending among Americans in early adulthood. *Victims & Offenders*, 15(4), 430–456. https://doi.org/10.1080/15564886.2020.1750517

Lu, M.C., & Halfon, N. (2003). Racial and ethnic disparities in birth outcomes: A life-course perspective. *Maternal and Child Health Journal*, 7(1), 13–30. https://doi.org/10.1023/A:1022537516969

MacKinnon, C.A. (1989). *Toward a feminist theory of the state*. Harvard University Press.

Mann, S.A. (2012). *Doing feminist theory: From modernity to postmodernity*. Oxford University Press.

March of Dimes. (2023). *March of dimes 2023 report card for United States*. www.marchofdimes.org/peristats/reports/united-states/report-card

Mariño-Ramírez, L., Jordan, I.K., Nápoles, A.M., & Pérez-Stable, E.J. (2022). Comparison of U.S. gun-related deaths among children and adolescents by race and ethnicity, 1999–2020. *Journal of the American Medical Association*, 328(23), 2359–2360. https://doi.org/10.1001/jama.2022

Mazerolle, P., Burton, V.S., Jr., Cullen, F.T., Eans, T.D., & Payne, G.L. (2000). Strain, anger, and delinquent adaptations: Specifying general strain theory. *Journal of Criminal Justice*, 28, 89–101.

McCarthy, A.M., Friebel-Klingner, T., Ehsan, S., He, W., Welch, M., Chen, J., Kontos, D., Domchek, S.M., Conant, E.F., Semine, A., Hughes, K., Bardia, A., Lehman, C., & Armstrong, K. (2021). Relationship of established risk factors with breast cancer subtypes. *Cancer Medicine (Malden, MA)*, 10(18), 6456–6467. https://doi.org/10.1002/cam4.4158

McCarthy, B., & Chaudhary, A. (2014). Rational choice theory. In G. Bruinsma, & D. Weisburd (Eds.), *Encyclopedia of criminology and criminal justice* (pp. 4307–4315). Springer. https://doi.org/10.1007/978-1-4614-5690-2_396

McDonald, D. (2000, July). Violence as a public health issue. *Australian Institute of Criminology: Trends and Issues in Crime and Criminal Justice*, 163, 1–6. www.aic.gov.au/publications/tandi/tandi163

McGough, M., Amin, K., Panchal, N., & Cox, C. (2023, July 18). *Child and teen firearm mortality in the U.S. and peer countries*. KFF. www.kff.org/mental-health/issue-brief/child-and-teen-firearm-mortality-in-the-u-s-and-peer-countries/.

Mercy, J.A., Rosenberg, M.L., Powell, K.E., Broome, C.V., & Roper, W.L. (1993). Public health policy for preventing violence. *Health Affairs*, 12(4), 8–29.

Messerschmidt, J.W. (1986). *Capitalism, patriarchy, and crime: Toward a socialist feminist criminology*. Roman & Littlefield.

Miller, W.B. (1958). Lower class culture as a generating milieu of gang culture. *Journal of Social Issues*, 14(3), 5–19.

Miro', F. (2014). *Routine activity theory*. The encyclopedia of theoretical criminology. John Wiley and Sons. https://doi.org/10.1002/9781118517390.wbetc198

Moffitt, T.E., & Caspi, A. (2001). Childhood predictors differentiate life-course persistent and adolescence-limited antisocial pathways among males and females. *Dev Psychopathol*, 13(2), 355–375. https://doi.org/10.1017/S0954579401002097

Muller, C., Sampson, R.J., & Winter, A.S. (2018). Environmental inequality: The social causes and consequences of lead exposure. *Annual Review of Sociology*, 44, 263–282. https://doi.org/10.1146/annurev-soc-073117-041222

Muro-Ruiz, D. (2002). The state of art: The logic of violence. *Politics*, 22(2), 109–117.

National Academies of Sciences, Engineering, and Medicine. (2018, April 6). *Addressing the social and cultural norms that underlie the acceptance of violence: Proceedings of a workshop—In brief. Division of behavioral and social sciences and education; health and medicine division; committee on law and justice; Board on children, youth, and families; board on global health; forum on global violence prevention.* Washington, DC. www.ncbi.nlm.nih.gov/books/NBK493719/. https://doi.org/10.17226/25075

National Center for Health Statistics. (2020, September). National health Interview Survey: 2019 Survey description.Division of Health Interview Statistics, National Center for Health Statistics. https://ftp.cdc.gov/pub/Health_Statistics/NCHS/Dataset_Documentation/NHIS/2019/srvydesc-508.pdf

National Center for Healthy Housing. (2023). Information and evidence: *Lead*. https://nchh.org/information-and-evidence/learn-about-healthy-housing/health-hazards-prevention-and-solutions/lead/.

National Center for Injury Prevention and Control. (2022). *The Social-Ecological Model: A framework for prevention*. Division of Violence Prevention, Centers for Disease Control and Prevention. www.cdc.gov/violence-prevention/about/?CDC_AAref_Val=https://www.cdc.gov/violenceprevention/about/social-ecologicalmodel.html

National Institute of Child Health and Human Development. (2021). Health: *Infant mortality*. www.nichd.nih.gov/health/topics/infant-mortality

National Institutes of Health. (n.d.). *NIH health disparities strategic plan fiscal years 2004–2008 volume I* (pp. 17–18). U.S. Department of Health and Human Services. https://www.ncbi.nlm.nih.gov/books/NBK57031/

National Institute of Justice (NIJ). (2016). *Children exposed to violence*. https://nij.ojp.gov/topics/articles/children-exposed-violence

National Institute of Mental Health (NIMH). (2023). Mental health information: *Mental illness*. www.nimh.nih.gov/health/statistics/mental-illness#part_2539

National Institute on Minority Health and Health Disparities. (2025). NIH-designated populations with health disparities.

Ndugga, N., & Artiga, S. (2023, April 12). *Disparities in health and health care: 5 key questions and answers*. KFF: The independent source for health policy research, polling, and news. www.kff.org/racial-equity-and-health-policy/issue-brief/disparities-in-health-and-health-care-5-key-question-and-answers/.

Noel, O.D., Stewart, E., Cress, R., Dall'Era, M.A., & Shrestha, A. (2023). Underutilization of intravesical chemotherapy and immunotherapy for high grade non-muscle invasive bladder cancer in California between 2006–2018: Effect of race, age and socioeconomic status on treatment disparities. *Urologic Oncology*, 41(10), 431.e7–431.e14. https://doi.org/10.1016/j.urolonc.2023.05.019

Oberschall, A. (1978). Theories of social conflict. *Annual Review of Sociology*, 4, 291–315.

Office of Juvenile Justice and Delinquency Prevention. (2020). Arrests by offense, age, and gender. https://ojjdp.ojp.gov/statistical-briefing-book/crime/faqs/ucr

Office of Policy Development and Research. (2016, Summer). Evidence matters: Transforming knowledge into housing and community development policy. *Neighborhoods and violent crimes*. U.S. Department of Housing and Urban Development. www.huduser.gov/portal/periodicals/em/summer16/highlight2.html

O'Grady, W. (2011). *Crime in Canadian context* (2nd ed., pp. 127–130). Oxford University Press.

Oliver, W., & Hairston, C.F. (2008). Intimate partner violence during the transition from prison to the community: Perspectives of incarcerated African American men. *Journal of Aggression, Maltreatment & Trauma*, 3(16), 258–276. https://doi.org/10.1080/10926770801925577

Olver, M.E., & Wong, S.C.P. (2015). Short- and long-term recidivism prediction of the PCL-R and the effects of age: A 24-year follow-up. *Personality Disorders*, 6(1), 97–105. https://doi.org/10.1037/per0000095

Or, P.P.L., Fang, Y., Sun, F., Poon, E.T.C., Chan, C.K.M., & Chung, L.M.Y. (2023) From parental issues of job and finance to child well-being and maltreatment: A systematic review of the pandemic-related spillover effect. *Child Abuse & Neglect*, 137, 106041. https://doi.org/10.1016/j.chiabu.2023.106041

Orcutt, J.D. (1973). Societal reaction and the response to deviation in small groups. *Social Forces*, 52(2), 259–267. https://doi.org/10.2307/2576380

Organisation for Economic Co-operation and Development (OECD). (2022a). *Income inequality chart*. https://data.oecd.org/inequality/income-inequality.htm

Organisation for Economic Co-operation and Development (OECD). (2022b). *Poverty gap*. https://data.oecd.org/inequality/poverty-gap.htm#indicator-chart

Organisation for Economic Co-operation and Development (OECD). (2022c). *Poverty rate chart*. https://data.oecd.org/inequality/poverty-rate.htm#indicator-chart

Paternoster, R., Jaynes, C.M., & Wilson, T. (2017). Rational choice theory and interest in the "fortune of others". *Journal of Research in Crime and Delinquency*, 1–22. https://doi.org/10.1177/0022427817707240

Perry, I. (2009) Violence: A public health perspective. *Global Crime*, 10(4), 368–395. https://doi.org/10.108017440570903

Petit, J.R. (2005). Management of the acutely violent patient. *Psychiatric Clinics*, 28(3), 701–711. www.antoniocasella.eu/archipsy/Petit_2005.pdf

Petrocelli, M., Piquerro, A.R., & Smith, M.R. (2003). Conflict theory and racial profiling: An empirical analysis of police traffic stop data. *Journal of Criminal Justice*, 31, 1–11.

Piquero, A.R., & Hickman, M. (2002). The Rational Choice implications of Control Balance Theory. In A.R. Piquero & S.G. Tibbetts (Eds.), *Rational choice and Criminal Behavior*. Routledge. Published as Chapter in Brunisma, D. and D. Weisburd (Eds) 2014. Encyclopedia of Crime and Criminal Justice . Springer. 1 Rational Choice Theory and Crime Bill McCarthy Ali R. Chaudhary Sociology, University of California Davis.

Ports, K., Ford, D., & Merrick, M. (2016). Adverse childhood experiences and sexual victimization in adulthood. *Child Abuse & Neglect*, 51, 313–322. https://doi.org/10.1016/j.chiabu.2015.08.017

Pulay, A.J., Dawson, D.A., Hasin, D.S., Goldstein, R.B., Ruan, W.J., Pickering, R.P., Huang, B., Chou, S.P., & Grant, B.F. (2008). Violent behavior and DSM-IV psychiatric disorders: Results from the national epidemiologic survey on alcohol and related conditiocs. *Journal of Clinical Psychiatry*, 69(1), 12–22. www.psychiatrist.com/wp-content/uploads/2021/02/18636_violent-behavior-dsm-iv-psychiatric-disorders-results.pdf

Quinney, R. (2001). *The social reality of crime*. Transaction Publishers Rowan, A. and McGuire, M. (2023). Introduction to Criminology. https://kpu.Pressbooks.pub

Reyes, M. (2020). The disproportional impact of COVID-19 on African Americans. *Health and Human Rights*, 22(2), 299–307. PMID: 33390715; PMCID: PMC7762908. www.ncbi.nlm.nih.gov/pmc/articles/PMC7762908/

Sallar, A.M., Williams, P.B., Omishakin, A.M., & Lloyd, D.P. (2010). Stroke prevention: Awareness of risk factors for stroke among African American residents in the Mississippi delta region. *Journal of the National Medical Association*, 102, 84–94. https://doi.org/10.1016/s0027-9684(15)30495-8

Sampson, R.J., & Raudenbush, S.W. (2001). *Disorder in urban neighborhoods: Does it lead to crime* (pp. 1–6). US Department of Justice, Office of Justice Programs, National Institute of Justice. National Institute of Justice Research Brief, NCJ 186049/. www.ojp.gov/pdffiles1/nij/186049.pdf

Schaeffer, K. (2020, February 07). 6 Facts about economic inequality in the U.S. Pew Research Center. www.pewresearch.org/short-reads/2020/02/07/6-facts-about-economic-inequality-in-the-u-s/.

Schmalleger, F. (2009). *Criminology today: An Integrative Introduction* (5th ed.). Pearson Education, Inc.

Schneider, M.J. (2000). *Introduction to public health*. Aspen Publishers.

Schwendinger, H., & Schwendinger, J. (1983). *Rape and inequality*. Sage.

Shichor, D. (1980). The new criminology: Some critical issues. *British Journal of Criminology*, 20, 29–48.

Siegel, L. (2009). *Criminology* (10th ed.). Thomason/Wadsworth.

Siegel, L.J. (2011). *Criminology* (11th ed.). Wadsworth Publishing.

Siegel, L.J. (2013). *Criminology: Theories, patterns, and typologies* (11th ed.). Cengage Learning.

Short, J.E., & Strodtbeck, F. (1965). *Group process and gang delinquency*. University of Chicago Press.

Simpson, S., Piquero, N., & Paternoster, R. (2002). Rationality and corporate offending decisions. In A. Piquero & S. Tibbetts (Eds.), *Rational choice and criminal behavior* (pp. 25–39). Routledge.

Substance Abuse and Mental Health Services Administration. (2022). Highlights by *race/ethnicity* for the 2022 *national survey on drug use and health*. www.samhsa.gov/data/sites/default/files/reports/rpt42731/2022-nsduh-race-eth-highlights.pdf

Talayero, S.M., Robbins, C., Smith, E., & Santos-Burgoa, C. (2023, August 1). The association between lead exposure and crime: A systematic review. *PLOS Glob Public Health*, 3(8), e0002177. https://doi.org/10.1371/journal.pgph.0002177. PMID: 37527230; PMCID: PMC10393136.

Taylor, I. (1971). Reviewed work: Criminality and economic conditions by William Bonger, Austin T. Turk. *The British Journal of Criminology*, 11(2), 198–201. Published by Oxford University Press.

Tessum, C. W., Paolella, D. A., Chambliss, S. E., Apte, J. S., Hill, J. D., & Marshall, J. D. (2021). PM2.5 polluters disproportionately and systemically affect people of color in the united states. *Science Advances*, 7(18). https://doi.org/10.1126/sciadv.abf4491

Thilakarathna, K.A. (2019). Classical School of criminology and its application in the Sri Lankan criminal justice system. *US-China Law Review*, 16(7), 271–280. https://doi.org/10.17265/1548-6605/2019.07.002

Thomson, N.D. (2019). Psychopathy and violent crime. In M. DeLisi (Ed.), *Routledge international handbook of psychopathy and crime* (1st ed., pp. 508–525). Routledge. https://doi.org/10.4324/9781315111476-33

Thornberry, T.P., & Farnworth, M. (1982). Social correlates of criminal involvement. *American Sociological Review*, 47, 505–517.

Tibbetts, S.G., & Hemmens, C. (2014). *Criminological theory: A text/reader* (2nd ed.). SAGE Publication Inc.

Tittle, C.R., & Villemez, W.J. (1977). Social class and criminality. *Social Forces*, 56, 474–503.

Title, C.R. (1980). Labeling and crime: An empirical evaluation. In W.R. Gove (Ed.), *The labeling of deviance: Evaluating a perspective* (2d ed., pp. 241–263). Sage.

Tolbert, J., Drake, P., & Damico, A. (2023, December 18). *Key facts about the uninsured population*. www.kff.org/uninsured/issue-brief/key-facts-about-the-uninsured-population/

Tsao, C.W., Aday, A.W., Almarzooq, Z.I., Anderson, C.A.M., Arora, P., Avery, C.L., Baker-Smith, C.M., Beaton, A.Z., Boehme, A.K., Buxton, A.E., Commodore-Mensah, Y., Elkind, M.S.V., Evenson, K.R., Eze-Nliam, C., Fugar, S., Generoso, G., Heard, D.G., Hiremath, S., Ho, J.E., Kalani, R., Kazi, D.S., Ko, D., Levine, D.A., Liu, J., Ma, J., Magnani, J.W., Michos, E.D., Mussolino, M.E., Navaneethan, S.D., Parikh, N.I., Poudel, R., Rezk-Hanna, M., Roth, G.A., Shah, N.S., St-Onge, M.-P., Thacker, E.L., Virani, S.S., Voeks, J.H., Wang, N.-Y., Wong, N.D., Wong, S.S., Yaffe, K., Martin, S. S., & American Heart Association Council on Epidemiology and Prevention Statistics Committee and Stroke Statistics Subcommittee. (2023). Heart disease and stroke statistics—2023 update: A report from the American Heart Association. *Circulation*. https://doi.org/10.1161/CIR.0000000000001123/. www.ahajournals.org/doi/epub/10.1161/CIR.0000000000001123

Turner, J. (1997). *The structure of sociological theory* (6th ed.). Wadsworth.

United States Accountability Office. (2022, June). GAO highlights of GAO-22-104737/ K-12 education: Student population has significantly diversified, but many schools remain divided along racial, ethnic, and economic lines. GAO- 22-104737 Highlights, K-12 EDUCATION: Student population has significantly diversified, but many schools remain divided along racial, ethnic, and economic lines.

United States Department of Health and Human Services (USDHHS). (n.d.a). *Neighborhood and built environment*. Healthy People 2030. Office of Disease Prevention and Health Promotion. https://health.gov/healthypeople/objectives-and-data/browse-objectives/neighborhood-and-built-environment

United States Department of Health and Human Services (USDHHS). (n.d.b). *Social and community context*. Healthy People 2030. Office of Disease Prevention and Health Promotion. https://health.gov/healthypeople/objectives-and-data/browse-objectives/social-and-community-context

United States Department of Justice, Office of Public Affairs. (2023, October 13). *Court finds that Galveston County Texas, redistricting plan violates the Voting Rights Act* [Press release]. www.justice.gov/opa/pr/court-finds-galveston-county-texas-redistricting-plan-violates-voting-rights-act

United States White House. (2022, July 12). *Excess mortality during the pandemic: The role of health insurance*. https://bidenwhitehouse.archives.gov/cea/written-materials/2022/07/12/excess-mortality-during-the-pandemic-the-role-of-health-insurance/

University of Southern California. (2023, November 17). *6 examples of health disparities and potential solutions*. https://healthadministrationdegree.usc.edu/blog/examples-of-health-disparities

Walsh, A., & Hemmens, C. (2013). *Introduction to criminology: A text reader*. Sage.

Walters, G.D. (2015). The decision to commit crime: Rational or nonrational? *Criminology, Criminal Justice Law, and Society*, 16(3), 1–18.

Weintraub, W.S. (2023). The economic burden of Illness. *JAMA Network Open*, 6(3), e232663. https://doi.org/10.1001/jamanetworkopen.2023.2663

White, R.J., Gondolf, E.W., Robertson, D.U., Goodwin, B.J., & Caraveo, L.E. (2002). Extent and characteristics of woman batterers among federal inmates. *International Journal of Offender Therapy and Comparative Criminology*, 46(4), 412–426. https://doi.org/10.1177/0306624X02464004

Wilcox, P., & Cullen, F.T. (2018). Situational opportunity theories of crime. *Annual Review of Criminology*, 1, 123–148. https://doi.org/10.1146/annurev-criminol-032317-092421

Wilkerson, I. (2010). *The warmth of other suns: The epic story of American's great migration*. Vintage Books.

Winter, R.S. (2020). *Is lead exposure a form of housing inequality?* Housing Perspectives: Research, trends, and Perspective from Harvard Joint Center for Housing Studies/Is Lead Exposure a Form of Housing Inequality? | Joint Center for Housing Studies (harvard.edu).

Wolff, N., & Shi, J. (2009). Contextualization of physical and sexual assault in male prisons: Incidents and their aftermath. *Journal of Correctional Health Care*, 15(1), 58–77. https://doi.org/10.1177/1078345808326622

Woolhandler, S., & Himmelstein, D. (2017). The relationship of health insurance and mortality: Is lack of insurance deadly? *Annals of Internal Medicine*, 167, 424–431. https://doi.org/10.7326/M17-1403

World Health Organization. (2002). *World Report on violence and health*. World Health Organization.

Wright, R., Brookman, F., & Bennett, T. (2006). Foreground dynamics of street robbery in Britain. *British Journal of Criminology*, 46(1), 1–15.

Zhong, S., Yu, R., & Fazel, S. (2020). Drug use disorders and violence: Associations with individual drug categories. *Epidemiologic Reviews*, 42(1), 103–116. https://doi.org/10.1093/epirev/mxaa006. PMID: 33005950; PMCID: PMC7879597.

3
DATA SOURCES FOR VICTIMIZATION

Introduction

Stumped after theorizing about violence and crime, Septh was reminded by several university colleagues that when considering public health issues, he should apply criminological as well as the public health perspectives. However, this is only part of what is needed since public health experts contend that reliable data are required to address violence. In public health, data are defined as individual facts, statistics, and other articles of information that are the result of data analysis that are collected for a given purpose typically from surveys or healthcare providers (Soucie et al., 2010). The process of data collection is referred to as surveillance and it serves to inform experts about public health issues that affect communities. For example, public health experts monitor the health status of Americans by compiling and analysing health data (Schneider, 2021). These data are taken from a variety of sources (e.g., individuals, the environment, and healthcare providers and families) and used to create health statistics. Schwalbe and colleagues (2020) report that data on medicine and public health are generated from sources such as individuals, public and private health systems, and health resources. Today, experts point out that these data are increasingly digitized and critical for new health interventions needed to improve health outcomes (p. 1).

Scholars contend that statistics play a vital role in assessing how healthy a community or population is since these data help to identify groups that are at risk, detect emerging health threats and trends, and assist in planning needed health programs. Moreover, statistics are required to evaluate program success as well as help prepare governmental budgets (Schneider, 2021). Health experts argue data without context do not provide insight. However, contextualized data from research literature provide helpful information since these studies reveal the methods and limitations found in scientific investigations. Others contend that numbers alone lack meaning until raw data are given context (Craig et al., 2018). In public health, researchers namely biostatisticians and epidemiologists rely on representative samples of the population to measure health issues. When this occurs, any finding that emerges from their investigation can become meaningful public health data. Consequently, health officials rely on epidemiologists, data scientists, data analysis, and

DOI: 10.4324/9781003373001-3

others to collect, measure, and communicate what is derived from data and research to the public. In fact, those using biostatistics help make predictions and control the spread of diseases and violence via the efficacy of public health interventions.

When monitoring the public's health, governmental officials, and others on the local, state, and federal levels collect statistics also known as raw data and use them for research that focuses on environmental health status, social and behavior status, and even what is occurring in the medical care system (Schneider, 2021). These data are quickly shared with all levels of public health. Perhaps the most recognized primary health statistics agency on the federal level that collects, analyses, and reports on the health status of Americans is the *National Centers for Health Statistics* (NCHS) which is part of the *Centers for Disease Control and Prevention* (CDC). Experts contend that NCHS collects data from states which transmit data compiled from local records including vital statistics. Moreover, NCHS surveys (e.g., the *National Health Interview Survey*) national representative samples of the population on matters such as health status, lifestyles, and health-related behaviors, onset, and diagnosis of trends in illness and disability, and use of medical care. It is important to reiterate that these surveys are conducted throughout the U.S. As a result, they are beneficial and useful to each state and local communities since they allow public health officials to track progress toward achieving national health objectives. NCHS also compiles statistical data that guide and inform action and policies necessary to improve the overall health of the population. While CDC is charged with leading the way to modernize data and surveillance infrastructure across the federal, state, tribal, and public health landscape, health experts also report that other federal agencies (e.g., *National Center for Emerging and Zoonotic Infectious Diseases, National Notifiable Diseases Surveillance System* and others) collect data for their own purposes and they typically share them with NCHS (Schneider, 2021).

The need for accurate and reliable health data cannot be overstated. In fact, public health officials argue that while the government collects large amounts of data on Americans, researchers argue that there can never be too much data since it is needed to inform the surveillance systems that influence public health practices as well as the quality of planning and evaluation required to keep Americans safe. Notwithstanding, they argue that what is needed is more consistent and detailed data from surveillance that can help identify risk factors that can be addressed through health intervention (Soucie, 2015). Research conducted by Blumenthal and Lurie (2023) is instructive in this regard. They report that during the *COVID-19* pandemic, access to good national data on matters that threaten the health of the nation was critical because of four reasons. First, these data can help to assess the nature and extent of any threat. Second, after the threat is established, a clear national estimate of the problem is necessary to determine what federal resources are needed (this suggests that during *COVID*, there was a lack of good data that accounted for a delay in the U.S. being able to detect the toll *COVID* had on marginalized people of color in the U.S.). Third, good national data are highly effective at assessing the success of interventions. As such, they attributed the U.S. failure of having good national data on *COVID* to several factors such as decentralization of public health in general, but on the fragmentation of how data are collected and shared. More specifically, Blumenthal and Lurie (2023) argued that each state and locality use a unique data system with its own definitions of critical terms and methods of collecting data. Consequently, federal authorities cannot impose any standards that require that data are consistent and is shared with other jurisdictions in a timely manner or if at all. The fourth issue that they attribute to data failure during *COVID* is the depletion of the U.S. public health infrastructure owing to years of neglect, especially gross underfunding at the state and local levels. The latter has resulted in some states and localities being unable to collect data using electronic formats and unfortunately, the computer software they use is inadequate (and slow as well as less secure) since it is dated or antiquated. They also observed that these states and localities lack the necessary infrastructure technology staff. As such, some are likely to rely on manual data entry which has historically been prone to error. This withstanding, the Health Information Management Systems Society (2022) reports that health experts estimate that modernizing state and local public health reporting systems can be achieved, but it comes with an expensive price that is estimated to cost the U.S. nearly $8 billion annually for ten years.

As stated earlier, public health researchers gather data from many sources that include, but is not limited to, insurance claims, medical records, vital records, surveys, and data that are published in academic literature (Schneider, 2021). Others contend that to fully address and prevent violence, public health researchers must also rely on data collected by crime and victimization sources such as agencies of justice, namely the Federal Bureau of Investigation's (FBI's) *Uniform Crime Reports* (UCR), the Justice Department and U.S. Census Bureau's *National Crime Victimization Survey* (NCVS), the Bureau of Justice Statistics' *National Incident-Based Reporting System* (NIBRS), and other victimization surveys (to be discussed in details later). In combination, these data can be used to paint a valid picture of the health status of the nation since they provide annual totals of the number of violent and property crimes that are reported to law enforcement agencies and researchers who interview victims of crime. While they do not account for every crime committed in the U.S., they can help contribute to our understanding of crimes that are violent in nature, the relationship, if any, between victims and offenders, regions of the country where the crime transpires, risk factors involved, what victim and offenders look like as well as other significant variables linked to the etiology of crime and violence (Siegel, 2011).

Soucie (2015) writes that data collected in public health surveillance include demographics, socioeconomics, and clinical characteristics of the population that is under surveillance. These data also provide outcomes such as disease complications and mortality. They include mitigating and aggregating behavior and risk factors. More specifically, these data offer the nature and extent of emerging health problems, and they reveal which groups of people are at risk of facing diseases and various levels of victimization from crime and violence. Despite these efforts, some experts contend that these are not perfect data, but rather, there are gaps in these data. For example, while CDC receives health data from a number of public health and healthcare sources, data collection methods are often imperfect and inconsistent and consequently reveal gaps and blind spots in the public health surveillance systems. This makes the picture of our national health status incomplete and unclear (Soucie, 2015). Similarly, the UCR data compilation was disrupted for certain periods during the *COVID-19* pandemic which highlights the need to continuously collect valid data on crime and victimization from justice agencies (Li & Ricard, 2023). Because incomplete and a lack of accurate data conspires to confound our understanding of crime and violence, and the ability to develop effective prevention strategies, health experts recommend that in order to address "dirty" data riddled with inaccuracies, health data must be periodically evaluated for accuracy, consistency, and completeness using standard data management protocols (e.g., electronic methods of filing that improves the quality of data). Efforts should also be made to protect public health data from natural disasters (e.g., pandemics) and improve data timeliness and accessibility. Experts also warn that because computers are used to analyse public health data, efforts must be made to protect against computer viruses, as well as protect data integrity (Schneider, 2021; Soucie, 2015). Needless to say, that the internet has also accelerated the accessibility and availability of public health information to public health workers and the general public (Thacker & Wetterhall, 1998).

Role of Public Health Data-Vital Statistics

In the U.S., all vital statistics start and are registered at the local level that report these data to the *NCHS*. In fact, many states have centralized vital records offices. Some estimate that there are over 6,000 local vital registrars throughout the U.S. (Schwartz, 2009). Experts argue that vital statistics are excellent sources of data that public health experts use to assess the overall health of a population since they examine characteristics of the population by periodically surveying vital statistics. For example, they can be used to study lifestyles, health-related matters, onset of violence, disease, injuries, and disabilities (Schneider, 2021). The purpose of these data are twofold: (1) "the legal registration of the record to prepare certified copies, and (2) to create an index for retrieving the records" (Swchwartz, 2009, p. 2).Vital statistics are data compilations on vital events such as births, deaths, marriages, divorces, termination of pregnancies, to name a few (Osterman et al., 2023; Schwartz, 2009). Vital records reveal that each year, there are an estimated 11 million vital events that are reported in the U.S. According to research by Sutton (2008) and MacDorman and colleagues (2007), in 2006, there were 4.3 million births, 2.4 million deaths, 26,000 fetal deaths, 2.1 million marriages, and 1.1 million divorces. There were also an estimated 1.2 million induced pregnancy terminations (*Guttmacher Institute*, 2008). Health experts contend that these data are highly reliable since they are legal documents that provide accurate demographics and medical data on virtually every birth, death, marriage, or divorce followed with a certificate being issued. In fact, where birth and death are concerned, the state health department is legally responsible for collecting these data and passing them on to the *NCHS* (Schneider, 2021). Vital statistics typically contain information about a person's health. For example, birth certificates provide a name, address, age of parent(s), race/ethnicity, state, and city. In addition, the hospital provides other information on medical health such as birth weight, medical risk factors, complications of labor or delivery, or if there were any abnormalities with the newborn. Recently, many states have started to include questions regarding the mother's use of tobacco during the pregnancy (Schneider, 2021; Osterman et al., 2023).

Experts argue that in public health research, the birth certificate provides data that can be used to detect features of the mother in general and whether her pregnancy in particular impacted the health of the child (Osterman et al., 2023). Similarly, death certificates can also be useful to public health officials, but they can be problematic. Chief among them is when no specific explanation is provided as an accurate cause of death. Experts are quick to report that in many cases, incorrect diagnoses are made, especially in the absence of an autopsy; the actual cause of death may never be discovered. The same experts contend that when several factors can be attributed to the death, it is challenging to determine what were the underlying compared with the immediate causes of death. Examples of deaths owing to AIDS and suicides have historically been misstated to avoid subjecting surviving family members to public ridicule and stigma associated with the circumstances of these deaths.

Other vital statistics are collected on marriages, divorces, sudden fetal deaths, and terminations of pregnancy (Schwartz, 2009). While records of marriages and divorces are important and accessible to those with an interest in reviewing them since these events must be reported, they are not often helpful to public health researchers. At best, they present a picture of the demographics of those who marry and divorce, the time frame of the marriage, the circumstances surrounding the divorce, but they lack information on the health status of either party. However, sudden or spontaneous fetal deaths and terminations of pregnancies provide researchers with public health data. For example, fetal deaths that occur because of a failure to carry to terms are typically viewed as unrecognized. At the same time, terminations of pregnancies are often unreported. Nevertheless, infant mortality is a very important public health issue to the extent that the *NCHS* has created a computer center that stores vital records on infants who died shortly after birth, especially those who do not survive the first year after birth. Health researchers who study and examine the causation of these deaths can compare information on the death certificates to detect factors that may have attributed to these untimely deaths (Schneider, 2021).

U.S. Census Data

Health experts argue that data collected from vital statistics and its systems must be converted into rates to be used for public health purposes. Consequently, health officials are concerned with the total number of people in the population as it relates to the likelihood of those who could be impacted by health concerns. Experts contend that population counts provide denominations that public health officials could and often use to determine disease prevalence rates (Cohen et al., 2019). However, to accomplish this, health officials rely on data collected by the *U.S. Census Bureau* (every ten years). Stated differently, public health officials look to census data for current and accurate demographic data on the U.S. population in order to calculate the number of people who may be impacted by a health risk. More specifically, census data are used to know and understand which group of people in the U.S. are impacted by vital statistics and other health concerns annually (e.g., violence, injuries, and diseases). Moreover, these data provide information on the growth of the population regarding race/ethnicity (as of 2022, there were 62,080.44 Hispanics or Latinos which compose 19.1% of the population), gender, age, income, and other salient characteristics that are important to public health data and research. As such, public health experts and researchers examine the demographics of the population, especially in relation to those who may be impacted or who are more susceptible to health risk or threat (Steinweg, 2023). For example, census data allow public health researchers to determine one's exposure to health risks by gender, race/ethnicity, age, and location. Furthermore, census data, along with the help of the *American Community Survey* (part of the decennial census), provides highly reliable data on the socioeconomic aspects of understanding the health of Americans since it allows health experts to contextualize peoples environmental circumstances (i.e., whether they live in poverty) when examining characteristics such as income earning, educational attainment, housing, and health insurance status (Steinweg, 2023; Cohen et al., 2019). Accurate census data are essential to many entities that range from healthcare providers, health insurance companies, government agencies, and others to make correct decisions regarding services that are provided. Census data also reveal which racial or ethnic groups have higher rates of disability due to arthritis, diabetes, hypertension, and other diseases. Despite the U.S. Constitution mandating that the census be taken every ten years, some health experts report that there are a number of factors that often challenge this task, namely budgetary constraints, a shift to online data collection, data security threats, and asking questions about race/ethnicity with questionable accuracy. The failure to adequately address these challenges will result in unreliable and inaccurate data that will be used to deny people the healthcare resources needed in their respective communities, especially in reducing social inequity in health care (Cohen et al., 2019).

Other Sources of Health Data that Provide Indicators of Lethal Violence in a Community

Experts emphasize that data are also needed to understand the circumstances surrounding incidents of violence and crime and how they impact the health of individuals and communities. Sponsored by the CDC, *the National Intimate Partner and Sexual Violence Survey (NISVS)* is the first national survey to collect data on intimate personal violence (IPV). The survey reveals that each year, millions of Americans are the victims of sexual violence (SV), stalking, and intimate partner violence. It was started in 2010 and is now an annual nationwide telephone survey that is used to collect data on the nature and extent of IPV. At its inception in 2010, the sample was composed of 9,086 women and 7,421 men. *NISVS* provides details regarding IPV, SV, and stalking (S) reported by men and women. This self-report survey allows respondents to identify their sexual orientation (e.g., heterosexual, lesbian, gay, and bisexual). As such, the survey addresses a neglected area of criminal justice, criminological, as well as public health research, that is, the extent and prevalence of *IPV, SV, and S* among special populations such as the *LGBQTI* community. These data provide the ages of victims who are 18 and older, gender, fear of safety concerns, and other important variables. They also indicate that despite the physical harm that is often associated with *IPV*, many victims also suffer emotionally as well as mentally. In fact, the impact of this violence transcends the individual person and affects economic costs associated with victimization (e.g., medical care, treatment, medications, loss of work, and the criminal justice system). Health researchers report that *IPV, SV, and S* are difficult to monitor given the sensitive and private nature of these victimizations. *NISVS* data are collected at the state and national levels. More specifically, *NISVS* regularly measures important health issues by focusing on lifetime and 12-month prevalence data. These data describe who is more likely to experience *IPV, SV, and S*, as well as how these victimizations adversely impact the health of its victims. *NISVS* data are composed of a representative sample of past year experiences with violence as well as one's lifetime experiences in the U.S. The survey is an important instrument that reveals the prevalence and indicators of lethal violence in each community. These data point to root causes of violence and can be helpful in determining how they impact community residents either directly or vicariously, and negative health consequences associated with being the victim of *IPV, SV, and S*. In the end, the *NISVS* provides data that help to better educate the community on the pervasiveness of these victimizations and resources that are available to assist victims. NISVS offers data that inform prevention efforts at the local, state, and national levels.

Because crimes such as sexual assaults, physical assaults, homicides, rapes, suicides, and others are commonplace and impact millions of Americans (personally and economically), many data sources are used to access the actual nature and extent of violence (Crosby et al., 2016). Another surveillance system that is used to collect information on violent deaths including suicide, homicide, unintentional firearm, child maltreatment, and undetermined injuries is called the *National Violent Death Reporting System* (NVDRS). Created in response to a 1999 report from the *Institute of Medicine* outlining the need for a national fatal intentional injury system, *NVDRS*, was implemented by the *CDC* in 2002. It emerged to provide the details and circumstances that precipitated violent deaths. The *NVDRS* reveals that in 2019, over 19,100 people were victims of homicide and more than 47,500 people committed suicide (Centers for Disease Control and Prevention [CDC], n.d.). These data are critical to developing prevention strategies to reduce the number of homicides and suicides committed annually because they link information about "who, when, where, and how" from data on violent deaths. Experts also argue they provide insight regarding "why" the death occurred (Crosby et al., 2016, p. 169). These data contain accurate information regarding the date, time, manner of death, narratives from medical examiners and police officers, as well as physical traits of victims. More specifically, *NVDRS* includes over 600 data elements that provide context about violent deaths. It provides data on the relationship between victims and suspects, location where the fatal act occurred, mental health problems and treatment, life stressors, toxicology results, whether victims had problems with employment, or physical health problems. It serves a threefold purpose: (1) collects detailed data on violent deaths committed in the U.S., including age, when, where, and method used, (2) links law enforcement data, vital statistics, and coroners'/medical examiners data into the reporting system, and (3) makes data available to public health officials, law enforcement, violence prevention groups and policymakers with the goal of helping to reduce violent deaths on the local, state, and national levels (Crosby et al., 2016).

NVDRS also serve as the basis for engaging in injury surveillance that informs violence prevention programs (Masho et al., 2016). More specifically, NVDRS data provide decision-makers with data on the pervasiveness, trends, patterns, and characteristics of violent deaths that occur in each community and state. Health experts favor these data because the NVDRS is linked from several sources such as death certificates, medical examiner records, crime incident reports and laboratory reports (CDC, 2014d). Health experts argue that *NVDRS* addresses what was missing in the past, especially in vital statistics death certificates, since it operates as a multi-state reporting system that provides details about violent deaths, links multiple source documents on violent-related deaths, and allows researchers to understand each death more comprehensively (Crosby et al., 2016). Despite their utility, the NVDRS has been criticized for being dated since these data are not offered in real time. Some experts argue that these data have about a three-year lag period (Masho et al., 2016).

Because homicide is the second leading cause of death among youth between the ages of 5 and 18, the *School-Associated Violent Death Surveillance System (SAVD-SS)* is another source of data that are used to measure the number of violent deaths (e.g., homicides, suicides, or legal intervention) that occur on school grounds, on the way to and from school, or at school-sponsored programs and events. The surveillance system includes violent deaths that occur at primary and secondary schools, in private as well as public schools. *SAVD-SS* monitors violent deaths that are linked to schools in the U.S. These data are typically taken from law enforcement agencies that investigate these fatal incidents and from media databases. Experts argue that while school-associated deaths make up less than 2% of the homicides that occur each year, *SAVD-SS* data can be used to reveal and assess national trends in fatally violent school shootings as well as help to inform prevention efforts. Data from *SAVD-SS* reveal that youth homicides typically involve a single victim, the victims are often a racial or ethnic minority, and the fatality occurred in an urban area. The firearm used in the school-associated homicide or suicide was taken from the perpetrator's home or from a relative or friend. In addition to *NCHS* efforts to collect data on the health of the U.S. population, public health experts contend that follow-back surveys, part of periodic studies, are also used to expand on vital statistics data (Pickett & Hanlon, 1990). For example, in 1988, *NCHS* selected a sample of birth certificates to further investigate the health of the mothers and babies.

NCHS sends questionnaires to doctors, mothers, and hospitals to collect more data on family traits, characteristics, as well as specific circumstances surrounding the pregnancies and births of those selected in the sample. More specifically, the National Center for Health Statistics (NCHS) (1999) reported that health researchers used an instrument called the *National Maternal and Infant Health Survey* to follow back on samples of fetal and infant deaths to examine practices that contributed to poor pregnancy outcomes. These surveys are also used to study cases of adult deaths. Schneider (2021) reveals that similar surveys are periodically used to conduct investigations into samples of death cases. When this occurs, the person who completed the death certificate is asked to respond to several questions that may include asking about the lifestyle and whether the deceased was taking any medication at the time of his or her demise. Furthermore, other instruments are often used to provide indicators of violence in a community. For instance, the *National Health Interview Survey* is used to assess the health of the population. The survey is given yearly to an estimated 50,000 households to collect data on health topics such as physical injuries, chronic conditions, injuries, impairments, illnesses, whether anyone in the home uses medical resources, and other health concerns (National Center for Health Statistics, 1999).

Data Allow Researchers to Monitor Changes in Fatal Violence Over Time

Health statistics reveal that youth violence can be fatal and is regarded as a major problem in the U.S. and remains the third leading cause of death for youth between the ages of 10 and 24. However, the same data show that it is the leading cause of death for Blacks between the ages of 10 and 24. Apart from this, the medical treatment associated with fatal violence and assault injuries costs the U.S. an estimated $17.5 billion annually (CDC, 2010, 2014, 2016, 2024). Mercy and colleagues (2002) reported that violence causes other concerns such as loss of productivity, disability, added burden to health and welfare services, fear, and community decay. Notwithstanding, because fatal violence possesses serious threat to public health, the need for better surveillance of violence cannot be overstated given that in order to create preventive steps, researchers and public health professionals must rely on a constant flow of accurate and up-to-date data to detect increases and decreases in levels of violence, along with newly emerging patterns of concern. As such, official as well as observational data collected from a variety of surveillance sources such as archival records from medical examiners, emergency room visits, police incident reports, ambulance pickups, juvenile justice intake, hospital discharges and others, can pinpoint and isolate locations regarding region, state, city, town, and where violence is occurring. Health data can also provide demographic characteristics about victims. Despite this, public health experts strongly encourage the use of local surveillance data to describe and monitor violence in the community (Masho et al., 2016). Through the systematic collection and analysis of data, violence can be routinely monitored, and interventions can be implemented so that health officials can determine the impact that their efforts are having on keeping communities safe from violence (Masho et al., 2016). As researchers monitor fatal violence, the *Department of Health and Human Services* makes reductions in violence-related morbidity and mortality a priority and typically places it among its goals (U.S. Department of Health and Human Services, 2013). When this occurs, Vivolo et al. (2011) report that the prevention wing of the CDC often establishes programs and initiatives including surveillance that monitors violence and research aimed at identifying risk and protective factors linked to violence to better inform those in public health so that effective interventions and policies can be implemented.

Identify Groups and Communities That Are at Risk to Violence

While surveillance data reveal violence effects every community in the U.S. and impacts millions of people, families, schools, and communities each year, it is the third leading cause of death and nonfatal injuries among adolescents and young adults between the ages of 1 and 45 (U.S. Department of Health and Human Services, 2014). However, it is the number one cause of death for Black Americans. In fact, Blacks are disproportionately impacted by firearm injuries and deaths. Statistics reveal that Blacks between the ages of 10 and 25 are nearly 20 times more likely than their White counterparts to be killed in a homicide (CDC, 2012). Moreover, statistics show that more than 86% of homicides in Black communities involve the use of firearms. The situation is so dire that public health officials at CDC reported that from 2018 to 2021, more Black men between the ages of 15 and 24 died from firearms-related homicides than unintentional injuries, suicide, heart disease, COVID-19, cancer, non-firearm homicide, diabetes, congenital abnormalities, police shootings, influenza, sepsis, chronic respiratory diseases, and others (Nguyen & Drane, 2023; Edmund, 2022). Surveillance data also link negative health outcomes to the conditions under which people live, work, and learn. Researchers interpret these data to mean that the conditions people experience are social determinants of their health.

According to homicide data from 2015, half of all gun homicides occurred in 127 cities in the U.S. that were under-resourced and racially segregated (Aufrichting et al., 2017). Moreover, health data indicate factors such as economic instability, poverty, bias, discrimination, limited education, and health inequities influence violence that impacts health outcomes. Consequently, communities that are disproportionately occupied by minorities experience more negative conditions and place residents at a greater risk of poor health outcomes. For example, surveillance data show that Blacks, American Indians, Alaskan Natives, and Latinx experience higher rates of violent assaults including homicides compared with their White counterparts. Some attribute this to a combination of factors such as weak gun laws, unequal access to safe housing, and living in areas that have historically suffered from disinvestments in public infrastructures and services (Edmund, 2022). Public health officials surmise that negative health outcomes have nothing to do with bad people, but rather, it has everything to do with the exposure to numerous risk factors (Center for Nonviolence and Social Justice, 2019). Therefore, health experts believe it is critically important to understand those specific factors that place groups of people and their communities at risk of becoming victims of violence. Data show that minority communities also disproportionately experience violence in the form of physical injuries and mental health conditions that often manifests into depression, anxiety, and post-traumatic stress disorders. It also has harmful effects on child development, the long-term health of affected populations, and the economic development of communities, especially those of color (Lead, 2018).

Research even suggests that after experiencing violence and the trauma that comes along with it, some victims face an elevated risk of developing chronic disease (e.g., hypertension, asthma, cancer, stroke) which are major causes of morbidity and mortality (Santaularia et al., 2014; Kung et al., 2008; Wilson et al., 2004). To some people, violence is a constant theme to the extent that the fear of being assaulted or killed has caused many people to alter their lifestyles by becoming socially isolated and forgoing activities that are healthy and routine to others such as going out at night, congregating with community residents, walking, and using parks and recreational spaces for exercise and relaxation (WHO, 2014). Public health professionals are also concerned with being able to identify risk factors in the community that influence people to commit acts of violence and crime. They contend that both are necessary in order to know where to place intervention efforts since community violence is a critical public health problem in the U.S. It presents in the form of homicides (which increased in many areas of the country in 2020 from 2019) and other acts of violence that cause harm (e.g., physical, emotional, and financial devastation) in communities nationwide, especially in neighborhoods characterized as being high in poverty.

Roles of Criminal Justice Data

While there are many sources of criminal justice data, when it comes to measuring the nature, extent, and types of crime and violence in the U.S., there are several primary sources of data. They are the *UCR*, *NIBRS*, *NCVS* and Self-Report Surveys (SRS) (Siegel, 2011; Senna & Siegel, 2000). These sources include information about crime that is reported to law enforcement agencies and that which is not reported to police for a variety of reasons. Researchers, criminal justice experts, as well as critics of justice data believe that these sources are complimentary to each other in that they provide official as well as unofficial crime data. In fact, critics argue that while official crime data sources such as the *UCR* and *NIBRS* can be used independently, they have limitations and because of that, they should be supplemented with *NCVS* and *SRS* data since in combination, they provide a fuller picture of the totality of crime that is committed in the U.S. For example, because many crimes are unreported to law enforcement agencies, they create what is known as the "dark figures" of crime or what experts refer to as the unknown numbers of crime. Since the *UCR* and the *NIBRS* are based on what is reported, they do not contain any information about crime that goes unreported by victims or offenders. As such, the *NCVS* and *SRS* are used to collect data on unreported crimes since the *NCVS* asks victims to report what crimes they have experienced but did not report to police, while *SRS* ask offenders to report the crime, they committed but were not arrested for committing or held criminally responsible. Both surveys are designed to measure the nature and extent of hidden crimes. While these data sources are different, they have enough similarities to assist criminal justice and criminological researchers in drawing conclusions about the severity of crime and violence in America. Taken together, they can also reveal if there is a crime problem, especially if rates reach epidemic proportions. This could indicate the need to use both criminal justice and public health approaches to respond to high levels of violence (Senna & Siegel, 2000; Rosenberg & Fenley, 1991). This is vitally important when attempting to calculate how much crime and victimization is occurring since criminal justice historians have long argued that survey data reveal that there is considerably more crime occurring than that which is officially known and gets reported to law enforcement officers and their respective agencies (Adler et al., 1996; Walker, 1998; Senna & Siegel, 2000).

Uniform Crime Reports (UCR)

Started in 1930, the *UCR* is an annual nationwide data compilation that is published by the *FBI* and the U.S. *Department of Justice*. Experts estimate that over 19,000 police agencies in the U.S. voluntarily provide reported crime data to the federal government. These reports reflect the offenses known by local, state, and federal agencies. It is believed that these law enforcement agencies cover 95% of the U.S. population (Gaines & Miller, 2009). This crime data is referred to as criminal statistics and is used in law enforcement administration, operation, and management as the most often cited source of aggregate criminal statistics (Wallace, 1998; Federal Bureau of Investigation [FBI], 1998). The *UCR* prepares an annual index that is composed of selected offenses used to determine changes in the overall rate of crime reported to all police agencies nationwide (Wallace, 1998). Some experts argue that the crime rate is based on a combination of *violent* and *property* crimes. More specifically, *UCR* data are used by law enforcement practitioners, media, politicians, citizens, and researchers who examine the trends and patterns associated with crime, especially the eight index crimes. The consumers of official police data must be aware that all crimes whether property or violent are not reported to police and added to its crime index. Nevertheless, these data are divided into two major categories: *Part One* and *Part Two*. Part One crimes are considered the most frequently committed and most serious offenses. They include murder, forcible rape, robbery, aggravated assault, burglary, larceny-theft, motor vehicle theft, and arson. Part Two crimes include less serious crimes and are referred to as misdemeanors (Gaines & Miller, 2009). The UCR data provide crime information that breaks down crimes committed by city, county, state, and standard metropolitan statistical area (Senna & Siegel, 2000). In essence, it gives the geographical distribution of crime along with the demographic characteristics (e.g., race/ ethnicity, gender, and age) of arrestees. These data are excellent in crime studies because they indicate how healthy the society is by the offering indicators of the trauma of violent crimes reported annually in the number of homicides, rapes, aggravated assaults, and other variables that reflect the health of the nation. Because these data have been collected since the 1930s, they lend themselves to longitudinal, as well as cross-sectional designs. Despite this, researchers caution that while these data are collected yearly, they are not perfect. In fact, they suffer in several areas such as citizens' reporting practices, law enforcement practices, and methodologically.

National Incident-Based Reporting System (NIBRS)

Because of the problems associated with the UCR, in the 1980s, *NIBRS* was created to address the UCR's shortcomings and to collect a better quality of crime data (Gaines & Miller, 2009). For example, unlike the UCR that collects data on eight index crimes, NIBRS requires that local agencies collect data on 22 categories of 46 specific crimes referred to as Group A offenses including the eight Part One crimes. More specifically, local agencies are asked to collect data on each single incident of crime. This effort is believed to generate a better quality of data since the UCR only indicated the number of crimes committed in the Type One category. The expansion in the number of offenses (compared to the eight offenses that the UCR primarily focused on) was designed to address many crimes that were previously ignored. They include many federal offenses such as drug offenses, bribery, blackmail, firearms violations, and embezzlement. Under NIBRS, local agencies provide details of a brief account of facts surrounding each crime. NIBRS also provides data on four datasets: victims, offenders, offenses, and arrestees (Siegel, 2011). While the switch has been ambitious, not all police agencies have readily embraced using NIBRS. In fact, most police agencies throughout the U.S. still collect crime data using the UCR since many departments lack the resources needed to make the conversion (Siegel, 2011). Similar to the UCR, NIBRS is also a good source of crime data for public health studies since it too offers crime data that reveals the number of violent crimes that occur each year, these data can also reveal crime victims, perpetrators, and where victimizations are more likely to occur. This can assist in crime mapping of places where intervention and prevention programs should be targeted the most.

National Crime Victimization Survey (NCVS)

While the *UCR* and *NIBRS* focus on reported crime, the *NCVS* is used to collect crime data about victims and victimizations that are not officially reported to law enforcement. Started in 1972 over growing concerns about the increasing crime rates and whether all crimes were being reported, the *National Crime Survey (NCS)* was created to calculate the total number of crime and victimizations that were occurring. Eventually, the NCS would be changed to the *NCVS*. The *NCVS* is conducted by the *U.S. Census Bureau* incorporation with the *Bureau of Justice Statistics* and the *U.S. Department of Justice* (Rennison, 1998). The *NCVS* estimates the number of offenses by collecting a sample of 40,000 households of 75,000 residents and asking them about their experience as victims over a three-year period. The sample is kept in a panel for three years. However, at every six-month intervals (or twice a year), residents are surveyed and asked whether they have experienced crime and victimizations such as rape, robbery, assault, larceny, burglary, and motor vehicle theft. When the three years expire, another panel is assembled, rotated into the panel and the surveying continues. These data allow researchers to measure whether there are increases in crime as well as victimization rates. More importantly, they can be used to isolate crime and violence that have an adverse impact on the community's public health since these data provide variations of crime rate by region, season, time of day, location, and other key variables. Moreover, the *NCVS* provides data on crime, offender, whether a weapon was used, number of offenders, perceived race/ethnicity of offender and victim, along with age (Blumstein et al., 1991). As previously stated, because many crimes go unreported, these data can help us measure what is reported and unreported. They are not affected by any bias law enforcement reporting and these data are not contingent on victims reporting crime to police (Gaines & Miller, 2009). Despite their use, there are several concerns that make some question the veracity of these data, namely that victims do not always report their criminal experiences for several reasons and chief among them is poor memory and the fear of reprisal from criminal offenders. Others point to the interval to which these data are reported and argue that they lead to erroneous reporting.

Self-Report Surveys (SRS)

Because of the problems associated with official crime data and victimization surveys, some researchers have sought to survey offenders about criminal behaviors they successfully got away with and where there is no criminal record that exists. By relying on SRSs, research participants are allowed to disclose information about their unknown criminal activities. When these surveys are used, participants are typically kept anonymous. Researchers believe that the promise of protection via confidentiality or anonymity ensures the likelihood that offenders will be honest and forthright as they share information about their law violations. As stated previously, SRS are used to collect data on the "dark figures" of crime or those crimes that are not included among reported official crime data. While these surveys are disproportionately used on juveniles because they are easy to survey since they can be approached at school where they congregate in large numbers (as captive audiences) and are expected to attend class during weekdays, they are also used to collect data on adult samples especially, prisoners, substance abusers, as well as other segments of the population. SRS data are used to calculate the actual number of adult offenders that are unknown to police, the crimes they commit without being charged or punished, and those who are repeat and chronic offenders. Similar to other surveys, including the NCVS, SRS data reveal that the number of people who violate the law is far greater than what is revealed in the UCR's official crime statistics (Hindelang, 1973). SRS also provides crime data about offenders that is not found among official statistics. Experts argue that when relying on UCR, NIBRS, NCVS, and SRS data, there should be convergence between officially reported crime, victims-reported crime, and self-reported criminal offenses, especially with respect to similarities regarding when and where crimes occurred and the demographical features of what victims and offenders look like (Siegel, 2011).

Needed Health Data on Injuries

Health experts are concerned about the number of fatal and nonfatal injuries that occur each year in the U.S. As such, they make efforts to collect these data. In fact, one such effort is the CDC's web-based injury statistics query and reporting system (WISQARS). This system is an online database that stores information on fatal and nonfatal injuries, violent deaths, and the costs that are associated with different types of injuries. These data are collected from reliable sources and used by health professionals, the media, and public health researchers. Some scholars report that WISQARS measures the economic burden linked to unintentional and violence-related injuries that occur annually. More specifically, WISQARS data assists researchers and others to ascertain information on whether injuries are intended or unintended, acts of violence such as a homicide or physical assault, suicide, or some other form of self-harm. It also provides the type of mechanism that was used in the injury such as a firearm, a fall, fire, auto accident, poisoning, or suffocation. It gives specific information on the area of the body where the injury occurred. For example, WISQARS data provides whether injury was sustained to the lower or upper extremities, torso, or traumatic brain injury. WISQARS data includes the nature of the injury and whether it was an open wound, internal injury, dislocation, fracture, burns, and even amputations. These data also provide researchers with the geographical location, as well as the demographical features of injured persons to include information on region of the country with respect to the state where the injured resides or lived and what injured persons look like with respect to race, ethnicity, and age.

Health experts report the benefits of WISQARS data are fourfold. First, these data provide the number of injury deaths and deaths by intent and mechanism used, along with the impact of injury-related deaths. They make distinctions between the impacts of premature deaths caused by injury compared with other leading causes of premature deaths. Second, these data provide a national estimate of the number of nonfatal injury reports taken from injuries treated in U.S. hospital emergency rooms. They provide intent and mechanism of injury by race and ethnicity, sex, and disposition upon release (e.g., status of injured party, treated, referred to specialized care, or hospitalized). Data also ranks the leading causes of nonfatal injuries treated by emergency room doctors. Fourth, WISQARS provides the estimated economic costs of injury deaths (for violent) and nonfatal injuries where patients were treated and later released from either an emergency room doctor or a hospital. Moreover, the economic costs include expenses associated with medical costs such as treatment and rehabilitation. They also include work loss costs such as loss of wages, benefits, and self-reported household services, and combined costs of medical and work loss. WISQARS data can be used to inform public health experts, researchers, and policymakers when efforts are needed to know the nature and extent of fatal and nonfatal injuries as well as identify risk factors that are associated with personal injuries. These data can also help to describe and compare trends associated with unintentional and violence-related injuries. This could invariably indicate newly emerging injury problems. In the end, policymakers can use these data to create reliable surveillance data for program and policy decisions.

Self-Reports of Attitudes, Beliefs, and Exposure to Violence

Health researchers and experts argue that attitudes toward violence are very important and have significant future implications. In studies that examined preschool children's attitudes and beliefs about intimate partner violence, Howell et al. (2012) reported that early exposure to domestic violence can impact children's acceptability toward violence. More specifically, in their research that used a sample of 92 preschool children, the study revealed that most developed at least one maladaptive attitude or belief about violence owing to their learned aggressiveness from maternal post-traumatic avoidance. This finding is consistent with what other research has found on childhood exposure to IPV and chronic impairment in children, especially among preschool children who appear to suffer the greatest harm from witnessing violent and aggressive behavior in the context of the home (Sternberg et al., 2006; Bevan & Higgins, 2002). Some other studies even suggest that when children are in the home when IPV occurs, they are exposed to it 95% of the time (see Fusco

& Fantuzzo, 2009). Behaviorists argue that when parents engage in violence, children may vicariously learn to contextualize and accept violence as a normal dispute resolution to address problems and disagreements. In fact, research conducted by Fosco and colleagues (2007) finds repeat exposure to family aggression often facilitates the development of internal beliefs and expectations about relationships that could increase the likelihood of aggression being accepted as normative behavior. Subsequently, research finds that violence and aggression learned at home may be revealed in behaviors with peers since children often imitate the violence witnessed at home (Guerra et al., 2003).

In a recent study, Copp and colleagues (2017) reported that social learning is a leading explanation of IPV. More specifically, in their study that examined the role of family violence and how it impacts the attitude of accepting IPV in a sample of 928 young men and women adults, the research concluded that the causal link between attitudes about violence is shaped by early exposure to family violence. This suggests that those exposed to violence while young will exhibit the behavior as adults since individuals often internalize cognitive scripts for violence and accept favorable attitudes toward IPV as they get older. However, the attitudes of violence are also influenced by other factors such as one's structural position which informs an attitudinal and cultural acceptance of violence that may be acquired not only from the family, but other institutions as well including one's school and neighborhood where one interacts with others who may also influence behavior. Moreover, the study revealed that females especially were more likely to exhibit an acceptance of the use of violence toward an intimate other. Another finding that their investigation revealed is that attitudes toward IPV are shaped by prior relationship experiences. In fact, some intimate violence experts find that former romantic relationships can serve as a reference of experiences that may structure future life courses trajectories for people, and it is through past violent relationships where some people learn an acceptance of IPV (Mannning et al., 2014; Raley et al., 2007).

Working from the view that exposure to aggressive behavior influences aggression in children, Spaccarelli and colleagues (1995) conducted research using a sample of 213 delinquent male adolescents (with a mean age of 16) to measure the effects of exposure to inter-adult family violence and physical abuse, attitudes toward aggression, self-reported competence, and coping strategies. In the investigation, the researchers relied on official juvenile arrest data (taken from the *Arizona Department of Youth Treatment and Rehabilitation*) and self-reports of violent behavior. The arrest data included demographical information such as ethnicity, date of birth, and age of first offense. The combined use of official and self-reported data enabled researchers to classify the subjects as either positive or negative for having a history of committing serious violent acts. Afterward, they categorized and divided the sample into four groups that included violent offenders (n=80), undetected violent offenders (n=56), violent deniers (n=23), and controls (n=54). The researchers relied on the *Conflict Tactics Scale* to measure the adolescent's exposure to violence, but it was modified, and two scales were created: one assessed inter-adult violence and the other assessed physical abuse. The adolescents' attitude toward aggression was also measured by an 18-item scale that asked questions about beliefs that supported aggression. The research established that the adolescents grouped as violent offenders and undetected violent offenders had higher rates of exposure to serious physical abuse involving weapons used by adults compared to those grouped as violent deniers and controls (Spaccarelli et al.,

1995). Interestingly, the study found that delinquent adolescents who were exposed to serious family violence were not as competent as those who were not exposed. They lacked self-esteem, self-control, autonomy, and dealt with stress by seeking to control others. In the end, the study concluded that exposure to family violence is a major risk factor for children later engaging in serious acts of interpersonal violence (Spaccarelli et al., 1995).

Costs of Treatment and Social Services

In 2021, health experts estimated that the U.S. spent more than $4.3 trillion (or an average of nearly $12,900 on each person) for health care. Researchers are quick to point out that the health of the nation comes at an expensive cost since studies reveal that 90% of the nation's healthcare expenditures are used to defray the cost for people suffering from chronic and mental health conditions. These and other diseases take a major economic toll on the system. Some studies show that strokes and heart diseases claim the lives of an estimated 877,500 Americans yearly. Some suggest that they cost the healthcare system an estimated $216 billion annually and attributed to $147 billion in loss of productivity (Benjamin et al., 2018). Another report found that each year in the U.S., an estimated 1.7 million people are diagnosed with cancer and 600,000 die from it. Health experts argue that the cost of treating patients with cancer is likely to continue to rise and by 2020, it is likely to reach $240 billion annually (Mariotto et al., 2020). Furthermore, the American Diabetes Association (2018) reports that more than 37 million Americans are diabetics and another 96 million are prediabetics. In 2017, the healthcare system paid an estimated $327 billion in medical costs and loss of productivity. Research also reveals that 20% of all children and 40% of adults in America suffer from obesity which costs the healthcare system nearly $173 billion each year (Ward et al., 2021). Moreover, arthritis affects an estimated 58.5 million adults in the U.S. In 2013, an estimated $303.5 billion was spent on medical expenses and indirect costs associated with lost earnings (Murphy et al., 2018).

Another disease that is becoming familiar to many Americans is Alzheimer. Medical experts report that it affects 5.7 million people, especially elderly Americans between the ages of 65 and older. As the population continues to gray, experts are concerned that this disease is likely to increase. In 2020, an estimated $305 billion was paid for healthcare treatment. Mental health experts project that by 2050, it will cost the system an estimated $1.1 trillion to provide for those with the disease (Alzheimer's Impact Movement and Alzheimer's Association, 2020). Research also finds that nearly 3 million adults and an estimated 470,000 children and teenagers suffer from epilepsy. In 2016, the healthcare system spent 8.6 billion in direct costs associated with treatment (Dieleman et al., 2020). Other health concerns that have been very expensive to the healthcare system include treating people affected by cigarette smoking and excessive alcohol use. For example, medical reports reveal that over 16 million Americans suffer from at least one disease caused by smoking. Consequently, the healthcare system spends an estimated $240 billion on treatment. Equally disturbing is that excessive alcohol use accounts for 140,000 deaths each year in the U.S. In 2010, it cost the economy $249 billion. These alarming statistics and their corresponding costs to the healthcare system far exceed that of other advanced nations. Health experts even report that despite the country's best efforts to treat and provide services, there is no evidence suggesting that the U.S. has received better healthcare outcomes. In fact, some reports find that the average cost of health care in many wealthy countries is about half as much spent in the U.S. with better results (Tikkanen & Abrams, 2020).

The cost of health care in the U.S. had been increasing long before the advent of COVID-19 struck. It only exacerbated what was already a rising U.S. expense. Moreover, economists report that healthcare costs have been on the rise since 1960. They contend that during that period, 5% of the gross national product (GNP) was spent on health care. However, as of 2021, 18% of the GNP is spent on health care. Healthcare experts attribute the increase in spending to two primary factors: an aging U.S. population and increasing costs of healthcare services. First, older Americans spend more on health care compared with any other demographic. More specifically, the number of people ages 65 and older has significantly increased over the years. This group increased from 13% in 2010 to 16% in 2021. Demographers estimate that their numbers are likely to increase to 20% by 2030. Furthermore, experts report that Americans who are 65 are eligible for Medicare. Currently, there are over 65 million and this number is growing substantially which will continue to increase the cost of Medicare over time. Second, health experts report the cost of healthcare services have increased faster than the cost for other goods and services. They argue that in the past 20 years, the *Consumer Price Index* (CPI) has increased at an average of 2.5%, while the CPI for medical care has grown to an average of 3.2 each year. This notwithstanding some attribute alarming healthcare costs to newly emerging healthcare technology, expensive procedures and products, and administrative waste in the insurance and provider systems.

Costs to the Healthcare System

Research shows that many Americans view the price of health care as a major concern since demographers report that the country is graying, and the cost of health care is beyond what most people can afford. Regardless of age, many Americans report that defraying the cost of health care is a burden and depending on the health care need, it can become a drain on their financial resources and life savings, especially medical care since it is arguably the biggest factor behind healthcare cost and accounts for 90% of all spending. This and the price of prescription drugs (experts estimate) will have increased by 136% from 2015 to 2025. More specifically, research studies reveal that half of U.S. adults report they have difficulties paying for healthcare costs. As such, they often delay or decide not to have a procedure done given the high cost of medical care (Montero et al., 2022). Chief among items that many Americans have delayed having done is dental work. Further, adults ages 65 and older indicated that they have put off getting hearing services, dental work, and having prescriptions filled when they are not covered by Medicare. Beyond the aged, other family members report that the cost of filling prescriptions has been so expensive that they have either not filled them, cut pills in half, or take dosages sporadically, especially minorities (e.g., Black, Latinx, and women) living in lower-income households (Montero et al., 2022). Moreover, research highlights that even among uninsured adults under 65, 85% report that they find the cost of health care difficult to afford. This is especially acute among those who are disproportionately impacted by the costs of health care such as uninsured Black and Hispanic adults and others living in poverty. Even Americans with health insurance and higher incomes face the burden of expensive health costs. In fact, nearly a third of insured adults report being worried about the affordability of monthly payments for insurance premiums and slightly under half expressed concerns about being able to afford their deductible before insurance pays. More alarming is the fact that 40% of Americans report being in debt owing to expenses attached to medical and dental services received along with money owed to credit cards, collection agencies, family members, and others for monies borrowed for health-related expenses, especially among the poor and uninsured. The situation is dire because prescription drugs play a major role in helping to prevent, manage, and cure many diseases and other health conditions (Montero et al., 2022).

Economists and public health experts report that health spending in the U.S. cost an estimated $4.3 trillion in 2021 or $12,914 per capita While this number seems astronomical, it is less than what was spent during the early *COVID-19* pandemic years because of the decline in pandemic government expenditures offsetting increased medical services that were not received by thousands of people in 2020. Nevertheless, healthcare costs are very expensive to the U.S. economy, especially when monies are allocated to pay for chronic or long-term medical conditions (e.g., cancer, obesity, heart disease, arthritis, and other often preventable health problems), the increase costs of new medicine, procedures, and technologies. It can be divided into separate categories such as hospital care (31.1%), physician services (14.9%), clinical services (5.4%), prescription drugs (8.9%), nursing care facilities (4.3%), home health care (2.9%), other personal healthcare costs (16.0%), government administration (1.2%), net cost of health insurance (6.0%), and government public health activities (4.4%). While many people in the U.S. are without insurance, experts have examined who pays the cost for health services in America. Data from 2021 revealed that the funding sources for care were composed of the following: private health insurance (28.5%), out of pocket (10.2%), Medicare (21.2%), Medicaid (17.2%), other health insurance programs (4.0%), government public health activities (4.4%), other federal programs (1.7%), other third-party players and programs (7.9%), and investment spending (4.9%) (U.S. Centers for Medical & Medicaid Services, 2022). Health experts posit that during COVID-19, the government invested large sums of resources to manage the pandemic. Its goals were to prevent and control public health concerns as well as provide and deliver health services.

Access to Health Care for Treatment and Social Services by Race and Income

Critics of the American health system have long argued that it is plagued with historical as well as structural racisms that account for disparities since some groups are not provided the same access to receive quality health services and treatments extended to others. The same critics examining race, income, and disparities in access to health insurance have called the matter concerning since *socioeconomic status* (SES) is a determinant that decides who gets access to health care in the U.S. (Becker & Newsom, 2003). As such, the poor and others with low incomes are likely to receive *Medicaid* or go without insurance. They are also likely to have poor quality health and seek health care only in emergencies (Swartz, 1994). Research shows that poor minorities report experiencing stress and anxiety from having to pay for doctors, hospital visits, and prescription drugs. Therefore, they often go without medical services and treatments (Becker & Newsom, 2003). Notwithstanding, some researchers report that physicians have a negative perception of Blacks and other minorities from low and middle SES compared with their White patients from upper SES when it comes to care and service delivery (van Ryan & Burke, 2000). Furthermore, some national opinion surveys reveal that Blacks and other minorities are more likely to rate the quality of the health services they receive as poor, or fair compared with their White counterparts. Scholars find that minority members' negative attitudes toward health and social institutions are based on their personal experiences with historical racial disparities in health care and other social institutions (Blendon et al., 1995). However, Ginzberg (1994) contends that these negative sentiments are also predicated on the fact that healthcare facilities in many minority communities, (especially inner-city areas) can be characterized as inferior or decreasing services, along with dwindling healthcare resources for low-income people.

Similarly, research conducted by Yearby et al. (2022) finds that racial and ethnic minorities in the U.S. have always suffered from health inequalities that may have been amplified by *COVID-19*. They report that these inequalities persist because of structural racism in healthcare policy which has created a two-tier system that is racially segregated or a healthcare system that provides access to high-quality care for Whites while denying racial and ethnic minority populations the same social services. In a report from the *Institute of Medicine*, several studies were presented that documented widespread racism in health care in the U.S. The studies reported that Whites are more likely than Blacks to receive a broader range of medical procedures, while Blacks are more likely to experience challenges with accessing the system and what to do when emergencies occur. They are also likely to receive undesirable interventions such as amputations (Becker & Newsom, 2003). Recently, there have been several studies devoted to addressing healthcare disparities in the U.S., namely the work of Lee et al. (2021) that revealed that income, race, and self-perceived health status finds racial identity is independently associated with a lack of health insurance and low income (minorities) with poor health had 68% less chances of having insurance compared with high income (Whites) with good health. Lee and colleagues (2021) conclude their findings could benefit health policymakers to direct and allocate their limited resources to the most vulnerable populations that need insurance coverage the most (e.g., those racial and ethnic minorities with low income and poor health).

Significant Limitations on Available Data

Currently, an abundance of data exists on violence and victimizations as well as healthcare matters. These data are gathered by surveillance systems in criminal justice and public health organizations. Some experts feel that these data can be problematic because they are collected by agencies, for agency purposes with definitions and meanings that may not be clear to many consumers of these data. Therefore, it bears mentioning that critics caution that these data are not perfect since they have historically been problematic owing to who is collecting these data and how they are collected. Some long-standing criticisms of the FBI's UCR data are that they are solely reported incidents of crime and not the total amount of crime that occurs annually since they are based on citizens reporting practices, law enforcement practices, and methodological techniques used by an estimated 19,000 police departments that participate in this data compilation. Consequently, this indicator of crime and violence is incomplete and leaves behind the issue of the "dark figures" of crime or what is referred to as the unknown cases of crime. Criminal justice historians argue that it was for this reason that NIBRS emerged because it addressed many of the shortcomings that were in the UCR. Another victimization surveillance system that is widely used but also has questionable validity about victimization is the NCVS. This data compilation is a panel study that uses a longitudinal design of three years. However, at every six-month interval, participants (e.g., *a national representative sample*) are surveyed to determine if they have experienced more victimization. Research experts have long discussed the problems associated with the use of surveys to collect data. Chief among them is that these data are only as good as the honesty of the respondents. Other concerns about survey data, especially the NCVS, is the timeframe used in the intervals of data collection since it could contribute to memory loss and *telescoping* since many people often fail to properly recall past events which confound data results. Health researchers reveal that medical records often lack the circumstances surrounding injuries. Furthermore, confidentiality typically prevents researchers from accessing medical records. Yet, some doctors report that surveys can provide more information regarding personal background and whether the patients were involved in crime and violence. However, they report that these data tend to be saturated with information suggesting the optimal treatment be given to patients. Another problem with surveys is that they can be contaminated with socially desirability responses. As such, researchers argue that the consumers of agency data (e.g., *both official and survey*) must be certain that they are valid and reliable measures of violence, victimizations, and matters of public health.

The Inevitability of "Big Data"

Because health data are generated and collected by many sources including individuals, researchers, and agencies, health records continue to grow and become part of *electronic health record systems*, *personal health records*, and *data created by digital health tools* (Dolley, 2018). Some health experts contend that the technology has morphed to the extent that healthcare data can be accessed via wearable medical devices and mobile health apps such as smart watches (*a digital health tool*) that can detect heart rates and abnormal breathing. Researchers have coined the phrase "big data" to express the emergence of massive amounts of complex health data stored in an extensive group of datasets that can be characterized as volumes, variety, or variability. These data are structured and unstructured. They are used to analyse health information that provides insight, trends, and patterns about the health status of Americans. Health experts posit that big data need a scalable architecture for storage, manipulation, and analysis (National Institute of Standards and Technology, 2015). They also argue that big data facilitate precision public health which allows easy prediction and understanding of public health risks that generates treatments for specific subpopulations since these data can help identify potential health problems before they occur. Health experts use this information to guide their decision-making when it comes to improving health outcomes, decrease health costs, and other salient matters. Big data relies on new data, technologies, and methods. According to Dolley (2018), big data can assist public health practitioners by offering volumes of data (e.g., structured and unstructured) that did not exist in previous years primarily because it is the culmination of data. Some experts argue that it is currently being used to widely disseminate research and trials on specific populations of at-risk segments with different health problems. Similarly, Lohr (2012) reports that big data is a new approach that has created innovation and new interventions in health care that goes beyond economic barriers. It is important to point out that big data give researchers access to very large amounts of data and methodologies used to collect data that can help improve the quality of life for Americans.

Do We Really Need an Abundance of Health Data?

Health researchers and policy experts report that data are the most important resources in health care since it could invariably lead to improved health outcomes (Zaldivar, 2023). To adequately make up a surveillance system that informs and guides health policy, accurate data are essential since they are required to assist health officials in assessing the level and magnitude of potential health threats that are either in the form of violence or disease. Data allow researchers to monitor or track public health for extended periods of time and provide a full picture of the health of the nation. Through health data, experts can properly assess and accurately diagnose emerging issues related to health. As such, statistics must continue to be collected by local, state, and federal agencies that monitor the public health since they provide data that indicate potential concerns and can be used to protect the public's health. Researchers indicate that data can identify trends in violence and disease across populations that point to specific indicators such as age, behavior, region of the country, and other salient factors. These could lead to prevention measures (Zaldivar, 2023). Health experts contend that it would be impossible to intervene in the absence of an analysis of existing data since problems are typically defined by surveillance data. The need of data to protect public health cannot be overstated because data and statistics identify problems that may require a public health response through intervention and evaluation to determine the effects of the intervention. Whether success is achieved will be reflected in statistics. Moreover, data and corresponding statistics provide invaluable insight into how the health system is performing nationally since it may reveal whether the public is at risk of experiencing another epidemic (Zaldivar, 2023).

Summary

Health experts and policymakers must rely on updated health surveillance data to measure the health of the nation. These data include a host of sources including vital statistics. U.S. census data are used to measure the nation's population as well as demographical characteristics with respect to SES. Other health data sources are used to measure indicators of lethal violence in communities throughout the nation. More specifically, the *National Intimate Partner and Sexual Violence Survey* is used to measure intimate personal victimizations on heterosexuals as well as the LGBTQI community. The NVDRS provides data on the method used in homicides, suicides, as well as accidental deaths. Health data allow researchers the ability to monitor changes that occur in fatal violence over time. Health experts, including epidemiologists, examine data to identify which groups and communities are at risk to violence and adverse health consequences. While health data are heavily used, criminal justice surveillance data are also used to measure the impact that violence has on the health of society. In fact, criminal justice sources such as the UCR, NIBRS, NCVS, and SRS measure the nature and extent of crime and victimization that occurs annually. These data sources have different units of analyses. For example, the UCR provides the number of reported crimes. The NIBRS was created to address shortcomings that are common to the UCR, and it includes more crime. The NCVS measures the amount and types of victimizations that occur in the U.S. It reveals whether there are increases in the amount of crime and victimization. SRS are self-reported accounts of crime as told by criminal offenders (where there is no official record). The UCR, NIBRS, NCVS, and SRS also provide the demographical and geographical features of crime, arrestees, offenders, and victims. These data can also be used to isolate those regions and cities that experience the most crime and victimization. They paint a picture of who is more at risk of this public health problem. Health researchers also investigate health data on injuries. In doing so, they typically rely on the CDC's WISQARS. These data provide fatal and nonfatal injuries, violent deaths, and cost of injuries from a variety of sources. Another data source on victimization includes self-reported attitude, beliefs, and behavior from those who were exposed to violence. They reveal the trajectories their lives have taken. Victimization data also reveals the costs of treatment and social services and what adverse health costs the healthcare system. Some health experts contend that there are healthcare disparities in access to treatment and social services based on race and SES that stems from historical and structural racism. Despite the availability of health and violence data, critics argue that there are concerns with these data that must not be ignored. Because of the many surveillance agencies collecting health data, it has led to the inevitability of "big data" that are needed to monitor the health of the nation.

Discussion Questions

1. What role does vital statistics play in health research?
2. How can official crime statistics be used to reveal the health of a nation?
3. What can survey data tell us about the health of a nation?
4. Why does it take public health and criminal justice data to measure the health of a nation?
5. What are some significant limitations on available data?
6. Define the evitability of big data.

References

Adler, F., Mueller, G.O., & Laufer, W.S. (1996). *Criminal justice: The core*. The McGraw-Hill Companies.

Alzheimer's Impact Movement and Alzheimer's Association. (2020). Alzheimer's disease facts and figures. Factsheet. https://aaic.alz.org/downloads2020/2020_Facts_and_Figure_Fact_Sheet.pdf

American Diabetes Association. (2018). Economic costs of diabetes in the U.S. in 2017. *Diabetes Care*, 41(5), 917–928.

Aufrichtig, A., Beckett, L., Diehm, J., & Lartey, J. (2017, January 9). Want to fix gun violence in America, Go Local. *The Guardian*. https://bit.ly/2i6kaKw

Becker, G., & Newsom, E. (2003). Socioeconomic status and dissatisfaction with health care among chronically ill African Americans. *American Journal of Public Health*, 93(5), 742–748.

Benjamin, E.J., Virani, S.S., Callaway, C.W., et al. (2018). Heart disease and stroke statistics-2018 update: A report from the American Heart Association. *Circulation*, 137, e67–e492.

Bevan, E., & Higgins, D.L. (2002). Is domestic violence learned?: The contribution of five forms of child maltreatment to men's violence and adjustment. *Journal of Family Violence*, 17(3), 223–245.

Blendon, R.J., Scheck, A.C., Donelan, K., et al., (1995). How white and African Americans view their health and social problems: Different experiences, different expectations. *JAMA*, 273, 341–346.

Blumenthal, D., & Lurie, N. (2023). A critical opportunity to improve public health data. *The New England Journal of Medicine*, 389(4), 289–291.

Blumstein, A., Cohen, J., & Rosenfeld, R. (1991). Trends and deviations in crime rates: A comparison of UCR and NCS data for burglary and robbery. *Criminology*, 29, 237–263.

Centers for Disease Control and Prevention (CDC). (n.d.). National Violent Death Reporting System (NVDRS). www.cdc.gov/nvdrs/about/index.html

Centers for Disease Control and Prevention (CDC). (2010). Youth risk behavior surveillance-U.S. 2009. *Mobility and Mortality Weekly Report*, 59(SS-5), 1–142.

Centers for Disease Control and Prevention (CDC). (2012). National center for injury prevention and control. Years of potential life lost from unintentional injuries among persons ages 0–19 years- United States, 2000–2009. www.cdc.gov/mmwr/preview/mmwrhtml/mm6141a2.htm

Centers for Disease Control and Prevention (CDC). (2014). National center for injury prevention and control. www.cdc.gov/injury-violence-prevention/index.html

Centers for Disease Control and Prevention (CDC). (2016). Youth violence: Facts at a glance. National Center of Injury Prevention and Control (U.S.). www.cdc.gov/violenceprevention

Center for Nonviolence and Social Justice. (2019). Healing hurt people. Available at: www.drexel.edu/cnsj/healing-hurt-people/overview/

Centers for Disease Control and Prevention (CDC). (2024). National Violent Death Reporting System (NVDRS). www.cdc.gov/nvdrs/about/index.html

Cohen, G.H., Ross, C.S., Cozier, Y.C., & Galea, S. (2019). Census 2020-A preventable public health catastrophe. *Promoting Public Health Research, Policy, Practice and Education*, 109(8), 1077–1078.

Copp, J.E., Giordano, P.C., Longmore, M.A., & Manning, W.D. (2017). The development of attitudes toward intimate partner violence: An examination of key correlates among a sample of young adults. *Journal of Interpersonal Violence*, 34(7), 1357–1387.

Craig, P., Di Ruggiero, E., Frohlich, K.L., Mykhalovskiy, E., & White M., on behalf of the Canadian Institutes of Health Research (CIHR)–National Institute for Health Research (NIHR) Context Guidance Authors Group. (2018). Taking account of context in population health intervention research: guidance for producers, users and funders of research. Southampton: NIHR Evaluation, Trials, and Studies Coordinating Centre.

Crosby, A.E., Mercy, J.A., & Houry, D. (2016). The National Violent Death Reporting System: Past, present, and future. *American Journal of Preventive Medicine*, 51(5S3), S169–S172.

Dieleman, J.L., Cao, J., & Chapin, A. (2020). U.S. Health care spending by payer and health condition, 1996-2016. *JAMA*, 323(9), 863–884.

Dolley, S. (2018). Big data's role in precision public health. *Frontiers in Public Health*, 6(68), 1–12.

Edmund, M. (2022). Gun violence disproportionately and overwhelmingly hurts communities of color: Fact Sheet. www.americaprogress.org/article/gun-violence-disproportionately-and-overwhelmingly-hurts-communities-of color/

Federal Bureau of Investigation (FBI). (1998). *Crime in the United States*. Government Printing Office.

Fosco, G.M., DeBoard, R.L., & Grych, J.H. (2007). Making sense of family violence: Implications of children's appraisals of interparental aggression for their short-and -long term functioning. *European Psychologist*, 12(1), 6–16.

Fusco, R.A., & Fntuzzo, J.W. (2009). Domestic violence crimes and children: A population-based investigation of direct sensory exposure and the nature of involvement. *Children and Youth Services Review*, 31(2), 249–256.

Gaines, L.K., & Miller, R.L. (2009). *Criminal justice in action: The core* (4th ed.). Thomson/Wadsworth.

Ginzberg, E. (1994). Improving health care for the poor: Lessons from the 1980s. *JAMA*, 271, 464–468.

Guerra, N., Huesmann, L.R., & Spindler, A. (2003). Community violence exposure, social cognition, and aggression among urban elementary-school children. *Child Development*, 74(5), 1561–1576.

Guttmacher Institute (2008, January). Facts on induced abortion in the United States. www.guttmac her.org/pubs/fb_induced_abortion.html

Health Information Management Systems Society. (2022). Public health information and technology infrastructure modernizing funding report: Core investments strategies to modernize and interoperate federal, state, and local, tribal pubic health systems. www.himss.org/sites/hde/files/media/file/2022/04/29/pubpolicydatamodernization_final.pdf

Hindelang, M. (1973). Causes of delinquency: A partial replication and extension. *Social Problems*, 20, 471–87.

Howell, K.H., Miller, L.E., & Graham-Bermann, S.A. (2012). Evaluating preschool children's attitudes and beliefs about intimate partner violence. *Violence and Victims*, 27(6), 941–956.

Kung, H.C., Hoyert, D.L., Xu, J., & Murphy, S.L. (2008). Deaths: Final data for 2005. In *National vital statistics reports* (Vol. 56). National Center for Health Statistics.

Lead, A. (2018). Violence is a public health issue: Public health is essential to understanding and treating violence in the U.S. American Public Health Association. www.apha.org/policy-and-advocacy/public-health-policy-briefs/policy-database/2019/01/28/violence-is-a-public-health-issue

Lee, D.C., Liang, H., & Shi, L. (2021). The convergence of racial and income disparities in health insurance coverage in the United States. *International Journal for Equity in Health*, 20(96). https://equityhealthj.biomedcentral.com/articles/10.1186/s12939-021-01436-z

Li, W., & Ricard, J. (2023). 4 reasons we should worry about missing crime data. The Marshall Project: Nonprofit journalism for criminal justice. www.themarshallproject.org/2023/07/13/fbi-crime-rates-data-gap-nibrs

Lohr, S. (2012). The age of big data. *NY Times*, 11:SR1. Available from: www.nytimes.com/2012/02/12/sunday-review/big-datas-impact-in-the-world.html

MacDorman, M.F., Munson, M.L., & Kirmeyer, S. (2007). Fetal and perinatal mortality, United States, 2004. National Vital Statistics Reports, 56(3). www.cdc.gov/nchs/data/nvsr56/nvsr56_03.pdf

Manning, W.D., Longmore, M.A., Copp, J.E., & Giordano, P.C. (2014). The complexities of adolescent dating and sexual relationship: Fluidity, meaning(s), and implications for young adults' well-being. In E.S. Lefkowitz & S.A. Vasulenko (Eds.), *New directions for child and adolescent development: Positive and negative outcomes of sexual behavior* (pp. 53–69). Jossey-Bass.

Mariotto, A.B., Enewold, L., Zhao, J., Zeruto, C.A., & Yabroff, K.R. (2020). Medical care costs associated with cancer survivorship in the United States. *Cancer Epidemiology, Biomarkers & Prevention*, 29, 1304–1312.

Mascho, S.W., Schoeny, M.E., Webster, D., & Sigel, E. (2016). Outcomes, data, and indicators of violence at the community level. *The Journal of Primary Prevention*, 37, 121–139.

Masho, S.W., Schoeny, M.E., Webster, D., & Sigel, E. (2016). Outcomes, data, and indicators of violence at the community level. *The Journal of Primary Prevention*, 37, 121–139.

Mercy, J., Butchart, A., Farrington, D., & Cerda´, M. (2002). Youth violence. In E.G. Krug, L.L. Dahlberg, J.A. Mercy, A.B. Zwi, & R. Lozano (Eds.), *The world report on violence and health* (pp. 25–56). World Health Organization.

Montero, A., Kearney, A., Hamel, L., & Brodie, M. (2022). Data note: America's challenges with health care costs. Washington, D.C. www.kff.org/health-costs/issue-brief/data-note-americans-challenges-health-care-costs/

Murphy, L.B., Cisternas, M.G., Pasta, D.J., Helmick, C.G., & Yelin, E.H. (2018). Medical expenditures and earning losses among U.S. adults with arthritis in 2013. *Arthritis Care Res (Hoboken)*, 70(6), 869–876.

National Center for Health Statistics (NCHS). (1999). National Health Interview Survey. Centers for Disease Control and Preventions. www.cdc.gov/nchs/nhis/index.html

National Institute of Standards and Technology. (2015). NIST Big Data Interoperability Framework: Volume 1, Definitions. U.S. Department of Commerce. http://dx.doi.org/10.6028/NIST.SP.1500-1

Nguyen, A., & Drane, K. (2023). *Gun violence in black communities*. To Prevent Gun Violence. www./giffords.org

Osterman, M.J., Hamilton, B.E., Martin, J.A., Driscoll, A.K., & Valenzuela, C.P. (2023). Births: Final Data for 2021. *National Vital Statistics Report*, 72(1), 1–10.

Pickett, G., & Hanlon, J.J. (1990). *Public health: Administration and practice*. Times Mirror/Mosby College Publishing.

Raley, K., Crissey, S., & Muller, C. (2007). Of sex and romance: Adolescent relationships in transition to adulthood. *Journal of Marriage and Family*, 69, 1210–1226.

Rennison, C.M. (1998). *Criminal victimization 1998 Changes 1997-1998 with trends 1993–98.* Bureau of Justice Statistics.

Rosenberg, M.L., & Fenley, M.A. (1991). *Violence in America: A public health approach.* Oxford University Press.

Santaularia, J., Johnson, M., Hart, L., Haskett, L., Welsh, E., & Faseru, B. (2014). Relationships between sexual violence and chronic disease: A cross-sectional study. *BMC Public Health*, 14(1286). www.biomedcentral.com/1471-2458/14/1286

Schneider, M.J. (2021). *Introduction to public health* (6th ed.). Jones and Bartlett Learning.

Schwalbe, N., Wahl, B., Song, J., & Lehtinaki, S. (2020). Data sharing and global public health: Defining what we mean by data. *Frontiers in Digital Health*, 2(61), 1–6.

Schwartz, S. (2009). The US Vital Statistics System: The role of state and local health departments. National Research Council (US) Committee on National Statistics. Washington, DC: National Academies Press./ www.ncbi.nlm.nih.gov/books/NBK219870

Senna, J.J., & Siegel, L.J. (2000). *Essentials of criminal justice* (3rd ed.). Belmont, CA: Wadsworth/ Thomson Learning.

Siegel, L.J. (2011). *Essentials of criminal justice* (7th ed.). Wadsworth Cengage Learning.

Soucie, J.M. (2015). Public health surveillance and data collection. General principles and impact on hemophilia Care. *Hematology*, 17(01), S144–S146.

Soucie, J.M., McAlister, S., McClellan, A., Oakley, M., & Su, T. (2010). The universal data collection surveillance system for rare bleeding disorders. *American Journal of Preventive Medicine*, 38(4), S475–S481.

Spaccarelli, S., Coatsworth, J.D., & Bowden, B.S. (1995). Exposure to serious family violence among incarcerated boys: Its association with violent offending and potential mediating variables. *Violence and Victims*, 10(3), 163–182.

Steinweg, A. (2023). Non-Hispanic blacks have higher rates of disability due to arthritis, diabetes, hypertension than non-Hispanic white adults. Racial/Ethnic Disparities in Disability by Health Condition. United States Department of Census Bureau. www.census.gov/library/stories/2023/07/disparities-in-disabilities.html

Sternberg, K.J., Baradaran, L.P., Abbott, C.B., Lamb, M.E., & Guterman, E. (2006). Type of violence, age, and gender differences in effects of family violence on children's behavior problems: A mega-analysis. *Developmental Review*, 26, 89–112.

Sutton, P.D. (2008). Births, marriages, divorces, and deaths: Provisional data for September 2007. National Vital Statistics Reports, 56(18). www.cdc.gov/pcd/issues/2004/oct/pdf/04_0074.pdf.

Swartz, K. (1994). Dynamics of people without health insurance: Don't let the numbers fool you. *JAMA*, 271, 64–67.

Thacker, S.B., & Wetterhall, S.F. (1998). *Data sources for public health in statistics in public health. Qualitative approaches to public health problems*, eds. D.F. Stroups and S.M. Teusch. New York: Oxford University Press, 39–57.

Tikkanen, R., & Abrams, M.K. (2020). US Healthcare from a global Perspective, 2019: Higher spending, worse outcome? (Commonwealth Fund, Jan).

U.S. Department of Health and Human Services. (2013). Announcement of solicitation of written comments on modifications of healthy people in 2020 objectives. Federal Register: The Daily journal of the United States Government. www.federalregister.gov/documents/2013/11/13/2013-27126/announcement-of-solicitation-of-written-comment-on-modifications-of-healthy-people-2020-objectives

U.S. Centers for Medical & Medicaid Services. (2022). National health spending grew slightly in 2021. https://www.cms.gov/newsroom/press-releases/national-health-spending-grew-slightly-2021#:~:text=The%202021%20National%20Health%20Expenditures,increase%20of%2010.3%25%20in%202020

U.S. Department of Health and Human Services. (2014). Child maltreatment 2014. Administration of Children, Youth and Families, Children's Bureau. Washington, DC. www.acf.hhs.gov/programs/cb/research-data-technology/statistics-research/child-maltreatment van Ryn, M. & Burke, J. (2000). The effect of patient race and socio-economic status on physicians' perceptions of patients. *Social Science & Medicine*, 50, 813–828.

Vivolo, A., Matjasko, J., & Massetti, G. (2011). Mobilizing communities and building capacity for youth violence prevention: The national academic centers of excellence for youth violence prevention. *American Journal of Community Psychology*, 48(1–2), 141–145. https://doi.org/10.1007/s10465-010-9419-5

Walker, S. (1998). *Sense and nonsense about crime and drugs: A policy guide* (4th ed.). West/Wadsworth.

Wallace, H. (1998). *Victimology: Legal, psychological, and social perspective*. Allyn & Bacon.

Ward, Z.J., Bleich, S.N., Long, M.W., & Gortmaker, S.L. (2021). Association of body mass index with heath care expenditures in the United States by age and sex. *PLoS One*, 16(3). https://doi.org/10.1371/journal.pone.0247307

Wilson, D.K., Kliewer, W., &Sica, D.A. (2004). The relationship between exposure to violence and blood pressure mechanisms. *Current Hypertension Reports*, 6, 321–326.

World Health Organization. (2014). Global status report on violence prevention. United Nations Office on Drugs and Crime. United Nations Development Programme. www.who.int/publications/i/item/978921564793

Yearby, R., Clark, B., & Figueroa, J.F. (2022). Structural racism in historical and modern US health care policy. *Health Affairs*, 41(2), 187–194.

Zaldivar, R. (2023). The benefits of using data in healthcare. Roger Zaldivar's Post. www.linkedin.com/pluse/benefits-using-data-healthcare-roger-zaldivar

4

ASSAULTIVE VIOLENCE AND PUBLIC HEALTH

Introduction

After the big rival game was played between two local high school football powerhouses, many fans left the stadium disappointed by the lack luster performance of their alma mater. Some were shocked and dejected by the lopsided score given the momentum that had been building all season between the two crosstown rivals. It was a classic story of the rich and poor given the geography of the teams: one from an affluent area and the other, in an impoverish area. However, the amount of talent on each team was the great equalizer this time since both teams were undefeated and the winner would go on to compete for the state championship title. The players, coaches, parents, and fanbase anticipated that many players on the winning team would be highly recruited by division 1 college football programs that would afford their children an opportunity to receive a first-rate education and possibly be drafted into the National Football League (NFL). Unfortunately, one father of a starting defensive player (on the losing team), whose son had earned All-American honors, did not respond well to the defeat since he believed it would jeopardize his son's chances of being recruited by a competitive football program since his performance in the game left many spectators wondering if he was the same player they had watched and cheered all season. Nevertheless, the players' father was inconsolable as he exited the parking lot of the rivalry game. As he drove away, he was overcome with anger and stress. He simply could not accept losing the game in such a horrific fashion and he knew that without a scholarship, he could not afford to send his son to any college. Consequently, to vent his anger, rage, and displeasure in the moment, he went out to his vehicle and removed his AK-47 from the trunk of his car. He concealed the firearm and returned to the stadium and opened fire on the opposing fans. Subsequently, he gunned down and killed 15 victims (e.g., 3 men, 4 women, and 8 teenagers) before police eventually shot and killed him. When reporters arrived on the scene and asked police if they could explain what happened, an officer simply stated while 15 people were killed, another 20 victims were rushed to the local hospital to be treated for various forms of gunshot wounds. He also revealed that assaultive violence (AV) in the area was on the rise and increasing throughout the city and state. He went on

DOI: 10.4324/9781003373001-4

to say that this was one of three mass shootings that he and other police officers were called to respond to in four weeks.

Assaultive Violence (AV) Defined

In the U.S., AV is defined as any incident that involves the use of force or threat of force that results in either nonfatal or fatal violence since it is intended to cause harm, injury, or death to another (Rosenberg & Mercy, 1991). However, the *World Health Organization (WHO)* provides a global definition of violence as

> the intentional use of physical force or power, threatened or actual, against oneself, another person, or against a group or community, that either results in or has a high likelihood of resulting in injury, death, psychological harm or maldevelopment or deprivation.
>
> *(World Health Organization [WHO], 1996, p. 2)*

Its definition of violence includes a psychological component that is important to public health given the trauma that AV causes. Both definitions suggest the effects of AV often result in negative health consequences such as psychological and social dysfunction, injury, and death (Rosenberg & Mercy, 1991). An observation made by researchers is that many forms of violence committed against women, the elderly, and children often do not manifest in physical injuries or death, but rather, they lead to physical, psychological, and social problems that remain with victims for extended periods of time long after the initial abuse (Krug et al., 2002). Experts contend that several pathways culminate in AV that include arguments between strangers, and acquaintances, domestic violence between spouses, and even robberies committed between strangers. Some health experts contend that each pathway that leads to AV can be linked to causal and risk factors found in several sources including psychological, cultural, structural, and community determinants. While AV receives more attention today compared to the past, experts argue that historically violence has been linked to physical action which has neglected other forms of violence, namely the non-physical varieties such as psychological violence, verbal violence, stalking, sexual harassment, and others (Outlaw, 2009). Because violence is a complex issue, researchers must work to create definitions that are inclusive of other victimizations. However, the UCR and other forms of official crime statistics list two categories of crime: violent and property crime. This chapter addresses violent crime which includes murder and nonnegligent manslaughter, rape and sexual assault, robbery, and aggravated assaults. It is important to note that aggravated assaults account for an estimated two-thirds of all violent crimes.

Nature and Extent of AV

AV is a serious problem in the U.S. since it affects millions of people annually including their families, schools, and communities. Therefore, both criminal justice and public health experts report that no one in society is completely immune from being the victim of AV since research, as well as health statistics show that victims of AV often range in age groups from infants to the elderly. Consequently, because of the sheer numbers of people directly and indirectly impacted by violence, it is a public health issue that requires both criminal justice and public health responses. As early as 1979, the *Surgeon General* recognized and identified violent crime as a major public health priority. As a result, in 1980, the CDC started to study and monitor patterns of AV. By 1992, it established the *National Center for Injury Prevention and Control* as the lead federal organization for violence prevention. As a public health problem, violence causes physical injuries and mental health issues such as depression, anxiety, and post-traumatic stress disorder. Moreover, health experts report that people living in violent communities face a higher risk of developing chronic diseases since they reside in places that are saturated with poor health outcomes. While this statement is true, criminal justice and health experts argue that AV mostly proliferates in impoverished areas, namely communities inhabited by people of color such as *Blacks, Hispanics, American Indians, and Alaskan Natives* who experience higher rates of homicide compared with other racial and ethnic groups. The same experts also report that even when lower-class residents survive violent crimes such as homicides, some may sustain disabilities, and other injuries that cause physical pain and health suffering that serve to diminish their quality of life. Other negative health outcomes that are disproportionately experienced by low-income neighborhoods include asthma, hypertension, cancer, stroke, and mental disorders.

Another aspect of violent victimization is related to gender. Some statistics reveal that where violent crime occurs, there is a gender nexus. Official data as well as victimization surveys support the notion that men account for the majority of AV cases except sexual assaults and intimate partner violence. Moreover, when men are victimized, it typically occurs in a public place, while women overwhelmingly experience violent crimes such as domestic violence and sexual assaults which occur in the home. The latter is supported by statistics that indicate that each year, an estimated 12 million men and women are victims of intimate partner violence.

In 2019, violent crime dropped by 1.7%. It especially impacted murder and nonnegligent manslaughter, reducing it by 6.1%. During this time, the UCR reported that 19,100 people in the U.S. were the victims of homicide. Moreover, rape and aggravated assaults dropped by 5.4% and 1.1%, respectively. However, robbery increased by 1.3% (Salter, 2023). Despite this, the CDC reported that the number of homicides increased significantly in 2020 to nearly 25,000 victims. At the same time, more than 1.4 million victims were treated in emergency rooms for assault-related injuries. In 2021, reports indicated that violent crime decreased slightly. This was a notable change from reports in 2020 when the murder rate increased by 29% during the pandemic. Some experts argue that because of changes in the way official data were collected during the pandemic (i.e., some law enforcement agencies did not provide their crime data to the FBI for inclusion in the UCR), data on violent crimes such as homicide, rape, robbery, and aggravated assault among others must be accepted and interpreted with caution since the FBI reported that the data collected in 2022 represented 83.3% of reported agencies that covered an estimated 93.5% of the U.S. population (Salter, 2023). Today, official statistics on violent crime reveal that as of 2022, they have decreased, but remain above pre-pandemic levels. More specifically, in 2022, the FBI reported that there were 380.7 violent crimes per 100,000 people. This constituted a 0.1 decrease from 2019. However, in 2020, the crime rate grew as high as 398.5 per every 100,000. In 2021, the estimate decreased to 387.0 per 100,000. In 2020, the number of murders and aggravated assaults increased slightly (Buchholz, 2023).

Types of Assaultive Violence

Crimes against Blacks

While Blacks have historically (dating back to slavery) experienced more violence than other groups in America relative to their representation in the population, the matter is exacerbated by the fact that Blacks are overwhelmingly victimized by people who share similar physical and background characteristics and who are similarly situated. Regarding assault violence, data on homicide indicate that among the 19,196 people in the U.S. who were murdered in 2022, 10,470 were Black (e.g., non-Hispanic Black person), 7,704 identified as White (e.g., non-Hispanic White person), 568 were of another race (e.g., American Indian, or Alaska Native), and 454 were of an unknown race (FBI, 2023). This is concerning to many scholars such as criminal justice experts and criminologists since Whites account for 75.5% of the U.S. population, while Blacks only comprise 13%. This suggests that Blacks are disproportionately more likely to be killed compared to their counterparts who factor more prominently in the population. Moreover, the *Bureau of Justice Statistics, NCVS* examined violent crimes such as rape/sexual assault, robbery, assault, aggravated assault, and simple assault for a five-year period from *2017 to 2021 and* reported that people identifying as White (19.8 violent victimizations per 1,000) experienced more than other groups (e.g., Asian, Native Hawaiian, Pacific Islander) except for Blacks. Furthermore, Blacks (2.8 per 1,000) and Hispanics (2.5 per 1,000) experienced higher rates of robbery victimization than Whites (1.6 per 1,000) and others (Thompson & Tapp, 2023). Crime experts argue that during this timeframe (including the advent of *COVID-19*), the overall violent victimization rate fell in the U.S. (Thompson & Tapp, 2023). However, in the past few years, there has been a surge in the number of reported hate crimes (Farivar, 2023). According to data from the FBI's *Hate Crime Statistics*, it revealed that the number of hate crimes reached its highest level in 12 years since 2008 when the number of incidents totaled 7,783. However, in 2022 that number increased to 11,634 hate crime incidents involving 13,337 offenses. More specifically, the FBI divided its hate or bias-motivated crimes into categories that included race/ethnicity/ancestry, religion, sexual orientation, gender identity, disability, and gender. It also reported these crimes left 13,278 victims. In its distribution of bias crimes, 59.1% were attributed to race, 17.3% were based on religion, 17.2% were for sexual orientation, 4% gender identity, 1.5% disability, and 0.9% for gender. These statistics show that Blacks were disproportionately the victims of hate-motivated crimes (Farivar, 2023). Others contend that Blacks experienced the largest amount of victimization since they were targeted in one-fifth of all hate crimes reported in major cities in the U.S. Survey data collected from 42 cities by the *Center for the Study of Hate and Extremism* found that in 2022, Blacks were the targets of 22% of biased crime. Experts contend the surge in racially motivated homicides over the last five years can be attributed to *the replacement theory* which is accepted by White supremacists and right-wing ideologues who believe that non-White immigrants are being brought to the U.S. to replace White people. To respond to this perceived threat, they target Black and Brown people for violence.

Crimes against Asians

Crime against the Asian community increased during the pandemic. Some contend that in 2020, crimes against Asian Americans and Pacific Islanders more than doubled (Barr, 2021;

Li & Lartey, 2023). Statistics reported by *Stop AAPI Hate*, a national coalition, evidenced that between 2020 and 2022, more than 11,400 hate crimes were committed against people of Asian descent (Rios, 2022). The organization tracks crimes committed against Asian Americans and Pacific Islanders. It discovered that since the start of the pandemic, racist sentiments from political officials and others led to scapegoating of Asians which has manifested into their continued harassment, verbal abuse, hate speech, physical attacks, and death (Li & Lartey, 2023; Rios, 2022). More specifically, two-thirds of the reported hate incidents received between 2020 and 2022 involved either verbal or written abuse and 40% occurred in public spaces. Physical assaults accounted for 17% of the incidents and 10% of the attacks occurred on public transit (Rios, 2022). Furthermore, in a national survey by *Stop AAHI Hate and Edelman Data and Intelligence*, results revealed that one in five Asian Americans and Pacific Islanders faced a hate encounter in the past two years which led to an increase in fear with more than half of the survey respondents reporting they experienced anxiety and depression (Rio, 2022). While in 2021, *Stop AAHI Hate* identified more than 9,000 hate incidents during the first year of the pandemic, the *Center for the Study of Hate and Extremism* reported that hate crimes against Asian Americans increased 339% nationally between 2020 and 2021 (Rios, 2022). According to the Department of Justice (2020), the FBI reported a 77% increase in anti-Asian hate incidents since 2019. California, with the largest population of Asian Americans and Pacific Islanders in the nation, reported the highest number of hate crime incidents at 4,000, followed by New York and Washington State. In the state of Ohio alone, the number of hate crimes increased from 159 incidents in 2019 to 279 by 2020. Researchers contend that an estimated 60% of all hate crimes are based solely on a person's race. However, FBI officials argue that these crimes are meant as an attack on the entire community. Crime experts argue that while most hate crimes are committed against Blacks, there has been an uptick in the number of anti-Asian motivated hate crimes premised on their alleged involvement with causing *COVID-19* (Barr, 2021).

Crimes against LGBTQIA

The NCVS reveals that unlike Blacks and Asians, those who identify as members of the LGBTQIA community are more likely to be the victims of hate crime based on sexual orientation or gender bias compared to non-LGBTQIA hate crime victims (Flores et al., 2022). More specifically, the survey reported that data collected from 2017 to 2020 allowed for a national representative sample to be compiled of people who identified as either LGBTQIA at ages 16 or older. The results revealed that they experienced significantly higher rates of victimization at 43.5 per 1,000 persons compared with non-LGBTQIA persons at 19.0 per 1,000 persons, respectively. Other reports suggest that LGBTQIA people are four times more likely to experience violence compared to heterosexuals. In fact, FBI data collected in 2019 support this contention (Heinze, 2021). All sources of data on hate crimes committed against members of the LGBTQIA community conclude that these crimes pose both negative physical and psychological impacts on the victims and they are challenging to overcome unless support and services are provided after victimization (Flores et al., 2022).

Unfortunately, emerging crime data show that the number of violent anti-LGBTQIA incidents has not abated, but rather, statistics reveal that these incidents have increased in recent years. Some contend that hate crime incidents are three times higher compared with 2020 and 2021 crime data. Migdon (2023) reported that the number of anti-LGBTQIA hate crimes increased sharply with a 19% jump since 2021. In fact, in 2022, there were an estimated 11,600 hate crimes reported to the FBI. While hate crimes encompass several protected classes (e.g., religion, race/ethnicity, sexual identity, disability, and others), sexual identity has become a common reason why people are targeted and victimized. Data reveal that those identifying as lesbians in 44% of cases reported being raped, experienced physical violence, and have been stalked by an intimate partner. Gay men reported being victims of hate crimes in 26% of cases; bisexual men reported in 37% of cases that they were the victim of physical violence and stalking. Bisexual women and trans men and women of color reported experiencing elevated risk of violence and death (NSVRC, 2021). In fact, the latter group has experienced grave threats of death, and in some cases, their plight has received media attention since the number of hate crimes and deaths has increased among the transgender population by 35% and accounted for 338 incidents. Similarly, Truman and Morgan (2022) reported that the rate of victimization among transgender persons was 51.5 per 1,000 persons which is much higher than the rate faced by heterosexuals at 20.5 per 1,000 persons.

Experts contend the increase in hate crimes can be attributed to anti-LGBTQIA sentiments flamed by political rhetoric, anti-LGBTQIA demonstrations and the Far Right's engagement in anti-LGBTQIA activities. Consequently, two-thirds of the community has experienced abuse and violence that include the use of weapons. For example, the reality is that members of the community are more likely than others to be victims of gun violence. Some experts report that the statistics are 4.6 compared with 11.5 per 1,000 persons in the U.S. In 2020, an estimated 45 transgender or gender nonconforming people, mostly women of color (i.e., Black and Latinx), were shot to death (The Human Rights Campaign, 2022). In eight out of every ten deaths of a Black trans woman, the weapon of choice was a handgun. Moreover, an estimated 16% of gay and lesbian youth have been threatened or injured at school by someone banishing a weapon compared to 7% of straight youths. Data reveal that 10% of bisexual youths have been threatened by someone with a handgun. Data also indicate that 50% of transgender people have been sexually assaulted. More shocking is an influx of reports that show transgender people are seven times more likely to experience violence and brutality at the hands of police compared to others. These reports also reveal that transgendered victims of human sex trafficking are treated like criminals, rather than being offered victim services by law enforcement officers (NSVRC, 2021).

Explaining the Roots of AV

As previously mentioned, AV is a serious public health problem in the U.S. because of the sheer numbers of people who are impacted by it as well as the consequences that it brings, mainly trauma. For example, to some victims, it affects them psychologically and contributes to social dysfunction along with injuries, suffering, and untimely deaths to only name a few. Altheimer and colleagues (2023) report that people who are exposed to chronic violence are more likely to experience several health-related problems. They also find that the health of the community is also diminished when it is saturated with violence. It is also important to note that AV has many manifestations (e.g., fear, anxiety, PTSD, mood swings, depression, sexual dysfunction, and others), and behavior pathways that are associated with a unique set of risk factors that are often found in the culture and structure where people live. Some research experts provide that the root cause of violence can be threefold: biological, psychological, and environmental. First, when AV is viewed as a biological factor, experts argue that perpetrators are influenced by genetics, hormones, brain structures, and neurotransmitters that predispose them to violence and crime. A popular view among those who subscribe to biological explanations is that specific genes influence brain chemicals such as serotonin and dopamine which affect impulse control and reactions to perceptions of being threatened. Second, psychological causes are attributed to mental health conditions combined with anger, impulsivity, delusions, or hallucinations that make some people more susceptible to violence. Third, environmental conditions where people live can be the stimulus to them engaging in AV. For example, economic and cultural conditions in one's environment have a pronounced presence in the criminological literature for being crime and violence generating. This is especially true when violence factors prominently in the family, with one's peers and is consumed by watching violent television programs. Many people living in violent environments often learn that violence is an acceptable behavioral response given the context one finds themselves. Because of this, experts argue that prevention efforts will require broad social changes as well as specific interventions from health and social services along with changes in the criminal justice system. They call for the implementation of holistic approaches to violence reduction (Altheimer et al., 2023).

What are the Risk Factors?

Experts contend that it is important to address acts of crime and violence for many reasons. However, it is equally important to be able to isolate what makes offenders engage in violence (Altheimer et al., 2023). To that end, Shaffer and Rubuck (2002) report several risk factors that enhance the prospect of AV occurring including one's gender, especially being a male, household socioeconomic status, depression, alcohol use, having a high level of physical development, drug use, violent offending, easy access to firearms, being a consistent drug user, a new drug user, and if one was a previous victim of violence a year earlier, it increased the likelihood that he will commit a violent crime a year later. Unfortunately, they conclude that repeat offending is more likely than repeat victimization. However, victims who receive support from significant others such as friends, parents, and teachers after being the victim of a violent crime are less likely to engage in crime (Shaffer & Rubuck, 2002). Some research investigations that relied on a retrospective cohort study revealed that a risk factor for being at a higher risk of victimization is having already experienced a firearm injury. This research focused on recurring firearm injuries (Pear et al., 2020). In fact, a few studies suggest that people who survive gunshot injuries later face more firearm injuries and the likelihood of death (Rowhani-Rahbar et al., 2015; Fahimi et al., 2016; Carter et al., 2015). Accordingly, Pear and colleagues (2020) report that data collected from the *National Center for Injury Prevention and Control* on the annual rate of firearm homicides in California from 2005 to 2013 found that the firearm homicide rate was greater than 60 times higher among people who had received a single nonfatal gunshot injury and more than 120 times greater among people with multiple injuries. Moreover, in a study that examined AV and the risk of PTSD, the authors concluded that having prior exposure to AV in the absence of PTSD did not increase the effects of trauma when no prior trauma existed (Breslau & Peterson, 2010).

Other research points to special risk factors for most AV cases, but especially in crimes regarding sexual assaults and homicides. Belle (1987), Merry (1981), and Steele and colleagues' research showed that minority women living in poverty face the greatest risk of violent and life-threatening victimizations. Despite this finding, current research finds that race and ethnicity alone do not determine whether one will be a victim of fatal or nonfatal violence. In fact, Koss and colleagues (1995) reported when considering factors such as family income and the husband's occupation, the rate of domestic violence cases for Black families is not statistically different compared to White families. This finding has led researchers to conclude that the increased risk of violence experienced by minority women is based on their economic situation since poor women are unable to secure their safety against violence or seek social services in communities that lack adequate resources. Consequently, in lower-class communities, cases of AV are high (Cardarelli, 1997).

Role of Inequity in AV

The research literature is replete with studies that find a robust relationship between income inequality and violence that emerges with remarkable consistency. Some scholars find it is the consensus among researchers in the academy that a clear link exists between poverty and violent crime (Elgar & Aitken, 2010; Messner & Rosenfeld, 1997; Hsieh-Ching & Pugh, 1993). This is not to suggest that poverty alone produces violence, but rather, studies that investigate the nexus between crime and income overwhelmingly find that income inequality is a much stronger predictor of violent crime than poverty (Daly et al., 2001). As such, the conventional wisdom is that relative poverty is a better predictor of violent crime than absolute poverty. Some experts even suggest that violent crime is produced by the unequal distribution of wealth and not the level of wealth in society that influences homicides. Comparative studies from other countries reveal that this relationship is universal (Elgar & Aitken, 2010). For example, cultural comparative studies reveal this nexus is also found in advanced as well as developing societies both between and within these countries. In fact, Daly and colleagues (2001) compared homicide rates and income between southern regions of the U.S. and several Canadian provinces. They reported that homicide rates in southern states were higher than rates in northern cities and those rates were influenced by income inequality. They also argued that rates of homicides are comparatively low because income differences are smaller in Canada. In another comparative study that examined the homicide rates of 50 countries, Lee and Bankston (1999) found that despite control measures used in different countries to lower homicide rates, the fact of the matter is that economic inequality is significantly related to homicide.

In research conducted by Shaw et al. (2005) that investigated homicide rates in Britain during the 1980s and 1990s, they observed an increase in murder rates that occurred simultaneously as the level of income inequality and relative deprivation increased among poor men. They attributed the increase in violence to income inequality that rendered many perpetrators feeling powerless, helpless, and hopeless while experiencing tension, anxiety, depression, and having no control over their lives. Similarly, comparative studies also cite evidence that suggests when crime reduction policies fail to reduce income inequality, they negate the potential to reduce the corresponding effect on homicides (Elgar & Aitken, 2010; Hsieh-Ching & Pugh, 1993). Likewise, Fajnzylber et al. (2002) reported that a small permanent decrease in income inequality in Spain to the level found in Canada would reduce its homicide rate by 20% and long-term robbery rates by 23.3%. Despite the pronounced nexus that studies find supporting the inequality and crime relationship, some scholars contend that the relationship is not as straightforward as some scholars suggest, but rather it defers, especially when it is focused on certain types of crime (Neumayer, 2005). To that end, Rufrancos et al. (2013, p. 8) argue in a time series study that income inequality better explains property crime since they are very strongly related to changing income inequality. However, they find mixed results when examining inequality and violent crime. They contend that the disparity could be the product of different levels of reporting certain crime; since violence such as homicide, robbery, and murder typically receive full coverage and higher rates of reporting and are sensitive to reasons that include income inequality, other violent crimes may not be reported with a similar amount of coverage and within the context of income inequality. This relationship can also be found in several cross-cultural studies (Rufrancos et al., 2013).

The Social-Ecological Model of Factors to Consider When Examining AV

Because researchers, as well as academics, work to prevent AV before it causes devastation to people and communities, they examine the factors that influence violence. Officials at the CDC employ a four-pronged model to grasp a better understanding of violence and what is needed to craft effective prevention strategies. Experts at the CDC use the social-ecological model which is a theoretical framework to isolate the dynamics and complexities that exist between individuals, relationships, community, and larger societal factors that place people at risk for engaging in violence and/or being the victims of violent crime (Delong & Reichert, 2019). They contend that these factors are not mutually exclusive of each other since each encompasses different experiences with violence and taken together, they allow researchers to acquire an in-depth understanding of how people interact with each other in their social environment and how it could invariably lead to AV. Stated differently, research scholars believe that violence results from a combination of multiple influences on one's behavior. Because of this, CDC officials argue that by addressing these factors, researchers will be able to identify people who are at risk to violence and reduce levels of victimization since they examine people, communities, as well as larger societal factors that influence violence. CDC officials have established that overlap is present in the four factors. Therefore, they are not independent of each other, and consequently, they overlap and influence each other (Delong & Reichert, 2019).

Individual Factors

The first level in the four-prong model focuses on individual factors that increase the likelihood of violence. These factors typically refer to one's biological characteristics, along with one's personal history, that increase the likelihood that one will either become a perpetrator or victim of violent crime (Dahlberg & Krug, 2002; Delong & Reichert, 2019). Individual-level attributes such as age, race/ethnicity, educational attainment, income, mental health, use of illegal substances, or history of abuse are major influencers or indicators. Public health and criminological research is replete with findings that link psychological development, biology (e.g., neurology, genetics, hormones, and others), and social processes with characteristics of perpetrators and victims of AV (Reichert et al., 2018). Age factors prominently among people who commit violence and crime as well as the victims of violence. One persistent finding is that younger people commit more crimes than older people (Steffensmeier & Streifel, 1991). Age is the strongest statistically determinant of crime and violence (Agnew,

2001). Both epidemiological and criminological research report that offenders and victims share similar race/ethnic makeup, lifestyles, and routine activities (e.g., out in public places) that place them either face to face or in close physical proximity with each other (Daday et al., 2005; Nagin & Paternoster, 2000). Moreover, the amount of education that perpetrators have is another factor that may increase the likelihood that they will engage in AV.

Official crime statistics and self-report surveys evidence that an overwhelming number of violent offenders do not acquire high levels of educational attainment. In fact, some studies report that because of a lack of education, many offenders turn to crime as an instrument to acquire what they cannot obtain legitimately. As previously stated, an established relationship exists between income and crime since violence proliferates in impoverished areas. Consequently, everyone living in the area is either directly or indirectly impacted by violence. Mental health research finds that for individuals who experience trauma and PTSD, it can lead to offending and violence, especially when they cause psychological distress and changes in cognition, mood, arousal, and reactivity. The research contends that those with PTSD and trauma history who experience persistent and intrusive distress have strong association with criminal justice involvement (Donley et al., 2012). Another individual factor that influences violence and crime is the use of illegal substances and having a history of substance abuse. Research reports show that many criminals have extensive experience with alcohol and drugs. It also suggests that drug abuse is a major factor in many violent and economic crimes (Dawkins, 1997; Gottfredson et al., 2008). Moreover, a national study revealed that known criminals tend to have long histories of substance abuse including polydrug abuse (Office of National Drug Control Policy, 2013).

Relationship Factors

The second level in the four-prong model focuses on close relationship factors that increase the likelihood of one becoming either a perpetrator or victim of violence (Dahlberg & Krug, 2002). The criminological literature has long established that important people (e.g., peers, partners, family, and others) and institutions (e.g., school, church, and others) that we interact with have significant influence and impact on our behavior since they are a part of our experiences. As such, negative relationships with people and institutions can have an adverse impact on the decisions we make. Social structural as well as social processing research that addresses one's experience in the lower-class culture (especially in socially disorganized areas), as well as the quality of socialization that people experience finds that negative socialization and destructive relationships with peers, or being reared by dysfunctional parents, or family members can influence one's decision-making process. Moreover, research suggests that children often yield influence over other children through peer pressure that often creates occasions when teenagers succumb to the pressure of engaging in inappropriate behaviors (e.g., violence, drug use, alcohol abuse, and crime) because they desire social acceptance from the clique or group. This phenomenon is universal and is more likely with peers who are also similarly situated in the same community and physical proximity (Watts et al., 2023). Consequently, this may lead teenagers to engage in violence (e.g., homicides, sexual assaults, robbery, and other crimes) to belong. Scholars have noted that with the increase in physical assault victimizations from bullying, victims are becoming aggressive and engaging in the same violent behavior against others to avoid continued victimization and appear strong as well as to protect themselves (Emler, 2009). Such finding has led researchers to conclude that early victimization experienced (either in the home or on the streets) during adolescence is a very strong predictor of future offending since these adverse experiences can be stressful and traumatic to some victims who later engage in violent crimes including intimate partner violence (Menard, 2012; Whitfield et al., 2003). Beyond this, family conflict and discord also have a pronounced presence on violence, especially when children either witness or have firsthand experiences with violent behavior displayed in the home. Researchers report that when family members accept and normalize violence by responding to strain or stressors with violent behavior instead of a peaceful dispute resolution, children are vicariously taught or socialized to believe that violence represents an acceptable behavioral response to life's stressors. As such, it contributes to the cycle of intimate personal violence as well as violence being used in other areas of their lives. Furthermore, a study by Oriol and colleagues (2017) found that exposure to violence in any form can lead to one engaging in violent behavior.

Community Factors

The third level in the four-prong model focuses on community factors that increase the likelihood of one becoming either a perpetrator or victim of violence. Unlike the others, this level examines the social settings where people find themselves such as schools, neighborhoods, and the workplace. It is also in these places that social relationships are forged for better or worse and how they influence one's chance of becoming a victim or perpetrator of crime since these environments can be toxic. More specifically, the community focus is on identifying and isolating specific characteristics that are linked to violence in terms of whether one will either become a perpetrator or victim (Dahlberg & Krug, 2002). Of the settings listed above, an area that most people fail to consider is how dangerous the workplace has become in recent times. The National Safety Council (NSC) (2018) reported a total of 900,380 incidents that caused employees to request days off from work including assault, nonfatal injuries, and illnesses. Surprisingly of that number, an estimated 20,790 incidents were owing to assault, both fatal and nonfatal assaults. NSC categorized work-related assaults as either threats and verbal assaults, strangulations, rape and sexual assault, shooting, hitting and stabbings, or bombing.

Researchers report that some community factors that may include a culture of violence, poverty, population density, access to illegal drugs and firearms, unemployment rates, and ease of transportation can influence crime, violence, and victimization (WHO, 2018a). These features are exacerbated in low-income communities where residents lack resources and access to help, and they fear assisting police in crime prevention and bringing fugitives to justice. Studies find that these residents refuse to assist police out of fear of reprisal in the form of retaliatory violence for snitching on perpetrators coupled with the lack of informal mechanisms (e.g., strong families, community leaders) that force people to confirm their behaviors to standards of the law or cultural norms. Unfortunately, many low-income areas are violent places where residents arm themselves for self-preservation if accosted at gunpoint by other residents who either intend to rob or harm them.

Because firearms and gunfire are constant themes in many lower-class communities, residents report that they are not shocked, outraged, or afraid when violence occurs. Many view it as a normal feature of their life circumstances (Messner & Rosenfeld, 2007). Research suggests that people who live in socially disorganized communities have become sensitized to violence and the carnage it brings. Since violence happens with such frequency, no one is surprised when it occurs. Consequently, some teenagers living in cultures of violence often seek membership in gangs for protection along with opportunities to earn money from the drug trade or underground economy. This invariably leads to more perpetrators, crime, violence, and victimization. According to Sacco and Kennedy (2002), by engaging in crime and associating with known offenders, one faces the prospect of increasing the likelihood that they will face future victimization and a reduced likelihood of being able to seek law enforcement assistance. Another byproduct of violence and teenagers joining a gang is that it also carries over into school since deviant and criminal value systems are often transmitted from one generation to the next starting early with youth and persisting over time (Howell, 2010; Nagin & Paternoster, 2000).

Societal Factors

The fourth level in the four-prong model focuses on societal factors that create and sustain a climate of violence. Some experts argue that these factors include social and cultural norms that encourage violence as an acceptable means of resolving conflict. They postulate that policies that promote disparities in access to health care, income, education, and social opportunities create a culture that causes more crime, offenders, and victims (Dahlberg & Krug, 2002). Others contend that societal factors that impact the social structure (e.g., social class arrangement) include its organizations and more broadly, its cultural norms that impact every aspect of the human experience, despite where people find themselves in the social order (Messerschmidt, 1997). Researchers explain that social norms are very compelling since most people readily accept them as normal, typical, or appropriate without question. Because of this, social norms often go unquestioned, unchallenged, and unspoken. In most cases, these norms signal to people how the broader society expects them to behave. Some experts contend that people follow social norms by falling in line or just to fit in with others around them. Some critical scholars argue it is taking these for granted as either being fair or that things have always been that way, and there is no need to change them. Furthermore, criminologists report that societal factors can explain the behaviors of people despite their socioeconomic status. Stated differently, the social norms (e.g., values, beliefs, attitudes) found in one's social class position or setting (whether lower class, middle class, or upper class) often influence the behavior they engage in whether it is acceptable or unacceptable. This often includes the practice and acceptance of racism, violent media constructions, disparate treatment, classism, homophobia, discrimination, sexism, and ableism (Bradley, 2022). Unfortunately, society creates a level of tolerance that makes violence and images of violent behavior acceptable to most people. Critical scholars also view institutions such as schools, church, government, and the justice system as institutions that are inherently patriarchal and racists to the extent that they work to maintain or reinforce the status quo including the inequalities that exist that further divide different segments of people. Societal factors may be more complex since they directly impact cultural norms that surround gender, race, class, and conflict resolution. Some research finds that men in general are more likely to engage in crime compared with their female counterparts because culturally and socially despite where they are positioned in society, they have been socialized to engage in aggressive behavior, display dominance, and respond to situations differently. Some studies even suggest that crime and violence are masculine enterprises and are resources used by men to construct their masculinity as well as do gender, race, and class (Messerschmidt, 1997). Consequently, men factor more prominently globally in crime statistics as revealed by every crime report measurement including the WHO, UCR, NCVS, and self-reported studies.

AV Is a Criminal Justice Issue

AV is a criminal justice issue because it encompasses crimes such as homicides, sexual assaults, intimate personal violence, robbery, and others that pose threats to community safety. When these crimes occur, the criminal justice system, especially police officers, is tasked with apprehending criminal suspects who often remain at large and victimize others in the community. The task of catching offenders can be challenging when community residents are committed to confirming to community informal norms such as not assisting police with bringing fellow residents to justice. Nevertheless, typically, after an act of AV is committed and the offense reported to police, it initiates the justice system's involvement in the crime since it is charged with dispatching an officer to investigate the crime and bring the perpetrator(s) to justice. When the perpetrator is apprehended, arrested, and taken into custody, he is read his constitutional rights, taken to the police station, and booked (e.g., a record is made of the facts that transpired, pictures and fingerprints). The suspect is then held in custody for an initial appearance before a judge (Gaines & Miller, 2010). It is at this brief period that the suspect is informed of the charges and given his constitutional rights (including to remain silent and right to an attorney) by the judge. Depending on the gravity of the criminality committed, the suspect may be released on bail (or their own recognizance) with the promise of reappearing to answer pending charges. After the initial appearance is completed and bail is set, the prosecutor must establish probable cause or that the suspect committed the crime with the evidence collected by police (Gaines & Miller, 2010). The next phase is the preliminary hearing. During this time, the suspect appears before a judge who must decide if the evidence is strong enough to prove guilt. When this is established, the case can proceed to trial. In most states, the grand jury determines whether *probable cause* exists to bind the suspect over for trial. When this occurs, the prosecutor goes before the grand jury to seek an indictment. If the grand jury finds that probable exists, it issues a true bill, and the trial date is set. If there is not a finding of probable cause, it issues a no bill (Gaines & Miller, 2010).

If a plea agreement is brokered behind closed doors between the prosecutor and defendant (or accused), the victim is often unaware and has no say in any plea negotiation (Gaines & Miller, 2010). If there is a trial, a surviving victim may be asked by a prosecutor to testify against an attacker in court. For many victims of violent crimes, the dissatisfaction is so distasteful that only 25% report crimes to police owing to having a lack of confidence in the system and fear of getting involved with police and the justice machinery will likely retraumatize them (Bradley, 2022). Unfortunately, for many victims of AV, this is the extent of the criminal justice system's reach since the justice system is not equipped or designed to provide victims with the services they need during and after their victimizations. Victims' advocacy groups in general, but the *Alliance for Safety and Justice* commissioned a national research report that included 1,500 crime victims from 50 states which concluded that the criminal justice system is failing most victims because they are not provided the help at critical periods they need in the aftermath of crime. In particular, the report provides three major concerns: nothing is being done to assist victims with short and long-term financial and health consequences, victims complain that few crimes are solved, and most victims wish that public safety would shift its focus from increasing arrests and incarceration efforts to addressing what causes violence and crime cycles (2022). Because of this, critics contend that the justice system is ineffective when addressing the harm and injuries associated with victims. These critics also argue that the justice system primarily focuses on punishing the perpetrators of crime and not treating or assisting crime victims (Bradley, 2022). In fact, some observers ponder if the criminal justice system was ever created to respond to victims since its name is its focus. After all, it is not named the victim's justice system.

AV Is a Public Health Issue

Public health officials contend the criminal justice system is not an effective forum to address AV. They argue that it is primarily because of its one-sided punitive approach and its inability to confront the many causal factors that perpetuate AV. Health officials also contend that each day in America, the justice system is bombarded with many challenges ranging from persistent high levels of crime and violence, newly emerging types of crime (e.g., identity theft, AI, and others), and its historical failure to discipline corrupt police officers not to mention adequately addressing the disproportionate amount of devastating AV that causes negative health consequences to minority communities, women, and children (Bradley, 2022). Other critics of the justice system list the many challenges that have rendered the justice system ineffective when dispensing justice and assisting crime victims to include being overburdened with heavy caseloads, insufficient funding for both material and a lack of human resources. Critics argue these challenges conspire to cause unreasonable delays in the justice process that have contributed to overuse of pretrial detention for extended periods, overcrowded prisons, and insufficient use of alternative sentencing options such as community-based initiatives to name a few. Perhaps their biggest concern is that crime victims are mostly left behind in the criminal justice system.

AV is a public health issue for several reasons, but chief among them are the negative health consequences that comes with victimizations from crimes that include, but not limited to child abuse, firearm violence, intimate partner violence, sexual assaults, elder abuse, and others. Victims may experience many health problems such as hypertension, stroke, mental disorders, and cancer (American Public Health Association [APHA], 2018). Some acts of AV often cause debilitating physical injuries, disease, and death (Centers for Disease Control and Prevention [CDC], 2021). In fact, research suggests that simply being exposed to violence can cause emotional and psychological trauma directly to victims and indirectly to the community at large (Metzler et al., 2017). Research literature also suggests that a strong relationship exists between adverse childhood experiences (ACEs) with violence that contributed to child engaging in lifelong participation in violence, negative health outcomes including many suffering from chronic disease and mental disorders (Metzler et al., 2017). Similarly, many research studies report that when children and adolescents are not the direct victims of violence, but are merely exposed to violence, they face a greater risk of suffering mental health problems such as depression, anxiety, post-traumatic stress disorders (Jones-Webb & Wall, 2008). As a result of AV, many victims often experience a diminished quality of life that may last for decades. Of great concern to public health officials is that when AV occurs in large numbers and effect many people (as it does in the U.S.), it is best viewed as an epidemic (like diseases that have spread throughout the population infecting many people) that requires epidemiological as well as public health approaches to prevent others from experiencing it. AV is a public health issue because of the sheer number of people who are impacted by it each year. Unfortunately, after the initial victimization, many victims will be hospitalized and require medical attention to address their injuries. Some victimizations such as violent physical assaults such as gunshot wounds and stabbings will require surgery. Even when this is complete, many survivors will have to stay in hospitals for extended periods for close observations of a physician. Upon discharge, it is common for some patients to receive rehabilitation services to return to their pre-victimization status. However, because of the trauma that violence brings, some victims will require emotional and psychological counseling as well as medications to help them cope in the aftermath of being victimized. According to Krug and colleagues (2002), while the victims of violence often endure the physical pain inflicted from their victimization, many also experience mental distress.

International Comparative Statistics

WHO has declared violence as a global problem with global consequences since it costs the lives of millions each year and leaves millions of others in need of health care to address nonfatal injuries either from a self-infliction, interpersonal, or collective violence (Krug et al., 2002). Experts agree that violence is among the leading causes of death globally among people between the ages of 15 and 44. While violence is an international problem that varies country by country (e.g., many European countries' violent crime rates are less than 1 incident per 100,000 peoples), it shares many common roots. Some experts argue that there are many factors that can influence the decision to engage in violent crime, and high levels of poverty and a lack of economic opportunities drive people worldwide to commit risky behavior typically out of desperation. In contrast, crime rates are lower in countries that are wealthy and people have favorable living conditions and a good quality of life. Some other variables that are related to crime that are also cross-cultural are age, law enforcement effectiveness, and access to firearms. International homicide statistics reveal that it is one of the leading causes of death globally. It is disproportionately committed by males living in poverty, and in places with easy access to firearms.

Examining comparative crime statistics between nations presents a challenge owing to different countries and regions using different definitions to list violent crime including unique methods of reporting and recording crime. Stated differently, it can be difficult to measure violent crime globally when different countries have different definitions of what constitutes a specific crime. Other barriers occur when some countries discourage and prevent certain people, especially women and young girls from reporting their victimizations. Comparative scholars also suggest that during times of large-scale conflict in some countries, it is difficult to discern AV related to the conflict from violent crime noncombatants. The matter is complicated more when there is no organization or agency designated to collect and publish crime data on a consistent basis that measures the nature and extent of its levels and rates of AV. Because these matters conspire to obstruct any accurate count of AV globally, the reality is that without updated crime data, it is impossible to know the true number of cases. However, when these data are available, researchers can make international comparisons of AV statistics. For example, WHO (2018) conducted a study analyzing data collected from 2000 to 2018 taken from 161 countries and areas on behalf of the *UN Interagency* work group on violence against women worldwide and found intimate personal violence to be a global problem, and a violation of women's human rights. Global data revealed that one in three (30%) women between the ages of 15 and 49 has been subjected to physical and/or sexual violence by an intimate partner or non-partner or both. Moreover, 38% of all murdered women involved someone the victim shared an intimate partner relationship. In only 6% of sexual assault cases, women reported the attacker was someone other than a partner. Comparative statistics show that estimates of lifetime intimate partner violence range vary by country. For example, WHO data show that the prevalence of lifetime violence is 20% in the Western Pacific, 22% in high-income countries in Europe, 25% in the WHO regions of the Americas, 33% in the WHO African region, 31% in the WHO Eastern Mediterranean region, and 33% in the WHO South-East Asia region (WHO, 2018).

Global statistics on homicides reveal that it is one of the leading causes of death (accounting for 475,000 people in 2019), for men and boys who are disproportionately (80%) its victims as well as perpetrators who live in poverty between the ages of 20 and 30 who are more at risk and those living in areas with easy access to firearms. Experts argue that availability alone is not the main determinant, but rather, weak oversight and control associated with impunity matters most. Women and girls are victims of homicide in 20% of all cases. However, they are mostly victims of homicides owing to a family member, or an intimate partner relationship. According to a 2022 global study on homicide conducted by United Nations Office on Drugs (UNODC) (2023) on intentional homicide trends and patterns worldwide, the continent of Africa recorded the highest number with an estimated 176,000 victims, followed by the Americas with a total of 154,000. The total number of intentional homicides in Asia was 109,000, while Europe had an estimated 17,000 followed by Oceania with 1,000. The study stated that this translates into people in Africa facing a rate of 12.7 victims per 100,000 population. While people in America face a rate of 15 victims per 100,000 population. Those living in Oceania face a rate of 2.9 victims per 100,000 population. People living in Asia face a rate of 2.3 victims per 100,000 population, and people in Europe face a rate of 2.2 victims per 100,000 population. Moreover, UNODC data reported that Africa accounted for 38% of all homicide victims, the Americas for 34%, Asian 24%, Europe 4%, and Oceania had less than 1% (UNODC, 2023).

Global statistics on child abuse are also alarming. According to Hillis and colleagues (2016), children worldwide face serious violence to the extent that it is a violation of human rights and a global health problem. To measure the magnitude of this international concern, they relied on data collected from 96 countries on reported cases that occurred the previous year. The data were used along with the size of the population of children to estimate the number of children in each region that experienced violence (Hillis et al., 2016). The statistics from their investigation revealed that at least 50% of children in Asia, Africa, and Northern America were the victims of violence in the past year. Among children between the ages of 2 and 17 that experienced the most severe forms of violence, 64% were from Asia followed by 56% from Northern America (but 61% experienced physical, sexual, and/or emotional abuse), 50% from Africa, 34% from Latin America (but 58% experienced physical, sexual, and/or emotional abuse), and 12% from Europe, respectively. Moreover, comparative data from United Nations Office on Drug Crime (2019) provide that homicide is the leading cause of death for children and youth, especially young men, and boys between the ages of 15 and 24. Furthermore, 38% of all Caribbean students and 26% of Central American students' report being involved in physical fights, and 32% and 30% of students from North and South America, respectively, report being bullied. While child sexual abuse data are limited, available data find that 16% of girls and 10% of boys in Honduras, 15% of girls and 8% of boys in Colombia, and 14% of girls and 3% of boys in El Salvador are victims of sexual violence before age 18. Alarmingly, an estimated 1 billion children between the ages of 2 and 17 worldwide are victims of violence each year (Hillis et al., 2016).

Public Health and Social Work

Intersection of Public Health and Social Work

The pervasiveness of violence requires extensive intervention efforts. While violence is typically discussed in terms of distinct types, "violence comes in many forms all containing similarities and dissimilarities, each independent from and dependent on the others" (Abt, 2017, p. 268). A typology of violence continuum indicates six forms of violence beginning with home/family violence on one end of the continuum followed by school violence, community violence, gang violence, organized violence, and ending with state violence (e.g., law enforcement and military). The intersection of public health and social work typically occurs in the middle—in the community (Abt, 2017).

Public health officials are trained to work with populations, especially communities. Social workers are also trained to work with communities to assess concerns and needs, build networks to create and expand resources, and organize and problem-solve by using community strengths, social capital, and collective wisdom (Brown & Stalker, 2023). Social work engages in community intervention to address AV, community violence, and violence in general, which occurs through the following strategies:

- Advocacy-based interventions using policy and awareness campaigns to bring to attention the community damage accruing through violence and the importance of violence prevention;
- Educational interventions teaching new skills through workshops for interpersonal communication, managing anger, and mediation;
- Direct services such as counseling, crisis intervention, and referral services such as group therapy for perpetrators of violence, support groups for violence survivors, crisis management, police and social work partnerships, and art therapy projects for children;
- Capacity-building which strengthens organizations' abilities to address community-level needs; and
- Community or neighborhood organizing and mobilization such as neighborhood-police anticrime efforts (Hardcastle et al., 2011; Association of Social Work Boards, 2025).

By working collaboratively, social work and public health goal is to improve the physical and social environment where people live, learn, work, and play. They strive to address structures leading to violence such as "neighborhood poverty, residential segregation and instability, [and] high density of alcohol outlets" (CDC, 2024). Community intervention is an "all hands-on deck" venture that requires the participation of many stakeholders: children and parents; community, business, and faith-based leaders; social service and health providers; and law enforcement and criminal justice agencies (Abt, 2017).

Health Disparities and Health Equities

AV encompasses many forms of violence and yet they all occur within the context of the community. Exposure to community violence (ECV) includes both witnessing and/or experiencing direct victimization by any number of violent community events impacting residents. For example, "street crimes are instructive in this regard since it often presents gang violence, physical assaults, rape, and many other adverse community conditions" (Lee et al., 2017, p. 69). Since these acts of violence are experienced both directly and indirectly, youth are most likely to be impacted (Finkelhor et al., 2010), which has led ECV to be considered a possible ACE (WHO, 2011). ACE involves experiencing violence, abuse, or neglect, witnessing violence in the home or community, having a family member attempt or die by suicide, and growing up in an environment with substance use and mental health problems, home conflict and parental separation, and incarcerated family members (Merrick et al., 2019). Additionally, community factors such as "poverty, unemployment, poor education, inadequate housing, poor public transportation, interpersonal violence, and decaying neighborhoods also contribute to health inequities" (Baciu et al., 2017, p. 1 of 23). In the U.S., communities of color experience more violence and that certain oppressed subgroups shoulder the burden of violence, namely women and those who identify as LGBTQ+ (APHA, 2018). Reducing violence in these communities and for specific targeted groups would substantially reduce violence-related health inequities such as "birth outcomes, life expectancy, and chronic disease," leading to healthier communities where people could thrive (APHA, 2018).

Merrick and colleagues (2019) evaluated ACE data provided by the Behavioral Risk Factor Surveillance System 2015–2017 from 25 states in the U.S. The results revealed that one in six adults surveyed (15.6%) reported four or more types of adverse ACE. This group comprised mostly younger persons (ages 18–24), women, American Indians and Alaska Natives (AI/AN), Blacks, and other racial minority groups. Approximately, 60.9% of those surveyed reported at least one ACE. For all groups, but particularly those experiencing four or more ACEs, the overall risk was shown to be elevated for developing coronary heart disease, stroke, asthma, chronic obstructive heart disease, and kidney disease and for becoming a smoker and/or heavy drinker. The highest risk appeared for developing depression. Health experts report that the impact of violence, or rather ACEs, is cumulative as exposure to violence and other traumatic events occur over time and exposure to six or more types of ACEs may decrease life expectancy by 20 years (Brown et al., 2009).

Negative Health Consequences of AV

While statistics reveal that crime and violence are more saturated in some communities compared with others for several reasons, it does not mean that other people and places are exempt from AV. The reality of violence is that it can affect anyone at any stage of their life course since, in many cases, it can be both random and intergenerational (Rivera et al., 2019). Research suggests that though rates of AV have decreased since the mid-1980s and early 1990s, when the U.S. waged war against the crack cocaine epidemic, the rates of homicides are once again on the rise which necessitates that criminal justice and public health policymakers have a broader understanding of the root causes of violence as well as its negative health consequences (Rivera et al., 2019). While this is not meant to be an exhaustive list of AV and its health consequences, since other forms and consequences are discussed throughout the book, it does provide examples of several types of AV that include childhood sexual abuse, intimate partner violence, elder abuse, sexual violence, bullying, other youth violence, and other adult interpersonal violence (for those ages 25 and older), and the health consequences that impact people who are directly affected by violence along with how others in the community are indirectly impacted by violence.

Research on the effects of physical and sexual abuse experienced during childhood is linked to an increased risk of mental illness throughout the life course, suicide attempts, substance use and abuse, obesity, sexually transmitted infections, and chronic diseases such as ulcers, migraines, and arthritis (Norman et al., 2012). Some studies report that child sexual abuse often leads to short- and long-term physical, mental, and behavioral health consequences that impact how children think, act, and feel over their life course including chronic conditions such as cancer and heart disease, and obesity. Other studies find that both males and females who experienced sexual abuse as children were also more likely to experience sexual victimization as young adults, but also engage in sexually aggressive behaviors toward others (Berger, 2017). A study conducted by Krause-Utz and colleagues (2021) found that females who experience sexual abuse are at 2–13 times greater risk of sexual violence as adults, and people who experience sexual abuse are at twice the risk for non-sexual intimate partner violence.

In a study by Smith and colleagues (2019) that examined the effects of intimate partner violence, it reported that both men and women are affected, but women are more likely to be severely victimized and sustain injuries that often require medical attention. In the aftermath of this type of violence, victims experience head and neck pain, elevated risk of experiencing asthma, gastrointestinal disorders, chronic pain, frequent headaches, and sexually transmitted infections. They also found that victims suffer mental health issues that include depression, anxiety, PTSD, and suicidality. In another study that examined how intimate personal violence affected children exposed to it, research reported that the consequences of violence go beyond the victims and have psychological, social, and cognitive consequences on adolescents that is linked to substance use, depression, suicidal behavior as well as chronic stress (Okuda et al., 2015).

In their investigation on elderly abuse, Yunus et al. (2019) reported that victims typically experience physical, psychological, and financial. More specifically, those who have been abused have higher levels of stress and depression compared to those who have not been abused. They also suffer an elevated risk of developing fear and anxiety, and suicide attempts. Many withdraw socially, which often exacerbates their physical and mental health. Research examining the effects of sexual violence finds many victims suffer from depression, anxiety, substance abuse, sleep disorders, and PTSD. Moreover, suicide attempts and completed suicides are four times higher for sexual assault victims compared with those in the general population (Rosellinin et al., 2017). Some researchers contend that the psychological consequences of being a victim of sexual violence are contingent on the quality of response received from one's social network including the medical community as well as the criminal justice system (Mason & Lodrick, 2013).

Bullying is often defined as any unwanted aggressive behavior by another young person or group where there is an observed or perception of an imbalance of power. It is also behavior that is repeated over time or is perceived to be repeated behavior (CDC, 2019). Research on bullying by Pozzoli (2013) finds that it affects victims' physical and emotional health including headaches, chronic abdominal pain, and sleep disturbances. Research conducted by Diliberti and colleagues (2019) report that victims of bullying experience the infliction of harm or distress that often includes physical, psychological, social, or educational harm. They also contend that it can be experienced through technology, referred to as cyberbullying. Other researchers report that those who are bullied face a greater risk of depression, anxiety, alcohol, and substance abuse. Similar to this finding, Moore and colleagues (2017) in their study using a meta-analysis of 55 studies on cyberbullying reported a strong association with victims experiencing depression, anxiety, self-esteem issues, and somatization. While some studies find support for the self-harm argument, others do not and argue instead that the correlation does not extend to isolated bullying, but rather, the likelihood of suicide is greater for people who have been long-term or chronic targets of bullying (Brunstein et al., 2019).

Youth violence is also of major concern in the U.S. to both criminal justice and public health officials since experts now report that it is the third leading cause of death among young people between the ages of 10 and 24. While it includes fighting, bullying, threats with weapons, and gang-related violence, it is the number one cause of death among young African-American males (David-Ferdon et al., 2021). What is more concerning is the fact that 88.9% of all homicides are committed with a firearm. Statistics show that a firearm is used in 94% of young African-American deaths. Moreover, Blacks are also more likely to be involved in fights that result in injuries and aggravated assaults compared with their counterparts (Sheats et al., 2018). Beyond the homicides, youths also experience gun-related injuries that often manifest in debilitating outcomes such as paralysis. Research also finds that youth who experience violence face an elevated risk of PTSD compared to those who are not exposed to or have direct encounters with violence. Research conducted by Coyle and colleagues (2017) reveal that youth who experience violent victimizations are more likely to abuse and develop a dependency on drugs and experience violence later in life, especially domestic violence and committing property or violent crimes. Public health officials report that youth violence often has a long-term impact on their health and well-being.

Unlike rates of violence for youth, research conducted on adult interpersonal violence finds that rates of violence are typically lower for adults ages 25 and older. People within this age group experience violent victimizations such as homicides as well as nonfatal assault-related injuries. Regarding homicide, epidemiologists estimate that in 2017, 13,667 adults within this age group were victims of violent homicide. They also report that a firearm was the weapon of choice in 72% of those deaths (CDC, 2019). Studies find that assault-related injuries are linked with a high risk of revictimization and negative health outcomes that may endure for short and long terms. For example, a study revealed that many people in this group who sustained a firearm injury were left with permanent disabilities that placed limitations on their ability to rejoin the workforce (Fowler et al., 2015). Moreover, victims who were hospitalized and treated for assault injuries were at a greater risk of experiencing

PTSD, depression, and sexually transmitted infections (Rahtz et al., 2017). Other research investigations report that adult violent offenders are more likely than others to die by suicide (Jokinen et al., 2017).

While violence has a direct impact on its victims, research suggests that it also impacts others in the broader community and invariably affects individual behavior. In their investigation, Lehrner and Yehuda (2018) reported that after someone in the community experiences violence, those people (friends, neighbors, family members) who are aware of the violence can also experience vicarious trauma that may have lasting effects. Considering recent shootings of unarmed young Black men by police officers, captured in real time and shown in 24-hour news cycles, researchers have identified negative health consequences that many residents in the Black community experience in the aftermath of police-inflicted violence. Research suggests that racial disparities exist in the rates of police-inflicted physical injuries, including death. It finds that Black men are injured and killed by police in a disproportionate manner compared with their White counterparts, and police violence against Blacks has a serious impact on the broader community that has created aggregated rates of chronic health conditions that most often manifest in mental health outcomes such as PTSD, depression, distress, suicidal behavior, and symptoms of psychosis (Devylder et al., 2022; Bor et al., 2018).

Criminal Justice Approaches to AV

Because the nature of the criminal justice system is reactionary, most of its efforts to combat or prevent AV occur after the fact, rather than proactively. Gebo (2022) describes the justice system's approach to addressing violence as working from the secondary and tertiary levels instead of making it its primary prevention focus. This often signals to observers that the system is focused on capturing and punishing offenders first, and prevention second, and hardly ever victims of AV (Potts, 2021; Sklansky, 2021). Gebo (2022) argued that the justice system places limited focus on advocating rehabilitation or restoration to the offender, victim, or community. Notwithstanding, some experts have attempted to address this historical shortcoming in the way police respond to crime. Therefore, to combat concerns about rising gun violence, increasing rates of homicide, as well as other types of AV, many in the law enforcement community have responded with several strategies to reduce violence that will not lead to similar mass incarceration strategies that were used in the 1980s and 1990s (Sklansky, 2021). Chief among them has been implementing problem-oriented policing (POP) techniques. Unlike past efforts, POP strategies take on a proactive role after police agencies identify long-term community problems including acts of AV, especially intimate personal violence, firearm-related violence, child abuse, and homicide. Those who advocate using POP contend that their effectiveness at reducing crime is contingent on whether police can mobilize community residents and service providers to respond to chronic crime conditions (Potts, 2021). As such, police departments are designating special units to address certain types of offenders (Siegel & Worrall, 2022).

POP strategies are typically used when police believe that AV is concentrated in hot spots, mainly in lower-income urban areas or at specific acts of violence (Siegel & Worrall, 2022). Sklansky (2021) suggests gun killings of non-intimates can be substantially reduced when violence reduction programs focus on small numbers of people, places, and social exchanges that are responsible for most street violence in a city. The example of *Operation Ceasefire*

(OC) is instructive in this regard since it is viewed as the model for others to replicate (Fox et al., 2015; Sklansky, 2021). OC was implemented in Boston as an intervention to reduce high rates of AV where firearms were used. More specifically, OC efforts were targeted at the increase in the number of teenage homicides that plagued the city. Research results revealed that after evaluating the program, OC was successful in reducing the number of violent youth homicides (by 60%) victimizations as well as other gun assaults in Boston (Fox et al., 2015). OC relied on coordination between police, several municipal agencies, and nonprofit groups, along with inner-city clergy members (Sklansky, 2021). Similarly, success was also found in Oakland when the city implemented OC; its adult homicide rates were reduced by 31%, and group-involved shootings or nonfatal shootings were reduced by 43%. As a result of their success, other jurisdictions around the country have tried to implement OC and POP strategies in their respective communities (Siegel & Worrall, 2022).

In their efforts to reduce gang violence, police in Jersey City, New Jersey used a variety of aggressive crime reduction strategies targeted at drug enforcement and community improvement techniques such as brightening dimly lit areas as well as cleaning dilapidated property in highly criminogenic areas (Braga et al., 2008). While research evaluations revealed that POP strategies are successful, some experts warn that this success should be accepted with caution since AV may disperse to other areas or locations that are not hot spots. Unfortunately, when arrests are made, they lead community residents to conclude that their problems with violence and crime have been effectively solved. However, Lawton and colleagues (2005) report that in most cases, POP efforts have a small deterrent effect that dissipates overtime owing to acts of AV being displaced to other areas that are not protected by police. Moreover, Potts (2021) reported that POP can be difficult and complexed to implement and be successful since it requires close coordination with multiple partners which can be challenging in hyperpolarized political environments. Experts suggest that for POP efforts to be successful: police agencies must not only focus on arrests, but rather, they should also prioritize preventing AV. Police must work with partners within the community, especially street outreach workers, service providers, and community residents. The partnership should facilitate information sharing about high-risk people and high-risk places (Potts, 2021).

Public Health Approaches

Public health focuses on the known causal factors of violence in its prevention efforts. The public health workforce plays a critical role in prevention through training, education, and analysis that emphasizes addressing inequities and reducing structural racism in societal institutions (Wren & Goodwin, 2016). Luby and colleagues (2005) suggest that public health violence prevention measures should follow disease prevention initiatives such as hand washing and vaccinations, but instead, encourage conflict resolution that could stop the transmission of violence. Public health and medical workers have many opportunities to interact with vulnerable populations such as domestic violence victims and persons diagnosed with mental illness, presenting opportunities for evaluation, screening, resource provision, and resilience-building programming (Gewirtz & Edelson, 2007). Public health approaches for violence prevention in homes and communities focus on building healthy relationships and justice-centered institutions (U.S. Department of Health and Human

Services, 2024), establishing healthier norms, and creating safe and protective environments (Center for Mental Health Services (U.S.), 2007).

To effectively initiate violence prevention in all parts of community life, public health calls on (1) local health departments to assess data collected on violence to improve health information related to violence and violence prevention models (APHA, 2018); (2) institutions funding community violence prevention to implement programs that detect and interrupt violence transmission; (3) health and academic institutions to train health professionals in identifying risks for violence victimization (Fischer et al., 2014), detecting the signs of violence, developing a trauma-informed response, connecting high-risk individuals with needed resources (Sumner et al., 2019); (4) local, state, and federal government agencies to invest in, adopt, and support evidence-based and promising public health approaches to violence prevention (APHA, 2018); and (5) the CDC, in conjunction with local and state department of public health, to establish or improve surveillance systems for violence occurring in communities (APHA, 2018).

Public Health and Social Work Approaches

Social work brings a trauma and violence-informed care (TVIC) perspective to violence prevention that attempts to minimize harm to those served. A trauma and violence-informed approach acknowledges the connection between "violence, trauma, negative health outcomes and behaviors" (Public Health Agency of Canada, 2018). TVIC approaches require policies and practices that are designed for persons who need services after experiencing violence. These approaches demand changes in system design, organizational function, and how practitioners view and engage with clients. The following key policy and practice TVIC principles are suggested:

1 Understand trauma and violence, and their impacts on peoples' lives and behaviors;
2 Create emotionally and physically safe environments;
3 Foster opportunities for choice, collaboration, and connection;
4 Provide a strengths-based and capacity-building approach to support client coping and resilience (Wathen & Mantler, 2022, p. 235).

Universal trauma precautions can provide a uniform and shared platform for integrating services within and across systems. In addition to the aforementioned principles, there are also the CDC's (2022) six tenets of trauma-informed care which social workers are encouraged to follow. They include the following:

1 Prioritizing clients' physical and emotional safety;
2 Building trust with the community through transparent communication;
3 Seeking peer support and encouraging clients to do the same;
4 Fostering collaboration and mutuality in their practices;
5 Empowering clients by giving them a voice and a choice; and
6 Considering broader contexts that impact client experiences, such as cultural, historical, and gendered influences.

Integrating Skills of Social Epidemiology to Address Disparities to Achieve Equity

Social epidemiologists work to identify social factors that are found among individuals and groups that can be used to better understand patterns that are linked to disparities in the types and incidents of diseases and health distributions found in neighborhoods, communities, and wider sections of a population (Knesebeck, 2015). This is necessitated by the fact that socioeconomics and racial inequalities in health typically factor prominently in the U.S. (Lathrop, 2020; Satcher & Higginbotham, 2008). Some social epidemiologists conduct studies designed to contribute to health services research when they examine social factors that impact adverse health. They contend that those factors or characteristics are not limited to merely influencing health, but rather, research reveals that these social factors are also strongly related to the quality of health care, or lack thereof, that people may or may not receive based on conditions they have no control over such as age, where they are born, grow, work, live, their quality health as well as life expectancy (Lathrop, 2020). To accomplish their goal, social epidemiologists integrate concepts such as *social inequalities, social relationships, social capital, and work stress* to study health disparities and determine how to achieve equity (Knesebeck, 2015; Wallerstein et al., 2011). First, social epidemiologists examine *social inequality* in society and look for factors or indicators such as income and education and focus on how they impact people having access to receive health care. They find that income inequality is a universal factor that impacts access to health care or quality healthcare systems that extends cross-culturally. Research reveals that the most prevalent health inequities are found where poverty exists. Second, social epidemiologists research *social relationships* mainly between social network and social support to determine if they have a positive influence on people's decision to seek medical treatment and avail themselves of health services and outcomes when they are available. Third, social epidemiologists look to determine if there is delivery of high-quality coordinated care. In doing so, they access *social capital* in healthcare organizations (e.g., social relations based on trusts, mutual understanding, common convictions, and shared values). Fourth, social epidemiologists study *work environments* of those who provide healthcare services, especially *work-related stress* and how it impacts the quality-of-service people receive. In the end, they conclude that these areas should be integrated when addressing disparities since they are significant social determinants of the quality of health care that people receive. As such, they should be included in research investigations that seek to better understand health disparities as well as to inform, develop, and implement interventions (Lathrop, 2020; Brazil et al., 2005).

In the early 1990s, researchers identified social epidemiology constructs as excellent targets for community empowerment. During this time, researchers argued that social epidemiology alone was not as effective as it could be when examining health disparities. However, success could be achieved if efforts were made to integrate social epidemiological skills to address health disparities with community-engaged intervention strategies given that both (social epidemiology and community-engaged researchers) have similar interests, namely the desire to reduce health inequalities (Wallerstein et al., 2011). Advocates argued that this would require an interdisciplinary collaboration that sought common research questions, models, and methods (Holmes et al., 2008). As such, relying on a transdisciplinary approach opened health disparities research to many questions. Moreover, social epidemiologists changed the scope of intervention research since collaborations enhanced evaluation designs and measures that better integrated both quantitative and qualitative approaches, while the results influenced both disciplines methods and measures, which enhanced their ability to better communicate findings to community partners that were translated into practice and policy (Wallerstein et al., 2011, p. 826). Scholars contend that this invariably led to an increase in social epidemiological community-engaged research that focused on community-engaged interventions to address health inequities (Berkman, 2004; Kaplan, 2004; Syme & Frohlich, 2002). Since epidemiology can be used to partner with others who target social determinants through health enhancing policies, practices, and interventions, it increases the likelihood that its research will be more successful compared with epidemiologists working alone. Moreover, it enriches the efforts for community-engaged researchers and others since it requires modifications to interventions, measurements of proper constructs, evaluations, and findings. In the end, it generates new theories and strategies to effect change that could help reduce health inequities which is necessary given its pervasiveness, unfairness because the people affected have very little control over the contributing factors and the issue of health equity can be addressed with viable policy solutions (Woodward & Kawachi, 2000; Wallerstein et al., 2011).

How Can AV Be Prevented?

Current statistics reveal that AV remains a persistent issue in the U.S. since it threatens the health, safety, and well-being of everyone because of the adverse emotional, physical, psychological, and debilitating injuries it brings that often span across time and relationships while adversely affecting others including family, friends, offenders, victims as well as the entire neighborhood (Smith & Cottler, 2018). Victimization data report each day someone either experiences or is indirectly impacted by a violent crime such as homicide, battery, sexual assault, intimate personal violence, robbery, workplace violence, and others. When violence occurs, the details surrounding the criminal episode often quickly emerge. They typically provide information on the number of people affected, who were impacted, and when and where violence transpired. Since violence creates many different types of hardships followed by needs that can be either financial, emotional, physical, psychological, medical, security, or a combination of these, victimologists postulate that caring for victimizations can easily exceed the resources of single individuals (Siegel & Worrall, 2022). Consequently, violence should be viewed as a community-wide problem and not an individual one. As such, it is incumbent on the entire community to assist assault victims in the aftermath of their victimization. To that end, residents and local agencies in the community should develop partnerships or collaborative efforts by combining their resources to make sure that victims receive the kind of treatment and services that are necessary to recover. They should also form alliances with public safety professionals to capture and bring perpetrators of violence to justice. Some violence prevention experts contend that violence reduction efforts should be implemented before and after AV occurs. With respect to the former, proactive measures can help to identify potential risk factors that address the root causes of AV. Therefore, violence experts argue that those in public safety professions, public health, and community organizations partner to implement strategies to prevent violence.

Public health efforts used to reduce violence are generally categorized into three types of activities: primary, secondary, and tertiary prevention. Primary efforts are designed to be proactive or stop violence before it occurs. These efforts are strategies that are placed on high-risk people and can be used to prevent violence within the entire community (e.g., bullying prevention programs at school that educate students on the harmfulness of violence). Secondary efforts are interventions that focus on minimizing the degree of harm sustained after the victimization occurs. These efforts can include community outreach programs that address the effects of being exposed to violence. Tertiary efforts are aimed at achieving long-term goals such as treating and rehabilitating offenders as well as victims to prevent the continuation and the negative health consequences that goes with AV (Rutherford et al., 2007). The public health approach relies on a four-step problem-solving strategy that includes the following: defining the problem, identifying risk and protective factors, developing, and testing prevention strategies, and assuring widespread adoption of successful outcomes (Mercy et al., 1993).

Because there are several factors that are believed to influence violence, namely individual, relationship, community factors, experts suggest that public health efforts to prevent AV should target these areas. First, public health officials at the CDC (n.d.) recommend that individual-level violence prevention strategies are used to provide offenders and victims with therapy, education, and skill training. More specifically, they argue cognitive behavioral therapy will help change attitudes and behaviors by educating at-risk people (*both perpetrators and victims*) to engage in prosocial and healthy ways to respond to situations and people in a non-violent or confrontational way since offenders and victims interact with each other and share the same routine activities and are often from the same community. Stated differently, if people who live in violent communities are influenced by their experiences to respond with violence, they can receive coping skills from anger management programs to use healthy behavioral responses to life stressors. Other efforts that can be addressed on the individual level are to provide income opportunities, alcohol and substance abuse treatment, and access to mental health and counseling to those suffering from poverty, addiction, trauma, and other forms of psychological distress. Second, research experts recommend that strategies can be implemented to help navigate the negative influences that people are exposed to either by peers, family, education, or other institutions where they have either been directly or indirectly socialized. This suggests that negative socialization can occur in any social class in the American system of stratification and income does not exempt people from being exposed to negative and destructive behaviors that may later impact their decision to engage in AV. However, when addressing prevention on the relationship level, experts recommend the use of educational programs that are designed to reeducate people to engage in healthy behaviors and work toward healthy relationships that will be displayed through positive interactions and exchanges starting in the home, and later in the neighborhood, with peers, school, and other institutions. Public health experts contend that families that exhibit violence can be encouraged to enroll in programs or classes that are family-focused and emphasize parenting and family therapy. In these classes, parents or caregivers will receive training in key areas such as conflict resolution, positive/negative reinforcement, and mentoring programs. Because of the nationwide increase in bullying, experts recommend aggressive anti-bullying campaigns at school can have a cost–benefit attached since they prevent future offending and the cycle of victim turning offender (Ttofi et al., 2011). Third, strategies can be implemented to address community-level factors that increase the number of offenders and victims of AV. As mentioned earlier, the social settings (e.g., violent homes, workplaces, schools, neighborhoods) where people find themselves can contribute to victimization, especially if there is a pervasive culture of violence, poverty, access to illegal drugs, and an availability of firearms. To that end, public health experts recommend several strategies designed to keep people safe and to empower them with economic resources. More specifically, they propose that AV can be prevented when efforts are made to increase school resources, create employment opportunities for those who face economic and health disparities, and create safe spaces in the community for recreational purposes (CDC, n.d.). With respect to preventing violence in the workplace, health experts recommend conducting a risk assessment, establishing clear responsibilities and communication channels, providing employee training and support, installing an effective surveillance system, installing panic button technology, implementing effective lockdown procedures, and offering mental health awareness training to employees. Fourth, societal factors are the last and most challenging level to address. Strategies used at the societal level must focus on improving complex systems such as the economy and education because of the well-established relationship between educational and economic disparities and their connection with AV. Consequently, policymakers and other government officials should invest resources in economically strained areas that need them most, especially poor neighborhoods and communities characterized by low levels of educational attainment, poverty, and social disorganization.

It is important to point out that the criminal justice system can and should be involved in violence prevention efforts aimed at individual, relationship, community, and societal factors that increase the likelihood that there will be more offenders and victims, especially when keeping people safe and removing offenders when they victimize others albeit this is only part of the solution. The impact that the justice system can have on the broader society is not to be minimized. For example, effective justice system efforts implemented nationally can have a pronounced effect on violence throughout society. In fact, some experts argue that it is not enough for public safety officials to simply apprehend and arrest perpetrators and someday return them to the same criminological community, but there must be collaborations between them and other agencies (including public health, community agencies, and other stakeholders), to create effective violence prevention interventions that removes the negative influences from the environment. Notwithstanding, many experts believe that criminal justice officials can assist in providing trauma-informed care units and rely on evidence-based programs to address what often happens in the aftermath of experiencing AV.

Policy Recommendations

Despite the negative consequences that are caused by AV, both criminal justice and public health experts agree that the behavior can be preventable if officials in public safety would form partnerships with public health agencies. While the former is more reactive and the latter proactive, the commonality that they share is that both groups are charged with keeping individuals, communities, and society safe from harm and injuries that often have devastating consequences that can be either short or long term. Because of this, researchers, policy experts, and others contend that there should be more partnerships formed with each other, along with community residents, community action groups, and other stakeholders to improve the quality of life and safety for those directly and indirectly exposed to AV. In those few cases that were cited in this chapter, the results revealed that through combined collaborative efforts with criminal justice agencies working in conjunction with public health organizations and others, the interventions proved successful in reducing AV in the targeted areas. Therefore, policy experts recommend that future research investigations should identify how these partnerships were successful and implement them in other areas when addressing AV. Furthermore, these efforts also revealed similar challenges that both agencies faced when addressing AV. As such, those challenges can inform further collaborations that mobilize more resources to confront violence on the individual, relationship, community, and societal level (Gebo, 2022).

On a broader scale, any strategy that is implemented to reduce AV must include elements that will allow for changes in attitudes and understanding about the causes and impact that it has on victims, and the community and society in general, since it has a "ripple effect" on those who are affected directly and others who are indirectly exposed to it. To that extent, some researchers have called for a paradigm shift in how we view and conceptualize AV including its perpetrators and victims. A better understanding of violence allows for specific interventions to occur before and after the fact by implementing strategies aimed at primary, secondary, and tertiary prevention efforts to address AV before a pattern of victimization is established or by working to minimize its consequences. As such, it means that those who work at violence prevention must engage in educational campaigns that are designed to provide victims with the support and services they need and develop programs to assist perpetrators to turn from violence. Either way, its consequences can prove expensive to everyone, but especially to those without access to education and economic resources since they are the least among us who can afford to defray the cost of the treatment and rehabilitation programs that are often needed after victimization (Rosenberg & Fenley, 1991).

Summary

Each day, many Americans (e.g., men, women, elderly, and children) are the victims of various forms of AV that typically include homicide, sexual assault, intimate personal violence, workplace violence, child physical and sexual abuse, and other victimizations that present negative health consequences often requiring either short- or long-term treatment and rehabilitation. When people either experience or become exposed to acts of AV, it sometimes manifests in physical, psychological, emotional, and social problems that in some cases may not result in injury, disability, or death, but rather, the need for therapeutic treatment programs that may last for decades depending on the type of AV experienced. Research reveals that the nature and extent of AV is pervasive and problematic in the U.S. as well as in other nations in the global community. While there are many types of AV such as homicides, nonfatal violence, sexual assaults, domestic violence, school violence including physical and cyberbullying, a few newly emerging types of AV are now receiving widespread media attention. They include crimes against Blacks, crimes against Asians, and crimes against members of the LGBTQIA community. Those who work toward violence prevention focus on understanding the many dimensions associated with AV and chief among them is to closely examine the root causes that can help to explain why AV occurs, who are its perpetrators and victims and what commonalities they share? This has led public health researchers to isolate risk factors that are linked to the former and latter. Consequently, violence experts examine factors that target the individual, relationship, community, and societal factors. Some experts even suggest that any feasible attempt to reduce violence must contain elements that address these risk factors. Because AV impacts many people, poses threats to individual safety, and are crimes prohibited by criminal law, it is a public safety issue requiring justice agencies to intervene to make arrests, hold offenders responsible, and keep the community safe. Those who criticize their efforts often point to the reactive role they play in the process and their emphasis on punishment. AV is a public health issue because of the negative health consequences that follow acts of violence, and the need victims have for receiving treatment, surgery, medication, or rehabilitation programs for either the short or long term. Unlike the justice system, public health officials are concerned with both perpetrators and victims. Therefore, it typically addresses AV by relying on primary, secondary, and tertiary prevention strategies to reduce the number of victims and perpetrators. As mentioned earlier, global statistics show that AV is also an international problem with similar root causes and negative health outcome to victims mainly the need for treating and caring for those in need of psychological, physical, emotional, and economic support in the aftermath of either experiencing or being exposed to AV. While experts argue AV is preventable, they believe that criminal justice approaches alone are not effective enough to address AV mainly because of its reactive nature, its historical neglect of victims, and its lack of resources including trained personnel to address the negative health consequences of victims. Because of this, public health researchers contend that public health approaches to violence prevention are more effective since they rely on wholistic approaches to crime prevention by enlisting the help of others through partnering with justice agencies, community residents, community action groups, and other stakeholders to improve the quality of life and well-being for communities facing issues of violence. Violence prevention researchers believe that success can be achieved in reducing violence by forming collaborative relationships with others in the fight against violence and relying on evidence-based research that has been proven to be effective at reducing AV.

Discussion Questions

1 What are some examples of assaultive violence?
2 How is the social-ecological model used to explain violence?
3 What are the differences between individual and community risk factors for violence?
4 Why is assaultive violence a public health issue?
5 Explain some negative health consequences linked to assaultive violence.
6 Why is the justice system ineffective when assisting the victims of violent crime?

References

Abt, T.P. (2017). Towards a framework for preventing community violence among youth. *Psychology, Health & Medicine*, 22(sup1), 266–285. https://doi.org/10.1080/13548506.2016.1257815

Agnew, R. (2001). *Juvenile delinquency: Causes and control*. Roxbury Publishing.

Alliance for Safety and Justice. (2022). New national survey of crime victims reveals critical insights into public safety debate. www.allianceforsafetyandjustice.org/press-release/new-national-survey-of-crime-victims-reveals-crticial-insights-into-public-safety-debate/

Altheimer, I., Tobey, A., D'Angelo, V., & Anto, J. (2023). *Violence as a public health issue*. College of Liberal Arts. Center for Public Safety Initiatives.

American Public Health Association (APHA). (2018). *Violence is a public health issue: Public health is essential to understanding and treating violence in the U.S.* Policy Number: 20185 www.apha.org/policies-and-advocacy/public-health-policy-statements/policy-database/2019/01/28/violence-is-a-public-health-issue#:~:text=Evidence%2DBased%20Interventions%20and%20Strategies,Examp les%20are%20outlined%20below.&text=The%20strategies%2

Association of Social Work Boards (ASWB). (2025). Examination guideline. www.aswb.org/wp-cont ent/uploads/2025/02/2025-ASWB-Examination-Pearson-VUE.pdf

Baciu, A., Negussie, Y., Geller, A., & Weinstein, J.N. (2017). Board on population health and public health practice, health and medicine division, national academies of sciences, engineering, and medicine, & committee on community-based solutions to promote health equity in the United States. In J.N. Weinstein, A. Baciu, A. Geller, & Y. Negussie (Eds.), *Communities in action: Pathways to health equity* (1st ed.). National Academies Press. https://doi.org/10.17226/24624

Barr, L. (2021). Hate crimes against Asians rose 76% in 2020 amid pandemic, FBI says. abcNews. www.abcnews.go.com/US/hate-crimes-asians-rose-76-2020-amid-pandemic/story?id=80746198

Belle, D. (1987). Gender differences in the social moderators of stress. In R. Barnett, L. Biener, & G. Baruch (Eds.), *Gender and stress* (pp. 121–143). Free Press.

Berkman, L.F. (2004). Seeing the forest and the trees: New visions in social epidemiology. *American Journal of Epidemiology*, 160(1), 1–2.

Bor, J., Venkataramani, A.S., Williams, D.R., & Tsai, A.C. (2018). Police killings and their spillover effects on the mental health of black Americans: A population based quasi-experimental study. *Lancet*, 392(10144), 302–310.

Bradley, J. (2022). The criminal justice system is retraumatizing victims of violent crime. *The Conversation.* https://theconversation.com/the-criminal-justice-system-is-retraumatizing-victims-of-violent-crime-193067

Braga, A.A., Pierce, G.L., McDevitt, J., Bond, B.J., & Cronin, S. (2008). The strategic prevention of gun violence among gang-involved offenders. *Justice Quarterly*, 25, 132–162.

Brazil, K., Ozer, E., Cloutier, M.M., Levine, R., & Stryer, D. (2005). From theory to practice: Improving the impact of health services research. BMC Health Services Research, 1–5.

Breslau, N., & Peterson, E.L. (2010). Assaultive violence and the risk of posttraumatic stress disorder following a subsequent trauma. *Behavior Research and Therapy*, 48, 1063–1066.

Brown, D.W., Anda, R.F., Tiemeier, H., Felitti, V.J., Edwards, V.J., Croft, J.B., & Giles, W.H. (2009). Adverse childhood experiences and the risk of premature mortality. *American Journal of Preventive Medicine*, 37(5), 389–396. https://doi.org/10.1016/j.amepre.2009.06.021

Brown, M.E., & Stalker, K. (2023). *Social work skills for community practice: Applied macro social work* (2nd ed.). Springer.

Brunstein-Klomek, A., Barzilay, S., Apter, A., Carli, V., Hoven, C.W., Sarchiapone, M., et al. (2019). Bi-directional longitudinal associations between different types of bullying victimization, suicide ideation/attempts, and depression among a large sample of European adolescents. *Journal of Child Psychology and Psychiatry*, 60(2). https://doi.org/10.1111/jcpp.12951

Buchholz, K. (2023). Violent crime: Violent crime rates fall in the U.S. www.statista.com/chart/31063/violent-and-other-crime-rates-us/

Cardarelli, A.P. (1997). *Violence between intimate partners: Patterns, causes, and effects.* Allyn & Bacon.

Carter, P., Walton, M., Roehler, D., Goldstick, J., Zimmerman, M.A., Blow, F.C., & Cunningham, R.M. (2015). Firearm violence among high-risk emergency department youth after an assault injury. *Pediatrics*, 135(5), 805–815.

Centers for Disease Control and Prevention (CDC). (n.d.). The social-ecological model: A framework for violence prevention. ww.cdc.gov/ViolencePrevention/pdf/SEM_Framework-a.pdf

Centers for Disease Control and Prevention (CDC). (2018). Youth risk behavior surveillance-United States, 2019. Morbidity and Mortality Weekly Report-Surveillance.

Centers for Disease Control and Prevention (CDC). (2019). *Fatal injury data.* CDC. www.cdc.gov/mmwr/volumes/70/wr/mm7048a2.htm

Centers for Disease Control and Prevention (CDC). (2021). Violence prevention. www.cdc.gov/violence-prevention/index.html

Centers for Disease Control and Prevention (CDC). (2022). 6 Guiding Principles to a Trauma Informed Approach Infographic. https://stacks.cdc.gov/view/cdc/138924/cdc_138924_DS1.pdf

Centers for Disease Control and Prevention (CDC). (2024, April 9). *About violence prevention.* www.cdc.gov/violence-prevention/about/index.html#

Center for Mental Health Services (U.S.). (2007). *Promotion and prevention in mental health: Strengthening parenting and enhancing child resilience: Report to congress requested in senate report 109-103 and conference report 109-337.* U.S. Dept. of Health and Human Services, Substance Abuse and Mental Health Services Administration, Center for Mental Health Services.

CNN. (2022). It took CNN anchors over 3 minutes to list all US cities that have has mass shootings this year. It's only May. www.cnn.com/videos/us/2022/05/16/us-mass-shootings-2022-new-day-sot-vpx.cnn

Coyle, K.K., Guinosso, S.A., Glassman, J.R., & Wilson, H.W. (2017). Exposure to violence and sexual risk among early adolescents in urban middle schools. *Journal of Early Adolescence*, 37(7), 889–909.

Daday, J.K., Broidy, L.M., Crandall, C.S., & Sklar, D.P. (2005). Individual, neighborhood, and situational factors associated with violent victimization and offending. *Criminal Justice Studies*, 18(2), 215–235.

Dahlberg, L.L., & Krug, E.G. (2002). Violence-a global public health problem. In E Krug, L.L. Dahlberg, J.A. Mercy, A.B. Zwi, & R. Lorano (Eds.), *World report on violence and health* (pp. 1–56). World Health Organization.

Dahlberg, L.L., Mercy, J.A., & National Center for Injury Prevention and Control (U.S.). (2009). *The history of violence as a public health issue.* Department of Health & Human Services, USA, Centers for Disease Control and Prevention.

Daly, M., Wilson, M., & Vasdev, S. (2001). Income inequality and homicide rates in Canada and the United States. *Canadian Journal of Criminology*, 43, 219–236.

David-Ferdon, Clayton, H.B., Dahlberg, L.L. et al. (2021). Vital signs: Prevalence of multiple forms of violence and increased risk behaviors and conditions among youth-United States, 2019. *MMWR Morb Mortal Weekly Report*, 70(5), 167–173. http://dx.doi.org/10.15585/mmwr.mm7005a4

Dawkins, M. (1997). Drug use and violent crime among adolescence. *Adolescence*, 32, 395–406.

Delong, C., & Reichert, J. (2019). The victim-offender overlap: Examining the relationship between victimization and offending. Illinois Criminal Justice Information Authority, Technical Report. www.researchgate.net/publication/330401733_The_Victim_Offender_Overlap_Explaining_the_Relationship_Between_Victimization_and_Offending

Department of Justice (2020). 2020 FBI hate crimes statistics. Community relations service. www.justice.gov/crs/highlights/2020-hate-crimes-statistics

Devylder, J.E., Anglin, D.M., Bowleg, L., Fedina, L., & Link, B.G. (2022). Police violence and public health. *Annual Review of Clinical Psychology*, 18, 527–552.

Diliberti, M., Jackson, M., Correa, S., & Padgett, Z. (2019). Crime, violence, discipline, and safety in U.S. public schools: Findings from the school survey on crime and safety: 2017–18 (NCES 2019-061). U.S. Department of Education. Washington, DC: National Center for Education Statistics. http://nces.ed.gov/pubsearch

Donley, S., Habib, L., Jovanovic, T., Kamkwalala, A., Evces, M., Egan, G., Bradley, B., & Ressler, K.J. (2012). Civilian PTSD symptoms and risk for involvement in the criminal justice system. *Journal of American Academy of Psychiatry and the Law*, 40(4), 522–529.

Elgar, F., & Aitken, N. (2010). Income inequality, trust, and homicide in 33 countries. *European Journal of Public Health*, 1–6. www.doi:10.1093/eurpub/ckq068

Emler, N. (2009). Delinquents as a minority group: Accidental tourists in forbidden territory or voluntary emigres? In F. Butera & J. Levine (Eds.), *Coping with minority status: Responses to exclusion and inclusion* (pp. 127–154). Cambridge University Press.

Fahimi, J., Larimer, E., Hamud-Ahmed, W., Anderson, E., Schnorr, C.D., Yen, I., & Alter, H (2016). Long-term mortality of patients surviving firearm violence. *Injury Prevention*, 22(2), 129–134.

Fajnzylber, P., Lederman, D., & Loayza, N. (2002). Inequality and violent crime. *Journal of Law and Economics*, 45, 1–39.

Farivar, M. (2023). Report: African Americans remain top target of hate crimes. www.voanews.com/a/report-african-americans-remain-top-target-of-hate-crimes/7246965.html

Finkelhor, D., Turner, H., Ormrod, R., & Hamby, S.L. (2010). Trends in childhood violence and abuse exposure: Evidence from 2 national surveys. *Archives of Pediatrics & Adolescent Medicine*, 164(3), 238–242. https://doi.org/10.1001/archpediatrics.2009.283

Fischer, K., Purtle, J., & Corbi, T. (2014). The affordable care act's medicaid expansion creates incentives for state medicaid agencies to provide reimbursement for hospital-based violence intervention programmes. *Injury Prevention*, 20(6), 427–430. https://doi.org/10.1136/injuryprev-2013-041070

Flores, A.R., Stotzer, R.L., Meyer, L.H., & Langton, L.L. (2022). Hate crime against LGBT people: National Crime Victimization Survey, 2017–2019. *PLOS One*, 17(12), e0279363. https://doi.org/10.1371/jurnal.pone.0279363

Fowler, K.A., Dahlberg, L.L., Haileyesus, T., & Annest, J.L. (2015). Firearm injuries in the United States. *Preventive Medicine*, 79, 5–14.

Fox, A.M., Katz, C.M., Choate, D.E., & Hedberg, E.C. (2015). Evaluation of the Phoenix TRUCE Project: A replication of Chicago Ceasefire. *Justice Quarterly*, 32, 85–115.

Gaines, L.K., & Miller, R.L. (2010). *Criminal justice in action* (5th ed.). Wadsworth/Cengage Learning.

Gebo, E. (2022). Intersectoral violence prevention: The potential of public health-criminal justice partnerships. *Health Promotion International*, 37, 1–11. https://doi.org/10.1093/heapro/daac062

Gewirtz, A.H., & Edleson, J.L. (2007). Young children's exposure to intimate partner violence: Towards a developmental risk and resilience framework for research intervention. *Journal of Family Violence*, 22(3), 151–163.

Gini, G., & Pozzoli, T. (2013). Bullied children and psychosomatic problems: A meta-analysis. *Pediatrics*, 132(4), 720–729.

Gonzalez, S. (2022). Houston's fight against crime sees progress under One Safe Houston. *Community Impact*. https://communityimpact.com/houston/heights-river-oaks-montrose/public-safety/2022/06/08/houstons-fight-against-crime-sees-progress-under-one-safe-houston/

Gottfredson, D., Kearley, B., & Bushway, S. (2008). Substance use, drug treatment, and crime: An examination of intra-individual variation in a drug court population. *Journal of Drug Issues*, 38, 601–630.

Hardcastle, D., Powers, P., & Wencur, S. (2011). *Community practice: Theories and skills for social workers* (3rd ed.). Oxford University Press.

Heinze, J.L. (2021). Fact sheet on injustice in the LGBTQ community. National Sexual Violence Resource Center. www.nsvrc.org/blogs/fact-sheet-injustice-lgbtq-community

Hillis, S., Mercy, J., Amobi, A., & Kress, H. (2016). Global prevalence of past-year violence against children: A systematic review and minimum estimates. *Pediatrics*, 137(3), 1–13.

Holmes, J.H., Lehman, A., Hade, E., Ferketich, A.K., Gehlert, S., Rauscher, G.H., Abrams, J., & Bird, C.E. (2008). Challenges for multilevel health disparities research in a transdisciplinary environment. *American Journal of Preventive Medicine*, 35(2), S182–S192.

Howell, J.C. (2010). *Gang prevention: An overview of research and programs.* Office of Juvenile Justice and Delinquency Prevention.

Hsieh-Ching, C., & Pugh, M.D. (1993). Poverty, income inequality, and violent crime: A meta-analysis of recent aggregate data studies. *Criminal Justice Review*, 18, 182–202.

Hunt, D., Chapman, M., Jalbert, S., Kling, R., Almozlino, Y., Rhodes, W., Flygare, C., Neary, K., & Nobo, C. (2014). ADAM II 2013 annual report: Arrestee drug abuse monitoring program II. Office of National Drug Control Policy. Washington, DC.

Jokinen, J., Forslund, K., Ahnemark, E., Gustavsson, J.P., Nordstrom, P., & Asberg, M. (2017). Karolinska interpersonal violence scale predicts suicide in suicide attempts. *The Journal of Clinical Psychiatry*, 71(8), 1025–1032.

Jones-Webb, R., & Wall, N. (2008). Neighborhood racial/ethnic concentration, social disadvantage, and homicide risk: An ecological analysis of 10 cities. *Journal of Urban Health: Bulletin of the New York Academy of Medicine*, 85(5), 662–676.

Kaplan, G.A. (2004). What's wrong with social epidemiology, and how can we make it better? *Epidemiologic Reviews*, 26, 124–135.

Knesebeck, O.V. (2015). Concepts of social epidemiology in health services research. *BMC Health Services Research*, 15, 357. www.doi.10.1186/s12913-015-1020-z

Koss, M.P, Goodman, L.A., Brown, A., Fitzgerald, L.F., Keita, G.P., & Russo, N.F. (1995). *No safe haven: Male violence against women at home, at work and in the community*. American Psychological Association.

Krahe, B., & Berger, A. (2017). Gendered pathways from child sexual abuse to sexual aggression victimization and perpetration in adolescence and young adulthood. *Child Abuse & Neglect*, 63, 261–272.

Krause-Utz, A., Dierick, J., Josef, T., Chatzaki, E., Willem, A., Hoogenboom, J., & Elzinga, B. (2021). Linking experiences of child sexual abuse to adult sexual intimate partner violence: The role of borderline personality features, maladaptive cognitive emotion regulation, and dissociation. *Borderline Personality Disorder and Emotion Dysregulation*, 8, 10. www.doi.10.1186/s40 479-021-00150-0

Krug, E.G., Dahlberg, L.L., & Mercy, J.A. (2002). *World report on violence and health*. World Health Organization.

Lathrop, B. (2020). Moving toward health equity by addressing social determinants of health. *Nursing for Women's Health*, 24(1), 36–44. www.doi:10.1016/j.nwh.2019.11.003

Lawton, B.A., Taylor, R.B., & Luongo, A.J. (2005). Police officers on drug corners in Philadelphia, drug crime, and violent crime: Intended, diffusion, and displacement impacts. *Justice Quarterly*, 22, 427–451.

Lee, E., Larkin, H., & Esaki, N. (2017). Exposure to community violence as a new adverse childhood experience category: Promising results and future considerations. *Families in Society*, 98(1), 69–78. https://doi.org/10.1606/1044-3894.2017.10

Lee, M.R., & Bankston, W. (1999). Political structure, economic inequality, and homicide: A cross-national analysis. *Deviant Behavior*, 19, 27–55.

Lehrner, A., & Yehuda, R. (2018). Trauma across generations and paths to adaptation and resilience. *Psychological Trauma*, 10(1), 22–29.

Li, W., & Lartey, J. (2023). New FBI data shows more hate crimes. These groups saw sharpest rise: Bias-related crime rose in 2021 to nearly 11,000 incidents. The Marshall Project. www.the marshallproject.org/2023/03/25/asian-hate-crime-fbi-black-lgbtq

Luby, S.P., Agboatwalla, M., Feikin, D.R., Painter, J., Billhimer, W., Altaf, A., & Hoekstra, R.M. (2005). Effect of handwashing on child health: A randomised controlled trial. *The Lancet (British Edition)*, 366(9481), 225–233. https://doi.org/10.1016/S0140-6736(05)66912-7

Mason, F., & Lodrick, Z. (2013). Psychological consequences of sexual assault. *Best Practice & Research Clinical Obstetrics & Gynaecology*, 27(1), 27–37.

Menard, S. (2012). Age, criminal victimization and offending: Changing relationships from adolescence to middle adulthood. *Victims and Offenders*, 7, 227–254.

Mercy, J.A., Rosenberg, M.L., Powell, K.E., Broome, C.V., & Roper, W.L. (1993). Public health policy for preventing violence. *Health Affairs*, 12(4), 7–29.

Merrick, M.T., Ford, D.C., Ports, K.A., Guinn, A.S., Chen, J., Klevens, J., Metzler, M., Jones, C.M., Simon, T.R., Daniel, V.M., Ottley, P., & Mercy, J.A. (2019). Vital signs: Estimated proportion of adult health problems attributable to adverse childhood experiences and implications for prevention—25 states, 2015–2017. *MMWR. Morbidity and Mortality Weekly Report*, 68(44), 999–1005. https://doi.org/10.15585/mmwr.mm6844e1

Merry, S. (1981). *Urban danger*. Temple University Press.

Messerschmidt, J.W. (1997). *Crime as structured action: Gender, race, class, and crime in the making*. Sage.

Messner, S.F., & Rosenfeld, R. (1997). Political restraint of the market and levels of criminal homicide: A cross national application of institutional anomie theory. *Social Forces*, 75, 1393–1416.

Messner, S.F., & Rosenfeld, R. (2007). *Crime and the American Dream* (4th ed.). Thomson/Wadsworth.

Metzler, M., Merrick, M.T., Klevens, J., Ports, K.A., & Ford, D.C. (2017). Adverse childhood experiences and life opportunities: Shifting the narrative. *Children and Youth Services Review*, 72, 141–149.

Migdon, B. (2023). FBI crime statistics show anti-LGBTQ hate crime on the rise. The Hill. www.theh ill.com/homenews/lgbtq/4259292-fbi-crime-statistics-show-anti-lgbtq-hate-crimes-on-the-rise/

Moore, S.E., Norman, R.E., Suetani, S., Thomas, H.J., Sly, P.D., & Scott, J.G. (2017). Consequences of bullying victimization in childhood and adolescence: A systematic review and meta-analysis. *World Journal of Psychiatry*, 7(1), 60–76.

Nagin, D., & Paternoster, R. (2000). Population heterogeneity and state dependence: State of the evidence and directions for future research. *Journal of Quantitative Criminology*, 16(2), 117–144.

National Safety Council (NSC). (2018). Injury facts: The complete reference source for safety statistics. www.ehstoday.com/safety/article/21919843/nsc-2018-nscs-injury-facts-now-include-workplace-section

Neumayer, E. (2005). Inequality and violent crime: Evidence from data on robbery and violent theft. *Journal of Peace Research*, 42, 101–112.

Norman, R.E., Byambaa, M., De, R., Butchart, A., Scott, J., & Vos, T. (2012). The long-term health consequences of child physical abuse, emotional abuse, and neglect: A systematic review and meta-analysis. *PLoS Medicine*, 9(11), e1001349.

Okuda, M., Olfson, M., Wang, S., Rubio, J.M., Xu, Y., & Blanco, C. (2015). Correlates of intimate partner violence perpetration: Results from a national epidemiologic survey. *Journal of Traumatic Stress*, 28(1), 49–56.

Oriol, X., Miranda, R., Amutio, A., Acosta, H.C., Mendoza, M.C., & Torres-Vallejos, J. (2017). Violent relationships at the social-ecological level; A multi-mediation model to predict adolescent victimization by peers, bullying and depression in early and late adolescence. *PLos One*, 12(3), e0174139.

Outlaw, M. (2009). No one type of intimate partner abuse: Exploring physical and nonphysical abuse among intimate partners. *Journal of Family Violence*, 24(4), 263–272.

Potts, J. (2021). Law enforcement strategies to reduce violence. Police 1. www.police1.com/chiefs-sheriffs/articles/law-enforcement-strategies-to-reduce-violence-wltHuxvLO0lHLEEk/

Public Health Agency of Canada. (2018). *Trauma and violence-informed approaches to policy and practice*. www.canada.ca/en/public-health/services/publications/health-risks-safety/trauma-violence-informed-approaches-policy-practice.html

Rahtz, E., Bhui, K., Smuk, M., Hutchison, I., & Korszun, A. (2017). Violent injury predicts poor psychological outcomes after traumatic injury in a hard-to-reach population: An observational cohort study. *BMJ Open*, 7(5), e014712.

Reichert, J., Gatens, A., Adam, S., Gleichert, L., Weisner, L., & Head, C. (2018). *Co-occurring mental health and substance use disorders of women in prison: An evaluation of the WestCare Foundation's Dual Diagnosis Program*. Illinois Criminal Justice Information Authority.

Rengifo, A., & Avila, L. (2022). The future of public safety: Exploring the power and possibility of Newark's Reimagined Public Safety Ecosystem" (Newark, NJ: Equal Justice USA, Newark Office of Violence Prevention and Trauma and Trauma Recovery, and Newark Community Street Team. www.newarksafety.org/wp-content/uploads/2023/02/TheFutureOfPublicSaf ety.pdf

Rios, E. (2022). Hate incidents against Asian Americans continue to surge, study finds. *The Guardian*. www.theguardian.com/us-news/2022/jul/21/asian-americans-hate-incidents-study

Rivera, F., Adhia, A., Lyons, V., Massey, A., Mills, B., Morgan, E., Smickes, M., & Rowhani-Rahbar, A. (2019). The effects of violence on health. *Health Affairs*, 38(10), 1622–1629. https://doi.org/10.1377/hlthaff.2019.00480

Rosellini, A.J., Street, A.E., Ursano, R.J. Chuiu, W.T., Heeringa, S.G., & Monahan, J., et al. (2017). Sexual assault victimization and mental health treatment, suicide attempts, and career outcomes among women in the US Army. *American Journal of Public Health*, 107(5), 732–739.

Rosenberg, M.L., & Mercy, J.A. (1991). Assaultive violence. In M.L. Rosenberg & A. Fenley (Eds.), *Violence in America: A public health approach* (pp. 1–15). Oxford University Press.

Rowhani-Rahbar, A., Zatzick, D., Wang, J., Mills, B.M., Simonetti, J.A., Fan, M.D., & Rivara, F.P. (2015). Firearm-related hospitalization and risk for subsequent violent injury, death, or crime perpetration: A cohort study. *Annals of Internal Medicine*, 162(7), 492–500.

Rufrancos, H.G., Power, M., Pickett, K.E., & Wilkinson, R. (2013). Income inequality and crime: A review and explanation of the time-series evidence. *Sociology and Criminology-Open Access*, 1, 103. https://doi.org/10.4172/scoa.1000103

Rutherford, A., Zwi, A.B., Grove, N.J., & Butchart, A. (2007). Violence: A glossary. *Journal of Epidemiology and Community Health*, 61(8), 676–680.

Sacco, V.F., & Kennedy, L. (2002). *The criminal event: Perspectives in space and time*. Wadsworth Publishers.

Salter, J. (2023). FBI report: Violent crime decreases to pre-pandemic levels, but property crime is on the rise. Associated Press. www.apnews.com/article/fbi-crime-report-violence-property-carjacking-murder-fa7c6e3879d3bf16f93bdfa42683b100

Satcher, D., & Higginbotham, E.J. (2008). The public health approach to eliminating disparities in health. *American Journal of Public Health*, 98(Suppl), S8–S11.

Shaffer, J.N., & Rubuck, R.B. (2002). Violent victimization as a risk factor for violent offending among juveniles. Office of Justice programs. Office of Juvenile Justice and Delinquency Prevention. Washington, DC.

Shaw, M., Tunstall, H., & Dorling, D. (2005). Increasing inequalities in risk of murder in Britain: Trends in the demographic and spatial distribution of murder, 1981–2000. *Health and Place*, 11, 45–54.

Sheats, K.J., Irving, S.M., Mercy, J.A., Simon, T.R., Crosby, A.E., Ford, D.C., Merrick, M.T., Annor, F.B., & Morgan, R.E. (2018). Violence-related disparities experienced by black you and young adults: Opportunities for prevention. *American Journal of Preventive Medicine*, 55(2), 462–469.

Siegel, L.J., & Worrall, J.L. (2022). *Introduction to criminal justice* (17th ed.). Cengage.

Sklansky, D.A. (2021). Addressing violent crime more effectively: Excessive punishment is the wrong response to rises in homicide rates. Brennan Center for Justice. www.brennancenter.org/our-work/analysis-opinion/addressing-violent-crime-more-effectively

Smith, N.D., & Cottler, L.B. (2018). The epidemiology of post-traumatic stress disorder and alcohol use disorder. *Alcohol Research*, 39(2), 113–120.

Smith, S.G., Zhang, X., Basile, K.C., Merrick, M.T., Wang, J., Kresnow, M., et al. (2019). *National intimate partner and sexual violence survey:2015 data brief-updated release*. Centers for Disease Control and Prevention. www.stacks.cdc.gov/view/cdc/60893

Steele, E., Mitchell, J., Graywolf, E., Belle, D., Chang, W., & Schuller, R.B. (1982). The human cost of discrimination. In D. Belle (Ed.), *Lives in stress: Women and depression* (pp. 109–119). Sage.

Steffensmeier, D., & Streifel, C. (1991). Age, gender, and crime across three historical periods: 1993, 1960, and 1985. *Social Forces*, 69, 869–894.

Sumner, S.A., Mercy, J.A., Dahlberg, L.L., Hills, S.D., Klevens, J., & Houry, D. (2015). Violence in the United States: Status, challenges, and opportunities. *JAMA*, 314(5), 478–488. www.doi:10.1001/jama.2015.8371

Syme, S.L., & Frohlich, K.L. (2002). The contribution of social epidemiology: Ten new books. *Epidemiology*, 13(1), 110–112.

The Human Rights Campaign. (2022). Fatal violence against the transgendered and gender non-conforming community in 2022. HRC Foundation. www.hrc.org/resources/fatal-violence-against-the-transgender-and-gender-expansive-community-in-2022

Thompson, A., & Tapp, T.N. (2023). *Violent victimization by race or Hispanic origin, 2008–2021.* Bureau of Justice Statistics. www.bjs.ojp.gov/library/publications/violent-victimization-race-or-hispanic-origin-2008-2021

Truman, J.L., & Morgan, R.E. (2022). *Violent victimizations by sexual orientation and gender identity.* U.S. Department of Justice, Bureau of Justice Statistics.

Ttofi, M.M., Farrington, D.P., Losel, F., & Loeber, R. (2011). The predictive efficiency of school bullying versus later offending: A systematic/meta-analytic review of longitudinal studies. *Criminal Behavior and Mental Health*, 21, 80–89.

United Nations Educational, Scientific and Cultural Organization. (n.d.). Violence against children. Pan American Health Organization. World Health Organization, Americas Region. www.paho.org/en/topics/violence-against-children

United Nations Office on Drug Crime (2019). Global study on homicide: Executive summary. www.unodc.org/documents/data-and-analysis/gsh/Booklet1.pdf

United Nations Office on Drugs (UNODC). (2023). World drug report. United Nations, Vienna, Austria.

U.S. Department of Health and Human Services (2024). Mental health. Substance abuse and mental health services administration. www.samhsa.gov/mental-health

Wallerstein, N.B., Yen, I.H., & Syme, S.L. (2011). Integration of social epidemiology and community-engaged interventions to improve heath equity. *American Journal of Public Health*, 101(5), 822–829.

Wathen, C.N., & Mantler, T. (2022). Trauma- and violence-informed care: Orienting intimate partner violence interventions to equity. *Current Epidemiology Reports*, 9(4), 233–244. https://doi.org/10.1007/s40471-022-00307-7

Watts, L.L., Hamza, E.A., Bedeway, D.A., & Moustafa, A.A. (2023). A meta-analysis study on peer influence and adolescent substance abuse. *Current Psychology*. https://doi.org/10.1007/s12144-023-04944-z

Wen, L.S., & Goodwin, K.E. (2016). Violence is a public health issue. *Journal of Public Health Management and Practice*, 22(6), 503–505. https://doi.org/10.1097/PHH.0000000000000501

Whitefield, C.L., Anda, F., Dube, S.R., & Felitti, V.J. (2003). Violent childhood experiences and the risk of intimate partner violence in adults: Assessment in a large health maintenance organization. *Journal of Interpersonal Violence*, 18(2), 166–185.

Widra, E. (2022). New data: LGBT people across all demographics are at heightened risk of violent victimization. Prison Policy Initiative. www.prisonpolicy.org/blog/2022/violentvictimization/

Wirtz, P.W., & Harrell, A.V. (1987). Assaultive versus nonassaultive victimization: A profile analysis of psychological response. *Journal of Interpersonal Violence*, 2(3), 264–277.

Woodward, A., & Kawachi, I. (2000). Why reduce health inequalities? *Journal of Epidemiology and Community Health*, 54(12), 923–929. www.doi:10.1136/jech.54.12.923

World Health Organization (WHO). (1996). Global consultation on violence and health. Violence: A public health priority. Geneva, World Health Organization (document WHO/EHA/SPI.POA.2).

World Health Organization (WHO). (2011). *Adverse childhood experiences international questionnaire.* Violence and Injury Prevention. www.who.int/violence_injury_prevention/violence/activities/adverse_childhood_experiences/en

World Health Organization (WHO). (2018a). The ecological framework. www.int/groups/violence-prevention-alliance/approach

World Health Organization (WHO). (2018b). Violence against women. www.who.int/news-room/fact-sheets/detail/violence-against-women#

Yunus, R.M., Hairi, N.N., & Choo, W.Y. (2019). Consequences of elder abuse and neglect: A systematic review of observational studies. *Trauma Violence Abuse*, 20(2), 197–213.

5

CHILD ABUSE AND PUBLIC HEALTH

Introduction

Lisa is a single mom with three children. Prior to her obtaining employment as a waitress, she was a stay-at-home mom who struggled to feed and care for her children. Due to financial stress, she at times, physically assaults her children by either slapping them in the face or burning them with a cigarette if they fail to wash dishes properly or take out the trash. During the evening hours, Lisa has to leave her children at home with the eldest child, who is ten serving as the guardian. Lisa has received a bonus on her job and can now afford a babysitter; however, the babysitter is an older female who sexually abuses young children. For most children, the family and caretaker/guardian are the primary means of socialization. Ideally, one's family provides endearing relationships, thus, providing emotional and financial support, as well as morals and values. However, there are instances in which family's caretakers/guardians fail to provide endearing relationships, but rather, neglect and abuse children physically, sexually, and emotionally. Thus, engaging in child abuse (CA) is a form of violence that has impacted every ethnicity, race, and socioeconomic background. A 2018 study revealed that there were nearly 700,000 child victims of nonfatal child maltreatment in the U.S. Of this number, approximately, 1,770 children died (U.S. Department of Health & Human Services, Administration for Children and Families, Administration on Children, Youth and Families, Children's Bureau, 2020).

Child Abuse Defined

According to the Leeb et al. (2008), CA and neglect also referred to as child maltreatment, is

> any act or series of acts of commission or omission by a parent or other caregiver (e.g., clergy, coach, teacher) that results in harm, potential for harm, or threat of harm to a child. Other definitions have also been provided for child abuse for example, the National Child Abuse and Neglect Data System (NCANDS) moves beyond a parent/caregiver and includes other persons as defined by State law who act or failure to act with a child

DOI: 10.4324/9781003373001-5

results in physical abuse, neglect, medical neglect, sexual abuse, emotional abuse, or an act or failure to act which presents an imminent risk of harm to a child.

(Administration for Children and Families [ACF], 2012)

World Health Organization (WHO) (2024) has a similar definition, but adds an age limit and states that child maltreatment is the abuse and neglect that occurs to children under 18 years of age. It includes all types of physical and/or emotional ill-treatment, sexual abuse, neglect, negligence, and commercial or other exploitation, which results in actual or potential harm to the child's health, survival, development, or, dignity in the context of a relationship of responsibility, trust or power.

The Child Abuse and Prevention and Treatment Act (CAPTA) in Sec. 3. GENERAL DEFINITIONS. [42 U.S.C. 5101, Note] state,

> In this Act— 1. the term "child" means a person who has not attained the lesser of— A. the age of 18; or B. except in the case of sexual abuse, the age specified by the child protection law of the State in which the child resides; At a minimum, any recent act or set of acts or failure to act on the part of a parent or caretaker, which results in death, serious physical or emotional harm, sexual abuse or exploitation, or an act or failure to act, which presents an imminent risk of serious harm.

This Act states to be entitled to receive funds under Section 106 of the act, "States must, at a minimum, include the conduct described in Section 3 in their State child abuse and neglect authorizing legislation." Moreover,

> federal law defines child abuse and neglect and identifies reporting requirements on tribal lands and on military installations); in some circumstances, state laws on child abuse and neglect reporting also apply to tribal lands and military installations. All 50 States, as well as American Samoa, the Commonwealth of Puerto Rico, the Commonwealth of the Northern Mariana Islands, the District of Columbia, Guam, and the Virgin Islands, have mandatory child abuse and neglect reporting laws that define the terms slightly differently for their jurisdiction and lay out the requirements for mandatory reporting.

(https://act.gov/sites/default/files/documents/cb/capta.pdf)

The many definitions of child maltreatment/abuse have posed problems for researchers since the 1970s (Giovannoni & Becerra, 1979; Finkelhor & Korbin, 1988; Ondersma et al., 2001). According to Laajasalo and colleagues (2023), these definitions limit research, policy formation, surveillance, and cross-country and cross-sector comparisons. Most definitions have not distinguished CA from child neglect. Therefore, Jud and Voll (2019) suggest that neglect may be more difficult to recognize and understand because it is based on acts of omission, rather than, commission. It may be difficult for researchers or policymakers to define neglect because poverty is widespread, and parents/caretakers cannot always be blamed for their socioeconomic condition. Other factors contributing to problems with the CA definition include jurisdictions having their own legal definitions and countries posing cultural differences (Raman & Hodes, 2012).

Leeb and colleagues (2011) suggest that the calculation of child victimization rates for abuse depends on how the definition of abuse is operationalized. The researchers further indicate the multiple sectors which include Child Protective Services (CPS), legal and medical communities, public health officials, researchers, practitioners, and advocates addressing this issue use their definitions, which limits communication across disciplines and hampers efforts to identify, assess, track, treat, and prevent CA and neglect effectively. Moreover, Leeb and colleagues report that victimization rates are often based on reports from a single source. For example, vital statistics or CPS (e.g., National Child Abuse and Neglect Data System [NCANDS]). What may be needed is the development of a uniform global definition of CA.

Nature and Extent of Child Abuse

Tarantola (2018) suggests that persons who have survived violence are likely to suffer negative short-and long-term health consequences. For Tarantola, CA brings about an expression of violence, due to the physical and psychological vulnerability of children and the severity of the impact their exposure to violence may have as they grow through adolescence and adulthood across generations. Fix and Nair (2020) suggest in a 2016 study that approximately, 3.4 million children were reported or suspected of experiencing CA. Most of these children were children of color.

Gilbert and colleagues (2009) suggested that the maltreatment of children was common and caused considerable health issues and educational and behavioral problems for children in the U.S. Likewise, Forston and colleagues (2016) stated that CA and neglect are a common problem with approximately, one in seven children experiencing abuse/neglect over the past year. They further suggest that CA/neglect rates were five times higher for children from families living in low socioeconomic conditions than those in higher socioeconomic brackets. Kim and colleagues (2017) and Wildeman and colleagues (2017) concluded that approximately, one in three children will have a maltreatment investigation as victims of CA before they reach the age of 18, and one in eight children will have experienced some form of CA or neglect during childhood. According to the U.S. Department of Health and Human Services (2020), 1,770 children died from abuse and neglect in 2018.

A study by Vachon and colleagues (2015) suggested that many children/adolescents experience co-occurrences of various types of abuse. For example, in a study of more than 2,200 school-aged children and adolescents who were maltreated, a small portion of the children experienced a single type of abuse; 1% were victims of sexual abuse, 4% were physically abused; 10% were emotionally abused; and 25% were neglected. The U.S. Department of Health and Human Services, Administration for Children and Families (2016 and 2020) contends that almost 676,000 children in the U.S. were regarded as victims of CA and neglect by Child Protective Services Systems (CPS) and approximately, 3.5 million children were referred for potential abuse and neglect. Moreover, the Department of Health and Human Services further indicated that the highest rates of maltreatment were experienced by American Indian/Alaskan Native (1.42%) and Black (1.39%) children.

The National Children's Alliance (NCA) (2022) reported that yearly, well over 600,000 children are abused in the U.S. It is possible that the number may be higher due to abuse that occurred during the restrictions of the COVID-19 pandemic when many cases went unreported. During this period, 3 million children of the 7 million children for which welfare authorities were charged with ensuring safety were investigated or received an alternative response from child protective service agencies. This number was down from previous years with explanations provided by several states which ranged from pandemic restrictions, a reduction in backlog, and screening and assessment policy changes.

Table 5.1 displays national statistics from Milner and Colleagues (2022) for the year 2022. According to the table, a total of 380,494 children were investigated for abuse. Per the table, there were 131,906 males, 246,954 females, and 2,771 who did not disclose their gender. The majority ages of children at first contact were 7 through 12 which accounted for 142,212 children. The total number of alleged offenders was 298,078 with parents accounting for 102,319. Sexual abuse was the largest type of abuse reported in the year 2022; and accounted for 247,543, followed by physical abuse which accounted for 80,246. The most abused children were White which represented 189,088 followed by 69,702 Black children which shows an increase from the U.S. Department of Health and Human Services report in 2018 (see Table 5.1 for NCA National Statistics, 2022).

According to the prevalence of CA, measuring child maltreatment is essential to determining the extent of physical, emotional, neglect, and sexual abuse in order to plan and evaluate public health interventions toward preventing it. Unfortunately, many children's cases never place limitations on determining the exact nature and extent of the abuse.

Types of Child Abuse

Zeanah and Humphreys (2018) suggest that the various types of CA and neglect pose major public health issues. Both the WHO (2022) and Leeb and colleagues (2008) identify four forms of child maltreatment physical abuse, emotional abuse, neglect, and sexual abuse. Children who suffer any type of abuse are prone to poor mental and physical health as adults, regardless of culture and geographical variations (Kumari, 2020). In fact, the global prevalence of CA was revealed in a worldwide meta-analysis which estimated rates of 12.7% for sexual abuse, 16.3% for physical neglect, 18.4% for emotional neglect, 22.6% for physical abuse, and 36.3% for emotional abuse (Stoltenborgh et al., 2015).

Physical Abuse

Fortson et al. (2016) define physical abuse as "the intentional use of physical force that can result in physical harm. Examples include hitting, kicking, shaking, burning, or other shows of force against a child." According to the (American Humane Society, 2003, p. 1–2):

> the most visible form of child maltreatment is physical abuse which has injuries that range from small bruises to brutal fractures or death that can be caused by punching, beating, kicking, biting, shaking, throwing, stabbing, choking, hitting with a hand, stick, strap or other object, burning, or otherwise harming a child.

Physical injury is considered as abuse whether the parent or guardian intended for it to occur. When examining a child to determine if he has been abused, Gonzalez and colleagues (2023) suggest rib fractures are found to be the most common finding associated with physical abuse. They further contend that child physical abuse (CPA) should be considered

TABLE 5.1 NCA National Statistics—PDF Report 2022

Race or ethnicity of total children seen:

White	189,088
Black/African-American	69,702
Hispanic/Latino	69,058
American Indian/Alaska Native	7,291
Asian/Pacific Islander	4,746
Other	22,757
Undisclosed	19,515

Number of the children receiving services:

Medical Exam/Treatment	89,058
Counseling Therapy	112,327
Referral to Counseling Therapy	113,709
Onsite Forensic Interviewing	260,105
Offsite Forensic Interviewing	7,435

Other services provided by CAC	*Children*	*Adults*	*Unknown Age*	*Total*
Case Management/Coordination	361,621	94,052	28,215	483,888
Prevention	1,071,949	364,449	161,607	1,598,005
Other Categories	187,856	149,183	596,468	933,507
Total number of children served:		380,494		

Gender of children:

Male	131,906
Female	246,954
Undisclosed	2,771

Age of children at first contact:

0–6 years	104,927
7–12 years	142,212
13–18 years	132,547
Undisclosed	2,206

Total number of alleged offenders:	298,078

Relationship of alleged offender child:

Parent	102,319
Stepparent	17,765
Other Relative	59,283
Parent's boyfriend/girlfriend	18,657
Other known person	71,795
Unknown	36,979

Age of alleged offender:

Under 13	17,222
Age 13–17	33,358
Age 18 +	193,194
Alleged Offender Age Undisclosed	61,184

(*Continued*)

TABLE 5.1 (Continued)

Types of abuse reported:	
Sexual Abuse	247,543
Physical Abuse	80,246
Neglect	30,748
Witness to Violence	26,957
Drug Endangerment	12,798
Other	27,263

when there is an injury to a nonverbal child; bruises on a child's torso, ear, or neck; burns to the genitalia; an injury to a non-ambulatory infant; or a caregiver who appears to be unconcerned about a child's injury.

Emotional Abuse

Emotional abuse involves acts that can damage a child's emotional well-being including behaviors that harm a child's self-worth or emotional well-being such as being called names, causing the child to feel shame in the presence of others, rejecting the child, failing to display love/affection, and threatening children (Forston et al., 2016). Stark (2015, p. 647) suggests that "emotional abuse is any kind of non-physical abuse imposed from one person to another. Victims of emotional abuse are subjected to repeated threats, manipulation, intimidation, and isolation that cause them to feel anxiety, fear, self-blame, and worthlessness." Emotional abuse can occur along with physical or sexual abuse, and it can occur in isolation. Victims of emotional abuse are those with the least power and resources, and the abuser exercises dominance over them.

Child emotional or psychological abuse is an elusive form of child maltreatment that it is difficult to define and measure (Black et al., 2001). Child emotional abuse is not explored as much as the other forms of abuse. However, it is the most common type of abuse to children. Likewise, Kumari (2020) contends that little societal or research attention has been given to emotional abuse either due to it being less visible than physical abuse or either due to cultural or regional differences regarding what constitutes emotional abuse (Gamma et al., 2021; Kumari, 2020). Emotional abuse often arises from the experiences of parents, teachers, guardians, and others who were abused themselves. They simply transmit abuse to children. Emotional abuse is often linked to neglect.

Neglect

There are examples of failure to act which can result in harm to children. WHO (2023) regards neglect as an act of omission in the care leading to potential or actual harm. WHO further suggests, that "neglect may include inadequate health care, education, supervision, protection from hazards in the environment, and unmet basic needs such as clothing and food." According to WHO, neglect is the most common form of CA. Likewise, Honor (2014) contends that while physical and sexual abuse are the most researched forms of abuse, neglect is the most common and deadliest form, but the least researched. According to the U.S. Department of Health and Human Services (2020), an estimated 1,750 children died from abuse and neglect during fiscal year 2020. This amounts to a rate of 2.38 per 100,000 children in the population. Of this number, 1,091 fatalities were attributed to neglect alone.

Brown and colleagues (2023) suggest that of the one in four children who are abused, 78% are neglected. "Physical examinations may not only demonstrate signs of physical abuse, but may show signs of neglect. A general examination may show poor oral hygiene with extensive dental cavities, malnutrition with significant growth failure, untreated diaper dermatitis, or untreated wounds" (WHO, 2023). Yet one must consider the family or caregiver's resources and whether they are able to adequately provide care that is in the best interest of the child. WHO (2023) cautioned that all healthcare providers are required to inform child welfare if there is a reasonable suspicion of abuse or neglect. For many children, this report may make the difference between life and death.

Sexual Abuse

The CDC (2022) defines:

> child sexual abuse as the involvement of a child, who is a person less than 18, in sexual activity that involves the laws or social taboos of society and that the child does not fully comprehend; does not consent to, or is unable to give informed consent, or is not developmentally prepared for and cannot give consent to.

According to the CDC, many children wait to report or never report sexual abuse. Therefore, only estimates can be provided about the number of children who have been abused. This notwithstanding, 1 in 4 girls and 1 in 20 boys in the U.S. have been sexually abused; and 91% of the sexual abuse was perpetrated by someone the child's family knew and trusted. Brown and colleagues (2023) suggest that of the one in four children who are abused, 9% are sexually abused. Sexual abuse involves inducing or coercing a child to engage in sexual acts this includes behaviors such as fondling, penetration, and exposing a child to other sexual activities (Forston et al., 2016). We will explore child sexual abuse (CSA) later in the chapter.

Explaining the Roots of Child Abuse

Greely (2012) concludes that the first evidence of injuries to be associated with CA can be attributed to Auguste Ambroise Tardieu, a French pathologist who authored, Forensic Study on Cruelty and the Ill Treatment of Children in 1860. Tardieu described acts of abuse in which children are victims of their parents, teachers, and those who have authority over them. Greely indicates that John Caffey in 1946 reintroduced CA when he described the cause of six infants suffering from chronic subdural hematomas and identified fractures from trauma.

Despite CA causing injury to children, it was not considered a deviant or criminal act in the U.S. prior to the 1960s. The investigation of CA as a crime was prompted when Stephen Pfohl revealed how pediatric radiologists examined X-rays of children in hospitals and discovered that the children had been abused (Lilly et al., 2019). However, beginning in 1962, criminal legislation was passed in all 50 states against the caretaker's abuse of children. An organized group of medical "interest" who were concerned with the "Battered

Child Syndrome" conducted a survey of how society responded to those who committed abusive behavior during the 1960s and the impact of reform movements such as the House of Refuge Movement, the Society for the Prevention of Cruelty to Children, and the establishment of the Juvenile Court would have on CA (Pfohl, 1977).

Kempe and colleagues (2007), published the article, "The Battered Child Syndrome;" which characterized children who had experienced physical abuse from a parent as being misdiagnosed and having either a rare brittle bone disease, a spontaneous case of subdural hematoma, or unexplained bleeding disorder, with the catch-all notion of "failure to thrive" by physicians who refused to believe that a parent could abuse a child. The use of X-rays alone to detect CA began to be challenged because X-ray images required a story that the child may be too young or too scared to provide. In essence, the images would not describe the social mistreatment or the political concerns of CA and the need for protection (Kempe et al., 1985). Medical personnel began to realize that explanations for CA extended beyond medical issues and would involve social workers, teachers, families, neighbors, policymakers, and the criminal justice system in safeguarding children.

Fromuth (1986) contends that stressful experiences in children, especially those who had suffered some form of abuse began to be studied during the early 1970s and 1980s. The study of child maltreatment continues to expand from case reports into reports of institutional experiences, database surveys, and literature syntheses (Greely, 2012). Various state and federal laws have been enacted with the goal of preventing child maltreatment and prevention data for CA has been provided by global case studies utilizing social science and medical literature. Despite these efforts, worldwide cases of CA continue.

What Are the Risk Factors?

Risk factors are characteristics that may increase the likelihood of experiencing or perpetrating CA and neglect; yet they may not be direct causes (CDC, 2024). The likelihood of a child being a victim of CA can be detected in some instances by examining the risk factors of the child or the caregiver's characteristics. NCANDS is responsible for collecting nationally standardized aggregate and case-level child maltreatment data. NCANDS reports as contained in the U.S. Department of Health and Human Services Child Maltreatment Report (2023) assert that risk factors can be difficult to accurately assess and measure and thus, may go undetected among many children and caregivers. Moreover, some states may lack the resources needed to gather information from other sources or agencies and may not have the ability to collect/store certain information in their child welfare system.

> In addition, some risk factors must be clinically diagnosed, which may not occur during the investigation or alternative response. If the case is closed prior to the diagnosis, the Child Protective Services agency may not be notified, and the information will not be reported to NCANDS.

Data for Federal Fiscal Year 2021, are provided for caregiver risk factors and the following NCANDS definitions of those factors:

- Alcohol abuse (caregiver): The compulsive use of alcohol that is not of a temporary nature.

- Domestic violence: Any abusive, violent, coercive, forceful, or threatening act or word inflicted by one member of a family or household on another. In NCANDS, the caregiver may be the perpetrator or the victim of domestic violence.
- Drug abuse (caregiver): The compulsive use of drugs that is not of a temporary nature.
- Financial problem(s): A risk factor related to the family's inability to provide sufficient financial resources to meet minimum needs.
- Inadequate housing: A risk factor related to substandard, overcrowded, or unsafe housing conditions, including homelessness.
- Public assistance: A risk factor related to the family's participation in social services programs, including Temporary Assistance for Needy Families; General Assistance; Medicaid; Social Security Income; and Special Supplemental Nutrition Program for Women, Infants, and Children (WIC).
- Caregiver disability: This category counts a victim with any of the six disability caregiver risk factors—Intellectual Disability, Emotional Disturbance, Visual or Hearing Impairment, Learning Disability, Physical Disability, and Other Medical Condition.

This chapter goes beyond risk factors for caregivers and views CA as a complex public health issue, with risk factors that range from the inequity in CA to individual, relationship, community, and social/cultural levels. These factors may assist in understanding additional causes of CA. We explain these risk factors below:

The Role of Inequality in CA

Inequality in CA can exist in the form of poverty, gender, and race.

Poverty

Poverty can exist due to parents/caregivers' inability to find employment or being underemployed. Research (Eckenrode et al., 2014; Kim & Drake, 2023) has revealed that people who live in marginalized communities are the victims of more health and social problems than those who live in more equal communities. CA can be added to these health and social problems. Eckenrode and colleagues (2014) conducted a study using the GINI Index (an index available for counties in the American Community Survey that is regularly done by the U.S. Census Bureau). Data specific to rates of child maltreatment were used from official reports submitted to each state's child protective services agency between 2005 and 2009 to study the relationship between county-level income inequality and the rates of CA. This study covered all 3,142 U.S. counties and linked higher risk of child maltreatment to localities where the gap between rich and poor is greatest; the findings revealed that as income inequality rises, so does CA and neglect regardless of average family income. Further findings revealed that the worst circumstance for children is to grow up in an extremely poor county where there is a great deal of income inequality.

Kim and Drake (2023) examined the county-level association from 2009 to 2018 in the U.S. between child poverty rates and child maltreatment report rates to determine if they changed over time. They examined overall child maltreatment report rates of all children in the county, as well as child maltreatment report rates that were specific to subgroups of children's sex, age, race/ethnicity, and maltreatment type for children and found that the county-level relationship between child poverty rates and child maltreatment report rates became stronger over time in the United States, not only overall, but also within most subgroups (child sex, age, race/ethnicity, and maltreatment type). These findings suggest that poverty may have become more detrimental to the parenting and safety of children.

Gender

Inequalities in gender can be perpetuated in cultures that view males as the superior sex and females as inferior and submissive. According to a cross-national analysis of data from 57 countries worldwide regarding the severe physical discipline of children (e.g., being hit, slapped or repeatedly beaten, or left without adult supervision). Kleven and Ports (2017) used data from surveys conducted by United Nations International Children's Emergency Fund (UNICEF) and Demographic and Health Surveys conducted by the United States Agency for International Development (USAID) from 2011 to 2015. Caregivers completed a face-to-face questionnaire regarding the type of discipline a child between the ages of 1 and 14 received from them. To investigate gender-based gaps, Kleven and Ports used three country-based indices of gender inequity; the Social and Institutional Gender Index or SIGI (which measures discrimination against women), the Gender Inequality Index or GII (which measures health economic and power inequities), and the Gender Gap Index or GGI (a measure of economic, education, health and political power).

The findings revealed that the rate of physical abuse of children varied between 1% and 43%, and the rate of child neglect was between 0.8% and 49%. The research indicated that rates of discrimination against women substantially influence the levels of CPA and child neglect. Moreover, Kleven and Ports found that all three gender inequity indices were significantly associated with physical abuse, and two of the three were significantly associated with neglect, after controlling for country-level development. Specifically, higher scores indicated greater levels of discrimination against women on the SIGI, greater gender inequity on the GII, and lower scores on the GGI indicated greater gender gaps are associated with higher rates of CPA and child neglect. Kleven and Ports conclude that reducing gender inequality might reduce CA and neglect.

According to Ma and colleagues (2022), gender inequality can lead to economic insecurity for women and violence. They conducted a study using data from over 420,000 households, from 51 countries, from the UNICEF Multiple Indicator Cluster Surveys and country-level indicators from the United Nations Development Program Human Development data and found that when economic problems cause distress for parents, it may increase violence against children. The study further noted that high levels of gender inequality and interpersonal violence can contribute to higher levels of physical abuse. Using an ecological perspective, the study examined the association of country-level gender inequality and household-level parental physical abuse and the moderating role of child gender in this association in low- and middle-income countries. The study's respondents answered questions regarding whether they hit, beat, or slapped the child in the face, head, or ears in the past month. A separate index collected by the UN measured levels of gender inequality. Using multiple variables, the researchers calculated the odds of CA and discovered that approximately, 8% of the children were exposed to physical abuse which occurred more often in circumstances where levels of gender inequality were higher. For those living in urban areas or having large members of the household, the level of CA was high. CA was lower for respondents who were not biological parents. Physical abuse was slightly higher for boys than girls when adult inequality was accounted for. Ma and colleagues contend that higher levels of gender inequality could be related to higher levels of violence against women or may be due to fewer opportunities for women. These findings indicate that macro-level interventions that reduce gender inequality are necessary to prevent and reduce CPA.

Race

Kim and colleagues (2017) contend that law enforcement may also explain the racial inequalities in the outcomes of the child welfare system. For example, police conduct surveillance of children in communities who may show signs of abuse and neglect and report this information to child welfare agencies. However, some families are singled out for maltreatment due to the officers' decisions regarding where to patrol. In other words, based on the officers' suspicions and the bias that exists in the criminal justice system, officers tend to patrol along racialized lines in communities where most members may have criminal records, which feeds into the officers' biased perceptions, irresponsibility, and unfitness to properly parent. As a result, children of color may be reported more frequently to child welfare services. Edwards (2019) suggests that in 2015, approximately, 9.7 police reports of child maltreatment were investigated per 1,000 Black children, about 4.3 per 1,000 American Indian–Alaska Native children, about 1.2 per 1,000 Asian–Pacific Islander children, about 4.7 per 1,000 Latino children, and about 5.1 per 1,000 white children. Black children were subject to 1.9 times more police-initiated maltreatment investigations than White children. American Indian–Alaska Native, Latino children, and Asian–Pacific Islander children were all subject to a lower rate of police reporting of maltreatment than their white counterparts.

Diyaolu and colleagues (2023) conducted a study of CA involving biased reports from physicians and nurses, which stated that Black children are victimized more than white children. This study drew from a national database of 798,353 traumatic injuries in children between the ages of 1 to 17 from 2010 to 2014, and from 2016 to 2017. The suspected CA victims accounted for 7,903 (1%) patients. Of these, 51% were White, 33% Black, 1% Asian, 0.3% Native Hawaiian/Other Pacific Islander, 2% American Indian, and 12% were identified as others. This study highlighted the decisions of doctors and nurses (i.e., individuals who are mandated to report their findings) of which injuries would be reported to Child Protective Services. Of the suspected abused children, white children were more likely than Black children to have worse injuries and be admitted to intensive care units. The problem with such reporting is that the under-reported white children may have been sent back to households where the abuse continued. Moreover, the over-reported Black children may be faced with the added stress of parental separation and the shame of having their parents placed in the criminal justice system.

Fix and Nair (2020) tested for disparate responses to minority children with reports of child physical and sexual abuse and examined how child and caregiver characteristics influence whether a case is substantiated (i.e., a case was founded or determined to have occurred by state law). Fix and Nair's study contained a total of 4,186,257 observations with 3,440,182 child IDs in the U.S. reported cases of maltreatment from the 2016 National CA and Neglect Data System. Excluded from the study were children over age 18, unborn children, and unknown/missing cases (0.74% unique child IDs). The child's race was influential in substantiating the decisions, with White and non-Latinx children being significantly more likely to have their cases substantiated than all other racial and ethnic groups. This effect was more pronounced for physical abuse than sexual abuse. Additionally, a unique subset of child and caregiver characteristics influenced child physical and sexual abuse outcomes. These factors differed somewhat between racial groups. Fix and Nair found that differentiating patterns of risk by type of abuse indicated the importance of separating out types of maltreatment in research that attempts to better understand what contributes to CA case substantiation. To address issues of disparity with race, Fix and Nair (2020) suggest using training and prevention efforts such as implicit bias awareness interventions for caseworkers and professionals who work with children.

Disability

Legano and colleagues (2021) suggest children with disabilities due to their intellectual limitations are often perceived as prime targets by predators and this may prevent them from being able to view the experience as abuse, and if their communication skills are impaired, they will not be able to inform others of the abuse. In addition, some forms of physical therapy may be painful, and the child may not be able to distinguish appropriate pain from abuse. Witt and colleagues (2011) and Romley and colleagues (2017) contend that children with disabilities can place additional financial, physical, and emotional stress on parents/caregivers who reach their breaking point and abuse the child.

Individual Factors

WHO (2024) provides several risk factors including individual/child, relationship individual parent/child relationship, and community/societal factors:

Individual/Child

WHO suggests that children are the victims and cannot be blamed for the abuse. Therefore, below are characteristics of a child that may increase the likelihood of abused:

- being either under 4 years old or an adolescent,
- being unwanted or failing to fulfill the expectations of parents,
- having special needs, crying persistently, or having abnormal physical features,
- having an intellectual disability or neurological disorder, and,
- identifying as or being identified as lesbian, gay, bisexual, or transgender.

Relationship Individual Parent/Child Relationship

Characteristics of the relationships within families or among intimate partners, friends, and peers that may increase the risk of child maltreatment include:

- family breakdown or violence between other family members,
- being isolated in the community or lacking a support network, and,
- a breakdown of support in child rearing from the extended family.

Community/Societal Factors

Characteristics of communities and societies that may increase the risk of child maltreatment include:

- gender and social inequality;
- lack of adequate housing or services to support families and institutions;
- high levels of unemployment or poverty;
- the easy availability of alcohol and drugs;
- inadequate policies and programs to prevent child maltreatment, child pornography, child prostitution and child labor;
- social and cultural norms that promote or glorify violence toward others, support the use of corporal punishment, demand rigid gender roles, or diminish the status of the child in parent–child relationships; and,
- social, economic, health, and education policies that lead to poor living standards, or to socioeconomic inequality or instability.

According to Milner and colleagues (2022), Stith and colleagues conducted the first meta-analysis of CPA risk factors in 2009, by reviewing literature from 1969 to 2003. Milner and colleagues provide an updated list of the Stith study risk factors which includes individual (caretaker), individual (child) relationship (interpersonal), community, and social/cultural factors. A replica of these factors is provided below (Figure 5.1):

All factors presented in this section can have a role in placing children at risk of CA.

Child Sexual Abuse Defined

A definition of CSA was provided earlier in this chapter by the CAPTA; however, other researchers and agencies have also provided definitions of the concept. WHO (1999) extended the definition of CSA beyond that which is perpetrated by a caregiver to suggest it is:

> The involvement of a child in sexual activity that he or she does not fully comprehend, is unable to give informed consent to, or for which the child is not developmentally prepared and cannot give consent, or that violate[s] the laws or social taboos of society. Child sexual abuse is evidenced by this activity between a child and an adult or another child who by age or development is in a relationship of responsibility, trust, or power, the activity being intended to gratify or satisfy the needs of the other person. This may include, but is not limited to the inducement or coercion of a child to engage in any unlawful sexual activity; the exploitative use of a child in prostitution or other unlawful sexual practices; the exploitative use of children in pornographic performances and materials.

As Murray and colleagues (2014) noted, the WHOs definition encompasses a broad array of behaviors, and they highlight the fact that children may not be aware of their victimization (e.g., being filmed or photographed) and that consent may not be given by the child. However, by definition, children are not of legal majority, and therefore, cannot give consent; thus, any sexual activity with a minor child falls under the definition of childhood

Individual (caretaker) level risk factors
Parent gender
Parent race
Parent age
Single parent
Non-biological parent/caretaker
Lower level of education
Unemployed
Lower socioeconomic status
Length of time in residence
Poor relationship with own parents
Childhood history of child neglect
Childhood history of child emotional abuse
Childhood history of child physical abuse
Childhood history of observing child maltreatment
Childhood history of observing marital violence
Experienced parents with mental health problems
Experienced unstable childhood family structure
Lacked childhood social support
History of criminal behavior
Unplanned pregnancy
Unwanted child
Poor prenatal care
Physical health problems
Psychophysiological reactivity
Neuropsychological problems
Cognitive limitations
Mental retardation
Psychopathology (other than those individually listed)
Psychosis Personality disorders (DSM-V, Cluster B: Antisocial PD, Borderline PD, Histrionic PD, Narcissistic PD)
Emotion-regulation difficulties
Lack of impulsive control
Aggressive
Lacks assertive skills
Trait anger
State anger
Trait anxiety
State anxiety
Hostility
Alexithymia (i.e., lacking emotional awareness, social attachment, and interpersonal relating)
Depression
Trauma symptoms (including PTSD)
Poor problem-solving skills
Parenting skill deficits
Poor general coping skills
More likely to use emotion-focused coping
Poor communication skills
Lack of communication with child
Adult attachment problems
Failure to bond with infant

FIGURE 5.1 Putative CPA Risk Factors Drawn from Perspective Models and Theories.

Adult attachment problems
Lack of social support
Social isolation
Loneliness
General stress
Personal stress
Parenting stress
Family stress
Feeling distressed
External locus of control
Lack of ego development
Low self-esteem/Poor ego-strength
Emotion recognition problems
Lack of empathy (dispositional)
Lack of empathy (child-related)
Parent perceives child as a problem
Negative child-related schema
Negative child-related attributions
Negative child-related affect
Lacks knowledge of child development
Unrealistic child-related expectations
Rigid child-related expectations
Negative expectations of child's behavior
Less likely to consider mitigating factors when evaluating a child's behaviors
Approval of corporal punishment
Greater use of harsh verbal discipline
Greater use of harsh physical discipline
Believes in punishment as retribution for child behaviors
More coercive child interactions
Less frequent positive (instrumental and emotional) child-directed behaviors
Maintains attitudes that support violence
Alcohol use/abuse
Substance abuse (illegal, prescription)

Individual (child) level risk (vulnerability) factors
Child gender
Child age
Prenatal problems
Premature infant
Postnatal problems
Adopted child
Foster child Infant attachment problems
Child disability/special needs child (physically handicapped/mentally handicapped)
Temperamentally difficult child
Child social competence
Child externalizing behaviors (e.g., impulsive, defiant, aggressive)
Child internalizing behaviors (e.g., fearful, withdrawn, depressed)

FIGURE 5.1 (Continued)

Relationship (interpersonal) level risk factors
Number of children in family
Family size
Transient caregivers in home
Unstable family structure
Marital discord
Lack of family cohesion
Lack of family support
Lack of family expressiveness
Lack of marital satisfaction
Inability to maintain supportive relationships
Family conflict
Spouse/intimate partner violence
Parents of abuser had mental health problems
Unemployed family members
Economic insecurity/lack of resources
Family residential instability
High family mobility
Socially isolated family
Fewer overall interactions with child
More negative parent-child interactions
More disruptive child interactions
Fewer synergistic child interactions
Less responsive/less modulation in response to their child's behaviors
Fewer helpful verbal instructions
More intrusive child directives
More negative feedback (e.g., disparaging, refusing to give help, threatening, teasing).
Less teaching (e.g., "showing, demonstrating, positioning")
Fewer positive parenting behaviors (instrumental and emotional support)
Less use of positive reinforcement (e.g., praise, rewards), especially for prosocial behavior

Community level risk factors
Neighborhood poverty
Neighborhood residential density
Neighborhood residential instability
Lack of employment opportunities
Lack of available childcare
Lack of community cohesion
Lack of community social connections
Availability of alcohol/drugs Level of neighborhood violence
Community tolerance of violence Lack of institutional support (from social welfare and judicial systems)

Societal/cultural level risk factors
Culturally sanctioned use of physical force
Cultural acceptance of corporal punishment of children
Cultural acceptance of violence
Cultural acceptance of exploitative interpersonal relationships
Devaluing children and other dependent individuals
Culture overvalues family privacy

FIGURE 5.1 (Continued)

Cultural values of competition versus cooperation
Individualistic versus collectivist systems
Inegalitarian/hierarchical social structures
Inequitable, alienating economic system (lack of equal opportunity)
Societal acceptance of permanent poor

Note: CPA = child physical abuse. Frequently, the CPA risk factors in this list overlap. However, each factor represents a risk factor described in a perspective, model, or theory. Therefore, overlapping CPA risk factors were included to be inclusive instead of selective.

FIGURE 5.1 (Continued)

sexual abuse. In 2018, WHO added the word "adolescent" to its definition of CSA and it reads:

> The involvement of a child or an adolescent in sexual activity that he or she does not fully comprehend and is unable to give informed consent to, or for which the child or adolescent is not developmentally prepared and cannot give consent, or that violates the laws or social taboos of society.

Putman's (2003) definition of CSA includes activities that constitute CSA such as intercourse, attempted intercourse, oral–genital contact, fondling of genitals directly or through clothing, exhibitionism or exposing children to adult sexual activity or pornography, and the use of the child for prostitution or pornography. Pulverman and colleagues (2018) note that:

> child sexual abuse can be defined as an unwanted sexual activity between an adult and a child, including vaginal, oral, and anal penetration. Besides, online child sexual abuse, including online sex, child pornography, and others, is also considered a vital type of child sexual abuse.

Fortson et al. (2016) define CSA as the involvement of a child (person less than 18 years old) in sexual activity that violates the laws or social taboos of society and that he does not fully comprehend; does not consent to or is unable to give informed consent to or is not developmentally prepared for and cannot give consent to. Daley and Gutovitz (2023) suggest that CSA is "the involvement of children or adolescents in sexual activities that he or she does not fully comprehend and can include exhibitionism, fondling, oral-genital contact, and rectal or vaginal penetration." Mathews and Collin-Vézina's (2019) definition of CSA is the unconscionability of the acts, which further indicates four types of activities such as the relationship of power between an adult and child, the child in the lower position facing inequality, the child's susceptibility is exploited based on their detriment, and truancy of true consent explains one of the inequality of CSA in that the child is in a lower position during CSA and has no recourse other than to be subjected to sexual abuse due to the power of the adult over the child.

Just as there are issues with defining CA, there are issues with defining CSA. Jud and Voll (2019) suggest that CSA has its own subtypes and definitional complexities and CSA definitions cover perpetrators beyond parents and caregivers while CA or maltreatment definitions assume a parent/caregiver as the perpetrator of physical abuse, neglect, and psychological maltreatment. According to Wild and colleagues (2020), there are different definitions of CSA. For example, sexual harassment can arise on a continuum of power and control, from non-contact sexual assault (such as exhibitionistic actions) to contact sexual assault (such as rape). Along with sexual harassment, internet sexual offending, and human trafficking are often not included in some of the definitions of CSA. This category concerns the distribution, acquisition, and possession of child sexual exploitation material, child grooming, and violent online contact with children for gratifying sexual desire (e.g., receiving sexually explicit images or cybersex). Singh and colleagues (2014) suggest that estimates of CSA can vary widely depending on the country under study and the definitions used for CSA. Therefore, this poses additional problems for researchers and policymakers. Perhaps, there needs to be a universal definition of CSA, given all its complexities.

Nature and Extent of Child Sexual Abuse

CSA occurs between family members, in dating, or in intimate relationships. According to the Fortson et al. (2016), many children wait to report or never report CSA. Therefore, the numbers listed below likely underestimate the true magnitude of the problem. Although estimates vary across studies, the research reveals that approximately, 1 in 4 girls and 1 in 20 boys in the U.S. experience CSA; 91% of CSA is perpetrated by an individual the child or his family knows and trusts. In 2015, the total lifetime economic burden for CSA in the U.S. was estimated to be at least $9.3 billion.

The Children's Advocacy Center (CAC) investigated 247,543 cases involving sexual abuse allegations in 2022, around 58% of all cases. While not all these cases resulted in a disclosure, charges, or conviction, it's an indication that the problem of sexual abuse may be much larger than federal statistics show. Daley and Gutovitz (2023) report that by adulthood, 26% of girls and 5% of boys experience sexual abuse.

CSA is not exclusively committed through physical contact which comes from molestation, rape, or masturbation. It also exists in the form of nonphysical contacts such as the internet, grooming, child pornography, or exhibitionism, In fact, most cases of CSA involve fondling and touching (Murphy et al., 2018). The assumption is that most CSA victims are female, but studies by Murphy and colleagues (2018) and Stemple and Meyer (2014) indicate there are more male victims or no significant difference in the gender of the victims. Saunders and Adams (2014) note that because national data surveys such as the National Crime Victimization Survey do not collect data on children younger than age 12, limited information is available about this age group.

Types of Child Sexual Abuse

There are several types of CSA including incest or intrafamilial abuse, indecent exposure, child grooming, and sexual exploitation which also impact the lives of children. These are discussed below:

Incest/Intrafamilial Abuse

Pusch and colleagues (2021) suggest intrafamilial sexual abuse is sexual abuse that occurs within the family. In this form of abuse, a family member involves a child in (or exposes a child to) sexual behaviors or activities. Seto and colleagues (2015) contend that all cultures display feelings of disgust regarding sexual relations with a close relative. Incest is associated with enormous negative consequences for the victims and for incestuously conceived children. In the U.S., a study by Finkelhor and colleagues (2014) found a lifetime prevalence rate for 17-year-old females of 5.5% for sexual abuse by a family member. Pusch and colleagues (2021) suggest that the main predictors of intrafamilial abuse are verbal and physical confrontation between the parents, accepted nudity between father and daughter, low maternal affection, and the presence of a nonbiological father in the household. Certain behaviors, such as sleeping or bathing together, are more common in abusive families. Moreover, incestuous families often show dysfunctional relationship patterns and a lack of affection between family members.

Indecent Exposure

Non-physical contact abuse has the highest prevalence estimates among cases of CSA. Indecent exposure accounts for approximately, 30% of these cases (Castro et al., 2021). Indecent exposure is a criminal act and its laws vary by jurisdiction. It involves the intentional exposure of one's genitals in a public area. In the majority of states, it is not required that someone actually observe the act, or see the perpetrator's private parts, for the perpetrator to face criminal charges.

Child Grooming

Grooming is the process by which a would-be abuser uses manipulative and coercive methods to entice and lure a child to engage in sexual activity (Jeglic & Calkins, 2018). Grooming tactics can include buying gifts or arranging special activities, which can further confuse the victim. Sexual grooming can occur from religious settings to sports activities. Jeglic and Calkins (2018) suggest that 99% of all sexual abuse involves a form of grooming.

Sexual Exploitation

Sexual exploitation occurs when a child or youth is coerced or manipulated into having sexual activity in exchange for items they may need or gifts or money. Child sexual exploitation can occur via the Internet and does not always involve physical contact. WHO defines sexual exploitation as any actual or attempted abuse of a position of vulnerability, differential power, or trust, for sexual purposes, including threatening or profiting monetarily, socially, or politically from the sexual exploitation of another (Task Team on SEA, 2017). Sexual exploitation of a child online might force the child to either send or post sexual images of themselves, film sexual activities, or engage in sexual conversations. Abusers may use and share videos or copies of conversations as threats and blackmail to force children/youth to engage in other sexual activity.

Globally, 1 in 5 girls and 1 in 13 boys have been sexually exploited or abused before reaching the age of 18 Some recent research suggests that online interaction is now so ubiquitous that it is likely to feature in some form in almost all cases of child sexual exploitation and abuse (CSEA). Increased internet penetration and advances in technology have allowed offenders to engage in CSEA in an unprecedented environment of secrecy and relative anonymity across the globe. While the full scope and extent of the threat of technology-facilitated CSEA remains unknown, global statistics show alarming increases in reported cases to national hotlines and clearing houses in recent years (United Nations International Emergency Children's Fund [UNICF], 2020).

What Are the Risk Factors of Child Sexual Abuse?

Although there is considerable uncertainty about the frequency and severity of child maltreatment, according to WHO (2022), an estimated 20% of women, and 5%–10% of men report being sexually abused as children. There are often various risk factors that cause sexual violence (CDC, 2024). We discuss risk factors that exist in the role of inequality in CSA and include the CDC's risk factors at the levels of individual, relationship, and community. Although the CDC has societal-level risk factors, we combine these with the risk factors for inequality in CSA.

For prevention efforts to be effective, clinicians need to accurately assess the risk of sexual victimization of a child, so that prevention is offered to those children identified as having a substantial risk for CSA victimization. In addition, to reduce the risk of future CSA, clinicians must determine what exactly should be addressed in these preventive efforts (Assink et al., 2019). Therefore, we discuss the role of inequity in CSA as a risk factor and include the CDC's risk factors for perpetration at the individual, relationship, community, and societal levels.

Role of Inequality in CSA

Risk factors involving the role of inequality in CSA include poverty, gender, race, and disability.

Poverty

The national child poverty rate was 16.9% in 2021, but there was considerable variation among states, ranging from 8.1% to 27.7% (Benson, 2022). Children who grow up in disadvantaged areas tend to experience high levels of crime and violence. Runarsdottir and colleagues (2019) note the 2010 research of Sedlak and colleagues who reported that children from families with low socioeconomic status were twice as likely to experience sexual abuse and three times as likely to be endangered than children from families with higher socioeconomic status. Runarsdottir and colleagues also mention a recent 2017 study by Lee and others which suggests that children who experience poverty have a higher risk of severe and multiple types of abuse including sexual abuse.

In poverty-stricken areas, there may also be societal norms that support sexual violence. For example, neighborhood disadvantage, which describes the percentage of single households with children below 18 years and households receiving public assistance, influences the high level of inconsistent condom use among high school students (Bauermeister et al., 2011). Moreover, studies show that higher poverty rates in the community are associated with early sexual experiences and having multiple sexual partners among adolescents and young adults (Brown et al., 2004, 2005; Dinkelman et al., 2008; Muchiri et al., 2017).

Race

Luken and colleagues (2021) conducted a study that examined geographical differences in racial disparities by identifying in which states, children from non-White communities were overrepresented in child protective services reports for child physical, sexual, and emotional abuse through exploratory mapping. The reports on child maltreatment came from the 2018 National CA and Neglect Data System as well as state-level population estimates from the U.S. Census Bureau. The maltreatment rates from these sources were calculated and the disparity ratios were computed with the U.S. Census population estimates. The researchers identified racial disparities in states with unequal proportions of reported child maltreatment among non-White child populations compared to the proportions among the white child populations. The results suggest that Black communities were the most overrepresented non-white community for CPA, CSA, and child emotional abuse. Luken and colleagues assert that these disparities indicate a "structural system" of racial oppression in the U.S. Moreover, Luken and colleagues suggest that although CA was declining due to funding allocated to each state to prevent it, it may be reasonable to suggest that these funds were not distributed equally to non-White communities which have higher rates of substance abuse, mental illness, and stress.

Gender

There are countries that support male dominance and sexual entitlement. Females in these countries are regarded as inferior and sexually submissive. Studies by Butler (2013) and Davies and Jones (2013) find that victims of CSA have been disproportionately female. Likewise, MacMillan and colleagues (2013) conducted a longitudinal Canadian study of Ontario children and youth which revealed that CSA was substantially higher among females than males. It is plausible that female children are viewed as powerless and submissive. Thus, easy prey for male or female sexual abusers. Historically, instances of women engaging in the act of sex offending date back to 27–66 A.D. when it was commonplace for women to stand around a bed clapping while young girls were raped (De Mause, 2008). In addition, intersecting vulnerabilities in children tend to increase risk. James and colleagues (2016) conducted a study of Indigenous sexual minorities in Canada and found that LGBTQI+ children who were members of Indigenous groups reported extremely high rates of physical and sexual violence. The study revealed that since the age of 15 years, 65% of the children had been sexually assaulted. Josenhans and colleagues (2020) and Hogan and Roe-Sepowitz (2023) identify LGBTQI+ status as a correlation or risk factor for CSA and exploitation. However, Capaldi and colleagues (2024) suggest that being LGBTQI+ is not in itself a causal factor of vulnerability to CSEA. The issue is how societal discrimination, stigma, and oppression as a result of LGBTQI+ status increase the risks of victimization.

Disability

According to Sullivan and Knutson (2000) children who have disabilities pose an increased risk of being sexually abused. Caldas and Bensy (2014) conducted a study of children between the ages of 6 and 17 in American school settings and examined the types of abuse, profiles of the victims of abuse, and profiles of the abusers. Their findings revealed that children with disabilities are at three times the risk of sexual abuse when compared with typically developing peers. Children with the greatest risk of abuse were children who had special education classroom support. One-half of these abused children were victimized by peers, and one-half were victimized by school personnel. Caldas and Bensy further found that such factors as the increased number of caregivers for disabled children, and limited access to information and training on personal safety and sexual abuse prevention contributed to the increased rate of sexual abuse among disabled children. According to the CDC (2022), risk factors are contributing factors. As such, they might not be direct causes of sexual abuse. Moreover, not everyone identified as being at risk becomes a perpetrator of violence. The following factors contribute to the risk of becoming a perpetrator of sexual violence. Understanding these factors can help identify opportunities for prevention:

The CDC's Risk Factors for Perpetration

Individual

- Alcohol and drug use
- Delinquency
- Lack of concern for others
- Aggressive behaviors and acceptance of violent behaviors
- Early sexual initiation
- Coercive sexual fantasies
- Preference for impersonal sex and sexual-risk taking
- Exposure to sexually explicit media
- Hostility toward women
- Adherence to traditional gender role norms
- Hyper-masculinity
- Suicidal behavior
- Prior sexual victimization or perpetration

Relationship

- Family history of conflict and violence
- Childhood history of physical, sexual, or emotional abuse
- Emotionally unsupportive family environment
- Poor parent–child relationships, particularly with fathers
- Association with sexually aggressive, hypermasculine, and delinquent peers
- Involvement in a violent or abusive intimate relationship

Community

- Poverty
- Lack of employment opportunities
- Lack of institutional support from the police and judicial system
- General tolerance of sexual violence within the community
- Weak community sanctions against sexual violence perpetrators

These risk factors have led to child abusers as well as the abused child engaging in crime.

Criminal Justice Issue

The criminal justice system responds to issues of CA primarily through its Office of Juvenile Justice and Delinquency Prevention (OJJDP). This agency governs and protects juvenile victims of crime and recognizes that CA may lead to a generational cycle of abuse and violence. OJJDP includes agencies such as law enforcement, criminal and civil court, child protection, child advocacy centers, victim services, and mental health agencies to assist CA victims. Moreover, cases of CA become criminal justice issues the moment a suspected perpetrator is arrested. If that suspected perpetrator is convicted, his case will be heard in either civil or criminal court. Courts will review the evidence and if the perpetrators are found guilty, they will be sentenced to payment of a fine, placed on probation, or incarcerated per the laws of the state.

The OJJDP provides support to its CACs across the country through the Victims of CA program by providing funding and subgrants to CACs. OJJDP awarded more than $43 million of funding to the Victims of CA Act Program which in addition to the CACs has under its umbrella, the Court Appointed Special Advocates (CASA) Training, Technical Assistance, and Subgrants Program; and the CA Training for Judicial and Court Personnel program (U.S. Department of Justice, 2023).

According to the DOJ (2023), the criminal justice system also assists law enforcement officers, due to the difficulty they have when investigating CA to determine if a child's injuries were caused by an accident or deliberately inflicted. To assist these officers, the OJJDP published, "Recognizing When a Child's Injury or Illness Is Caused by Abuse" which outlines questions that assist officers in making the correct decision. Moreover, police officers often interact with families and children, and in all U.S. states, police are required to report suspected CA and neglect to local child protection agencies. In 2015, police filed 4,00,000 reports to child welfare agencies alleging abuse or neglect. This was nearly one-fifth of the national total (Children's Bureau, 2017).

CA can have profound effects on children's behavior and lead to involvement in either delinquent or criminal behavior. Edwards (2019) suggested that the Federal Bureau of Investigation (FBI) data showed a national arrest rate in 2015 of about 45 arrests per thousand adults, an incidence rate similar to the per capita rate of CA and neglect reporting. According to the National Institute of Justice (2017), CA and neglect increase the risk of antisocial behavior such as violence perpetration and criminal activity in adulthood. Edalati and Nicholls (2019) suggest exposure to child maltreatment, especially in the form of CPA and CSA is the most significant predictor of involvement with the criminal justice system through arrests, imprisonment, and criminal activities. For example, Thornberry and Henry's (2013) research demonstrates that children who have been abused or victimized are more likely to engage in violence with family members, especially children or an intimate partner. Widom and colleagues (2015) found that 11% of adults with documented histories of CSA had an official child protective services report for the sexual abuse of their offspring, compared to 3% of non-abused comparison adults. Therefore, CA is a criminal justice issue.

National Institute of Justice (NIJ) (2017) contends that it is not well known how being abused as a child can lead to involvement with criminal behavior, but cite research findings by Herrenkohl and colleagues that assist in addressing this gap in the literature. Herrenkohl's study involved participants who were drawn from the Lehigh Longitudinal Study, which examined the long-term effects of CA and neglect which started in the 1970s and tracked

450 children from preschool to adulthood. The study collected reports of CA from Child Protective Services records and parental reports of abusive parenting when the children were 18 months to 6 years of age and linked the reports to self-reported criminal involvement three decades later. The report also measured antisocial behavior in the intervening years during mid-childhood and adolescence. The findings revealed that childhood abuse increased the risk of adulthood crime by promoting antisocial behavior during childhood and adolescence. It also showed that those who were abused developed relationships with antisocial romantic partners and peers in adulthood. Additional findings from a subset of participants with histories of childhood physical and emotional abuse revealed that female participants were more likely to exhibit problems with depression, social withdrawal, and anxiety during mid-childhood, which in turn, increased the risk of adult crime. The male participants were more likely to exhibit behavioral problems such as aggression, hostility, and delinquency during mid-childhood, which led to adult criminal behavior.

NIJ (2017) suggests that in Herrenkohl and colleagues' research, individuals with proven histories of child maltreatment were more likely to perpetrate sexual and physical intimate partner violence in adulthood compared to their non-maltreated peers. The research did not examine the processes by which child maltreatment leads to violence perpetration in adulthood. While these studies examined data regarding the involvement of CA victims in criminal behavior, more research needs to be done to further narrow the gap in the literature on how being abused as a child can lead to criminal behavior as an adult.

Public Health Issue

Of the 4 million children who were involved in maltreatment investigations in 2020, more than 618,000 of them were victims of abuse (U.S. Department of Health and Human Services, 2020). The Department of Health and Human Services reports that there were approximately, 1,750 children's deaths from abuse or neglect in 2020. This was a rate of about 2 per 100,000 children. The rate per 100,000 for children's deaths from abuse or neglect has remained steady since 2005. However, almost half of the victims were younger than one year old.

According to WHO (2024), CA has short- and long-term physical, sexual, and mental health consequences which include head injuries, severe disability, post-traumatic stress, anxiety, depression, and sexually transmitted infections. For the adolescent females, Finkler and colleagues (2015) suggest that at least one in seven children experienced CA or neglect in the past year in the U.S., although several cases are unreported. In 2021, 1,820 children died of abuse and neglect in the U.S. (U.S. Department of Health and Human Services, 2023). According to Gilbert and colleagues (2009), childhood abuse and neglect are important from a public health perspective because it has long-lasting effects on adult mental health, drug and alcohol misuse, and obesity. Similarly, WHO suggests that due to CA being associated with substance abuse and smoking, it can cause cardiovascular diseases and cancer. CA poses trauma to children and studies have shown that it causes problems such issues as depression, post-traumatic stress disorder (PTSD), depression, and anxiety which can be carried into adulthood.

Just as CA has long-lasting effects on adults, so does CSA. CSA is associated with various negative health outcomes which come from abusers from every segment of the population.

According to Lindert and colleagues (2014) and Nanni and colleagues (2012), abused children suffer from depression, physical health issues, and suicidal tendencies. Noll and others (2019) suggest that children who have been sexually abused have problematic sexual behavior. Nagtegaal and Boonmann (2022) contend that CSA is related to sexual, health, and psychological problems. According to the Young Women's Christian Association (YWCA) (2017), approximately, 500,000 children face sexual abuse yearly. A report by the UNICEF (2020) revealed that more than 120 million individuals worldwide face forced sexual acts during their childhood. Most are females (89%), and 11% are males.

Both WHO and CDC recognize CA as a public health issue. The number of children's deaths each year from abuse, and the growing percentages of children who suffer from neglect and sexual abuse coupled with the short and long-term mental and physical illnesses that linger into adulthood account for CA being viewed as a public health issue that must be prevented.

International Comparative Statistics

CA is a global phenomenon that causes injury and death to children. Estimates from the UNICEF reveal that approximately, 400 million children under 5 or 6 in 10 children of that same age group globally experience psychological aggression or physical punishment in the home regularly. Of this, 330 million are punished by physical means (UNICEF, 2025). An October report by the UNICEF further found that one in 5 women and 1 in 7 men reported having been sexually abused as a child (UNICEF, 2025). According to WHO, CA/maltreatment has data that is missing from several low and middle-income countries, but global data indicate that child maltreatment poses life-long consequences for abused children (WHO, 2022). Regarding death, WHO (2022; 2024) reports that yearly, there are an estimated 40,150 homicides of children under the age of 18 and some include children who have been abused. However, WHO cautions that the true numbers of children's deaths are underestimated and deaths from CA are often attributed to falls and burns. WHO similar to Singh and colleagues (2014) suggests that CA is complex and difficult to study, and estimates vary depending on the research method used by a country. These estimates depend on (1) the definition of child maltreatment used; (2) the type of child maltreatment studied; (3) the quality and coverage of official statistics; and (4) the quality and coverage of surveys that request self-reports from victims, parents, or caregivers.

WHO (2021) suggests that physical punishment of children is a global occurrence that happens in homes and schools. Approximately, 60% of children aged 2–14 are physically punished by their parents or caregivers. WHO also reported data from the United National International Children Emergency Fund which contained representative surveys from 56 countries from 2005 through 2013 that revealed almost 6 out of 10 children ranging in age from 2 to 14 had experienced corporal punishment from adults in their homes within the past month. The report suggests that on average, 17% of children experienced severe physical punishment in some countries and this figure was exceeded by 40% in other countries. The punishment ranged from being hit on the head, face, or ears (WHO, 2021).

In 2018, WHO reported that approximately, 150 million girls and 73 million children younger than 18 had been victims of violence and sexual exploitation during childhood. WHO (2022) later reported that one in 5 women and 1 in 13 men report having been sexually abused as a child aged 0–17 years. This organization also reports that 120 million girls and young women under 20 years of age have suffered some form of forced sexual contact.

Push and colleagues (2021) cite a 2015 article by Neutze and Osterheider who conducted a gender-representative anonymous online survey of 7,909 young adults in Germany regarding sexual abuse. A total of 8.5% of the participants reported having suffered sexual abuse in childhood and as a youth. Push and colleagues also cite a 2018, German study conducted by Witt and others which compared the data sets of two surveys on CSA from the years 2010 with 2,504 participants and 2016 with 2,510 participants each. In 2010, 12.6% (n = 316) of the participants reported having experienced sexual abuse. Using the screening version of the Childhood Trauma Questionnaire, abuse experiences were rated as mild or moderate in 6.3% (n = 158), moderate to severe in 4.4% (n = 111), and severe to extreme sexual abuse in 1.9% (n = 48) of the participants. In 2016, a total of 13.9% (n = 349) individuals reported sexual abuse in childhood, with 6.3% (n = 159) grading the abuse slight to moderate, 5.3% (n = 133) moderate to severe, and 2.3% (n = 58) severe to extreme. This study revealed that two-thirds of the youth and young adults had not informed anyone of their abuse before they participated in the study, and only 1% of those who had been abused reported the incident to authorities. Push and colleagues further indicate that Neutze and Osterheider found that two-thirds of the affected youths and young adults had not told anybody about the abuse before they participated in the study. Only 1% of the experiences of abuse had been reported to the authorities.

Public Health and Social Work

Intersection of Public Health and Social Work

Social workers play a critical role in preventing CA since they are often front-line workers employed by departments of health and social services, emergency departments, schools, and mental health and substance abuse treatment facilities (U.S. Bureau of Labor Statistics, 2024). Licensed clinical social workers can treat CA victims as well as perpetrators of the behavior (Ennis et al., 1995). Because they are often the first service provider to contact children and families experiencing abuse, social workers *identify risk factors* such as family conflict, financial strain, mental health issues, substance use, and other types of abuse such as domestic violence. They also identify early signs of abuse, provide crisis intervention, family and child counseling and support services, create safety plans, and coordinate response systems when needed to place children or an abused parent/caregiver in a safe placement.

Social work and public health often intervene in their CA prevention functions. Both social work and public health can assist in designing and providing targeted interventions for high-risk families and children by implementing programs that include home visitation and support groups (Lee, 2024). For example, in a study involving public health nurses doing home visits, the nurses created a specific process for reporting suspected CA that "maximized child safety, highlighted maternal strengths, and created opportunities to maintain the nurse-client relationship" (Jack et al., 2021, p. 1). Public health workers can also play a role in prevention by assisting victims with finding intervention services and rehabilitation programs for offenders.

Health Disparities and Health Equities

The CA literature has established a link between abuse and negative outcomes in childhood, adolescence, and adulthood. It suggests that abuse that occurs early in life with a long duration has the greatest effects on development (Dunn et al., 2018). CA and neglect increase the likelihood of developing psychiatric disorders such as depression and bipolar disease (Anand et al., 2015; Chapman et al., 2004). Where bipolar disorder is concerned, childhood maltreatment is associated with a more destructive disease course, with a greater number and intensity of mood episodes, and a more severe psychosis (Agnew-Blais & Danese, 2016; Daruy-Filho et al., 2011; Povlova et al., 2018). Moreover, abuse experienced during childhood is also linked to a greater vulnerability to anxiety disorders, PTSD, substance use disorders, and an increased risk of suicide (Withers et al., 2013). The reasons for marked susceptibility to mental health disorders are related to persistent biological alternations such as systemic inflammation (Danese et al., 2007; Toft et al., 2018), increased plasma CRP levels, and increased body mass index (Aas et al., 2016), alterations of the hypothalamic–pituitary–adrenal (HPA) axis and corticotropin-releasing factor (CRF) circuits, and the role that genetics plays in the development of mood disorders following childhood stressors (Nemeroff, 2016). Early life abuse also has a demonstrated link to high-risk health behaviors such as smoking, alcohol consumption, and drug use (Hughes et al., 2017; Shin et al., 2016) with a progression toward heavy polysubstance use (Hyucksun, 2012) and substance use disorders (Garami et al., 2019; Lei et al., 2018). In addition to a reduction in life expectancy (Sachs-Ericsson et al., 2017), CA is also correlated with the increased likelihood of experiencing certain medical conditions that include coronary artery disease, myocardial infarction, cerebrovascular disease and stroke, type II diabetes, asthma, as well as certain types of cancer (Nemeroff, 2016).

Negative Health Consequences of Child Abuse

Children who are abused and neglected may not only suffer physical injuries, but may also suffer from emotional and psychological problems such as post-traumatic stress and anxiety (Leeb et al., 2011). CA and neglect can also affect broader health outcomes, mental health, social development, and risk-taking behavior into adolescence and adulthood. Strong evidence confirms that childhood violence increases the risks of injury, sexually transmitted infections, including HIV, mental health problems, delayed cognitive development, reproductive health problems, involvement in sex trafficking, and noncommunicable diseases, which, in turn, can cause damage to the nervous, endocrine, circulatory, musculoskeletal, reproductive, respiratory, and immune systems.

The physical abuse of children is likely to cause behavioral, emotional, and psychological issues (Fayaz, 2019). Fayaz mentions that studies conducted in 2003 by Gover and Mackenzie; Harden; and Kilpatrick and others discovered that CPA is a predictor of depression. Buctchart and others (2006) suggested that in non-fatal cases of CA, direct physical injury causes less morbidity to the child than the long-term impact of the violence on the child's neurological, cognitive, emotional development, and overall health. Fayaz (2019) contends that other indicators of CPA are poor school performance, substance abuse, and engaging in criminal/delinquent behavior.

Children who suffer from neglect may have short and long-term problems. These children may find it difficult to maintain relationships with others, and as they become older with their own children. Neglected children may experience depression, and PTSD (Fayaz, 2019). They may also experience cognitive disorders such as impaired memory, abuse of substances, and running away from home (Child Welfare Information Gateway, 2009).

A child who has been sexually abused might experience symptoms such as genital bleeding, vaginal/urethral discharge, urinary tract infection, sexualized behavior, depression, eating disorders, impaired ability to cope with stress, and suicidal tendencies (Allnock et al., 2009; Lo iocabo et al., 2021). Studies by Devries and colleagues (2014), Windom and colleagues (2012), Ports and colleagues (2016), and Wild (2020) have found linkages between a child's having a history of CSA and negative health outcomes such as mental health problems, drug and alcohol abuse, suicide and self-harming behaviors, re-victimization, poor educational attainment, physical health dysfunctions, and decreased life satisfaction. Other negative health consequences of sexual abuse have been identified by Tang and colleagues (2018), and include injuries, unintended pregnancy, and genital infections. Essabar and colleagues (2015); as well as Moaris and colleagues (2018) found that individuals who were sexually abused in childhood were more inclined to develop behavioral and psychological problems which ranged from sleep disturbance, eating disorders, self-esteem issues, and fear and anxiety. Vrolijk-Bosscheart and colleagues (2018) assert that CSA harms the physical health of children and can lead to genital pain, genital bleeding, and incontinence.

Pandey and colleagues (2020) suggest that there is growing literature in countries with high and low income that indicates that emotional abuse possibly has the most negative mental health impact of all types of childhood abuse. Emotional abuse for children is associated with symptoms of depression and can bring on substance abuse and suicidal risk (Martins et al., 2014). Children who suffer from emotional abuse often have psychological, social, and moral development problems, are normally aggressive, exhibit antisocial behaviors, act older than they are, are unhappy, frightened, and distressed, are low achievers, are frequently absent from school, exhibit low academic performance levels, do not make friends easily, their ability to feel and express emotions is impaired, and either show signs of physical neglect or complain of physical symptoms (Stark, 2015).

Criminal Justice Approaches

Many police departments have special units that handle CA and neglect. Police handle noncriminal maltreatment investigations in some jurisdictions (Cross et al., 2015). Regardless of jurisdiction, police conduct surveillance of children for signs of abuse and neglect. They produce information about the fitness of an adult to parent through the application of criminal stigma, and they create both short- and long-term crises of care when they incapacitate caregivers. Law enforcement officers are charged with the identification and regulation of unlawful and deviant behavior. In addition, the juvenile justice system is charged with acting in the best interest of children if parents are no longer able or unwilling.

Many agencies are required by law in all states to conduct investigations in reports of child maltreatment and to offer treatment to families where CA and neglect have taken place or are likely to take place. Many jurisdictions differ in their approach to responding to child maltreatment, but most follow the pattern of identification, reporting, intake and investigation, assessment, case planning, treatment, evaluation of how the family is progressing, case closure, involvement of juvenile or family court, termination of parental rights, and prosecution of parents (Bartollas & Schmalleger, 2013). This process is outlined below:

Identification

- Individuals who observe the family and children on a regular basis and are likely to identify the abuse can consist of teachers, nurses/physicians, police officers, individuals from social services, probation officers, child-care workers, clergy, friends, and neighbors.

Reporting

- The initial report of abuse is made to child protective services or law enforcement.

Intake and Investigation

- A decision is made to either support or substantiate the allegation of abuse or there is insufficient evidence to support the allegation.
- A decision may be made to remove the child from the home.

Assessment

- Protective services personnel must identify factors that contribute to the abuse and address the most critical need(s).

Case Planning

- Plans are developed by protective services, other treatment providers, and the family to alter the conditions and/or behaviors that result in CA or neglect.

Treatment

- A treatment plan is implemented for the family by protective services and other treatment providers.

Evaluation of Family Progress

- Protective services, after implementing the treatment plan, will evaluate the family to see if there are changes in the behavior and conditions that led to child maltreatment.

Case Closure

- Cases may be closed due to progress made in the home and others are closed when a determination is made that the family will not protect the child. At this point, the child is removed from the home and parental rights may be terminated so that permanent alternatives can be found for the child.

Involvement of Juvenile or Family Court

- The case is referred to juvenile court when an adjudication (fact-finding) hearing is held if a petition of abuse or neglect has been filed by the Department of Social Services.
- States vary in the standards of proof needed to substantiate allegations of CA and neglect. Some states rely on the caseworker's judgment, some on credible evidence, some on the preponderance of evidence, and others have no official reporting means.

Termination of Parental Rights

- In serious cases, the state moves to terminate parental rights and place the child up for adoption.

Prosecution of Parents

- Cases most likely to be terminated are those in which the child is seriously injured or killed (Finkelhor et al., 2005).

In addition to this process, the Department of Homeland Security (DHS) serves as a global leader in combating CA and exploitation through its Child Exploitation Investigations Unit (CEIU) which is part of the Homeland Security Investigations (HSI) Cyber Crimes Center. This unit leads the nation in the fight against online CSA. CEIU detects and apprehends producers and distributors of CSA material and perpetrators of transnational CSA; identifies and rescues child victims around the world; and trains domestic and international law enforcement partners in cutting-edge investigative practices. CEIU partners with agencies from the U.S. Secret Service to the Science and Technology directorate to combat the abuse and exploitation of children in 2021. In 2021 HSI identified and rescued 1,177 victims in child exploitation investigations during this same period, CEIU arrested 3,776 individuals for crimes involving the sexual exploitation of children and helped to secure more than 1,500 convictions. In addition, CEIU's Angel Watch Center issued 1,722 notifications regarding international travel of convicted child sex offenders resulting in more than 600 denials of entry by foreign nations (Department of Homeland Security [DHS], 2022). All areas of law enforcement and child protective services work together in responding to child maltreatment. Beyond criminal justice approaches to addressing child maltreatment, there are also public health approaches.

Public Health Approaches

The primary goal of a public health approach to CA is prevention. Higgins (2015) suggests that there is a growing consensus that communities are served best using a public health approach to child protection. The goal of public health approaches for protecting children from maltreatment is early intervention and prevention strategies. Peden and colleagues (2008) contend that within a global public health framework, CA and neglect can be conceptualized as a four-step process with the goals of: (1) defining the problem through data collection and surveillance efforts; (2) uncovering possible causes of abuse and neglect through identifying risk and protective factors; (3) developing and testing interventions to discover the most efficient means of addressing the problem; and (4) implementing and monitoring prevention and control strategies. Higgins suggests four steps for a public health approach:

1 **Surveillance** serves as the first step toward the control and prevention of an identified health threat. Higgins (2015) uses Thacker and colleagues' definition of surveillance as the ongoing collection, analysis, and interpretation of outcome data for use in the planning, implementation, and interpretation of population health. Higgins further states that public health surveillance efforts are initiated to detect and describe a problem that can then be monitored for geographic and temporal trends in its occurrence.

2 **Identification of Risk and Protective Factors Surveillance** provides ongoing information as to the magnitude of the health threat. According to Higgins, the next step in a public health framework involves identifying those factors that place individuals at risk and those that serve to protect them. Higgins states that public health relies on ecological models that allow risk and protective factors to be considered at both the individual and contextual levels.

3 **Development and Testing of Interventions after Surveillance.** In this stage, efforts are used to define the scope of the problem. It identifies risk and protective factors. The public health framework in this stage involves developing and testing preventive strategies. Higgins contends that public health is focused on the health of the entire population, and prevention programs are targeted at different segments of the population. Primary prevention programs are directed at the general population. Secondary prevention programs are more narrowly targeted toward populations identified as having one or more risk factors associated with the problem. Tertiary prevention efforts focus on individuals experiencing the problem with the goal of minimizing negative effects and preventing its recurrence.

4 **Implementation of Effective Prevention and Control Strategies.** This step involves the implementation of effective programs at the community level. Higgins contends that the features are dissemination and continued surveillance which are required over time. Within this framework, the cycle returns to surveillance after the widespread adoption of a prevention program in order to assess its efficacy across the entire population.

Higgins and colleagues (2019) suggest child protection systems have become inadequate and cite the 2014 work of Price-Robertson and colleagues which described two systems; the "child protection" orientation which is found in Australia, Canada, the U.K., and in America, and the "family service" orientation found in Belgium, Sweden, and Denmark. Higgins and colleagues further suggest that a third system, "informal community care systems" are found in countries where formal protective systems are limited. These countries use familial, community, and cultural networks. The Higgins study outlined some of the problems inherent in previous child protection systems that a new public health system would need to address. These issues are not limited to:

• Poor engagement with services—either because of their lack of availability or the fact that families have to be "reported" to child protection to get referred to the services they need to address the issues underlying the parenting capability concerns (particularly mental health, substance misuse, and family violence);

- Instability in care (frequent placement breakdowns resulting in children having multiple carers throughout their childhood);
- The complex link between domestic and family violence and child protection, and the risk of "mother blaming" in child protection responses to situations of family violence;
- Addressing both maltreatment that has occurred, and concerns about the future;
- Overrepresentation of Indigenous/Aboriginal children—particularly in countries with a colonial history like Australia, New Zealand and Canada;
- A far stronger role and involvement for citizens in ground-up, community-based initiatives that mobilize informal helping networks and resources; and,
- Integrated service systems and collaborative organizational approaches.

Public Health and Social Work Approaches

A core component of public health approaches to CA prevention is centered around understanding and assisting in ameliorating or eliminating inequities that are risk factors for CA (Lee, 2024). These conditions include inequities that lead to parental substance use, domestic violence, financial distress, and familial social isolation. Public health is also in a unique position to employ methods that enhance protective factors for children and families on a large scale, such as creating opportunities for growing social connections, improving access to health care, mental health services and community resources, data collection, and educating the public on a large-scale about the signs of CA and reporting protocols. This model also requires large-scale efforts and multidisciplinary infrastructure to bring evidence-based parenting programs that nurture children to the public and political forefront (Herrenkohl et al., 2015). Social workers can work alongside public health officials to offer family education, carry out community outreach such as awareness campaigns and resource distribution, and collaborate with schools to offer child personal safety training, counseling, support, and teacher/staff training to identify the signs of abuse and how to report abuse. Collaboratively, public health and social work can advocate for children's rights, systems improvement, and resources for building community resilience (Lee, 2024).

Integrating Skills of Social Epidemiology to Address Disparities and Achieve Equity

There are hidden disparities based on victims of CA's socioeconomic status, race, and gender that unfairly determine a child's future after the abuse has occurred. These disparities include over-representation of children of color in clinical evaluations, substantiation of abuse and neglect cases from clinicians and physicians, foster care placement, and criminal prosecution. The National Crimes against Children Investigators Association (NCACIA) (2024) has proposed strategies for alleviating poverty for children who experience CA. This is a holistic approach that involves the collaboration between CA professionals, social workers, policymakers, healthcare providers, and community organizations. The strategies include the following:

1 **Providing Economic Support for Families:** Policies and programs that offer financial relief to low-income families can have a significant impact on reducing child maltreatment. Some examples include child tax credits, rental assistance, food assistance programs,

and access to affordable health care. These measures can reduce parental stress and give families the stability they need to care for their children.

2 **Accessing Quality Childcare and Early Education:** Affordable, high-quality childcare and early education programs can help mitigate the impact of poverty on children's development. These programs not only provide children with safe and nurturing environments, but also offer parents the opportunity to work or pursue education and lift families out of poverty. Additionally, early education programs can serve as a protective factor by providing children with supportive relationships and developmental opportunities.

3 **Strengthening Community Support Networks:** Building strong, connected communities can help reduce the risk of abuse by providing families with a safety net of support. Community centers, parenting support groups, and accessible mental health services can give parents the resources needed to cope with stress and build positive parenting skills. Community outreach efforts can also help families feel less isolated and more empowered to seek help when needed.

4 **Trauma-Informed Interventions:** Professionals working with families in poverty must adopt the trauma-informed approach, that recognizes that poverty and abuse are intertwined. Trauma-informed care involves understanding the impact of trauma on behavior and responding in ways that promote healing and resilience. This approach can help professionals build trust with families and work collaboratively to create safer and more stable environments for children.

5 **Education and Job Training Programs:** Breaking the cycle of poverty requires opportunities for education and employment. Job training and educational programs can empower parents to secure stable, higher-paying jobs, reducing the economic stress that contributes to abuse and neglect. These programs can also be coupled with parenting classes to help parents develop skillsets that promote healthy family dynamics.

The NCACIA has also implemented a public health model that involves:

1 **Raising Awareness and Educating the Public:** Public awareness campaigns are a cornerstone in primary prevention. These initiatives educate the public about the signs of CA, how to report concerns, and the importance of creating safe environments for children. These campaigns can also challenge harmful societal norms, such as the normalization of harsh physical punishment, and promoting positive parenting practices. Schools, community centers, and healthcare providers can be encouraged to spread awareness and provide education. By informing the community, we create a culture where CA is less likely to be tolerated and more likely to be prevented.

2 **Strengthening Economic Supports for Families:** Addressing socioeconomic factors that contribute to CA is essential. Policies that provide economic relief, such as tax credits, affordable childcare, and paid family leave, can help reduce parental stress and the risk of maltreatment. Communities can advocate for systemic changes that support families and promote their economic well-being, recognizing that financial stability is a powerful protective factor.

3 **Providing Early Support to Families in Need:** Programs such as home visiting services for at-risk families offer crucial secondary prevention. Home visitors can teach parents about child development, connect them to resources, and provide emotional support. Similarly,

family resource centers can offer counseling, parenting classes, and crisis intervention services, that create a safety net for vulnerable families. Healthcare professionals play a pivotal role in early identification. Routine screenings for risk factors such as parental mental health issues or intimate partner violence, can help identify families in need of support. When identified early, appropriate interventions can be implemented to prevent abuse.

4 **Building Community Resilience:** Strong, communities are safer for children. Community-based initiatives that foster relationships and reduce isolation can have a significant impact on its well-being. Some examples include neighborhood parenting groups, mentorship programs for youth, and community centers that offer recreational and support services. When families are supported and have a network to rely on, the risk of abuse decreases. Faith-based organizations, schools, and local businesses can also partner in building community resilience. By working together, communities can create a network of protective factors that keep children safe.

5 **Data Collection and Research:** To effectively prevent CA, we need to understand the scope of the problem and the effectiveness of prevention strategies. Collecting data on CA cases, analyzing trends, and evaluating prevention programs are crucial steps. Public health officials and researchers can collaborate with CA practitioners and other professionals to ensure that prevention efforts are evidence-based and effective. Continuous evaluation allows communities to adapt their strategies to meet changing needs, ensuring that prevention efforts remain relevant and impactful.

Last, NCACIA (2024) states that public policy plays a major role in addressing CA; therefore, the agency suggests the following strategies to create a more effective system and eliminate disparities:

1 **Funding Limitations:** Many CA prevention and survivor support programs are underfunded, which limits their reach and effectiveness. Public policy must prioritize funding child protective services, mental health care, and early intervention programs to ensure that all children and survivors receive the support they need. Policies that streamline funding to high-need areas and ensure efficient use of resources are essential for expanding the capacity of these programs.

2 **Disparities in Access to Services:** Geographic, racial, and socioeconomic disparities often impact a child's or survivor's ability to access the services and programs they need. For example, children living in rural areas have limited access to mental health services, and marginalized communities face barriers to receiving adequate support due to systemic inequalities. Public policies must address these disparities by expanding access to services in underserved areas, improving cultural competency among service providers, and reducing economic barriers to care. Policies that address these inequalities ensure that all children and survivors, regardless of their background, receive equal protection and support.

3 **Coordination between Agencies:** Public policy should promote better coordination between agencies involved in child protection, such as child welfare services, law enforcement, schools, and healthcare providers. Effective interagency collaboration ensures that children and survivors do not fall through the cracks and fail to receive comprehensive care. The creation of multidisciplinary teams and Child Advocacy

Centers are examples of policy initiatives that encourage collaboration between agencies, improving outcomes for children and survivors by streamlining communication and response efforts.

Similarly, the CDC's pamphlet, Essentials for Childhood (2024), provides goals and strategies for preventing CA and neglect. This document is useful for anyone who desires to promote positive change for children and families. It contains strategies that are organized into four sections focused on a specific goal and related steps that build the foundation for safe and nurturing relationships and environments. These goals and strategies are as follows:

Goal 1: Raise awareness and commitment to promote safe, stable, nurturing relationships and environments, and prevent CA and neglect.

- Adopt the vision of "assuring safe, stable, nurturing relationships and environments to protect children from child abuse and neglect"
- Raise awareness in support of the vision
- Partner with others to unite behind the vision

Goal 2: Use data to inform actions.

- Build a partnership to gather and synthesize relevant data
- Take stock of existing data
- Identify and fill critical data gaps
- Use the data to support other action steps

Goal 3: Create the context for healthy children and families through norm changes and programs.

- Promote community norms that protect shared responsibility for the well-being of children
- Promote positive community norms about parenting programs and acceptable parenting behaviors
- Implement evidence-based programs for parents and caregivers

Goal 4: Create the context for healthy children and families through policies.

- Identify and assess which policies may positively impact the lives of children and families in your community
- Provide decision makers and community leaders with information on the benefits of evidence-based strategies and rigorous evaluation.

Goal 1 suggests that providing safe and nurturing environments and relationships requires partnering with individuals or groups—in government, the public, community organizations, leaders, decision makers, and media to promote awareness, and to change beliefs, attitudes, behaviors, norms, programs, systems, and policies. Partners or stakeholders must be committed to this vision and willing to act. To observe an impact on CA and neglect, there must be commitment combined with comprehensive data, effective programmatic strategies, and policy approaches.

Goal 2 involves gathering data that provides a foundation for engaging partners, building commitment, informing decision makers, and helping partners focus and monitor prevention efforts. Moreover, obtaining data assists in understanding how prevalent and impactful CA and neglect are in the community, the behaviors and conditions that increase the occurrence of the abuse, and the policies that create and recreate these conditions. Data also provides critical information that supports the other goals. These data may come from vital statistics, health records, criminal justice records, childcare and welfare, and education records.

Goal 3 advocates promoting parents and caregivers in providing safe, stable, and nurturing relationships and environments. The CDC suggests that communities can help change policies in support of families, increase access to quality childcare and education, develop safe places or neighborhood activities where children are monitored and supervised, and families can come together, interact, and get to know each other. This provides caregivers with parenting programs that introduce new skills and behaviors that teach caregivers positive child-rearing and child-management practices to facilitate safe, stable, nurturing relationships and environments. In this goal, the community supports all caregivers by providing access to evidence-based parent training programs such as Nurse-Family Partnerships, which focus on improving maternal and child health, and early head start that helps parents build skills to assist their child's development, increase family literacy, and promote healthy parent-child relationships.

Goal 4 posits that creating policies that provide safe, stable, nurturing relationships and environments requires efforts from public and private organizations, which include state and local health departments, the media, and community organizations. There should be an awareness of the societal factors that help children thrive and policies that support healthy child development and resources that support the long-term implementation and evaluation of policies. The policies must have reliable data and evidence-based effectiveness.

Using strategies from NCACIA and the goals of the CDC will assist in preventing and detecting CA. With individuals, communities, governmental agencies, and advocacy groups working together to improve the quality of life for children and their families, the cycle of abuse can be broken and children regardless of socioeconomic status, race, or gender will have the opportunity to live in safe, nurturing, and supportive environments.

How Can Child Abuse Be Prevented

According to the CDC (2024), CA and neglect are serious public health problems that can have a long-term impact on health, opportunity, and well-being. CDC's goal is to prevent CA and neglect from occurring. Therefore, a pamphlet of prevention resources was compiled by the CDC based on the best strategies to assist in preventing CA and neglect (Fortson et al., 2016). They include strengthening economic support for families, changing social norms to support parents and positive parenting; providing quality care and early education;

enhancing parenting skills to promote healthy child development; and intervening to reduce harm and prevent future risk (Forston et al., 2016):

- **Strengthening Economic Support to Families**
  An increase in family income may provide improvements in the child's development, reductions in CPA, reductions in adolescent risky health behavior, reductions in chronic disease, poor academic achievement, and poor health. Family-friendly work policies that allow parents to provide for their children's needs by reducing the risk factors of stress and depression can be found in programs such as the Temporary Assistance for Needy Families program and state Supplemental Nutrition Assistance Program (SNAPS). In addition, employers can provide paid leave which replaces income while families are caring for newborns or recovering from an illness. Flexible work schedules can be provided by employers to allow adaptability during work hours.
- **Change Social Norms to Support Parents and Positive Parenting**
  Two approaches are used to inform the public about CA and neglect and how to prevent it. They include public engagement and education campaigns, and legislative approaches to reduce corporal punishment. Public engagement uses various channels of communication to educate and inform the public via town hall meetings, mass or social media, and neighborhood screenings. Legislative approaches are used to eliminate corporal punishment and use effective discipline strategies. This approach can help establish effective discipline strategies to reduce the harms of harsh physical punishment to children not only in the home, but some states that have outlawed corporal punishment in daycare facilities, after-school care, schools, juvenile detention facilities, and foster care. Changing social norms to support parents and positive parenting can increase public support for policies supportive of children and families, reduce the notion that corporal punishment is appropriate for children, reduce reported acts of corporal punishment, and increase the idea that nurturing children is appropriate at all ages.
- **Provide Quality Care and Education Early in Life**
  Programs such as Early Childhood and Child Parent Centers are preschool programs with family engagement that have documented positive impacts on children's cognitive skills, school achievement, social skills, and conduct problems and are effective in reducing CA and neglect. Also, quality licensed and accredited childcare provides a caring and nurturing environment for children. This strategy produces fewer encounters with child welfare services, rates of out-of-home placement are reduced, and juvenile delinquency rates are lessened.
- **Enhance Parenting Skills to Promote Healthy Child Development**
  Strategies used to prevent CA and neglect are early childhood home visitation and parenting skills and family relationship approaches. Early childhood home visitation programs provide training to parents about caring for children, and providing caregiver support, and child health through home visits. Parenting skills and family relationship programs provide behavior management and positive parenting skills. Among the outcomes of both approaches are reductions in the perpetration of CA and neglect, reductions in risk facts; increased nurturing from parents; fewer visits to the emergency room; and reductions in criminal behavior.
- **Intervention to Lessen Harms and Prevent Future Risk**

Many approaches serve to intervene to reduce harm and prevent future risks posed by CA and neglect exposure or its associated risk factors:

o *Enhanced primary care may be used to identify and address psychosocial problems in the family that serve as risk factors for child abuse and neglect.* Here, primary care providers can address such things as substance abuse, parental depression, intimate partner violence, and harsh punishment.

o *Behavioral parent training programs may reduce the recurrence of child abuse and neglect while teaching parents specific skills to build a safe, stable, nurturing relationship with their children.* Topics covered in these programs often range from parent-child interactions and relationship enhancement skills to child behavior management and discipline skills.

o *Treatment for children and families to reduce the harms of abuse and neglect exposure.* Therapeutic treatment can mitigate the health consequences of abuse and neglect exposure, decrease the risk for other types of violence later in life, and decrease the likelihood that individuals will abuse their own children. These treatments are typically delivered by trained professionals in a 1–1 or group setting and over the course of 12 or more sessions. Treatment is often provided to children at varying ages and stages of development. As such, may engage both the child and parent in the treatment process.

o *Treatment for children and families to prevent problem behavior and later involvement in violence.* Therapeutic treatments are typically delivered by highly trained professionals in a 1–1 or group setting and over the course of several months. Given the focus on youth and the role of parents and caregivers in monitoring and guiding the child's behavior, parents and caregivers are often included in the treatment process or the child's entire social network may be engaged. Children of all ages may participate in these programs, although the specific age of children targeted often depends on the specific program being implemented.

Potential outcomes for these strategies include: reductions in abuse and neglect perpetration; reductions in short- and long-term trauma-related symptoms of the child; including internalizing (e.g., post-traumatic stress, depression, anxiety) and externalizing (e.g., sexualized behaviors, aggressive behavior) symptom; improved parent-child interactions, parenting behaviors, and family functioning; reductions in parental depression, emotional distress, and substance use; decreased number of and time spent in out-of-home placements; reductions in substance use among youth; reductions in re-offending (Forstein et al., 2016).

According to WHO (2025), a multisectoral approach starting early in a child's life is needed to prevent and respond to CA. This intervention will improve a child's cognitive development behavior, social competence, and educational attainment. For society, it results in reduced crime and delinquency. These interventions include the following:

• *Support from parent/caregiver:* This involves providing information and skill-building sessions to support the development of nurturing, non-violent parenting delivered by nurses, social workers, or trained legal workers through a series of home visits or in a community setting.

- *Education and life skills approaches*:
  - o Increasing enrollment in quality education so that children acquire knowledge, skills, and experiences that build resilience and reduce risk factors for violence;
  - o Initiating programs to prevent sexual abuse that build awareness and teach skills to help children/adolescents understand consent, avoid and prevent sexual abuse and exploitation, and to seek help and support; and
  - o Interventions to build a positive school climate and violence-free environment, and strengthening relationships between students, teachers, and administrators.
- *Norms and values approaches*: Programs to transform restrictive and harmful gender and social norms around child-rearing, child discipline, and gender equality and promote the nurturing role of fathers.
- *Implementation and enforcement of laws*: laws to prohibit violent punishment and to protect children from sexual abuse and exploitation.
- *Response and support services*: Early case recognition coupled with ongoing care of child victims and families to help reduce the recurrence of maltreatment and lessen its consequences.

WHO (2025) further recommends increasing the effectiveness of prevention and care interventions should be delivered as part of a four-step public health approach:

- defining the problem;
- identifying causes and risk factors;
- designing and testing interventions aimed at minimizing the risk factors; and
- disseminating information about the effectiveness of interventions and increasing the scale of proven effective interventions.

Policy Recommendations

CA is a global public health problem that can and has caused psychological, emotional, physical, neurobiological deficits, and behavioral problems which can last into adulthood for millions of children. While many organizations have come to the aid of children, much more needs to be done until child maltreatment of any kind is better detected and eliminated. In a series of studies on the prevalence worldwide of CA, Stoltenborgh and colleagues (2015), found an overall estimated prevalence ranging from 12.7% (for sexual abuse) to 36.3% (for emotional abuse) in self-report studies, and a prevalence ranging from 0.3% (for physical abuse and emotional abuse) to 0.4% (for sexual abuse) in studies using informants. Given the rising statistics of CA, CSA, and neglect, we offer the following policy recommendations:

1 Because CSA is a serious public health issue with negative health consequences that can adversely impact its victims, it is incumbent on law enforcement and public health agencies to prevent the behavior. This requires multifaceted and comprehensive intervention programs (Kewley et al., 2021).
2 While programs/policies such as home visitation programs for at-risk mothers; family-friendly work policies, increasing TANF and SNAPSs; paid family leave; and flexible consistent work schedules have been somewhat effective, more needs to be done to prevent CA. Experts also suggest that media campaigns should be used to promote knowledge

of child sexual offenders. Campaigns using multifaceted methods have been proven to increase awareness and understanding and help facilitate the public to take preventive measures (United Nations Children's Fund, 2020). Those seeking to prevent CA and CSA must realize that preventing the behavior requires both criminal justice and public health approaches with a commitment from all stakeholders and policymakers and long-term funding for preventing the maltreatment of children. These efforts should also include state and federal funding for more research in this area (Kewley et al., 2021; Lee et al., 2007).

3 Early CA Education Programs. Policy implementations should be proactive and embedded into school curriculums to prevent CA. Such courses start at the primary level and continue at the secondary level and focus on games or role-playing instead of traditional teaching students are engaged by taking an active role. For example, a study by Gubbel and colleagues (2021) reported on the effect of body safety training and lessons led by classroom teachers reading from a script that prompts them to ask children questions, practice skills, and use encouraging language. This study found that programs focusing on strengthening social–emotional skills of children, avoiding self-blame, using puppets, and using games or quizzes yielded larger effects on CA-related knowledge. Program effectiveness could possibly be improved by integrating these components and techniques into these programs. Such programs should be embedded into the educational curriculum worldwide to increase children's knowledge of abuse, and the preventative measures children can take toward self-protection. WHO (2018) suggests that few school-based programs are offered in European countries. It is also questionable if such programs are utilized or offered in rural community schools or in marginalized neighborhood schools in the U.S.

4 If the situation warrants it, child abusers should be apprehended, arrested, and held criminally responsible. Criminal justice practitioners must recognize that not only CA, but CSA is a growing problem. Therefore, offenders should be given treatment, that includes individual therapy, and cognitive behavioral treatment, in correctional settings to reduce the risk of the offender recidivating once released. The treatment approach should confront the initial thoughts and beliefs that lead to antisocial behavior and offer offenders opportunities to model and engage in prosocial skills.

5 Access to Safe, Affordable Child-Care. To assist working parents with safe and affordable childcare as opposed to leaving children under the supervision of older children, relatives, or neighbors, child-care centers should be established in neighborhoods. These centers should be facilitated by trained personnel who are sworn to report abuse and act in the best interest of the child. In addition, the centers should provide a homelike nurturing environment. Maternal depression is an important risk factor for CA and neglect. Therefore, such a center may reduce maternal depression and improve CA outcomes.

6 Eliminate bias when responding to suspicions in reporting and evaluating CA to promote equity. Clinicians, social workers, and law enforcement officers are sworn to report suspicions of CA. As such, they often engage in inequitable practices and overreport CA in marginalized families and underreport abuse in families with higher socioeconomic status. Efforts need to be made to ensure that those who are sworn to report receive training in implicit biases so that unconscious attitudes, judgments, and prejudices can be controlled.

Concerning law enforcement officers, critics report that implicit biases are found in the nature of their work since the work brings them in contact with people (in their respective communities) whom they see as suspicious, dangerous, or undesirable. This suggests that whether officers are racists is influenced by the implicit biases they acquire from society in general, and their work, in particular (Devine, 1989). To eliminate implicit biases, experts encourage policymakers and law enforcement management teams to diversify their law enforcement agencies and provide training programs such as intergroup contact; counter-stereotypic exemplars; stereotype negation training; and multifaceted interventions. First, a meta-analysis of intergroup contact with non-negative contact with out-group members found a reduction in bias. Second, exposure to outgroup members who controvert group-based stereotypes can also reduce bias (Park & Glaser, 2011). Third, refraining from using stereotypes in training by rejecting stereotypical sayings was found to reduce the activation of stereotypes in future behavior. Last, counter-stereotype imaging, individuation, and increasing opportunities for intergroup contact helped to reduce implicit racial bias (Devine et al., 2012). It is important to note that while most law enforcement departments offer training in cultural competency, the addition of implicit bias training can help reduce the effect of cultural biases and stereotypes that often influence decisions. This argument is not limited to law enforcement officers, but rather, it can be made for every professional that has contact or encounters with minorities.

The prevention of CA, CSA, and neglect will require collaborations that bring public health, government, education, social services, and justice agencies together to develop strategies to detect, monitor, and treat the behavior. To achieve success, public health strategies require that each community rely on a range of resources (e.g., billboards, radio, public service announcements) to educate the public about the danger and pervasiveness of child sexual offending and the resources of the existing programs to assist those needing help. There must be an understanding that it is vitally important to prevent future child abusers and child sex offenders from committing their first offense and ultimately reoffending. The failure to do so will inevitably mean more children will experience this traumatic and at times violent type of victimization.

Summary

Children by nature are vulnerable, which can result in those with power/authority abusing them. CA including CSA is a major public health issue that places children globally at risk for the development of health as well as negative mental health problems. It has both short-term and long-term implications for its victims ranging from obesity, relationship problems, depression, teenage pregnancy, and mental health issues, to name a few. CA presents itself in various forms: physical, emotional, neglect, or sexual abuse. While children are never the reason for abuse, they pose factors that lower their defenses against abuse which limit their abilities to protect themselves and seek help. These factors are referred to as risk factors which may serve as clues to the potential for abuse or further abuse. Risk factors occur at the levels of inequalities, individuals, relationships, and communities. Epidemiologists can use this information to plan and evaluate strategies that are designed to provide intervention and ultimately prevent abuse. However, epidemiologists do not always capture the true percentages of abused children in a population due to disproportionality in physicians and other clinicians reporting cases of abuse to child protective services as well as to those cases that go unreported by children. Within and across systems of care, practitioners, policymakers, and decision makers must make concerted efforts to reduce and prevent CA by addressing the underlying causes. Therefore, researchers must continue to investigate these risk factors, especially those that involve the role of inequality, so that through interventions and preventative methods, strategies can be developed that have the potential to ensure that children and families have a better awareness and understanding of the impact of CA on the health and wellness of the victim, the family, and society.

Discussion Questions

1 A scenario was presented at the beginning of this chapter regarding Lisa, please describe the types of child abuse that occur in the scenario.
2 Discuss child abuse and its prevalence.
3 Describe some criminal justice approaches used in response to child abuse.
4 Discuss the various types of child sexual abuse.
5 What are some of the risk factors that can predict child abuse?
6 Discuss the negative health consequences of child abuse.

References

Aas, M., Andreassen, O.A., Aminoff, S.R., Færden, A., Romm, K.L., Nesvåg, R., Berg, A.O., Simonsen, C., Agartz, I., Melle, I. A. (2016). A history of childhood trauma is associated with slower improvement rates: Findings from a one-year follow-up study of patients with a first-episode psychosis. *BMC Psychiatry*, 16(126), 2–8.

Administration for Children and Families (ACF). (2012). Child maltreatment, 2011 report. Washington, DC: U.S. Department of Health and Human Services. https://acf.gov/sites/default/files/documents/cm2012_0.pd

Agnew-Blais, J., & Danese, A., (2016). Childhood maltreatment and unfavourable clinical outcomes in bipolar disorder: A systematic review and meta-analysis. *The Lancet Psychiatry*, 3(4), 342–349. https://doi.org/10.1016/S2215-0366(15)00544-1

Allnock, D., Bunting, L., Price, A., Morgan-Klein, N., Ellis, J., Radford, L., & Stafford, A. (2009). *Sexual abuse and therapeutic services for children and young people: The gap between provision and need (Executive summary)*. NSPCC. www.pure.ed.ac.uk/ws/files/13314420/K200908.pdf

American Humane. (2003). Fact sheet, 1–2. Retrieved from https://projectlifeline.us/wp-content/uploads/2020/09/Child-Physical-Abuse.pdf

Anand, A., Koller, D.L., Lawson, W.B., Gershon, E.S., Nurnberger, J.I., & BiGS Collaborative. (2015). Genetic and childhood trauma interaction effect on age of onset in bipolar disorder: An exploratory analysis. *Journal of Affective Disorders*, 179, 1–5. https://doi.org/10.1016/j.jad.2015.02.029

Assink, M., van der Put, C.E., Meeuwsen, M.W.C.M., de Jong, N.M., Oort, F.J., Stams, G.J.J.M., & Hoeve, M. (2019). Risk factors for child sexual abuse victimization: A meta-analytic review. *Psychological Bulletin*, 145(5), 459–489.

Bartollas, C., & Schmalleger, F. (2013). *Juvenile delinquency*. Pearson.

Barrios, Y.V., Gelaye, B., Zhong, Q., Nicolaidis, C., Rondon, M.B., Garcia, P.J., Sanchez, P.A.M., Sanchez, S.E., & Williams, M.A. (2015). Association of childhood physical and sexual abuse with intimate partner violence, poor general health and depressive symptoms among pregnant women. *PLoS One*, 10, e0116609. https://doi.org/10.1371/journal.pone.0116609

Bauermeister, J.A., Zimmerman, M.A, & Caldwell, C.H. (2011). Neighborhood disadvantage and changes in condom use among African American adolescents. *Journal of Urban Health*, 88(1), 66–83. https://doi.org/10.1007/s11524-010-9506-9

Benson, C. (2022). *Poverty rate of children higher than national rate, lower for older populations*. U.S. Census Bureau. www.census.gov/library/stories/2022/10/poverty-rate-varies-by-age-groups.html

Black, D.A., Heyman, R.E., & Slep, A.M. (2001). Risk factors for child physical abuse. *Aggression and Violent Behavior*, 6(2–3), 121–188.

Brown, C.L., Yilanli, M., & Rabbit, A.L. (2023). In StatPearls Publishing. www.ncbi.nlm.nih.gov/books/NBK470337/

Browning, C.R., Leventhal, T., & Brooks-Gunn, J. (2004). Neighborhood context and racial differences in early adolescent sexual activity. *Demography*, 41(4), 697–720. https://doi.org/10.1353/dem.2004.0029

Browning, C.R., Leventhal, T., & Brooks-Gunn, J. (2005). Sexual initiation in early adolescence: The nexus of parental and community control. *American Sociological Review* , 70(5), 758–778. https://doi.org/10.1177/000312240507000502

Butchart, A., Phinney Harvey, A., Kahane, T., Mian, M., & Furniss, T. (2006). Preventing child maltreatment: A guide to action and generating evidence. World Health Organization and International Society for Prevention of Child Abuse and Neglect.

Butler, A.C. (2013). Child sexual assault: Risk factors for girls. *Child Abuse & Neglect*, 37, 643–652. https://doi.org/10.1016/j.chiabu.2013.06.009

Caldas, S.J., & Bensy, M.L. (2014). The sexual maltreatment of students with disabilities in American school settings. *Journal of Child Sex Abuse*, 23(4), 345–366.

Capaldi, M., Schatz, J., & Kavenoh, M. (2024). Child sexual abuse/exploitation and LGBTQ1+ children: Context, links, vulnerabilities, gaps, challenges, and priorities. Vol.1. J. Chipro. https://doi.org/10.1016/j.chipro.2024.10000

Castro, A., Moreno, J.D., Maté, B., Ibáñez-Vidal, J., & Barrada, J.R. (2021, April 27). Profiling children sexual abuse in a sample of university students: A study on characteristic of victims, abusers, and abuse episodes. *International Journal of Environmental Research and Public Health*, 18(9), 4610. https://doi.org/10.3390/ijerph18094610. PMID: 33925293; PMCID: PMC8123693. www.nspcc.org.uk/what-is-child-abuse/types-of-abuse/child-sexual-exploitation/

Centers for Disease, Control and Prevention (CDC). (2024, May 16). A public health approach to child abuse and neglect. Child Abuse and Neglect Prevention.

Chapman, D.P., Whitfield, C.L., Felitti, V.J., Dube, S.R., Edwards, V.J., & Anda, R.F. (2004). Adverse childhood experiences and the risk of depressive disorders in adulthood. *Journal of Affective Disorders*, 82(2), 217–225. https://doi.org/10.1016/j.jad.2003.12.013

Child Welfare Information Gateway. (2009). Understanding the effects of maltreatment on brain development (PDF). Washington, D.C.: United States Department of Health and Human Services.

Child Welfare Information Gateway. (2016). *Racial Disproportionality and Disparity in Child Welfare*. US Department of Health and Human Services, Children's Bureau. www.govinfo.gov/content/pkg/GOVPUB-HE-PURL-gpo159394/pdf/GOVPUB-HE-PURL-gpo159394.pdf

Cross, T.P., Chuang, E., Helton, J.J., & Lux, E.A. (2015). Criminal investigations in child protective services cases: An empirical analysis. *Child Maltreatment*, 20(2), 104–114.

Daley, S.F., & Gutovitz, S. (2023). *Child sexual abuse*. StatPearls Publishing. www.ncbi.nlm.nih.gov/sites/books/NBK470563/

Danese, A., Pariante, C.M., Caspi, A., Taylor, A., & Poulton, R. (2007). Childhood maltreatment predicts adult inflammation in a life-course study. *Proceedings of the National Academy of Sciences – PNAS*, 104(4), 1319–1324. https://doi.org/10.1073/pnas.0610362104

Daruy-Filho, L., Brietzke, E., Lafer, B., & Grassi-Oliveira, R. (2011). Childhood maltreatment and clinical outcomes of bipolar disorder. *Acta Psychiatrica Scandinavica*, 124(6), 427–434. https://doi.org/10.1111/j.1600-0447.2011.01756.x

Davies, E.A., & Jones, A.C. (2013). Risk factors in child sexual abuse. *Journal of Forensic and Legal Medicine*, 20, 146–150. https://doi.org/10.1016/j.jflm.2012.06.005

De Mause, L. (2008). Infanticide, child rape and war in early states. In L. De Mause (Ed.), *The origins of war in child abuse*. Available from ttps://psychohistory.com/books/the-origins-of-war-in-child-abuse/chapter-8-infanticide-child-rape-and-war-in-early-states/

Develop Services Group, Inc for Administration on Children, Youth, and Families. (2015). Promoting protective factors for in-risk families and youth: A brief for researchers. Children's Bureau, 1–8. https://dsgonline.com/acyf/PF_Research_Brief.pdf

Devine, P.G. (1989). Stereotypes and prejudices: Their automatic and controlled components. *Journal of Personality and Social Psychology*, 56(1), 5–18.

Devine, P.G., Forscher, P.S., Austin, A.J., & Cox, W.T.L. (2012). Long-term reduction in implicit bias: A prejudice habit-breaking intervention. *Journal of Experimental Social Psychology*, 48(6), 1267–1278.

Devries, K.M., Mak, J.Y., Child, J.C., Falder, G., Bacchus, L.J., Astbury, J., Watts, C.H. (2014, May). Childhood sexual abuse and suicidal behavior: A meta-analysis. *Pediatrics*, 133(5), e1331–e1344. https://doi.org/10.1542/peds.2013-2166. Epub 2014 Apr 14. PMID: 24733879.

Dinkelman, T.L., Lam, D., & Leibbrandt, M. (2008). Linking poverty and income shocks to risky sexual behaviour: Evidence from a panel study of young adults in cape town. *South African Journal of Economics*, 76(1), s52–74. https://doi.org/10.1111/j.1813-6982.2008.00170.x

Diyaolu, M., Ye, C., Huang, Z., Han, R., Wild, H., Tennakoon, L., Spain, D., Chao, S. D. (2023). Disparities in detection of suspected child abuse. *Journal of Pediatric Surgery*, 58(2), 337–343. https://doi.org/10.1016/j.jpedsurg.2022.10.039

Dunn, E.C., Nishimi, K., Gomez, S.H., Powers, A., & Bradley, B. (2018). Developmental timing of trauma exposure and emotion dysregulation in adulthood: Are there sensitive periods when trauma is most harmful? *Journal of Affective Disorders*, 227, 869–877. https://doi.org/10.1016/j.jad.2017.10.045

Eckenrode, J., Smith, E.G., McCarthy, M.E., & Dineen, M. (2014, March). Income inequality and child maltreatment in the United States. *Journal of Pediatrics*, 133(3), 454–461. https://doi.org/10.1542/peds.2013-1707. Epub 2014 Feb 10. PMID: 25415511.

Edalati, H., & Nicholls, T.L. (2019). Childhood maltreatment and the risk for criminal justice involvement and victimization among homeless individuals: A systematic review. *Trauma, Violence & Abuse*, 20(3), 315–330. www.jstor.org/stable/27010969

Edwards, F. (2019). Family surveillance: Police and the reporting of child abuse and neglect. *RSF: The Russell Sage Foundation Journal of the Social Sciences*, 5(1), 50–70. https://doi.org/10.7758/RSF.2019.5.1.03

Ennis, J., Williams, B., & Kendrick, A. (1995). Working with perpetrators of child sexual abuse: Issues for social work practice. *Child Care in Practice: Northern Ireland Journal of Multi-Disciplinary Child Care Practice*, 2(1), 60–70. https://doi.org/10.1080/13575279508412877

Essabar, L., Khalqallah, A., & Benjelloun, B.S. (2015). Child sexual abuse: Report of 311 cases with review of literature. *Pan African Medical Journal*, 20. https://doi.org/10.11604/pamj.2015.20.47.4569

Fayaz, I. (2019). Child abuse: Effects and prevention measures. *The International Journal of Indian Psychology*, 7, 871–884.

Finkelhor, D., Cross, T., & Canter, E., (2005). The justice system for juvenile victims: A comprehensive model of case flow. *Trauma, Violence, & Abuse*, 6(2), 83–102. https://doi.org/10.1177/1524838005275090

Finkelhor, D., & Korbin, J. (1988). Child abuse as an international issue. *Child Abuse & Neglect*, 12, 3–23. https://doi.org/10.1016/0145-2134(88)90003-8

Finkelhor, D., Shattuck, A., Turner, H.A., & Hamby, S.L. (2014). The lifetime prevalence of child sexual abuse and sexual assault assessed in late adolescence. *The Journal of Adolescent Health*, 55(3), 329–333. https://doi.org/10.1016/j.jadohealth.2013.12.026

Finkelhor, D., Turner, H.A., Shattuck, A., & Hamby, S.L. (2015). Prevalence of childhood exposure to violence, crime, and abuse: Results from the National Survey of Children's Exposure to Violence. *JAMA Pediatrics*, 169(8), 746–754. https://doi.org/10.1001/jamapediatrics.2015.0676

Fix, R. L., & Nair, R. (2020). Racial/ethnic and gender disparities in substantiation of child physical and sexual abuse: Influences of caregiver and child characteristics. *Children and Youth Services Review*, 116, 105186.

Fortson, B.L., Klevens, J., Merrick, M.T., Gilbert, L.K., & Alexander, S.P. (2016). *Child abuse and neglect prevention resource for action: A compilation of the best available evidence*. National Center for Injury Prevention and Control, Centers for Disease Control and Prevention.

Fortson, B.L., & Mercy, J. (2012). Violence against children. In J.M. Rippe (Ed.), *Encyclopedia of lifestyle medicine and health* (pp. 2818–2829). Sage.

Fromuth, M.E. (1986). The relationship of childhood sexual abuse with later psychological and sexual adjustment in a sample of college women. *Child Abuse & Neglect*, 10(1), 5–15.

Gama, C.M.F., Portugal, L.C.L., Gonçalves, R.M., de Souza Junior, S., Vilete, L.M.P., Mendlowicz, M.V., Figueira, I., Volchan, E., David, I.A., de Oliveira, & L., Pereira, M.G. (2021). The invisible scars of emotional abuse: A common and highly harmful form of childhood maltreatment. *BMC Psychiatry*, 21, 156. https://doi.org/10.1186/s12888-021-03134-0

Garami, J., Valikhani, A., Parkes, D., Haber, P., Mahlberg, J., Misiak, B., Frydecka, D., & Moustafa, A.A. (2019). Examining perceived stress, childhood trauma and interpersonal trauma in individuals with drug addiction. *Psychological Reports*, 122(2), 433–450. https://doi.org/10.1177/003329411 8764918

Gilbert, R., Widom, C.S., Browne, K., Ferguson, D., Webb, E., & Janson, S. (2009). Burden and consequences of child maltreatment in high-income countries. *Lancet*, 373(9657), 68–81. PMID:19056114.

Giovannoni, J., & Becerra, R. (1979). *Defining child abuse*. Free Press.

Gomez, A.M. (2011, September). Sexual violence as a predictor of unintended pregnancy, contraceptive use, and unmet need among female youth in Colombia. *Journal of Women's Health*, 20(9), 1349–1356. https://doi.org/10.1089/jwh.2010.2518. Epub 2011 Jul 8. PMID: 21740193.

Gonzalez, D., Bethencourt Mirabal, A., & McCall, J.D. (2023, July 4). Child Abuse and Neglect. In: StatPearls [Internet]. Treasure Island (FL): StatPearls Publishing; Available from: www.ncbi.nlm.nih.gov/books/NBK459146/

Greely, C.S. (2012). The evolution of the child maltreatment literature. *Pediatrics*, 130(2), 347–348. https://doi.org/10.1542/peds.2012-1442

Gubbels, J., van der Put, C.E., Stams, G.J.M., & Assink, M. (2021, September). Effective components of school-based prevention programs for child abuse: A meta-analytic review. *Clinical Child and Family Psychology Review*, 24(3), 553–578. https://doi.org/10.1007/s10567-021-00353-5. Epub 2021 Jun 4. PMID: 34086183; PMCID: PMC8176877.

Hanson, R.F., & Wallis, E. (2018). Treating victims of child sexual abuse. *American Journal of Psychiatry*, 175(11), 1051–1150.

Herrenkohl, T.I. (Eds). *Re-Visioning Public Health Approaches for Protecting Children* (Vol. 9). Child maltreatment. Springer. https://doi.org/10.1007/978-3-030-05858-6_1

Herrenkohl, T.I., Higgins, D.J., Merrick, M.T., & Leeb, R.T. (2015). Positioning a public health framework at the intersection of child maltreatment and intimate partner violence: Primary prevention requires working outside existing systems. *Child Abuse & Neglect*, 48, 22–28. https://doi.org/10.1016/j.chiabu.2015.04.013

Higgins, D., Lonne, B., Herrenkohl, T.I., & Scott, D. (2019). The successes and limitations of contemporary approaches to child protection. In B. Lonne, D. Scott, & D. Higgins (Eds.). Re-visioning public health approaches for protecting children. *Child Maltreatment*, 9, 3–17. Springer, Cham. https://doi.org/10.1007/978-3-030-05858-6_1

Higgins, D.J. (2015). A public health approach to enhancing safe and supportive family environments for children. *Family Matters*, 96, 39–52.

Hogan, K.A., & Roe-Sepowitz, D. (2023). LGBTQ+ homeless young adults and sex trafficking vulnerability. *Journal of Human Trafficking*, 9(1), 63–78. https://doi.org/10.1080/23322 705.2020.1841985

Honjo, K. (2004, September). Social epidemiology: Definition, history, and research examples. *Environmental Health and Preventive Medicine*, 9(5), 193–199. https://doi.org/10.1007/BF0 2898100.

Honor, G. (2014). Child neglect: Assessment and intervention. *Journal of Pediatric Health Care*, 28(2), 186–192.

Hughes, K., Bellis, M.A., Hardcastle, K.A., Sethi, D., Butchart, A., Mikton, C., Jones, L., & Dunne, M.P. (2017). The effect of multiple adverse childhood experiences on health: A systematic review and meta-analysis. *The Lancet Public Health*, 2(8), e356–e366. https://doi.org/10.1016/S2468-2667(17)30118-4

Jack, S.M., Gonzalez, A., Marcellus, L., Tonmyr, L., Varcoe, C., Van Borek, N., Sheehan, D., MacKinnon, K., Campbell, K., Catherine, N., Kurtz Landy, C., MacMillan, H.L., & Waddell, C. (2021). Public health nurses' professional practices to prevent, recognize, and respond to suspected child maltreatment in home visiting: An interpretive descriptive study. *Global Qualitative Nursing Research*, 8. https://doi.org/10.1177/2333393621993450

James, E., Herman, J., Rankin, S., Keisling, M., Mottet, L., & Anafi, M. (2016). The report of the 2015 U.S. Transgender Survey, National Center for Transgender Equality. https://transequality.org/sites/default/files/docs/usts/USTS-Full-Report-Dec17.pdf

Jeglic, E.L., & Calkins, C.A. (2018). *Protecting your child from sexual abuse: What you need to know to keep your kids safe*. Skyhorse Publishing.

Josenhans, V., Kavenagh, M., Smith, S., & Wekerle, C. (2020). Gender, rights and responsibilities: The need for a global analysis of the sexual exploitation of boys. *Child Abuse & Neglect*, 110(Pt 1). https://doi.org/10.1016/j.chiabu.2019.104291

Jud, A., & Voll, P. (2019). The definitions are legion: Academic views and practice perspectives on violence against children. *Sociological Studies of Children and Youth*, 25, 47–66. https://doi.org/10.1108/S1537-466120190000025004

Kelley, B., Thornberry, T., & Smith, C. (1997). *In the wake of childhood maltreatment*. Youth development series bulletin. U.S. Department of Justice, Office of Juvenile Justice and Delinquency Prevention, NCJ 165257.

Kempe, A. (2007). *A good knight for children: C. Henry Kempe's quest to protect the abused child* (e-book). Booklocker.com, Inc.

Kempe, C.H., Silverman, F.D., Steele, B.F., Droegemuller, W., & Silver, H.K. (1985). The battered child syndrome. *Child Abuse and Neglect*, 9, 143–154.

Kewley, S., Mhlanga-Gunda, R., & Van Hount, M.C. (2021). Preventing child sexual abuse before it occurs: Examining the scale and nature of secondary public health prevention approaches. *Journal of Sexual Aggression*. https://doi.org/10.1080/13552600.2021.2000651

Kim, H., & Drake, B. (2023, September). Has the relationship between community poverty and child maltreatment report rates become stronger or weaker over time? *Child Abuse and Neglect*, 143, 106333. https://doi.org/10.1016/j.chiabu.2023.106333. Epub 2023 Jun 26.PMIDF: 37379728; PMCID:PMC10651183

Kim, H., Wildeman, C., Jonson-Reid, M., & Drake, B. (2017). Lifetime prevalence of investigating child maltreatment among US children. *American Journal of Public Health*, 107, 274–280. https://doi.org/10.2105/AJPH.2016.303545

Klevens, J., & Ports, K.A. (2017). Gender inequity associated with increased child physical abuse and neglect: A cross-country analysis of population-based surveys and country-level statistics. *Journal of Family Violence*, 2017. https://doi.org/10.1007/s10896-017-9925-4

Kumari, V. (2020). Emotional abuse and neglect: Time to focus on prevention and mental health consequences. *British Journal of Psychiatry*, 217(5), 597–599. https://doi.org/10.1192/bjp.2020.154. PMID: 32892766; PMCID: PMC7589986.

Laajasalo, T., Cowley, L.E., Otterman, G., Lamela, D., Rodrigues, L.B., Jud, A., Alison, K., Naughton, A., Hurt, L., Soldino, V., Ntinapogias, A., & Nurmatov, U. (2023). Current issues and challenges in the definition and operationalization of child maltreatment: A scoping review. *Elsevier*, 140. https://doi.org/10.1016/J.chiabu.2023.106187

Lee, D.S., Guy, L., Perry, B., Sniffen, C.K., & Mixson, S.A. (2007). Sexual violence prevention. *The Prevention Researcher*, 14(2), 15–20.

Lee, M. (2024a). *The impact of poverty on child abuse and neglect*. The National Crimes against Children Investigators Association. www.ncacia.org/post/the-impact-of-poverty-on-child-abuse-and-neglect

Lee, M. (2024b). *The role of public policy in preventing child abuse and supporting survivors*. The National Crimes against Children Investigators Association. www.ncacia.org/post/the-role-of-public-policy-in-preventing-child-abuse-and-supporting-survivors

Lee, M. (2024c). *Using a public health approach to address and prevent child abuse*. National Crimes against Children Investigators Association.

Leeb, R.T., Lewis, T., & Zolotor, A.J. (2011). A review of the physical and mental health consequences of child abuse and neglect and implications for practice. *American Journal of Lifestyle Medicine*, 5(5), 454–468.

Leeb, R.T., Paulozzi, L., Melanson, C., Simon, T., & Arias, I. (2008). Child maltreatment surveillance: Uniform definitions for public health and recommended data elements. Centers for Disease Control and Prevention, National Center for Injury Prevention and Control, Version 1.0. (1–135).

Legano, L.A., Desch, L.W., Messner, S.A., Idzerda, S., Flaherty, E.G., & AAP Council On Child Abuse and Neglect, AAP Council On Children With Disabilities. (2021). Maltreatment of children with disabilities. *Pediatrics*, 147(5), e2021050920.

Lei, Y., Xi, C., Li, P., Luo, M., Wang, W., Pan, S., Gao, X., Xu, Y., Huang, G., Deng, X., Guo, L., & Lu, C. (2018). Association between childhood maltreatment and non-medical prescription opioid use among Chinese senior high school students: The moderating role of gender. *Journal of Affective Disorders*, 235, 421–427. https://doi.org/10.1016/j.jad.2018.04.070

Lilly, R., Cullen, F.T., & Ball, R. (2019). *Criminological theory: Context and consequences* (7th ed.). Sage.

Lim, Y.Y., Wahab, S., Kumar, J, Ibrahim, F., & Kamaluddin, M.R. (2021). Typologies and psychological profiles of child sexual abusers: An extensive review. *Children (Basel)*, 8(5), 333. https://doi.org/10.3390/children8050333

Lindert, J., von Ehrenstein, O.S., Grashow, R., Gal, G., Braehler, E., & Weisskopf, M.G. (2014). Sexual and physical abuse in childhood is associated with depression and anxiety over the life course: Systematic review and me-ta-analysis. *International Journal of Public Health*, 59, 359–372. https://doi.org/10.1007/s00038-013-0519-5

Lippard, E.T.C., & Nemeroff, C.B. (2020). The devastating clinical consequences of child abuse and neglect: Increased disease vulnerability and poor treatment response in mood disorders. *The American Journal of Psychiatry*, 177(1), 20–36. https://doi.org/10.1176/appi.ajp.2019.19010020

Liu, J., He, Y., & Luo, X. (2017). Letter to the editor "Childhood maltreatment severity is associated with elevated C-reactive protein and body mass index in adult with schizophrenia and bipolar diagnoses". *Brain, Behavior, and Immunity*, 65, 362–362. https://doi.org/10.1016/j.bbi.2017.07.007

Lo, I.L, Trentini, C., & Carola, V. (2021). Psychobiological consequences of childhood sexual abuse: Current knowledge and clinical implications. *Front Neurosci*, 2, 15, 771511. https://doi.org/10.3389/fnins.2021.771511

Luken, A., Nair, R., & Fix, R.L. (2021). On racial disparities in child abuse reports: Exploratory mapping the 2018 NCANDS. *Child Maltreatment*, 26(3), 267–281. https://doi.org/10.1177/10775595211001926

Ma, J., Grogan-Kaylor, A., Lee, S., Pace, G., & Paxton Ward, K., (2022). Gender inequality in low- and middle-income countries: Associations with parental physical abuse and Moderation by Child Gender. *International Journal of Environmental Research and Public Health*. https://doi.org/10.3390/ijerph191911928

MacMillan, H.L., Tanaka, M., Duku, E., Vaillancourt, T., & Boyle, M.H. (2013). Child physical and sexual abuse in a community sample of young adults: Results from the Ontario Child Health Study. *Child Abuse & Neglect*, 37, 14–21. https://doi.org/10.1016/j.chiabu.2012.06.005

Martins, C.M., Von Werne Baes, C., Tofoli, S.M., & Juruena, M.F. (2014). Emotional abuse in childhood is a differential factor for the development of depression in adults. *Journal of Nervous and Mental Disease*, 202(11), 774–782.

Mathews, B., & Collin-Vézina, D. (2019). Child sexual abuse: Toward a conceptual model and definition. *Trauma Violence Abuse*, 20(2), 131–148. https://doi.org/10.1177/1524838017738726

Matta Oshima, K.M., Jonson-Reid, M., & Seay, K.D. (2014). The influence of childhood sexual abuse on adolescent outcomes: The roles of gender, poverty, and revictimization. *Journal of Child*

Sexual Abuse, 23(4), 367–386. https://10.1080/10538712.2014.896845. PMID: 24641766; PMCID: PMC4047823.

Melmer, M.N., & Gutovitz, S. Child Sexual Abuse and Neglect. [Updated 2023 Aug 28]. In: StatPearls [Internet]. Treasure Island (FL): StatPearls Publishing; 2024 Jan. Available from: www.ncbi.nlm.nih.gov/books/NBK470563/

Merrick, M.T., Fortson, B.L., & Mercy, J.A. (2015). The epidemiology of child maltreatment. In P.D. Donnelly & C.L. Ward (Eds.), *Oxford textbook of violence prevention: Epidemiology, evidence, and policy* (pp. 19–26). Oxford University Press.

Milner, J., Crouch, J.L., McCarthy, R.J., Ammar, J., Dominguez-Martinez, R., Thomas, C.L., & Jensen, A.P. (2022). Child physical abuse risk factors: A systematic review and a meta-analysis. *Aggression and Violent Behavior*, 66. https://doi.org/10.1016/j.avb.2022.101778

Morais, H.B., Alexander, A.A., Fix, R.L., & Burkhart, B.R. (2018). Childhood sexual abuse in adolescents adjudicated for sexual offenses: Mental health consequences and sexual offending behaviors. *Sexual Abuse*, 2018, 30. https://doi.org/10.1177/1079063215625224

Muchiri, E.O., Odimegwu, C., Banda, P., Ntoimo, L., & Adedini, S. (2017). Ecological correlates of multiple sexual partnerships among adolescents and young adults in Urban Cape Town: A cumulative risk factor approach. *African Journal of AIDS Research*, 16(2), 119–128.

Murray, L.K., Nguyen, A., & Cohen, J.A. (2014). Child sexual abuse. *Child and Adolescent Psychiatric Clinics of North America*, 23(2), 321–337. https://doi.org/10.1016/j.chc.2014.01.003

Nagtegaal, M.H., & Boonmann, C. (2022). Child sexual abuse and problems reported by survivors of CSA: A meta-review. *Journal of Child Sexual Abuse*, 31(2), 147–176.

Nanni, V., Uher, R., & Danese, A. (2012). Childhood maltreatment predicts unfavorable course of Illness and treatment outcome in depression: A meta-analysis. *The American Journal of Psychiatry*, 169, 141–151. https://doi.org/10.1176/appi.ajp.2011.11020335

National Institute of Justice (NIJ). (2017, October 11). Pathways between child maltreatment and adult criminal involvement. nij.ojp.gov: https://nij.ojp.gov/topics/articles/pathways-between-child-maltreatment-and-adult-criminal-involvement

Nemeroff, C. (2016). Paradise lost: The neurobiological and clinical consequences of child abuse and neglect. *Neuron (Cambridge, MA)*, 89(5), 892–909. https://doi.org/10.1016/j.neuron.2016.01.019

Noll, J.G., Guastaferro, K., Beal, S.J., Schreier, H.M.C., Barnes, J., Reader, J.M., & Font, S.A. (2019). Is sexual abuse a unique predictor of sexual risk behaviors, pregnancy, and motherhood in adolescence? *Journal of Research on Adolescence*, 29(4), 967–983.

Noll, J.G., Trickett, P.K., Long, J.D., Negriff, S., Susman, E.J., Shalev, I., Li, J.C., & Putnam, F.W. (2016). Childhood sexual abuse and early timing of puberty. *Journal of Adolescent Health*, 60. https://doi.org/10.1016/j.jadohealth.2016.09.008

Norman, R.E., Byambaa, M., De, R., Butchart, A., Scott, J., & Vos, T. (2012). The long-term health consequences of child physical abuse, emotional abuse, and neglect: A systematic review and meta-analysis. *PLoS Medicine*, 9(11), e1001349. https://doi.org/10.1371/journal.pmed.1001349

Okeafor, C.U., Okeafor, I.N., & Tobin-West, C.I. (2018). Relationship between sexual abuse in childhood and the occurrence of mental illness in adulthood: A matched case–control study in Nigeria. *Sexual Abuse: Journal of Research and Treatment*, 30, 438–453. https://doi.org/10.1177/1079063216672172

Ondersma, S., Chaffin, M., Berliner, L., Cordon, I., Goodman, G., & Barnett, D. (2001). Sex with children is abuse: Comment on Rind, Tromovitch, and Bauserman (1998). *Psychological Bulletin*, 127, 707–714. https://doi.org/10.1037//0033-2909.127.6.707

Pandey, R., Gupta, S., Upadhyay, A., Gupta, R.P., Shukla, M., Mishra, R.C., Arya, Y.K., Singh, T., Niraula, S., Lau, J.Y.F., Kumari, V. (2020). Childhood maltreatment and its mental health consequences among Indian adolescents with a history of child work. *Australian and New Zealand Journal of Psychiatry*, 54, 496–508.

Park, S.H., & Glaser, J. (2011). Implicit motivation to control prejudice and exposure to counter-stereotypic instances reduce spontaneous discriminatory behavior. *Korean Journal of Social and Personality Psychology*, 25(4), 107–120.

Pavlova, B., Perroud, N., Cordera, P., Uher, R., Alda, M., Dayer, A., & Aubry, J. (2018). Anxiety disorders and childhood maltreatment as predictors of outcome in bipolar disorder. *Journal of Affective Disorders*, 225, 337–341. https://doi.org/10.1016/j.jad.2017.08.048

Peden, M., Oyegbite, K., Ozanne-Smith, J., Hyder, A., Branche, C., Rahman, A., Rivara, F., & Bartolomeo, K. (2008). *World Report on Child Injury Prevention*. World Health Organization. UNICEF.

Pfohl, S. (1977). The "discovery" of child abuse. *Social Problems*, 24(3), 310–323. https://doi.org/10.2307/800083

Ports, K.A., Ford, D.C., & Merrick, M.T. (2016, January). Adverse childhood experiences and sexual victimization in adulthood. *Child Abuse & Neglect*, 51, 313–22. https://doi.org/10.1016/j.chiabu.2015.08.017. Epub 2015 Sep 19. PMID: 26386753; PMCID: PMC4713310.

Pulverman, C.S., Kilimnik, C.D., & Meston, C.M. (2018). The impact of childhood sexual abuse on women's sexual health: a comprehensive review. *Sexual Medicine Reviews*, 6(2), 188–200. https://doi.org/10.1016/j.sxmr.2017.12.002

Pusch, S.A., Ross, T., & Fontao, M.I. (2021). The environment of intrafamilial offenders – A systematic review of dynamics in incestuous families. *Sexual Offending: Theory, Research, and Prevention*, 16, Article e5461. https://sotrap.psychopen.eu/index.php/sotrap/article/view/5461.

Putnam, F.W. (2003). Ten-year research update review: Child sexual abuse. *Journal of the American Academy of Child and Adolescent Psychiatry*, 42, 269–78. Available from: www.jaacap.com/article/S0890-8567(09)60559-1/abstract

Raman, S., & Hodes, D. (2012). Cultural issues in child maltreatment. *Journal of Paediatrics and Child Health*, 48, 30–37. https://doi.org/10.1111/j.1440-1754.2011.02184.x

Roberts, D.E. (2014). Child protection as surveillance of African American families. *Journal of Social Welfare Family Law*, 36(4): 426–437.

Romley, J.A., Shah, A.K., Chung, P.J., Elliott, M.N., Vestal, K.D., & Schuster, M.A. (2017). Family-provided health care for children with special health care needs. *Pediatrics*, 139(1), e20161287.

Runarsdottir, E., Smith, E., & Arnarsson, A. (2019, May 20).The effects of gender and family wealth on sexual abuse of adolescents. *International Journal of Environmental Research and Public Health*, 16(10), 1788. https://doi.org/10.3390/ijerph16101788

Sachs-Ericsson, N.J., Sheffler, J.L., Stanley, I.H., Piazza, J.R., & Preacher, K.J. (2017). When emotional pain becomes physical: Adverse childhood experiences, pain, and the role of mood and anxiety disorders. *Journal of Clinical Psychology*, 73(10), 1403–1428. https://doi.org/10.1002/jclp.22444

Saladino, V., Eleuteri, S., Zamparelli, E., Petrilli, M., & Verrastro, V. (2021, May 14). Sexual violence and trauma in childhood: A case report based on strategic counseling. *International Journal of Environmental Research and Public Health*, 18(10), 5259. https://doi.org/10.3390/ijerph18105259. PMID: 34069273; PMCID: PMC8156533.

Saunders, B.E., & Adams, Z.W. (2014). Epidemiology of traumatic experiences in childhood. *Child and Adolescent Psychiatric Clinics of North America*, 23, 167–184.

Seto, M.C., Babchishin, K.M., Pullman, L.E., & McPhail, I.V. (2015). The puzzle of intrafamilial child sexual abuse: A meta-analysis comparing intrafamilial and extrafamilial offenders with child victims. *Clinical Psychology Review*, 39, 42–57. https://doi.org/10.1016/j.cpr.2015.04.001

Shevlin, M., Murphy, S., Elklit, A., Murphy, J., & Hyland, P. (2018). Typologies of child sexual abuse: An analysis of multiple abuse acts among a large sample of danish treatment-seeking survivors of childhood sexual abuse. *Psychological Trauma: Theory, Research, Practice, and Policy*, 10, 263–269. https://doi.org/10.1037/tra0000268

Shin, S.H. (2012). A longitudinal examination of the relationships between childhood maltreatment and patterns of adolescent substance use among high-risk adolescents. *The American Journal on Addictions*, 21(5), 453–461. https://doi.org/10.1111/j.1521-0391.2012.00255.x

Shin, S.H., Chung, Y., & Rosenberg, R.D. (2016). Identifying sensitive periods for alcohol use: The roles of timing and chronicity of child physical abuse. *Alcoholism, Clinical and Experimental Research*, 40(5), 1020–1029. https://doi.org/10.1111/acer.13038

Singh, M.M., Parsekar, S.S., & Nair, S.N. (2014). An epidemiological overview of child sexual abuse. *Journal of Family Med Prim Care*, 3(4), 430–435. https://doi.org/10.4103/2249-4863.148139

Stark, S. (2015). Emotional abuse. In *Psychology & behavioral health* (4th ed., Vol. 1, pp. 647–650). Salem Press.

Stemple, L., & Meyer, I.H. (2014). The sexual victimization of men in America: New data challenge old assumptions. *American Journal of Public Health*, 104. https://doi.org/10.2105/AJPH.2014.301946

Stith, S.M., Liu, T., Davies, L.C., Boykin, E.L., Alder, M.C., Harris, J.M., Som, A., McPherson, M., & Dees, J.E.M.E.G. (2009). Risk factors in child maltreatment: A meta-analytic review of the literature. *Aggression and Violent Behavior*, 14(1), 13–29. https://doi.org/10.1016/j.avb.2006.03.006

Stoltenborgh, M., Bakermans-Kranenburg, M.J., Alink, L.R.A., & van IJzendoorn, M.H. (2015). The prevalence of child maltreatment across the globe: Review of a series of meta-analyses: Prevalence of child maltreatment across the globe. *Child Abuse Review*, 24(1), 37–50.

Sullivan, P.M., & Knutson, J.F. (2000). Maltreatment and disabilities: A population-based epidemiological study. *Child Abuse & Neglect*, 24(10), 1257–1273.

Tang, K., Qu, X., Li, C., & Tan, S. (2018). Childhood sexual abuse, risky sexual behaviors and adverse reproductive health outcomes among Chinese college students. *Child Abuse & Neglect*, 84. https://doi.org/10.1016/j.chiabu.2018.07.038

Tarantola, D. (2018). Child maltreatment: Daunting and universally prevalent. *American Journal of Public Health*, 108(9), 1119–1120. https://doi.org/10.2105/AJPH.2018.304637

Task Team on SEA. (2017). Glossary on sexual exploitation and abuse: Thematic glossary of current terminology related to sexual exploitation and abuse (SEA) in the context of the United Nations second edition. United Nations.

Tatem, B., & Haskins, P. (2021, August 10). Dual system youth: At the intersection of child maltreatment and delinquency. nij.ojp.gov. https://nij.ojp.gov/topics/articles/dual-system-youth-intersection-child-maltreatment-and-delinquency

The National Child Traumatic Stress Network. (2009, April). Coping with the shock of intrafamilial sexual abuse – Information for parents and caregivers. www.NCTSN.org

Thornberry, T.P., & Henry, K.L. (2013). Intergenerational continuity in maltreatment. *Journal of Abnormal Child Psychology*, 41(4), 555–569. https://doi.org/10.1007/s10802-012-9697-5

Toft, H., Neupane, S.P., Bramness, J.G., Tilden, T., Wampold, B.E., & Lien, L. (2018). The effect of trauma and alcohol on the relationship between level of cytokines and depression among patients entering psychiatric treatment. *BMC Psychiatry*, 18(1), 95–95. https://doi.org/10.1186/s12888-018-1677-z

United Nations International Children's Emergency Fund (UNICEF). (2020a). For every child, reimagine. UNICEF Annual Report 2019. United Nations Children's Fund (UNICEF).

United Nations International Emergency Children's Fund (UNICF). (2020b). Action to end child sexual abuse and exploitation: A review of the evidence. UNICEF Child Protection Section Programme. www.unicef.org/media/89096/file/CSAE-Report-v2.pdf

United Nations International Emergency Children's Fund (UNICF). (2024, October). When numbers demand action: Confronting the global scale of sexual violence against children, UNICEF. https://data.unicef.org/topic/child-protection/violence/sexual-violence/#status

United Nations International Emergency Children's Fund (UNICF). (2025, June). Measuring technology-facilitated violence against children in line with the International Classification of Violence against Children, UNICEF, New York. www.unicef.org/press-releases/nearly-400-million-young-children-worldwide-regularly-experience-violent-discipline

U.S. Bureau of Labor Statistics. (2024). Occupational outlook handbook. www.bls.gov/ooh/community-and-social-service/social-workers.htm

U.S. Centers for Disease, Control and Prevention (CDC). (2020). Preventing child abuse & neglect. National Center for Injury Prevention and Control.

U.S. Centers for Disease Control and Prevention (CDC). (2024a). Sexual violence prevention. www.cdc.gov/sexual-violence/risk-factors/index.html

U.S. Centers for Disease Control and Prevention (CDC). (2024b). Child abuse and neglect prevention. www.cdc.gov/child-abuse-neglect/about/index.html

U.S. Department of Health and Human Services. (2020). Children maltreatment 2018. www.acf.hhs.gov/cb/research-data-technology/statistics-research/child-maltreatment

U.S. Department of Health and Human Services. (2020). Children maltreatment 2020. www.acf.hhs.gov/cb/data-research/child-maltreatment

U.S. Department of Health and Human Services, Administration for Children and Families. (2016 and 2018). Administration for Children and Families.

U.S. Department of Health and Human Services, Administration for Children and Families, Administration on Children, Youth and Families, Children's Bureau. (2020). Child Maltreatment 2018. Available from www.acf.hhs.gov/cb/research-data-technology /statistics-research/child-maltreatment

U.S. Department of Health and Human Services, Administration for Children and Families, Administration on Children, Youth and Families, Administration on Children, Youth and Families, Children's Bureau. (2023). Children Maltreatment 2021. www.acf.hhs.gov/cb/data-research/child-maltreatment

U.S. Department of Health and Human Services, Administration for Children and Families, Administration on Children, Youth and Families, Children's Bureau. (2025). Child Maltreatment 2023. Available from www.acf.hhs.gov/cb/data-research/child-maltreatment

U.S. Department of Homeland Security. (2022). Fact sheet: DHS efforts to combat child exploitation and abuse. www.dhs.gov/archive/news/2022/04/04/fact-sheet-dhs-efforts-combat-child-exploitation-and-abuse

U.S. Department of Justice. (2020). Child abuse: Special feature. Office of Justice Programs.

U.S. Department of Justice. (2023). National strategy for child exploitation, prevention and interdiction: A report to Congress, 1–391. www.justice.gov/psc/publications-resources

Vachon, D.D., Krueger, R.F., Rogoscho, F.A., & Cicchetti, D. (2015). Assessment of the harmful psychiatric and behavioral effects of different forms of child maltreatment. *JAMA Psychiatry*, 72, 1135–1142.

Varahachaikol, A. (2024). Prevention: The 10 signs of child abuse you need to know. National Children's Advocacy Center Statistics. National Children's Alliance. www.nationalchildrensalliance.org/the-10-signs-of-child-abuse-you-need-to-know/

Vrolijk-Bosschaart, T.F., Brilleslijper-Kater S.N., Benninga, M.A., Lindauer, R.J., Teeuw, A.H. (2018). Clinical practice: Recognizing child sexual abuse—What makes it so difficult? *European Journal of Pediatrics*, 177, 1343–1350. https://doi.org/10.1007/s00431-018-3193-z

Widom, C.S., Czaja, S.J., Bentley, T., & Johnson, M.S. (2012). A prospective investigation of physical health outcomes in abused and neglected children: New findings from a 30-year follow-up. *American Journal of Public Health*, 102(6), 1135–1144. https://doi.org/10.2105/AJPH.2011.300636

Widom, C.S., Czaja, S.J., & DuMont, K.A. (2015). Intergenerational transmission of child abuse and neglect: Real or detection bias? *Science*, 347(6229), 1480–1485. https://doi.org/10.1126/science.1259917

Wild, T.S., Müller, I., Fromberger, P., Jordan, K., Klein, L., & Müller J.L. (2020). Prevention of sexual child abuse: Preliminary results from an outpatient therapy program. *Frontiers in Psychiatry*, 11(88). https://doi.org/10.3389/fpsyt.2020.00088

Wildeman, C., Emanuel, N., Leventhal, J.M., Putnam-Hornstein, E., Waldfogel. J., & Lee, H. (2014). The prevalence of confirmed maltreatment among US children, 2004 to 2011. *JAMA Pediatrics*, 168, 706–713. https://doi.org/10.1001/jamapediatrics.2014.410

Withers, A.C., Tarasoff, J.M., & Stewart, J.W. (2013). Is depression with atypical features associated with trauma history? *The Journal of Clinical Psychiatry*, 74(5), 500–506. https://doi.org/10.4088/jcp.12m07870

Witt, W.P., Litzelman, K., Mandic, C.G., Wisk, L.E., Hampton, J.M., Creswell, P.D., Gottlieb, C.A., & Gangnon, R.E. (2011). Healthcare-related financial burden among families in the U.S.: The role of childhood activity limitations and income. *Journal of Family and Economic Issues*, 1, 32(2), 308–326. https://doi.org/10.1007/s10834-011-9253-4

World Health Organization (WHO). (1999). *Report of the consultation on child abuse prevention.* WHO [cited 2018 Jul 12]. Available from: http://apps.who.int/iris/handle/10665/65900#sthash.lclqbNv9.dpuf [Google Scholar].

World Health Organization (WHO). (2003). *Guidelines for medico-legal care for victims of sexual violence* [cited 2018 Jul 12]. Available from: https://iris.who.int/bitstream/handle/10665/42788/924154628X.pdf

World Health Organization (WHO). (2018). *European status report on preventing child maltreatment.* World Health Organization.

World Health Organization. (2021). Corporal punishment and health. www.who.int/news-room/fact-sheets/detail/corporal-punishment-and-health

World Health Organization (WHO). (2022, 19 September). Child maltreatment. https://iris.who.int/bitstream/handle/10665/361272/9789240048737-eng.pdf?sequence=1

World Health Organization. (2024). Child Maltreatment. www.who.int/news-room/fact-sheets-detail/child-maltreatment

World Health Organization. (2025). Framework to implement a life course approach in practice.

Wright, K.A., Turanovic, J.J., O'Neal, E.N., Morse, S.J., & Booth, E.T. (2019). The cycle of violence revisited: Childhood victimization, resilience, and future violence. *Journal of Interpersonal Violence*, 34(6), 1261–1286. https://doi.org/10.1177/0886260516651090

Young Women's Christian Association (YWCA). (2017). Child sexual abuse facts. www.worldywca.org/wp-content/uploads/2020/11/Week-Without-Violence-2018.pdf

Zeanah, C.H., & Humphreys, K.L. (2018, September). Child abuse and neglect. *Journal of the American Academy of Child and Adolescent Psychiatry*, 57(9), 637–644. https://doi.org/10.1016/j.jaac.2018.06.007

6

RAPE AND SEXUAL ASSAULT AND PUBLIC HEALTH

Introduction

Natalie and Christopher were from the same hometown, graduated from the same high school, and had recently matriculated at the local university. They met for the first time at a study session for an anthropology course they took together during a spring semester. About two months after knowing each other, Natalie and Christopher realized they had more in common than anthropology and other courses. While they never officially dated, they were often seen together. Some classmates and students in their study sessions thought they were a couple. One Friday, after their anthropology class, Christopher asked Natalie if she would attend a party with him, and she gladly accepted. Christopher picked up Natalie from her dormitory and drove to the party. At the party, Natalie noticed that Christopher was becoming more intoxicated as the night went on. In fact, on several occasions, she asked him if he had had enough to drink already, and he laughed and said, "This is the last one." It dawned on Natalie that maybe she did not know Christopher as well as she had thought, and perhaps, he had a substance abuse problem. After returning Natalie to her dormitory, Christopher noticed that her roommate was not there, and he started acting aggressively toward her. He ridiculed her for withholding emotional and sexual attention throughout their relationship. She was shocked by his behavior because they were platonic friends who shared a class and the same study group. Christopher overpowered Natalie and held her down on the sofa and forced her to have intercourse with him. While this occurred, she froze and was unable to speak or resist his intrusion. After he finished, he stayed and made small talk with her before leaving. She remained quiet the entire time and sat on the floor crying before showering and going to bed. The next morning, her roommate asked for the details on what she had hoped was a fun and exciting night for her. Natalie started to cry and ask her roommate if she thought she had been raped. In the next few weeks, Natalie began exhibiting signs of depression, and she subsequently withdrew from the university and returned home, where she never revealed what happened during her freshman year at college.

DOI: 10.4324/9781003373001-6

Rape and Sexual Assault Defined

The terms rape and sexual assault are often used interchangeably, but they are different. Under common law, rape is defined as the carnal knowledge of a female by force and against her will. Under this definition, rape occurred only when a man engaged in non-consensual sexual intercourse with a woman. Consequently, sexual acts that men inflicted on other men or sexual acts that women inflicted on other women were not considered rape under common law (Krahe' et al., 2003). However, today, most sex abuse researchers as well as the Federal Bureau of Investigation (FBI) view the act of rape as a form of sexual violence directed at both men and women. Sexual assault is a crime of violence and aggression that manifests in a variety of behaviors that could include either of the following: unwanted touching, grabbing, oral sex, anal sex, sexual penetration with an object, being made to perform sex acts, or sexual intercourse (Keith & Skidmore, 2024). Moreover, because critics viewed the legal or common law definition of rape as restrictive and limited, most people prefer the use of sexual assault because it is broader in scope and includes more people and behaviors (e.g., spouses, attempted rape, rape of men, same-sex rapes) that were traditionally excluded from the definition of rape. Not to mention, the emphasis that the former placed on the use of force directed at a victim (Peak & Everett, 2017; Rosenberg & Fenley, 1991). The Centers for Disease Control and Prevention (CDC) defines sexual violence as any sexual act or an attempt to acquire a sexual act from a person's sexuality using coercion, regardless of an existing relationship with the victim, and committed in any setting, including the home or workplace (Federal Bureau of Investigation [FBI], 2013). The definition includes the element of coercion, which is important when examining the different levels of force or lack thereof often involved in sexual assaults. Coercion can be physical, psychological, or blackmail, or occur when facing the threat of losing one's economic situation, either in the form of termination or being denied employment owing to the failure to render sexual favors. Coercion also exists when the victim is incapable of giving consent, especially in cases where the victim is intoxicated, drugged, asleep, or mentally unsound and lacks an understanding of what is occurring (FBI, 2013). In the past, the element of force was a requirement that had to be established in every jurisdiction to establish a showing of physical force or coerced penetration of the vagina, anus, or mouth using a penis, other body parts, or an object (Peak & Everett, 2017).

Nature and Extent of Rape and Sexual Assault

Because of the hidden nature of rape and sexual assault, researchers are challenged with the difficult task of estimating the actual number of occurrences with accuracy. Rates often vary based on who is collecting the data. For example, it could be a governmental agency, police department, private researcher, or a victim assistance agency. As such, these data may be impacted by the person or agency collecting them and the methods they use to compile them. Typically, rape and sexual assault data are collected using official and survey data. Some researchers report that when rape or sexual assault data are collected from surveys, the victims are more likely to reveal their experiences compared to when victims report sexual assault to police, which makes up official crime statistics (Schram & Tibbetts, 2014). The reluctance and refusal to report a rape to police has much to do with the private nature of sexual victimization, guilt, and shame associated with the experience, not wanting others to know, or the fear of reprisal from the rapist or their friends and family. These reasons are why most sexual assault cases go either unreported or underreported (Jones et al., 2009). However, existing statistics reveal that every 73 seconds, an American is the victim of a sexual assault. Moreover, recent violent victimization statistics from the National Crime Victimization Survey (NCVS) on the prevalence of rape and sexual assault from 2018 to 2022 show that they decreased from 734,630 (rate 2.7 per 1,000) to 459,310 (rate 1.7 per 1,000) in 2019. They continued to decrease to 319,950 (rate 1.2 per 1,000) in 2020. Then they increased to 324,500 (rate 1.2 per 1,000) in 2021 and by 2022, they reached a reported 531,810 (rate 1.9 per 1,000) incidents (U.S. Department of Justice, 2023). However, according to Uniform Crime Reports (UCR) data, the number of citizens reports to police regarding rape and sexual assault included 143,765 and 139,815 from 2018 to 2019, respectively (FBI, 2019). Despite the data, experts in public safety and public health argue that rape and sexual assaults are pervasive in the U.S. to the extent that it is referred to as a public health problem since some sources reveal that millions of people (e.g., men, women, and children) are affected by these behaviors each day.

While rape and sexual assault can impact everyone, women are disproportionately the targets for this victimization at a ratio of 91% female to 9% male, respectively (Rennison, 2002). Research conducted by Smith et al. (2017) found that an estimated 1.47 million rape-related assaults were committed against women from 2010 to 2012. They reported that one in five (or an estimated 23 million) U.S. women surveyed reported that they had either experienced being raped or they were the victim of an attempted rape during their lifetime. More alarmingly is that 80% of the women surveyed shared that they were first raped before age 25, and 41% revealed being raped before age 18 (Smith et al., 2017). Regarding lifetime chances of being raped, literature shows that women of color, especially Black and Indigenous women, experience higher prevalences of rape and attempted rape compared with other groups of women (Kilpatrick et al., 2007; West & Johnson, 2013). The demographical characteristics for women experiencing rape at some point in their lives by race demonstrate the following: 32% of multiracial women, 29% of American Indian/ Alaska Native women, 21% of non-Hispanic Black women, 20% of non-Hispanic White women, 15% of Hispanic women, and 10% of Asian Pacific Islander women (Smith et al., 2017). A third of women reporting being raped before age 18 later experienced rape again as an adult. While statistics also reveal that men are victims of rape and sexual assaults, they, like many women, are less likely to report their sexual victimizations owing to gender-specific stigma and socially constructed stereotypes about masculinity and sexuality (Stemple & Meyer, 2014; Kimerling et al., 2002). Nevertheless, some sources report that one in every ten rapes targets a male victim and about 3% of men in the U.S. have either been the victim of rape or experienced an attempted rape. Male sexual assault statistics report that each year, an estimated 2.78 million men are the victims of sexual assault or rape. Research conducted by Smith et al. (2018) reports that nearly 25% of men have experienced sexual violence during their lifetime, with only 3.5% reporting what happened in 2017. According to an investigation, 26% of gay men and 37% of bisexual men experience rape compared with 29% of heterosexual men. According to a study by Krebs et al. (2007), one in every 16 college men has experienced being sexually assaulted. Black et al. (2011) find that 27.8% of men who were raped or sexually assaulted were 10 or younger when first raped.

Research into sexual assaults committed against LGBT and gender diverse people reveals an increase in their levels of victimization, surpassing those experienced by heterosexuals.

A report from the Department of Justice examining sexual orientation from 2017 to 2020 revealed that LGB people experience rape and sexual assault at a higher rate compared to heterosexuals at 3.1 and 27.6 compared to 1.5 of every 1,000 persons aged 16 and older (Truman & Morgan, 2022). Another report focused on the sexual victimization of non-heterosexual shows that 21% of TGON (*transgender, genderqueer, nonconforming*) college students have been sexually assaulted compared with 18% of non-TGON females and 4% of non-TGON males. Nationally, data were collected between 2016 and 2017 using the National Intimate Partner and Sexual Violence Survey (NISVS), which found that bisexual women reported having greater rates of experiencing lifetime sexual violence compared with heterosexual and lesbian women. The study also discovered that gay and bisexual men reported experiencing greater rates of sexual violence over their lifetime compared with heterosexual men (Chen et al., 2023). A 2015 national study relying on the *U.S. Transgender Survey* findings reported that almost 50% of trans survey respondents revealed being sexually assaulted at some point in their lives, and of that number, 10% faced victimization within the past year (James et al., 2016).

Data from watchdog organizations reveal that many immigrants and women (80%) and men (30%) with disabilities are especially vulnerable and face greater rates of rape and sexual assaults compared with able-bodied people. Sorensen (2000) and Valenti-Hein and Schwartz (1995) find that between 50% and 59% of intellectually challenged women have been assaulted more than ten times. Statistically, women with intellectual disabilities are 12 times more likely to experience rape and sexual assault compared with women without disabilities. Valenti-Hein and Schwartz also report that more than 90% of those with intellectual challenges will experience sexual abuse during their lifetime. Children with developmental challenges are also among rape victims since studies find that they are three times more likely to be sexually abused compared with their counterparts without developmental challenges. When these sexual assaults occur, they are often committed in healthcare environments such as facilities and home care. Other places include hospitals, general practitioners' offices, and therapy sessions. Sadly, only 3% of rapes involving people with intellectual and developmental disabilities will be reported (Valenti-Hein & Schwartz, 1995).

Where age is concerned, those between the ages of 12 and 34 face the greatest likelihood of being rape victims, while people aged 65 and older are 92% less likely than those between the ages of 12 and 24 years old to be victims of rape and sexual assault, and 83% less likely than those between the ages of 25 and 49 (Department of Justice, 1997, 2014). This suggests that, like adult women, young girls face the highest rates of sexual violence (Moody et al., 2018). Data report that 82% of juvenile rape victims are female, and 90% of victims are adult females (Department of Justice, 2000). Research conducted by *Rape, Abuse and Incest National Network* (RAINN) revealed that younger people also face a high risk of victimization. RAINN reported that in 2014, younger people between the ages of 12 and 17 accounted for 15% of all rapes (Department of Justice, 2014). Finkelhor et al. (1990) reported that one in every four girls and one in six boys will be sexually abused before reaching the age of 18. Other research reveals that 12.3% of women were 10 years old or younger when they experienced rape or sexual assault, and an additional 30% were raped between the ages of 11 and 17 (Black et al., 2011). Data collected in 2017 revealed that an estimated 58,000 cases of child sexual abuse occurred in the U.S., which resulted in an incidence rate of 78 per 100,000 children (Department of Health and Human Services, 2017).

Typologies of Rape and Sexual Assault

Rape and sexual assaults are complex and, therefore, must be viewed with wide lenses. Researchers argue that rape typology is multifaceted because some are based on the victim–offender relationship, offender motivation, degree of force or coercion used, and level of planning used to commit the crime (Friis-Rodel et al., 2021). Rape experts and researchers argue that sexual assault is often caused by the need to dominate and exercise power and control over others. These actions also have elements of time, location, and circumstances since different typologies include spousal, stranger, acquaintance, workplace, statutory, campus, jails, prison, and military.

Spousal/Partner Rape

Spousal rape is also referred to as partner or marital rape. It occurs between those who were either married or still married. Experts argue that of the different types of rape, spousal rape is often misunderstood by many in the U.S. and is more common than stranger rape (Wallace, 1999). Family violence experts contend that it was once commonly believed that a man had a right to have sex with his spouse (Wallace, 1999). Several types of partner rape include the following: battering rape, force-only rape, and obsessive/sadistic rape. Decades ago, courts in America did not intervene when wives filed rape charges against a spouse. Today, husbands can be charged for raping and sexually assaulting their spouse (Wallace, 1999). Finkelhor and Yllo (1985) categorized marital rapes into three areas: force-only, battering rapes, and obsessive rapes. Battering rape consists of both physical and sexual violence aimed at degrading and humiliating the wife, often occurring when violence is used during sexual acts to injure or hurt the spouse. Second, force-only rape involves dominance and the use of power and control over another. Some associate this with a spouse being forced to perform oral and anal sex without regard to spousal feelings about these activities. Third, obsessive/sadistic rape involves the use of torture and committing perverse sexual acts on an unwilling spouse such as demanding that the spouse engage in sexual intercourse with friends and coworkers (Finkelhor & Yllo, 1985; Wallace, 1999).

Stranger Rape

Stranger rape occurs among people who are unknown to each other. Of the typologies, it is the most stereotypical and socially constructed of any form of rape or sexual assault since it has been perpetuated by *Hollywood* and widely discussed among people and social institutions. Experts report that compared with the other types, it is disproportionately depicted in most rape scenes on television programs including infotainment docudramas. Moreover, media critics have long argued that depictions of stranger-only rapes continue to perpetuate cultural stereotypes and myths about the dynamics that exist between victims and offenders and have aided in diminishing most people's social reality of sexual assault to the extent that many in the U.S. view stranger rape as the only "real" form of sexual assault. This suggests that because of historical and cultural stereotypes, many men and women have not defined the other types of rape as criminal law violations. Oddly, stranger rapes are not as common as most people believe since research shows that most rapes are committed by someone who is known to the victim, and girls older than 12 years of age are more likely to experience a violent victimization from someone close to them. Stanger rapes are also considered more threating and violent compared with others (Friis-Rodel et al., 2021; Brownstein, 2000).

Acquaintance/Date Rape

Acquaintance rape, also known as date rape, is a serious problem in the U.S. that shows no signs of abating unless boys are socialized into viewing females as their equals and not as objects to chase, conquer, and dominate (Wallace, 1999). It occurs between two people who know each other. Women are more likely to experience being sexually assaulted by an acquaintance. It typically occurs between people who share a social relationship, such as a friend, classmate, relative, or coworker. Because of the way these rapes are committed, many victims of acquaintance rape and others in the U.S. do not recognize this type of rape as "real" rape because the perpetrator is not a stranger and may even be dating the victim (Pollard, 1995). In some cases, rather than using force, rapes are often carried out using manipulation or coerced sexual contact. Hence, many victims view the uninvited sexual intercourse or sex on demand as something that happens within the context of dating. Statistics reveal that 80% of rape victims know the offender.

Statutory Rape

Statutory rape occurs when an adult has sexual intercourse with a minor or someone who is not in the age of majority and who cannot legally consent to have sex. Where the law is concerned, the use of physical force or threat is unimportant and not included as an element that must be established to charge someone for having intercourse with a minor. The simple fact that the person is a teenager or minor is enough to charge an adult. The age of consent to have sexual intercourse varies from state to state. For example, in most states, the age is 16–17, and in others, it is 18. Sometimes, states may have an exception to statutory rape: when the couple is legally married or near the same age (cannot be more than three years older than the person having intercourse). Nevertheless, statutory rape is also common in the U.S. In 2016, *Child Protective Services* agencies nationwide reported that strong evidence established that 57,329 children were sexually assaulted by men (in 88% of the cases), women (in 9% of cases), and unknown (in 3% of cases) (U.S. Department of Health and Human Services, 2013, 2018). Another report revealed that one in every nine girls and one in every 20 boys under the age of 18 were the victims of sexual assault, while 82% of minor victims were females (Department of Justice, 2000). Females between the ages of 16 and 19 are four times greater than people in the general population to experience rape, attempted rape, or sexual assault (Department of Justice, 1997).

Campus Rape

Campus rapes are acts of forced sexual intercourse that occur at any institution of learning. While rapes occur at elementary schools, junior high schools, or high schools, sexual assaults and rapes are common at colleges and universities and are mostly identified as acquaintance rape. Statistics indicate that among undergraduate students, 26.4% of females and 6.8% of males reported being raped. Among graduate and professional students, 9.7% of females and 6.8% of males reported being raped by physical force, violence, or incapacitation. Furthermore, 23.1% of transgender, genderqueer, nonbinary (TGQN) college students have been sexually assaulted (Cantor et al., 2020). The average age of college victims is 18.5 years old. A national survey of more than 6,000 students at 32 U.S. colleges and universities reported the following: one in every four women reported either experiencing rape or have been the victim of an attempted rape, 84% knew the attacker, 57% of the rapes occurred while the victim and offender were on a date, and only 27% of the victims believed they were raped. Only 42% of the women told someone that they were raped, and only 5% reported the crime to police (Bohmer & Parrot, 1993).

Military Rape

Data show that members of the nation's armed forces are not exempted from being raped or sexually assaulted. Statistics from 2016 show that rape in the military was pervasive since 14,900 active military personnel reported experiencing victimization. LGBTQ women reported a victimization rate of 27.5%, and LGBQT men reported a rate of 18.3%, and 4.3% among those who do not identify as LGBTQ. Of that number, many were sexually assaulted multiple times, which resulted in an estimated 41,000 incidents (Department of Defense [DoD], 2016). Most victims were women (8,600) and men (6,300) and the perpetrators were not strangers, but rather, they were known to victims since they often served in the same company. A recent report finds that the Army experienced an increase of 25.6% from 2020 to 2021, but now, it has experienced a 13% increase in sexual assault reports. The Navy reported a 9.2% increase, while the Air Force and Marines experienced a 2% increase (Liebermann et al., 2022).

Jail/Prison Rape

Another type of rape and sexual assault that often gets ignored is that occurring in jails and prisons between inmates and correctional staff. Since correctional institutions are closed to the public, people are unaware of what occurs in such places. Despite the U.S. promise to eliminate prison rapes with the creation of the *Prison Rape Elimination Act* of 2003, places of confinement continue to experience sexual victimizations. According to the *Bureau of Justice Statistics*, correctional administrators reported that in 2018, an estimated 27,826 rape allegations were made by inmates in U.S. correctional settings. This number represents a 14% increase compared with the 24,514 rapes that occurred in 2015 (Buehler, 2021). Of those allegations substantiated, 58% were considered as inmate-on-inmate violence, and the remaining 42% were committed by correctional staff on inmates (Buehler, 2021). Despite the number of reported rape and sexual assault claims made by inmates, correctional investigations into these matters often find it difficult to confirm or corroborate inmates' claims of rape. For example, a nationwide investigation into inmates claims of being raped from 2016 to 2018 was successful at establishing that only 55% occurred (Buehler, 2021).

Explaining the Roots of Rape and Sexual Assault

Because sexual assault varies and can be complex, researchers believe that prevention requires understanding the underlying root causes. They argue that no single factor can be pointed to as a trigger that causes sexual violence or an act of aggression. Some scholars argue that theories on rape and sexual assault are expected to explain why some people engage in these behaviors, but must also explain why some people do not commit rape and acts of sexual aggression and why violence directed at women takes on a sexual nature (Baumeister et al., 2002; Lowell, 2010). While several theories can explain sexual aggression toward women (e.g., psychological, biological, machoism, and others), perhaps the most common theories include the feminist theory, social learning theory, self-control theory, and the evolutionary theory.

Radical Feminist Theory

Although rape and sexual assault appear to be sex crimes, researchers have compiled decades of evidence that refutes the notion that they are committed to achieve sexual gratification, or due to lust or a high sex drive, but rather, radical feminist theory postulates that rapists are influenced by aggression, violence, and dominance they use to subordinate, intimidate, and frighten women (Kalra & Bhugra, 2013). A commonly held view among radical feminists is that rape is an act that men use to exert power and control over women, and to some men, sex is another commodity they wish to acquire (Simpson, 1989; Baker, 1997). Early studies by radical feminists linked male sexual aggression to patriarchal power and control or unequal distributions of power since men have historically dominated all social institutions (e.g., family, workplace, education, church, government, military, justice system, others) in capitalist societies in terms of power relations. Because in patriarchal societies, men have always been more powerful and women powerless, they have also controlled what is culturally accepted and expected regarding gender roles, and attitudes toward sexual relations (Kalra & Bhugra, 2013). Some theorists contend that women's double marginality has increased the likelihood that they will experience more violent victimizations such as rape (Chapman, 1990). Alternatively, some also suggest that in capitalist societies, the need to feel empowered and to control something or someone has led lower-class men to commit rape and sexual assault. Consequently, some radical feminists view rape as men doing "class and gender" on women (Messerschmidt, 1993). McPhail (2015) contends that the feminist theory sees rape as a gender-based crime that supports patriarchal structures. For radical feminists, rape is caused by hostility that men have toward women, and it manifests in the form of rape (Melani & Fodaski, 1974). Similarly, Brownmiller (1975) reported that rape is a display of male domination and female degradation used by all men to keep women in a perpetual state of fear. Moreover, radical feminists argue that the sexual victimization of women, including rape and sexual assault, is a function of male socialization that teaches young males to react toward females in an aggressive and exploitive way, especially on college campuses, where males often have friends and same-sex peer groups that encourage the use of violence against women. They are typically protected from retribution by a code of secrecy. While some may be critical of the radical feminist position, a national survey by the *Center for Research on Women* at *Wellesley College* supported their argument. According to results from the Center, 90% of adolescent girls reported experiencing sexual harassment in school, 30% reported being pressured to engage in some form of sexual behavior, and 10% reported being forced to commit a sexual act (Center for Research on Women, 1993).

Social Learning Theory

Albert Bandura's social modeling theory provides the most plausible explanation for why men commit rape and sexual assault. According to the theory, aggressive tendencies are not innate but are learned behavior from exposure to violence and are later modeled. Bandura suggests that exposure to violence can come directly from one's friends, family members, or strangers. Being exposed to violence can also come from the mass media, especially violent depictions in television programming, violent pornography, and violence that occurs in popular culture (Barkan, 2006). This suggests learning is complex and can be influenced by many sources. Therefore, one can learn acts of aggression both directly and indirectly, and that aggression is acceptable. After being exposed to violence, people often model or imitate what they have seen or witnessed. However, Bandura (1973) argued that learning aggressive behavior is more likely to occur when there are no observed consequences for committing the behavior. For example, when children are reared in abusive homes characterized by physical, sexual, and emotional violence, and the abusive parent is not punished and held responsible for the behavior. Consequently, the cycle of violence continues generationally (Barkan, 2006).

Experts examining rape and sexual assault contend that individual, community, and societal acceptance of violence against women increases the likelihood of more violence against women. The regularity of violent depictions of women as victims of rape in movies, television, and pornography serves to desensitize people to the harsh reality of violence (Kennedy-Bergan & Bogel, 2000). Pornography has become accepted globally and grosses an estimated $100 billion annually. However, in the U.S. alone, it is a $13 billion a year industry with depictions and images of women and others engaging in gang bangs, rapes, bondage, and pain. Critics of violent porn argue that this genre leads consumers to normalize forced sex, misogyny, humiliation, rape culture, and pain (Vera-Gray et al., 2021). Research finds that these socially constructed images and views about women and sex are especially true on college campuses where there are groups, cliques, and cultures that promote aggression against women. Some studies reveal that college students in fraternities face pressure from their frat brothers to acquire many sexual conquests to the extent that they receive encouragement and support for taking advantage of girls too intoxicated to refuse sex or who have passed out. Because the group culture often devalues girls, these practices and norms are passed on to fraternity members (Schwartz & Nogrady, 1996; Martin & Hummer, 1989). This is exacerbated when colleges fail to punish men for committing rape and when students do not report them, increasing the likelihood that fraternity members will develop attitudes favorable toward rape and engage in violence against women.

Self-Control Theory

Some researchers report evidence to suggest that when men have insatiable, uncontrollable sexual desires, this could explain why they engage in rape and sexual assault. This category of rapists does not believe they are responsible for their behavior, given they have more sexual energy compared with other men and the women they target play a direct role in their decision. This form of victim-blaming holds that the rape is precipitated by women who withhold intercourse from hypersexual men struggling to satisfy their sex drive (Polaschek & Ward, 2002). This view is influenced by Gottfredson and Hirschi's low self-control theory, holding that all crime, including rape and sexual assault, occurs because perpetrators are selfish and lack self-control. Since rapists suffer from low self-control, it forces them to have their need for immediate gratification quickly satisfied, since they cannot work at investing in healthy human relationships with others where sexual relations may be a natural part of a nurtured courtship or marriage (Gottfredson & Hirschi, 1990). Studies on rapists find that many possess lower empathy, lower attachment, and stronger sexual dominance motives compared with non-rapists (Abbey et al., 2007, p. 1574). Similarly, data from a sample of 69 repeat sex offenders, committing two or more sexual offences against a stranger, revealed that sexual offenders with a low level of control exhibited behaviors that were consistent with low self-control theory (Katherine & Beauregard, 2016). Behaviors included impulsive, risky, insensitive, short-sighted, and physically aggressive behavior during various stages of sexual offending.

Evolutionary Theory

Evolutionary theory is also known as a biological explanation for rape. While the theory is heavily criticized and runs counter to the power and control argument, Ellis (1989) and Siegert and Ward (2002) provide that evolutionary theory posits rape is an extreme response to natural selection in which some males attempt to copulate with as many women sex partners as possible even if it must be accomplished by use of force. Evolutionary theorist Thornhill (1999) contends that men who rape women can procreate and reproduce more efficiently and have children who shared their traits. Thornhill provides that rape has a positive effect on rapists' reproductive success and research supports that some men have a psychological adaptation to engage in rape that is specific to committing a certain type of rape on a certain woman. For these theorists, sex is about gratification and being able to pass on one's genes through rape (Chisholm & Burbank, 1991). Evidence also shows that rape removes the struggle that exists between women and men about a choice mate. Women may prefer protective mates with status, resources, and specific physical features, because they often weigh the option of selecting a mate that can obstruct the evolutionary process from moving rapidly. Thus, the rapist gets the women without social resources or being attractive (Chisholm & Burbank, 1991). Therefore, rape is a residual of men's quest to have causal sex without the commitment attached (Thornhill, 1999).

Culture of Violence Theory

The culture of violence theory, also referred to as the intergenerational transmission of violence theory, holds that violence is deeply ingrained in the American culture, arguing that the culture legitimizes the use of violence as seen throughout the country's history. Some theorists contend that the culture is responsible for intergenerational violence that manifests in different forms, such as child abuse, intimate personal violence, and other violent crimes, since early childhood exposure to violence in the household influences violent patterns of behavior later in life. Put differently, children who are the victims or witnesses to child abuse or domestic violence by a parent are more likely to grow up and react in the same manner. What is more alarming is that the child survivor of abuse develops a predisposition to violence in their own family, which may become generational. According to Wallace (1999), violence is learned in the family and is generational. Experts also contend that many factors contribute to the continuation of violence among individuals and on a societal level. Kalra and Bhugra (2013) echo this sentiment by reporting that sexual violence is saturated in cultures perpetuating the belief in male superiority and female inferiority. Research shows as early as the 1970s, some theorists argued that the American culture and its tolerance for violence fostered a rape culture or a pervasive ideology that supported or excused rape and sexual assaults against girls and women. They attributed sexual violence against women to the culture by contending that U.S. boys are socialized to believe it is normal to be sexually aggressive, and girls are taught it is proper to be sexually passive. This cultural acceptance of rape or sexual aggression can be interpreted as an extreme example of sanctioned intercourse between males and females, but a normal practice (Johnson & Johnson, 2021).

What Are the Risk Factors?

Any person can become a victim of sexual aggression (Krug et al., 2002). Experts contend that there is overlap between the different types of rape and sexual assault. Multiple factors increase the likelihood of rape and the risk of someone being forced into sex as well as factors in the individual and his or her social environment that influence the occasion of rape. Studies suggest one or more risk factors can increase the likelihood that someone will either become a perpetrator or a victim of abuse. Research finds that while risk factors should be considered causal, the more risk factors people are exposed to, the greater the likelihood that sexual violence will occur, since these factors contribute to violence. Risk factors are not meant to convey that victims are responsible for their victimization (Corbin et al., 2001). Researchers and policymakers are interested in understanding risk factors to prevent the number of rape and sexual assault cases that occur since they can inform what prevention strategies need to target or identify opportunities for prevention, especially for high-risk groups and places. The CDC has presented several individual, relationship, community, and societal risk factors that contribute to rape and sexual violence.

Individual Factors

In their report, Tharp et al. (2013) identify several individual risk factors that influence sexual violence. They include alcohol and drug use, delinquency, lack of concern for others, early sexual initiation, coercive sexual fantasies, exposure to sexually explicit media, hostility toward women, hypermasculinity, suicidal behavior, prior sexual victimization, adherence to traditional gender role norms, preference for impersonal sex and sexual risk taking, and an acceptance of aggressive and violent behavior. Dahlberg and Krug (2002) reported that other individual risk factors are age, education, income, substance use, and history of abuse. The presence of any one or more of these risk factors can influence rape and sexual assault. For example, Carey et al. (2015) reported that rapes on college campuses have reached epidemic proportions and student risky drinking behavior is one of the main factors. Moreover, research using a survey to measure sexual assault on college campuses found that the use of drugs and alcohol has a pronounced presence at many sexual assault scenes (Corbin et al., 2001).

Relationship Factors (Friends/Family)

While there are individual factors that increase the likelihood of rape and sexual assault, experts also link relationships such as those with family members and friends as contributing factors. They contend that a person's closest inner circle of friends, partners, and family members often impact their behavior and influence decision-making (Dahlberg & Krug, 2002). They argue that characteristics such as having a family history of conflict and violence, a childhood history of physically, sexually, or emotionally unsupportive parents, use of drugs and alcohol by parents, and poor parent–child relations can impact rape and sexual assault. They also find that one's peers and friends have a binding impact on their behaviors. For example, one's chances are greater for committing rape or sexual assault or being the victim if one's associates are sexually aggressive, hypermasculine, or delinquent (Tharp et al., 2013).

Community Factors

Studies show that even if one does not have individual or relationships with significant others placing them at risk for sexual violence, the community where one lives, including its schools, workplaces, and neighborhoods, can expose them to attitudes and values that accept and embrace rape and other forms of sexual aggression. One can be introduced to attitudes shared by many people in the community who are rapists or have misogynistic ideas about the role and place of women in the family, community, and broader society. Some studies reveal that criminogenic neighborhoods lacking economic resources and are characterized by poverty tend to be fertile grounds for crime including predatory behaviors such as rape and sexual assault (Tharp et al., 2013). Beyond economic disparities, these areas often lack employment opportunities and suffer social disorganization that renders informal mechanisms of social control (e.g., family, school, peers, church) ineffective, thereby weakening the neighborhood's ability to make residents conform to normative behavior. When apathy becomes pervasive in these neighborhoods, with an acceptance of "no snitching," they become places where lawlessness and violence proliferate since most people lack confidence in police or the judicial system. Unfortunately, residents develop a tolerance for sexual violence by turning a blind eye to sexual perpetrators (Tharp et al., 2013; Jewkes et al., 2002).

Societal Factors

Macro-level factors that impact rape and sexual assault must be viewed within a wider framework since institutional and societal practices have historically influenced them and created a climate that has allowed them to sustain themselves (Dahlberg & Krug, 2002). For example, feminist theorists argue that in patriarchal societies, there has always existed an acceptance of societal norms that support sexual violence, male superiority, and sexual entitlement. These social and cultural norms have perpetuated hypersexualization among young people and put more women at risk of sexually aggressive behavior. They also believe that societal norms defining traditional gender roles have worked to maintain the belief that women are inferior and sexually submissive, rendering women powerless and open to historical victimization (World Health Organization [WHO], 2010; Jewkes et al.,

2002). Sexist social norms have been reinforced by weak laws and policies in the areas of health, economics, education, and social arenas (created by men), failing to adequately punish sexual violence and gender inequality. Rather, they have fostered high levels of crime and other forms of violence against women (Tharp et al., 2013; Dahlberg & Krug, 2002). Feminists view patriarchal societies and their structures as oppressive to girls and women since all social institutions are dominated by men including those responsible for creating and constructing rape laws and those who judge those committing sexual assault. They also view the dominant consciousness as a construct perpetuated by men using the mass media and other mechanisms to reinforce power and control over gender relations (Bailey, 1999).

Role of Inequity

Research reveals that socioeconomic status has a historical presence in rape and sexual assault statistics. In a study on the geographical clusters of reported rape cases in the U.S., researchers find poverty and rape are associated (Amin et al., 2015). For many, poverty is universally one of the greatest factors that increase the risk of sexual violence against poor girls and women since it confronts them in daily routine activities, such as walking home from work or receiving less parental supervision when not in school. They can also be forced into occupations that elevate the risk of sexual violence. Impoverished women also experience intimate partner violence that often includes sexual violence (Krug et al., 2002; Heinze, 2021). Stated differently, poverty and economic loss lead to an increase in the number of rape and sexual exploitation cases (Bailey, 1999; Heinze, 2021). Feminists contend that because of the gender relations found in patriarchal systems producing gender socioeconomic inequality, impoverished men or those who face harsh economic times experience levels of frustration and diffuse aggression that are often acted out on the women they encounter. Therefore, the economy can produce supplies of offenders and victims, and gender socioeconomic inequality contributes to sexual violence against women (Schwendinger & Schwendinger, 1983; Bailey, 1999).

Sexual assault is more likely to occur among impoverished women because their economic insecurity lessens their ability to secure safe living arrangements (Bailey, 1999). Research examining a cross-city examination of determinants of forcible rape in major cities from 1980 to 1990 supports this contention. A study reported that female income was the only significant determinant in rape cases. More specifically, the investigation revealed that in cities where women reported having higher income levels, they experienced less forcible rapes and other violent crimes compared with women in cities with high concentration of poverty and high rates of crime including rap. The study concluded that living in areas where income is higher affords women a degree of safety, and they avoid encounters with men experiencing frustration and aggression owing to their economic plight (Bailey, 1999). Other studies find that on the individual level, women who experience housing insecurity may be two or four times more likely to face sexual violence or exploitation since predatory landlords are propositioning women. At the community level, vulnerable women living in poverty face an elevated risk of being raped and sexually assaulted. On the societal level, those women who live in areas with higher unemployment rates or financial desperation also risk experiencing higher rates of sexual violence (Yodanis, 2004; Heinze, 2021).

Rape and Sexual Assault Are Criminal Justice Issues

Rape and sexual assault are criminal justice issues because the system is charged with ensuring community safety and investigating crimes after they are reported (Gaines & Miller, 2010). Next to homicide, rape is the second most serious offense regardless of victim gender, racial or cultural background, age, religion, or social economic status (Whelan, 2020). Rape is listed among violent crimes in Part One offenses in the UCR collected annually by the FBI on known crimes committed in the U.S. (Gaines & Miller, 2010). Despite this, critics argue that among all crimes, the number of rape and intimate personal violence cases are the most underreported. Some critics and victim's advocacy groups contend that the justice system has historically failed victims of rape and sexual assault nationwide given its dismal arrest rates of offenders and successful prosecutions. Justice officials, namely police officers as first responders to rape cases are required to follow procedures, ensuring the safety of victims and minimizing the guilt and shame they experience. However, this is not always achieved. Police often exacerbate the matter by adding to rape victim's stress, anxiety, and silence around rape (New York State Coalition against Sexual Violence, 2003; Whelan, 2020). This often occurs when victims finally muster the courage to come forward, only to have their case not taken seriously because of evidence issues, long periods before a case gets heard, or to be asked if they precipitated their victimization. Furthermore, prosecuting attorneys often fail to inform the victims of crimes about the existence of victims' compensation programs and applications for monies available to assist crime victims who agree to assist in the criminal prosecution. For many victims, they interpret the justice system's mishandling or rejection of their case as an affront to their credibility as well as dignity (Parent et al., 1991).

Spohn and Tellis (2014) reported that a study into *Los Angeles Police Department, Los Angeles Sheriff Department*, and the *Los Angeles District Attorney* office, examining police response and prosecution's response to sexual assault allegations discovered that because many cases were submitted to the DA's office before suspects were arrested, it created a higher level of proof needed to make an arrest. Additionally, law enforcement agencies used pre-arrest charges to screen out cases they considered difficult to prove if they determined the victim engaged in risky behavior. Some researchers have collected evidence suggesting that serial rapists often target vulnerable victims that the justice system has failed since in many cases, the criminal justice system places the onus on sexual assault victims to ensure a successful outcome in rape cases. Research reveals that because participating in the justice process is traumatic and creates a second victimizations for many rape victims and victim-blaming, most victims either refuse to participate in the justice process or to opt not to report the crime (Lovell et al., 2021).

Rape and Sexual Assault Are Public Health Issues

After the justice process is complete, the effects of rape or sexual assault still linger. Therefore, CDC experts contend that criminal justice is a small aspect of criminal victimization since the justice system's response to violence is not designed to address the health needs of survivors. These experts argue that the justice system emphasizes apprehending perpetrators and bringing them to justice. Waechter (2021) reports that sexual violence has maintained prevalence for a very long time in society because of slow prevention efforts. Consequently, victims of rape and sexual assault feel as though the system is focused on protecting and safeguarding the constitutional rights of suspects and not a victim's well-being throughout the justice process and in the aftermath of the crime. As such, criminal justice and public health concede that a harsh reality is that most rape victims will never fully return to their pre-victimization status. The experience of rape transcends criminal justice and is also regarded as a public health problem requiring public health responses since victims often need treatment and services that are provided by public health and healthcare professionals such as emergency clinical services, crisis counseling, and long-term specialized therapy to name a few (Freire-Vargas, 2018; Rosenberg & Fenley, 1991). Because public health officials are concerned about prevention, they contend that treatment must also be extended to offenders since violence impacts the entire community. More specifically, they recommend that healthcare providers who treat rapists must be trained specialists using the group treatment approach rather than one-on-one sessions because the former structure allows a way to confront offenders who are highly manipulative and untrustworthy. This is believed to increase the likelihood that they will receive effective therapeutic sessions that may help change their behavior (Groth, 1979).

Public health issues threaten the health of people and their communities. Unlike health care, which is individualized, public health targets the entire population regarding matters such as infectious disease, unsafe air, and water quality that poses a threat to individuals, communities, national environment, or they can also be toxic levels of violence, including rape and sexual assault especially when it has reached epidemic levels. Experts at the Institute of Medicine (US) (1988, p. 40) defined public health's mission as "the fulfillment of society's interest in assuring the conditions in which people can be healthy." Public health views violence as a disease that affects people in different ways, and depending on the severity, it could lead to death, injury, along with short- and long-term pain and suffering. Like a disease, it goes beyond the individual and could affect others in the community, especially when efforts are not taken to prevent it and it reaches epidemic proportions (Freire-Vargas, 2018). According to officials at the *CDC, FBI, NCVS,* and researchers, the number of people in the U.S. impacted by rape and sexual assault can never truly be known given the personal nature of the crime, as well as it being one of the most underreported crimes chiefly due to the lack of trust in the justice system and victims not wanting others to know about their victimization (Cohn et al., 2013; Meadows, 2004; Freire-Vargas, 2018). The reported sexual assault cases that are known are believed to reach epidemic proportions in the U.S. This, along with the profound consequences that they bring to victims, makes them a public health issue.

International Comparative Statistics

Unlike the U.S., many countries lack national data reporting systems or clearinghouses that store crime data, such as the UCR, National Incident-Based Reporting System (NIBRS), or the NCVS, either because of culture, economics, or other reasons, such as not wanting the world to know about the crime that exists within their borders. Despite this, WHO (2021) statistics show that violence against women including rape and sexual assault are not exclusive to any given society (e.g., advanced or developing) but are a global problem that effect an estimated 736 million women since one in three women worldwide are believed to experience them during their lifetime by either an intimate partner or from a non-partner. Similarly, Amnesty International (2018) reported that though an estimated

9 million women between the ages of 15 and older in the *European Union* (EU) have been raped, the number is grossly underreported. Moreover, data from an EU wide survey show that women and girls who are especially challenged to assert a rape claim are sex workers, transgendered women, those living in rural areas, homeless women, asylum seekers, those with questionable immigration status, and those suffering mental health illnesses and substance issues. Because of this, public health experts argue that violence against women has reached epidemic proportions globally with its extent varying by country and culture but includes crimes such as murder, assault, battery, sexual assault, rape, robbery, and other crimes linked to use of force by their male counterparts. Nevertheless, when it comes to measuring rape and sexual assault cases globally, researchers are confronted with many challenges that confound collecting accurate rape statistics. The evidence suggests that the cases are still highly underreported, arguably because of victim embarrassment, fear of reprisal, lack of trust in the justice system, and insufficient laws. Additionally, researchers often face the following: (1) high rates of underreporting that could be more than 90% since in some countries rape victims are either ostracized by their families or killed as a form of honor killing and (2) definitions and tracking methods of rape vary by country. For example, in some countries, spousal rape is not a crime and every occurrence or rape between the same two people, if reported, is only one single offense, despite the number of times it occurred.

While some countries may consider any non-consensual sex as a rape, others only count forced vaginal penetration during sexual intercourse, while other countries consider unwarranted penetration of the mouth, anus, or vulva with a body part or object. Some countries may track rapes that are between male-on-female only, while others consider those that are female-on-female, female-on-male, and male-on-male. Furthermore, some countries count gang rapes as a single incident despite the number of people involved, while other countries count gang rape as multiple incidents. Most sexual assault experts agree that in some countries, the laws prohibiting rape are insufficient, inconsistent, or not enforced. Thereby, discouraging victims from taking steps toward reporting their victimization, believing the matter as counterproductive. Because these matters conspire to render rape statistics questionable at best, the United Nations (2021) ranks each country by its number of rapes and sexual assaults per 100,000 people in the population, we present the ten highest and the ten fewest for illustrative purposes. According to data collected by the *United Nations*, those countries with the highest rape rates are ranked as follows: (1) Botswana at 92.93; (2) Lesotho at 82.68; (3) Bermuda at 67.29; (4) Sweden at 63.54; (5) Costa Rica at 36.70; (6) Grenada at 30.63; (7) Australia at 28.60; (8) Belgium at 27.92; (9) U.K. at 27.29; and (10) U.S. at 27.31. Conversely, those countries with the fewest number of rapes and sexual assault include the following: (1) Egypt at 0.11; (2) Azerbaijan at 0.17; (3) Mozambique at 0.19; (4) Lebanon at 0.46; (5) Tajikistan at 0.53; (6) Serbia at 0.73; (7) Albania at 0.75; (8) Nepal at 0.75; (9) Yemen at 0.75; and (10) Guinea at 0.98. It is important to note that while some countries appear to have low rates of rapes and sexual assaults, this should be taken within a broader social context and could be a product of several factors that include male guardianship whereby single women are prohibited by law from living on their own, renting an apartment or traveling anywhere without being accompanied by a male. In some countries, women under age 25 are not allowed to travel unless they receive permission from a male guardian (e.g., father, husband, or brother). Even more troubling is the fact that in some cultures, women who are raped or sexually assaulted may no longer be considered desirable for married. Therefore, some cultures have resorted to preserve the integrity of the victim and her family by requiring the rapist to marry her and this union excuses the rape or restoring the family honor may require that the raped victim become an outcast or murdered (Mercy, 1993). Consequently, they may not report the matter to their family or local authorities.

Public Health and Social Work

Intersection of Public Health and Social Work

Social workers intersect with victims of rape and sexual abuse in a myriad of professional roles and places of employment. They often intervene with survivors at women's shelters, emergency departments, rape crisis clinics, community mental health clinics, physician offices, and in private therapy. Rape and sexual assault survivors often need immediate support and referrals for services such as health care, access to safety, and connections with support groups and legal advocacy which social workers can provide through casework practice (Socialworkin, 2022). Because sexual assault and rape are likely to cause detrimental health and emotional consequences, survivors can benefit from trauma-focused therapy provided by licensed clinical social workers and psychiatrists, or counseling provided by trained crisis response personnel. These are therapies that may be beneficial for treating post-traumatic stress disorder (PTSD), trauma-related depression, and anxiety (Bisson & Andrew, 2007). They include cognitive processing therapy, in vivo or imaginal exposure-based therapy, and eye movement desensitization and reprocessing (EMDR) (Regehr et al., 2013). According to Lamade and Okanlawon (2020), therapies for treating perpetrators of sexual assault include the risk needs responsivity (RNR) model, the Good Lives Model (GLM), Motivational Interviewing (MI), and Relapse Prevention (RP). Social workers and public health officials often collaborate in prevention efforts such as community education, targeting potential victims, about consent, healthy relationships, safety planning, and available resources for utilization both before and after victimization (Wilson & Jiminez, 2023).

Health Disparities and Health Equities

While people living in a state of vulnerability (e.g., women, children, persons with disabilities, and the elderly) face an elevated risk of rape and its consequences, research reveals that Black women are especially burdened with risk factors linked to rape (e.g., poverty and child sex abuse), and therefore, are at a heightened susceptibility to its long-term consequences (Bryant-Davis et al., 2010; West & Johnson, 2013). This includes an increased likelihood of developing PTSD and contracting sexually transmitted infections. This may be exacerbated by the fact that, unlike White women, research reports that Black women may be less likely to seek and receive care after an assault due to racial bias that exists in the criminal justice and healthcare systems (Hakimi et al., 2018; Iverson et al., 2011). Therefore, they may experience more negative physical and psychological effects owing to the matter going undiagnosed and untreated, especially when it comes to developing PTSD (Jacques-Tiura et al., 2010).

When research controls for race, age, and education, studies find that women who experience rape, compared to women without a history of rape, those who have experienced rape have a higher risk of developing asthma, irritable bowel syndrome, frequent headaches, chronic pain, difficulty sleeping, activity limitations, poor physical health, poor mental health, and the need for specialized medical equipment such as wheelchairs. The greatest risk was for poor mental health. Men who are raped and who are "made to penetrate" (MTP) also have higher levels of negative health consequences compared with males who are not assaulted or MTP (Smith et al., 2022). *MTP* is defined by Basile and colleagues (2022, p. 1) as:

> Being made to vaginally penetrate a female using one's own penis; being made to penetrate a female's vagina or anus with their mouth; being made to anally penetrate a male or female; or being made to receive oral sex from a male or female.

Smith and colleagues (2022) analyzed data from 8,032,000 males who experienced rape only, MTP assault only, or both to measure levels and types of impacts. Health conditions measured included those mentioned above, with women experiencing sexual assault: asthma, irritable bowel syndrome, frequent headaches, chronic pain, difficulty sleeping, activity limitations, poor physical health, poor mental health, the need for specialized medical equipment such as wheelchairs, and high blood pressure. After controlling for age, race, education, and other forms of violence, it was discovered that men with a history of rape were significantly more likely to report limitations of activity and require the use of special medical equipment. Victims of MTP were significantly more likely to report frequent headaches, chronic pain, sleep difficulties, limitation of activities, needing the use of specialized medical equipment, and poor mental health. One in three men who reported rape and MTP by a single perpetrator were also more likely to report physical injuries.

Negative Health Consequences of Rape and Sexual Assault

Officials at the Centers for Disease Control and Prevention (CDC) (n.d.) report that because physical force is not used in every rape, the consequence of sexual violence often varies. For example, a small number of rapes result in pregnancy and death to victims (Krug et al., 2002). However, the most common consequences are physical and psychological; in some cases, they can be chronic since survivors often experience PTSD, and recurring gastrointestinal, cardiovascular, and sexual health problems. Health experts contend that sexual violence can have a lifelong impact on the health of victims (e.g., all genders, orientations, and ages) as well as others in the community, especially feelings of insecurity and a diminished quality of life (CDC, n.d.). Moreover, the victims of sexual violence can also experience reproductive problems, genital injuries, as well as sexually transmitted infections such as *HIV/AIDS*, herpes, syphilis, and gonorrhea (Krug et al., 2002). Some experts even argue that being raped could impact the survivor's behavior since research shows that many survivors are more likely to smoke, abuse alcohol, use drugs, engage in risky sexual activity, and entertain suicidal thoughts in the aftermath of their sexual assault. As such, health experts contend that rape and sexual assault survivors have needs that far exceed holding their perpetrators criminally responsible for the harm they inflicted. These experts argue that while rape survivors respond to traumatic events differently, what is commonly observed in the aftermath of their victimization is that they typically experience short-term or long-term trauma. Neelam and Gasparini (2023) research revealed that being raped or sexually assaulted can present long-term health consequences that often manifest in adverse physical and mental health. They provide that people with a history of sexual assault and trauma suffer poorer health compared with others and tend to display symptoms such as headaches, fatigue, difficulty sleeping, nausea, and difficulty concentrating. They also endure conditions that include chronic pelvic pain and urinary tract infections, menstrual disturbances such as pain with menstruation, irregular menstrual cycles, multiple yeast infections, pelvic inflammatory diseases, fibromyalgia, and gastrointestinal disorders. Regarding mental health, Neelam and Gasparini (2023) find that people with a history of sexual assault experience a variety of mental health disorders that require support from professionals trained to address these issues. They argue that many survivors of rape display depression that include feelings of hopelessness and sadness, sleep disturbances, loss of interest in routine activities, and change in appetite. The researchers warn that these are not meant to be an exhaustive list of negative physical and mental health conditions that some survivors experience that require a public health response.

Criminal Justice Approaches to Rape and Sexual Assault

As previously mentioned, the criminal justice system has been widely cited for its historical neglect of rape victims while focusing its aim, in most cases, on apprehending and punishing suspects when the evidence points to their guilt (Seidman & Pokorak, 2011). In the U.S., this reactionary approach has been highly criticized by victims, family members, as well as victim advocacy groups that contend it discourages victims from reporting their victimization and it makes victims distrust police since caring for victims is not the goal of the criminal justice system (Seidman & Pokorak, 2011). Experts also argue that one of the main reasons that victims often do not report being raped, or pursue justice, is because they lack support after experiencing sexual assault. Early research by Holmstrom (1985) and Harrell et al. (1985) reported after rape, victims experience a range of emotions that are grounded in fear, anxiety, and mood states. As such, police should develop protocols to help victims regain their sense of well-being and since police occupy a critical role in handling sexual assault cases, reforms should focus on developing an audit trail to track cases, use female police officers in rape cases, treat victims as an ally in these cases, and advise victims on how to be effective witnesses. Victims of rape report experiencing a second victimization at the hands of the justice system in general, but from police, prosecutors, judges, and juries in particular who tend to be influenced by myths, stereotypes, and misogynistic attitudes about the sexual assault of women (LeDoux & Hazelwood, 1985; Bartol & Bartol, 2017). While efforts have changed over the years to improve how rape victims are treated by the public, medical, and criminal justice systems, victims and victim advocacy groups believe some justice officials still have attitudes and behaviors that reflect a general reluctance to believe rape victims (Barkan, 2006; Rousseau, 2019). One positive step in the right direction has been that most states have passed "shield laws" to protect women from being subjected to embarrassing and degrading cross-examinations from defense attorneys who put their prior sexual history on trial and force them to prove they did not give consent. Experts contend that the enactment of shield laws and its protection of women's privacy has encouraged some women to report their sexual assault, but it is still not enough to adequately address rape and sexual assault (Gaines & Miller, 2010; Barak, 2006). Because of this, some criminal justice experts suggest that police departments practice victim-centered approaches, rather than, focusing on quickly closing rape and sexual assault cases.

Critics observe that many rape cases do not proceed to trial for several reasons and chief among them is the quality of evidence that investigating officers collect from victims typically comes down to her words against his. When this occurs, the prosecutor needs strong enough evidence to bring charges against a suspect and win a criminal conviction. In their investigation, Westera and colleagues (2016) argue that the hidden nature of sexual assaults presents challenges for victims to achieve justice. More specifically, their research suggests that if the criminal justice system desires to improve the quality of evidence police can obtain in the aftermath of sexual assaults, it requires a better utilization of police interviewing methods in these difficult cases. They contend video recording the testimony of the complainant and suspect being interviewed shortly after the crime about their thoughts and emotions can offer credible and believable testimony that could contradict stereotypes of rape and sexual assault that decision-makers and juries are prone to accept as a true reflection of rape (Westera et al., 2016).

Another area of concern that criminal justice professionals have expressed is the need for mandatory victim trauma training for police officers and advanced training for detectives and prosecutors who process rape and sexual assault cases. It is vitally important moving forward in the different stages of the justice process that someone addresses the needs of the victim of rape trauma. Given that reports indicate that in 2017, only an estimated 32% of all rape cases in the U.S. were closed and many police department declared rape cases as unfounded (Mustian & Sisak, 2018). Justice officials have recognized the need to clear more rape cases since this neglect often signals to victims that they are not a primary concern of the justice system. In another effort to best respond to rape victims, Human Rights Watch (2013) officials interviewed sex crime detectives from four cities that included *Austin, Texas; Philadelphia, Pennsylvania; Kansas City, Missouri; and Grand Rapid Michigan* to determine the most effective criminal justice responses to sexual assault. These cities were selected because of their efforts to re-examine their approach to sexual assault investigations.

While six recommendations emerged from the *Human Rights Watch* report, it was determined that the best approaches are victim-centered. The report revealed that when police investigations are victim-centered, it leads to successful victim interviewing, which often produces better outcomes. First, the report showed that after a sexual assault, victims suffer trauma that impacts the quality of statements they make during the interview, and, unfortunately, sometimes they provide police with inconsistent or incomplete statements about what transpired. If officers are untrained in dealing with trauma, it creates suspicion and disbelief. Therefore, officers, especially first responders, should be trained to address the traumatic aspects of rape and the impact it has on victims. These officers should collect a limited amount of information from the sexually assaulted victim immediately after the assault. Second, the report provides that the preliminary interview should be conducted with compassion in a nonjudgmental environment, which requires officers to be trained not to judge the victim's behavior and to tell them that nothing they may have done can justify the sexual assault. Third, officers should also explain the importance of not withholding information lest they risk having their credibility questioned later. Fourth, the report found that recording the interview is helpful since it allows investigators to focus on the exchange and avoid inconsistencies in the victim's testimony. Interestingly, it found that using trained, compassionate investigators is more important than the gender of the investigating officer. This challenges the notion that women officers are always more sensitive than their male counterparts when it comes to rape investigations. This notwithstanding, if the victim requests a female officer, it should be provided if possible. Fifth, the report recommends addressing one of the most frustrating aspects that victims describe in rape cases, the lack of contact with police regarding the status of their case. Therefore, police should keep victims informed about their case since it is good for their emotional recovery and increases the likelihood that they will continue in the process. Sixth, rape victims should have an advocate to assist them with navigating the criminal justice process. Advocates should be trained to explain the esoteric nature of the justice process and to lend moral support to minimize victims' stress (Human Rights Watch, 2013). Even with these approaches, scholars report that the criminal justice system alone cannot be expected to prevent violence (Donzinger, 1996).

Public Health Approaches to Rape and Sexual Assault

Because rape and sexual assault are criminal justice and public health issues, experts argue they need more than just a criminal justice framework. Given the gravity of these victimizations, they also require a public health response. Public health officials argue that criminal justice approaches are limited, and their efforts have failed to show reductions in the number of rape cases and recidivism levels among perpetrators. These experts contend that criminal justice policies alone may cause more harm to victims and offenders since the cycle of violence continues and more people are impacted (Shield & Feder, 2016). Health experts at CDC (2022) *National Center for Injury Prevention, Division of Violence Prevention* recently reported that the suffering of large numbers of rape victims and potential victims remains a widespread and devastating public health U.S. crisis. Similarly, others posit that sexual violence is a critical public health problem in communities that manifests in physical, mental, and behavioral consequences negatively impacting individuals, families, and communities (Shield & Feder, 2016). The CDC's report found that almost 9.5 million women and 4.5 million men experienced sexual violence in the past year (CDC, 2022). These victimizations are exacerbated by the human suffering that victims can experience. It is for these and other reasons why rape and sexual assault is highly important for public health officials to address, especially since evidence suggests there are mounting negative health consequences (some have short-term and others long-term impact) associated with these crimes as well as the recovery rate for these victims compared with other victims of different types of crime. Research reveals that for victims of rape and sexual assault, recovery tends to be slower. Health experts report that in sexual assault cases, recovery is never easy; it takes time and can be a painful process as victims often suffer from PTSD, depression, and physical injuries that could last for decades (Rosenberg & Fenley, 1991).

Unlike criminal justice efforts, public health focus is directed at the populations' overall health, safety, and well-being. It requires collaborative efforts from agencies that include health, education, social services, justice, policy, and the private sector (Schneider, 2020). Rape and sexual assault present a health problem to everyone: those affected directly and others who are vicariously impacted including men, women, children, elderly, incarcerated inmates, military personnel, members of *LGBTQI* community, and others, respectively. Statistics on sexual violence reveal that no one in society (nationally or globally) is exempt or immune from this devastating victimization since it can happen to anyone, anywhere, and at any time. Rape statistics also show that sexual violence is not distributed equally regarding race, ethnicity, gender, income, power, and access to health care (Armstrong et al., 2018). Research estimates that one in three women globally will experience physical or sexual assault over their lifetime, committed at the hands of a partner or stranger (WHO, 2021; Wong et al., 2022). Because of the pervasiveness of rape and sexual assault globally, public health officials believe it is incumbent on society to create violence prevention programs and policies aimed at the individual, relational, community, and society levels to educate the public about the prevalence, myths, devastation, and consequence of rape to prevent it from occurring and to treat both offenders and victims in hope to break the cycle of violence. They argue that using a public health approach to address sexual violence allows experts to focus on its root causes and to work toward prevention instead of solely acting by focusing on punishing perpetrators after these acts of violence are committed. Public health experts argue that a comprehensive approach is needed to adequately address prevention strategies, including shared risk factors and protective factors found in each community. These will enable community residents as well as practitioners to recognize factors that can influence one's chance of becoming a victim or perpetrator of sexual violence.

Since rape and sexual assault present negative health consequences for its victims and others, a range of interventions at the individual, community, and societal levels are needed to address and prevent these victimizations. Public health officials contend that in the aftermath of sexual violence, victims are in desperate need of counseling, therapy, and help from support groups to survive these victimizations since many victims often blame themselves and experience psychological damage that negatively impacts their decision to participate in the justice system and to have healthy recoveries (Meyer & Taylor, 1986). In some cases, victims require short-term counseling after a rape occurs. In other cases, victims may need long-term therapy from a skilled therapist with experience working with raped victims. Beyond this, they will also need the services of a trained staff member to accompany them to the hospital to seek medical attention and provide DNA evidence after the assault. A trained staff member can also assist victims with making better decisions about reporting the assault to police (Rosenberg & Fenley, 1991). Furthermore, victims need help from family and community members. Barlow and Wolfe (1981) report that family, friends, and others in a victim's social network experience stress in rape cases that are particularly gruesome. As a result, they may require intervention to help with the stressors and post-traumatic link to how they received, stored, and processed the news about the violent assault. Other individuals in need of treatment are the perpetrators who commit sexual violence. Experts argue that the few programs that target perpetrators in rape cases tend to overwhelmingly focus on men who often deny committing these violent acts. These experts believe that by collaborating with victim support service programs, the perpetrators can be treated if they are willing to accept responsibility for their actions and that these matters are known in the community (Kaufman, 2001). Public health officials also emphasize that treating sexual offenders is an important part of community healing since failing to treat them can lead to more of the same behavior, and others in the community can become exposed to risk factors that could affect their decision to become perpetrators.

On the community level, residents and action groups must engage in massive educational programs that promote awareness about gender issues, *STI* prevention, and problems with sexual and physical violence against women. These community-based efforts are designed to change public attitudes toward sexual violence by using billboards, public radio, television, and public transportation to reach large numbers of people who either tune in, listen to, or read as they travel (Krug et al., 2002). Another community effort that could impact men is the creation of initiatives for men that are designed to sensitize them to violence against women, specifically sexual violence. These groups also teach and promote types of masculinity constructions that are non-violent and promote gender equality (Flood, 2001). On the societal level, all health professionals, especially case workers who interact with victims of sexual violence, need more training in issues and awareness of sexual abuse. Experts contend that health service staff, including psychiatrists and counselors, should be trained to quickly recognize and handle cases of abuse with the degree of sensitivity the situations require. They argue that in the U.S., healthcare professionals should adopt comparative practices that are used in countries such as the Philippines, where public health providers are taught the root causes of violence within the context of culture, gender, and other social aspects. They should also be able to identify high-risk situations within the context of the family or home that increase the likelihood of violence.

Public Health and Social Work Approaches

Public health's population approach to rape and sexual assault prevention is not dissimilar to macro approaches used by social workers. Public health methods include intervening upon environmental conditions that can lead to violence, such as community norms around violence and gender-based inequality (Jacoby et al., 2018) and the vicious cycle of community violence that enables individual violence (Bingenheimer, 2005; Buka et al., 2001). Social work believes that one way to protect vulnerable people is to ensure that their basic needs are met and that they encounter people "who have the cultural knowledge, skills, and attitudes to help them" (Wilson & Webb, 2018, p. 9). They advocate for the Office on Violence Against Women to include provisions in the Violence Against Women Act that endorse prevention programming for the LGBTQ+ community. Similar to public health, social work supports national standards for rape and sexual assault reporting. As with other types of violence, both social work and public health lobby for policy and structural changes to modify the risks for rape and sexual assault, as with alcohol-related policy (DeVocht et al., 2017), and protective and restraining order policies (Wilson & Webb, 2018).

Integrating Skills of Social Epidemiology to Address Disparities and Achieve Equity

Social epidemiology is concerned with identifying social factors that affect patterns of diseases and the health distribution of the population (von dem Knesebeck, 2015). Research reveals that epidemiologists engage in a systematic analysis of concepts such as social inequalities, social relationships, social capital, and work stress to determine how they can be used in health services research since they intersect with the health of the population and are related to the quality of healthcare services people receive. Social factors are also linked to different health outcomes (von dem Knesebeck, 2015). For example, social inequality typically refers to unequal distribution of goods, services, and opportunities that some groups have access to compared with other groups. Social epidemiologists use indicators such as education, income, and occupation to reference social inequity since they have a pronounced effect on whether people have access to treatment and health care (Siegrist & Marmot, 2006). This is especially true for most victims of rape and sexual assault both nationally and globally who are disproportionately from lower socioeconomic or impoverished backgrounds, lacking access to health care, and are in need of healthcare services and treatments immediately after victimization. Similarly, social relationships in general, but the degree of support from those with whom people interact, often influence whether victims and perpetrators will seek help for their victimization or offense, respectively. For example, will victims of rape or sexual assault receive social support from others (e.g., family, friends, colleagues) to seek out emotional help as well as treatments needed in the aftermath of their victimization? Comparatively, will the perpetrators of rape and sexual assault seek community interventions to affect a certain outcome? Similarly, social capital via healthcare organizations is required to deliver quality health care to people. Some contend that it refers to people working in social networks to deliver what is needed by the collective (Kawachi & Berkman, 2000). However, most acts of rape or sexual assault take place in areas in need of economic resources to provide quality healthcare services to victims and perpetrators. According to social epidemiologists, social inequity can fundamentally determine one's health, while other risk factors, such as social relationships and social capital, are in the pathway between social inequality and health outcome (WHO, 2008).

Epidemiologists examine risk factors within the population and view them as an opportunity for intervention. Simultaneously, community-engaged interventionists focus on the community rather than the broader population. Notwithstanding, community researchers are tasked with considering whether identified risk factors should be a priority for the community. More specifically, they are concerned with whether community priorities can be changed and how to use community strengths to create that change (Wallerstein et al., 2011). Scholars contend that when social epidemiologists and community-engaged researchers collaborate to formulate common research questions, models, and methods, they can receive results like other successful interdisciplinary approaches have achieved (Holmes et al., 2008). These collaborations can enhance the contributions that both will bring to translating results into actionable knowledge that can be put into practice to reduce health inequities, including the occurrences of rape and sexual assault.

How Can Rape and Sexual Assault Be Prevented?

Because rapes and sexual assaults threaten the health and well-being of Americans and people worldwide, it is incumbent on society, especially public health researchers and policymakers, to create viable strategies to prevent the continuation of more sexual perpetrators and rape and sexual assault victims along with the negative health consequences they cause. Though originally passed by Congress in 1994, the *Violence Against Women Act* was reauthorized in 2022. The Act allocates monies to support the creation of *Rape Prevention and Education* (RPE) programs to develop comprehensive sexual violence prevention strategies. The

CDC endorses the use of RPE programs because these programs are designed to create collaborative efforts with diverse stakeholders and other state agencies that partner to determine whether their state is making progress toward preventing sexual violence. To that extent, RPE programs provide funding so that every U.S. state, including the District of Columbia, Puerto Rico, the U.S. Virgin Islands, and state, territorial, and tribal sexual assault coalitions, can implement and effectively evaluate the success of their RPE program (CDC, 2024). To ensure their success, the CDC also provides financial support through research of RPE programs. More specifically, the CDC provides training, tools, and technical assistance with the implementation and evaluation of each state's RPE programs, practices, and policies that are evidence-based. Research suggests that the main objective of RPE is to address primary prevention efforts such as preventing first-time occurrences of sexual assault, reducing risk factors, and increasing protective factors associated with sexual violence, using the best evidence to plan, implement, and evaluate programs. Research conducted by Simon et al. (2012) agrees that primary prevention is a critical and necessary component of any strategy that is aimed at preventing revictimization as well as recidivism and reducing the negative consequences of sexual violence. Additionally, RPE programs aim to implement comprehensive strategies that target individual, relationship, community, and societal factors that impact sexual violence. They also analyze community and state data to inform program decisions and to identify trends. RPE programs evaluate prevention efforts and use the results to improve future programs (CDC, 2024).

Criminal justice prevention strategies primarily focus on responding to rape and assault violence after harm is inflicted. Public health officials argue that an effective strategy is to target this form of assaultive violence before it occurs and to quickly treat the behavior before it manifests into short-term or long-term or more serious injuries (DeGue et al., 2012). They argue that prevention can be achieved through *primary*, *secondary*, and *tertiary* prevention efforts. While the three elements are essential to prevention, some believe that policymakers, researchers, and nongovernmental organizations should view *primary* prevention as playing a more critical role since it requires knowing what works to prevent, for example, sexual violence, and implementing effective strategies which are informed by research findings and evidence-based solutions (DeGue et al., 2014; Lee et al., 2007; Krug et al., 2002). Instead of simply providing services to survivors, it is essential to know what services are needed and if they are effective. The CDC refers to this as a technical package to prevent sexual violence. It contends that community policymakers and other stakeholders should create sexual violence prevention strategies and approaches that are informed by the best available data. Therefore, CDC (n.d.) officials have examined prevention programs and determined from evidence-based research that the most effective approaches to preventing sexual assault impact the behavior of individuals, relationships, family, schools, community, and societal factors influencing risk and protective factors. A fivefold approach is recommended that includes (1) promoting social norms that protect against violence, (2) teaching skills to prevent sexual violence, (3) providing opportunities to empower girls and women, (4) creating protective environments, and (5) supporting victims and survivors to reduce harm (CDC, n.d.). First, efforts must be made to practice social norms that promote viewing violence as unacceptable, rather than normative behaviors that are acceptable. This requires mobilizing boys and men as allies since they are often the perpetrators of abusive violence. Second, since violence is regarded as learned behavior, health officials argue that people can be taught not to engage in violence. This requires teaching and promoting mutual respect, healthy ideas about sexuality, healthy, and safe dating practices to everyone regardless of age and gender, social–emotional learning, and training both males and females to feel and become empowered. Third, since impoverished women are more likely to experience sexual violence, society should work to provide them with opportunities to become empowered. Experts report that this can be achieved by offering girls and women economic and leadership opportunities (Basile & Smith, 2011). Fourth, protective environments are needed, especially in settings such as schools, workplaces, and the community, where people often feel vulnerable. Fifth, health experts recommend that support should be given to victims/survivors to help reduce the impact of injuries and harm inflicted. Research reveals that victims need immediate treatments, services, and programs after experiencing a sexual assault because of the trauma, stress, and anxiety associated with these victimizations. They typically need victim-centered services, treatment for the negative health consequences linked to sexual violence, and treatment for other at-risk people either in the home or community from becoming a victim or perpetrator (CDC, 2016).

Similarly to recommendations provided by the CDC, officials at World Health Organization (WHO) and the UN contend that growing evidence suggests that violence against women in general, including sexual assault, can be prevented with the implementation of several strategies in a framework that includes relationship strengthening, empowerment of women, services ensured, poverty reduced, enabling environments created, child and adolescent abuse prevented and transformed attitudes, beliefs, and norms (RESPECT). More specifically, RESPECT is aimed at policymakers to implement via interventions on several levels targeting individual, relational, family, community, and the broader society in areas characterized by low and high resources. They argue that promising interventions are those that provide women who have survived intimate personal violence with psychological and psychosocial support, economic empowerment programs to those with low or no income, cash transfers, the creation of community mobilization programs designed to address unequal gender norms, assisting couples to opt for peaceful resolutions such as better and effective communication skills, education programs designed to protect children and teenagers that increase school safety and challenge traditional curriculum that perpetuate gender stereotypes by teaching equality in relationships, and group-based educational activities with men and women that promote discussions on power relationships. RESPECT believes its recommendation can be most effective when these strategies are implemented to address multiple risk factors that lead to violence and sexual assault early in the life course (WHO, 2021).

Policy Recommendations

Since rape and sexual assault is a criminal justice and public health issue, experts contend that policy recommendations must come from both areas. First, the criminal justice system can be more effective at reducing sexual assaults if it brings perpetrators to justice by working to get higher conviction rates, keeping recidivism rates low, treating victims with respect, compassion, and dignity, especially since immediately after sexual violence, victim's advocacy groups report it is the most critical time that rape survivals decide whether they will go forward in the justice process (since many do not file an assault report if they feel as though they are experiencing a second victimization from justice officials). Survivors need to be believed, and many are not. Because they often feel ashamed, embarrassed, or fear reprisal and retaliation from perpetrators, many do not report. Consequently, justice officials should be properly trained to interview assault victims with objectivity and professionalism without implying they are not credible or that they may have precipitated their sexual victimization either by acting in a provocative manner or by sending mixed signals. Because millions of people are the victims of sexual assault, it is incumbent on the justice system to investigate these cases seriously. Second, public health officials are keenly aware of the justice system's failure owing to its reactionary role. Therefore, it focuses on prevention, rather than taking punitive measures to address this devastating public health problem. To public health officials, the risk and causal factors are many, but so too are the number of protective factors that can be used to prevent rape and sexual assault, along with the negative health consequences that they present. Public health officials believe that risk and protective factors occur at every level of the ecological model, existing in a complex interplay on multiple levels. This approach allows researchers to explore relationships between people and contextual factors regarding where they are situated in the social structure. They argue that violence prevention can be successful if efforts are made to address it at the individual, relational, community, and societal levels since it impacts lifelong health, and the emotional and psychological well-being of every community, people of all genders, sexual orientations, and ages.

When prevention efforts use a public health approach, researchers make interventions on three levels: primary prevention, secondary prevention, and tertiary prevention efforts. As previously stated, most experts agree that of the three levels of intervention, *primary* is considered the most important. *Primary prevention* is a proactive intervention designed as a preemptive approach to prevent the targeted behavior from occurring. It is also premised on the notion that if primary prevention is successful, there is no need to treat the negative health consequences of the behavior. *Secondary prevention* is a reactive intervention given to victims and perpetrators designed to reduce the impact of their victimization or offending behavior. *Tertiary prevention* is an intervention effort to lessen the long-term disability caused by a disease or victimization. Since sexual assault prevention efforts must focus on the individual, relational, community, and societal levels, prevention strategies should include the following: educational programs as forms of *primary* intervention that target the individual level, especially children and teenagers who are enrolled in middle school, high school, and college given that many sexual assault victims are within a certain age group, vulnerable, and have friends with similar experiences and attitudes. It is at the individual level where efforts must be made to dispel stereotypes about rape myths and the realities of sexual assault should be shared with young males and females. Educational programs on sexual assault prevention should also promote and teach teenagers respect for cultural sensitivity and gender equality. School curricula should be transformed to reflect and promote gender equity. Some experts contend that the sooner *primary* prevention occurs, the better, given that sexual victimization occurs early. Research suggests that half of girls are raped while still minors, and four in five before age 25. This could also address the social and cultural attitudes that the young have been taught about rape and sexual assault.

On the relational level, friends, peers, and cliques, especially among high school and college age males, where ideas about sexuality and sexual practices become entrenched, educational campaigns are needed to reeducate them on the realities of sexual violence and other disparities that intersect with gender, race, and income inequality could offer a better explanation for sexual violence. It is hoped that educational programs are provided in the school system that can mitigate and filter into students' respective communities and have a prosocial and positive impact on their attitudes and behaviors. At the same time, concerning their relationship with family members, educational programs that teach and define the different types of sexual assaults as unlawful and unacceptable may encourage victims to seek help and get treated for the negative health consequences linked to the assault. Where the community is concerned, educational programs designed to provide instructions in healthy child-rearing practices may be needed, as well as support services for both victims and perpetrators of sexual assault, as an attempt to prevent recidivism as well as an increase in both groups. Because many victims are adversely impacted by sexual violence in several ways, each community must work to change its views and attitudes about sexual violence, gender equitable-masculinity, and power relations, since a failure to do so will mean that it devalues safety and vicariously perpetuates more sexual violence. As part of its educational campaign, public health approaches rely on the media, billboards, television, and radio broadcasting systems to increase public awareness about issues that pose a threat to the health and overall wellness of the public, including sexual violence. Any of these efforts can reach thousands or millions of viewers and listeners while serving as a primary, secondary, or tertiary prevention effort since each provides information on the prevalence, danger, and consequences of behavior. These public service announcements also inform those impacted by the issue where to find help and where to direct others in need of assistance.

On the societal level, efforts must be made to create programs that are designed to view, treat, and equitably respect women either through massive educational programs, training, or the allocation of resources designed to socially and economically empower women to have the right to self-determination since a relationship exists between gender, socioeconomic inequality, and sexual violence. Feminist scholars believe that when there is gender parity, there will be fewer rapes. Another societal effort that could facilitate a paradigm shift in how girls and women are viewed and treated could occur if *Hollywood* and the movie industry pledge to become socially responsible in their depictions, presentations, use of imagery, and social constructions of how girls and women are presented for public consumption. Feminist scholars and some media critics have argued that when women are devalued, denied the same economic opportunities as their male counterparts, presented as sexual objects, and treated in a misogynistic manner, it has a lasting impact on the attitudes, cultural norms, and corresponding behavior of everyone in society. Health officials argue that anyone can experience or perpetrate sexual violence. Therefore, it uses massive educational campaigns to reeducate everyone on the nature, extent, and pervasiveness of sexual violence and the toll that it takes on public health and the well-being of everyone in society. Beyond this, it provides strategies to prevent the continuation of this form of violence.

Summary

Rape and sexual assault vary depending on how each state defines the behavior. Despite that, sexual violence is pervasive in the U.S. as well as in the rest of the world. Several data sources are used to measure the nature and extent of rape and sexual assault, namely the *UCR, NCVS, NIBRS, WHO, CDC,* and *Amnesty International* to name a few. While statistics differ regarding the actual numbers of rape victims, each data source agrees that the numbers are much higher than what is officially reported owing to several reasons. The latter is the case when one examines sexual violence reported nationally as well as globally. These data also reveal commonalities such as most victims are disproportionately women, young, minorities, and poor. Nevertheless, anyone in society can be a victim of sexual violence, including men, those who are mentally and physically disabled, women, the elderly, children, members of the *LGBTQIA* community, and others. Research shows that there are different typologies, such as spousal/partner, stranger, acquaintance, statutory, campus, military, and prison sexual assaults. There are many reasons why sexual violence occurs. Feminist scholars contend that rape and sexual assault is not about sexual gratification, but rather, it occurs because men desire to exert power and control over women. They also argue that relegating women to positions of powerlessness in society perpetuates the behavior. Learning theorists argue that all behaviors are learned; therefore, boys and men are socialized into devaluing girls and women via societal norms. Moreover, their personal experiences with others who share beliefs and attitudes serve to promote sexual violence and misogyny against women. Some contend that rape and sexual assault occurs because young and older men lack self-control and are unable to suppress the need to control their desire to possess women sexually. Evolutionary theory posits that the nature of most men is to have as much sexual intercourse with as many women as possible to reproduce. In contrast, the culture of violence theory holds that being exposed to a culture of violence, especially where sexual violence is permitted, will invariably create or produce more of the same behavior. While examining sexual violence, public health officials consider the risk factors associated with rape and sexual assault. They point to individual factors, relationship factors, community factors, societal factors, and the role of inequality and how these factors intersect. Rape and sexual assault are criminal justice and public health issues, given the number of people impacted, as well as the negative health consequences caused to victims and others. As previously mentioned, sexual violence is commonplace worldwide. In its aftermath, survivors experience a range of adverse health conditions that may include depression, STIs, PTSD, panic attacks, and other concerns that require a variety of services. While criminal justice responses are reactive, they are vital in assisting and encouraging crime victims to pursue justice. Public health responses are proactive and focus on prevention on three levels: primary prevention, secondary prevention, and tertiary prevention. Experts agree that while sexual violence can be devastating to victims, families, and others in the community, it can be prevented when efforts are made that are directed at individual factors, relational factors, community factors, and societal factors.

Discussion Questions

1 Why is sexual violence a public health issue?
2 Explain some negative health consequences linked to rape and sexual assault.
3 According to feminist theory, why does rape and sexual assault occur?
4 List and explain the risk factors associated with rape and sexual assault.
5 What are some public health approaches that can be used to address rape and sexual assault?
6 What do global statistics suggest about sexual violence?

References

Abbey, A., Parkhill, M., Clinton-Sherrod, A., & Zawacki, T. (2007). A comparison of men who committed different types of sexual assault in a community sample. *Journal of Interpersonal Violence*, 22(12), 1567–1580.

American Public Health Association. (2010). Special issue on the science of eliminating health disparities. *American Journal of Public Health*, 100 (Suppl 1), S1–S280.

Amin, R., Nabors, N.S., Nelson, A.M., Saqlain, M., & Kulldorff, M. (2015). Geographical clusters of rape in the United States: 2000–2012. *Statistics and Public Policy*, 2(1), 1–6. http://dx.doi.org/10.1080/2330443X.2015.1092899

Amnesty International (2018). Let's talk about yes. www.amnesty.org

Armstrong, E.A., Gleckman-Krut, M., & Johnson, L. (2018). Silence, power, and inequality: A intersectional approach to sexual violence. *Annual Review of Sociology*, 44, 99–122. https://doi.org/10.1146/annurev-soc-073117-041410

Bailey, W.C. (1999). The socioeconomic status of women and patterns of forcible rape for major U.S. cities. *Sociological Focus*, 32(2), 43–63.

Baker, K.K. (1997). Once a rapist? Motivational evidence and relevancy in rape law. *Harvard Law Review*, 110(3), 563–624.

Bandura, A. (1973). *Aggression: A social learning analysis*. Prentice Hall.

Barkan, S. E. (2006). *Criminology: A sociological understanding* (3rd. ed.). Prentice Hall.

Barlow, D.H., & Wolfe, B.E. (1981). Behavioral approaches to anxiety disorders: A report on the NIMH-SUNY-Albany research conference. *Journal of Consulting and Clinical Psychology*, 49, 448–454.

Bartol, C., & Bartol, A. (2017). *Criminal behavior: A psychological approach* (11 ed.). Pearson Press.

Basile, K.C., & Smith, S.G. (2011). Sexual violence victimization of women: Prevalence, characteristics, and the role of public health. *American Journal of Lifestyle Medicine*, 5. 407–417.

Basile, K.C., Smith, S.G., Chen, J., & Zwald, M. (2021). Chronic diseases, health conditions, and other impacts associated with rape victimization of U.S. women. *Journal of Interpersonal Violence*, 36(23–24), NP12504–NP12520. https://doi.org/10.1177/0886260519900335

Basile, K.C., Smith, S.G., Kresnow, M., Khatiwada, S., & Leemis, R.W. (2022). *The National Intimate Partner and Sexual Violence Survey: 2016/2017 Report on sexual violence*. Atlanta, GA: National Center for Injury Prevention and Control, Centers for Disease Control and Prevention. The National Intimate Partner and Sexual Violence Survey: 2016/2017 Report on Sexual Violence.

Baumeister, R., Catanese, K., & Wallace, H. (2002). Conquest by force: A narcissistic reactance theory of rape and sexual coercion. *Review of General Psychology*, 6(1), 92–135.

Bingenheimer, J.B., Brennan, R.T., & Earls, F.J. (2005). Firearm violence exposure and serious violent behavior. *Science (American Association for the Advancement of Science)*, 308(5726), 1323–1326. https://doi.org/10.1126/science.1110096

Bisson, J., & Andrew, M. (2007). Psychological treatment of post-traumatic stress disorder (PTSD). *Cochrane Database of Systematic Reviews*, 3(CD003388). https://doi.org/10.1002/14651858.CD003388.pub3

Black, M.C., Basile, K.C., Breiding, M.J., Smith, S.G., Walters, M.L., Merrick, M.T., & Stevens, M.R. (2011). The National Intimate Partner and Sexual Violence Survey 2010 summary report. Centers of Disease Control and Prevention. National Center for Injury Prevention and Control. www.cdc.gov/nisvs/documentation/nisvsReportonSexualViolence.pdf

Bohmer, C., & Parrot, A. (1993). *Sexual assault on campus*. Lexington Books.

Brownmiller, S. (1975). *Against our will: Men, women, and rape*. Simon and Schuster.

Brownstein, H.H. (2000). *The social reality of violence and violent crime*. Allyn & Bacon.

Bryant-Davis, T., Ullman, S.E., Tsong, Y., Tillman, S., & Smith, K. (2010). Struggling to survive: Sexual assault, poverty, and mental health outcomes of African American women. *American Journal of Orthopsychiatry*, 80(1), 61–70. https://doi.org/10.1111/j.1939-0025.2010.01007.x

Buehler, E.D. (2021). Sexual victimization reported by adult correctional authorities, 2016–2018. Bureau of Justice Statistics. https://bjs.gov/library/publications/sexual-victimization-reported-adult-correctional-authorities-2016-2018

Buka, S.L., Stichick, T.L., Birdthistle, I., & Earls, F.J. (2001). Youth exposure to violence: Prevalence, risks, and consequences. *American Journal of Orthopsychiatry*, 71(3), 298–310. https://doi.org/10.1037/0002-9432.71.3.298

Cantor, D., Fisher, B., Chibnall, S., Townsend, R. et al. (2020). Report on the AAU Campus Climate Survey on Sexual Assault and Sexual Misconduct. Association of American Universities.

Carey, K.B., Durney, S.E., Shepardson, R.L., & Carey, M.P. (2015). Incapacitated and forcible rape of college women: Prevalence across the first year. *Adolescent Health Brief*, 56, 678–680.

Center for Research on Women (1993). *Secrets in public: Sexual harassment in our schools*. Wellesley College.

Centers for Disease Control and Prevention (CDC). (2016). Preventing multiple forms of violence: A strategic vision for connecting the dots. Atlanta, GA: National Center for Injury Prevention and Control, Centers for Disease Control and Prevention.

Centers for Disease Control and Prevention (CDC). (2022). New sexual violence data from the CDC confirms: Sexual violence remains a widespread and devastating public health crisis. https://hopehealgrow.org/new-sexual-violence-data-from-the-cdc-confirms-a-widespread-anddevastinf-public-health-criris/

Centers for Disease Control and Prevention (CDC). (2024, November 15). Program: Rape prevention and education program. www.cdc.gov/sexual-violence/programs/index.html#

Centers for Disease Control and Prevention (CDC). (2024). Preventing sexual violence. www.cdc.gov/sexual-violence/prevention/index.html

Chapman, J.R. (1990). Violence against women as a violation of human rights. *Social Justice*, 17, 54–71.

Chen, J., Khatiwada, S., Chen, M.S., Smith, S.G., Leemis, R.W., Friar, N.W., Vasile, K.C., & Kresnow, M. (2023). The National Intimate Partner and Sexual Violence Survey: 2016/2017 report on victimization by sexual identity. National Center for Injury Prevention and Control, centers for Disease Control and Prevention, 16 www.cdc.gov/nisvs/documentation/nisvsReportonSexualIdentity.pd

Chisholm, J.S., & Burbank, V.K. (1991). Monogamy and polygyny in Southeast Arnhem Land: Male coercion and female choice. *Ethology and Sociobiology*, 12, 291–313.

Cohn, A.M., Zinzow, H.M., Resnick, H.S., & Kilpatrick, D.G. (2013). Correlates of reasons for not reporting rape to police: Results from a national telephone household probability sample of women with forcible or drug-or-alcohol facilitated/incapacitated rape. *Journal of Interpersonal Violence*, 28(3), 455–473.

Corbin, W., Bernat, J., Calhoun, K., McNair, L., & Seals, K. (2001). Role of alcohol expectancies and alcohol consumption among sexually victimized and nonvictimized college women. *Journal of Interpersonal Violence*, 16, 297–311.

Dahlberg, L.L., & Krug, E.G. (2002). Violence: A global public health problem. In E. Krug, L.L. Dahlberg, J.A. Mercy, A.B. Zwi, & R. Lozano (Eds.), *World report on violence and health*. World Health Organization.

DeGue, S., Simon, T.R., Basile, K.C., Yee, S.L., Lang, K., & Spivak, H. (2012). Moving forward by looking back: Reflecting on a decade of CDC's work in sexual violence prevention, 2000–2010. *Journals of Women's Health*, 21(12), 1211–1218.

DeGue, S., Valle, L.A., Holt, M.K., Massetti, G.M., Matjasko, J.L., & Tharp, A.T. (2014). A systematic review of primary prevention strategies for sexual violence perpetration. *Aggression and Violent Behavior*, 19(4), 346–362. https://doi.org/10.1016/j.avb.2014.5.004

Department of Defense (DoD) (2016). Inspector general, evaluation of the separation of service members who made a report of sexual assault, 3–21. www.apps.dtic.mil/sti/tr/pdf/AD1013629.pdf

Department of Health and Human Services (2017). Administration on children, youth, and families, Children's Bureau. Child maltreatment 2017. Washington, DC: HHS: 2017. www.acf.hhs.gov/cb/research-data-technology/statistics-research/child-maltreatment

Department of Justice (1997). Sex offenses and offenders. Office of Justice Programs, Bureau of Justice Statistics.

Department of Justice (2000). Sexual assault of young children as reported to law enforcement. Office of Justice Programs, Bureau of Justice Statistics.

Department of Justice (2014). Crimes against the elderly: 2003-2013. Office of Justice Programs, Bureau of Justice Statistics.

Department of Justice (2020). National crime victimization survey 2019. Sex offenses and offenders. Office of Justice Programs, Bureau of Justice Statistics.

De Vocht, F., Heron, J., Campbell, R., Egan, M., Mooney, J.D., Angus, C., Brennan, A., & Hickman, M. (2017). Testing the impact of local alcohol licencing policies on reported crime rates in England. *Journal of Epidemiology and Community Health (1979)*, 71(2), 137–145. https://doi.org/10.1136/jech-2016-207753

Donzinger, S.R. (1996). *The real war on crime: The report of the national criminal justice commission.* Harper Perennial.

Edemekong, P.F., & Tenny, S. (2022). Public health – StatPearls. *National Institutes of Health (NIH).* ww.ncbi.nlm.nih.gov/books/NBKA470250/

Elflein, J. (2023). Covid19 deaths worldwide as of May 2, 2023, by country and territory. www.statista.com

Ellis, L. (1989). *Theories of rape: Inquiries into the cause of sexual aggression.* Hemisphere Publishing Corporation.

Federal Bureau of Investigation (FBI). (2013). Summary reporting system (SRS) user manual version 1.0. Criminal Justice Information Services (CJIS) division, Uniform Crime Reporting (UCR) program. Washington, DC: FBI. https://ucr.fbi.gov/nibrs/summary-reporting-system-srs-user-manual

Federal Bureau of Investigation (FBI). (2019). Crime in the United States 2019. Criminal Justice Information Services Division, Uniform Crime Reporting Program. www.ucr.fbi.gov/crime-in-the-u.s/2019/crime-in-the-u.s.-20

Finkelhor, D., Hotaling, G., Lewis, I.A., & Smith, C. (1990). Sexual abuse in a national survey of adult men and women: Prevalence, characteristics, and risk factors. *Child Abuse & Neglect*, 14, 19–28. https://doi.org/10.1016/0145-2134(90)90077-7

Finkelhor, D., & Yllo, K. (1985). *License to rape.* Holt, Rinehart, & Winston Press.

Flood, M. (2001). Men's collective anti-violence activism and the struggle for gender justice. *Development*, 44, 42–47.

Freire-Vargas, L. (2018). Violence as a public health crisis. *AMA Journal of Ethics*, https://journalofethics.ama-assn.org/article/violemce-public-health-crisis/2018-01

Friis-Rodel, A.M., Leth, P.M., & Astrup, B.S. (2021). Stranger rape; distinctions between the typical rape type and other types of rape. A study based on data from center of victims of sexual assault. *Journal of Forensic and Legal Medicine*, www.sciencedirect.com/science/article/abs/pii/S175292 8X21000445

Gaines, L.K., & Miller, R.L. (2010). *Criminal justice in action: The core* (5th ed.). Wadsworth.

Gottfredson, M., & Hirschi, T. (1990). *A general theory of crime.* Standard University Press.

Groth, A. N. (1979). *Men who rape: The psychology of the offender.* Plenum Press.

Hakimi, D., Bryant-Davis, T., Ullman, S.E., & Gobin, R.L. (2018). Relationship between negative social reactions to sexual assault disclosure and mental health outcomes of black and white female survivors. *Psychological Trauma*, 10(3), 270–275. https://doi.org/10.1037/tra0000245

Harrell, A.V., Smith, B.E., & Cook, R.F. (1985). *The social psychological effects of victimization* (Final report to the National Institute of Justice). Institute for Social Analysis.

Heinze, J.L. (2021). *Economics as a factor in sexual violence.* National Sexual Violence Resource Center. www.nsvrc.org/blogs/economics-factor-sexual-violence

Holmes, J., Lehman, A., Hade, R. et al. (2008). Challenges for multilevel health disparities research in a transdisciplinary environment. *American Journal of Preventive Medicine*, 35(2 Suppl), S182–S192.

Holmstrom, L.L. (1985). Criminal justice system's response to the rape victim. In A.W. Burgess (Ed.), *From rape and sexual assault* (pp. 189–198). Garland Publishing.

Human Rights Watch (2013). Improving police response to sexual assaults. www.hrw.org/reports/improving_sa_investigations.pdf

Institute of Medicine (US). (1988). *Committee for the study of the future of public health: The future of public health*. National Academy Press.

Iverson, K.M., Gradus, J.L., Resick, P.A., Suvak, M.K., Smith, K.F., & Monson, C.M. (2011). Cognitive-behavioral therapy for PTSD and depression symptoms reduces risk for future intimate partner violence among interpersonal trauma survivors. *Journal of Consulting and Clinical Psychology*, 79(2), 193–202. https://doi.org/10.1037/a0022512

Jacoby, S.F., Dong, B., Beard, J.H., Wiebe, D.J., & Morrison, C.N. (2018). The enduring impact of historical and structural racism on urban violence in Philadelphia. *Social Science & Medicine (1982)*, 199, 87–95. https://doi.org/10.1016/j.socscimed.2017.05.038

Jacques-Tiura, A.J., Tkatch, R., Abbey, A., & Wegner, R. (2010). Disclosure of sexual assault: Characteristics and implications for posttraumatic stress symptoms among African American and caucasian survivors. *Journal of Trauma & Dissociation*, 11(2), 174–192. https://doi.org/10.1080/15299730903502938

James, S.E., Herman, J.L., Rankin, S., Keisling, M., Mottet, L., & Anafi, M. (2016). *The Report of the 2015 U.S. Transgendered Survey*. National Center for Transgender Equality. https://transequality.org/sites/default/files/docs/usts/USTS-Full-Report-Dec17.pdf

Jewkes, R., Sen, P., & Garcia-Moreno, C. (2002). Sexual violence. In E.G. Krug, L.L. Dahlberg, J.A. Mercy, A. Zwi, & R. Lozano-Ascencio (Eds.), *World report on violence and health* (pp. 147–181). World Health Organization.

Johnson, N.L., & Johnson, D.M. (2021). An empirical exploration into the measurement of rape culture. *Journal of Interpersonal Violence*, 36(1–2), NP70–NP95. https://doi.org/10.1177/0886260517732347

Jones, J.S., Alexander, C., Wynn, B.N., Rossman, L., & Dunnuck, C. (2009). Why women don't report sexual assault to police: The influence of psychological variables and traumatic injury. *The Journal of Emergency Medicine*, 36(4), 417–424.

Kalra, G., & Bhugra, D. (2013). Sexual violence against women: Understanding cross-cultural intersections. *Indian Journal of Psychiatry*, 55(3), 244–249. https://doi.org/10.4103/0019-5545.117139

Katherine, O., & Beauregard, E. (2016). Sex offending and low self-control: An extension and test of general strain theory of crime. *Journal of Criminal Justice*, 47, 62–73.

Kaufman, M. (2001). Building a movement of men working to end violence against women. *Development*, 44, 9–14.

Kawachi, I., & Berkman, L.F. (2000). Social cohesion, social capital, and health. In L.F. Berkman & I. Kawachi (Eds.), *Social epidemiology* (pp. 174–190). Oxford University Press.

Keith, J., & Skidmore, C. (2024). *Sexual assault experienced as an adult*. PTSD: National Center for PTSD. www.ptsd.va.gov/professional/trat/type/sexual_assault_adult.asp

Kennedy-Bergen, R., & Bogle, K.A. (2000). Exploring the connection between pornography and sexual violence. *Violence and Victims*, 15(3), 227–234.

Kilpatrick, D.G., Resnick, H.S., Ruggiero, K.J., Conoscenti, L.M., & McCauley, M.S. (2007). Drug-facilitated, incapacitated, and forcible rape. A national study. Medical University of South Carolina (MUSC), National Crime Victims Research Treatment Center, www.ncjrs.gov/pdffiles1/nij/grants/219181.pdf

Kimerling, R., Rellini, A., & Learman, L.A. (2002). Gender differences in victim and crime characteristics of sexual assaults. *Journal of Interpersonal Violence*, 17(5), 526–532.

Krahe', B., Scheinberger-Olwig, R., & Bieneck, S. (2003). Men's report of nonconsensual sexual interactions with women: Prevalence and impact. *Archives of Sexual Behavior*, 32, 165–176.

Krebs, C.P., Lindquist, C., Warner, T., Fisher, B., & Martin, S. (2007). The campus sexual assault (CSA) study: Final report. www.ojp.gov/ncjrs/virtual-library/abstracts/campus-sexual-assault-csa-study

Krug, E.G., Dahlberg, L.L., Mercy, J.A., Zwi, A.B., & Lozano, R. (2002). *World report on violence and health*. World Health Organization.

Lamade, R., & Okanlawon, A. (2020). Treatment interventions for perpetrators of sexual violence. In R. Geffner, J.W. White, L.K. Hamberger, A. Rosenbaum, V. Vaughan-Eden, & V.I. Vieth (Eds.), *Handbook of Interpersonal Violence and Abuse Across the Lifespan*. Springer. https://doi.org/10.1007/978-3-319-62122-7_213-1

LeDoux, J., & Hazlewood, R. (1985). Police attitudes and beliefs toward rape. *Journal of Police Science and Administration*, 13, 211–220.

Lee, D.S., Guy, L., Perry, B., Sniffen, C.K., & Mixon, S.A. (2007). Sexual violence prevention. *The Prevention Researcher*, 14(2), 15–20.

Liebermann, O., Kaufman, E., & Starr, B. (2022). Reports of sexual assault in the US military increased by 19%. www.cnn.com/2022/09/01/politics/sexuaal-assault-military-report/index.htmi

Lovell, R., Overman, L., Huang, D., & Flannery, D.J. (2021). The bureaucratic burden of identifying your rapist and remaining "cooperative": What the sexual assault kit initiative tells us about sexual assault case attrition and outcomes. *American Journal of Criminal Justice*, 46, 528–553. https://doi.org/10.1007/s12103-020-09573-x

Lowell, G. (2010). A review of rape statistics, theories, and policy. *Undergraduate Review*, 6, 158–163. https://vc.bridgew.edu/undergrad_rev/vol6/iss1/29

Martin, P.Y., & Hummer, R. (1989). Fraternities and rape on campus. *Gender & Society*, 3(4), 457–473.

McPhail, B.A. (2015). Feminist framework plus: Knitting feminist theories of rap etiology into a comprehensive mode. *Trauma, Violence, & Abuse*, 1–16. https://doi.org/10.1177/1524838015584367

Meadows, R.J. (2004). *Understanding violence and victimization* (3rd ed.). Pearson/Prentice-Hall.

Melani, L., & Fodaski, L. (1974). The psychology of the rapist and his victim. In N. Connell & C. Wilson (Eds.), *Rape: The first sourcebook for women* (pp. 82–93). New American Library.

Mercy, J.A. et al. (1993). Intentional injuries. In A.Y. Mashaly, P.H. Graitcer, & Z.M. Youssef (Eds.), *Injury in Egypt: An analysis of injuries as a health problem* (pp. 65–84). Rose El Youssef New Press. www.cnn.com/2022/09/01/politics/sexual-assault-military-repor

Messerschmidt, J. (1993). *Masculinities and crime: Critique and reconceptualization of theory*. Rowman & Littlefield.

Meyers, C.B., & Taylor, S.E. (1986). Adjustment of rape. *Journal of Personality and Social Psychology*, 50, 1226–1234.

Moody, G., Cannings-John, R., Hood, K., & Robling, M. (2018). Establishing the international prevalence of self-reported child maltreatment: A systematic review by maltreatment type and gender. *BMC Public Health*, 18(1), 1164. https://doi.org/10.1186/s12889-018-6044-y

Mosher, D., & Anderson, R. (1987). Macho personality, sexual aggression, and reactions to guided imagery of realistic rape. *Journal of Research in Personality*, 20, 77–94.

Mustian, J., & Sisak, M. (2018). Despite #MeToo, rape cases still confound police. Associated Press. www.apnews.com/article/6fd581bO3bf343cd8724543bc555eed9

Neelam, R.K., & Gasparini, D. (2023). *Long term effects of sexual assault*. www.charliehealth.com/post/long-term-effects-of-sexual-assault

New York State Coalition Against Domestic Violence (NYSCASV). (2003). Albany, New York. www.nyscadv.org

Parent, D.G., Auerbauh, B., & Carlson, K.E. (1991). *Compensating crime victims: A summary of policies and practices*. US Department of Justice, National Institute of Justice.

Peak, K.J., & Everett, P.M. (2017). *Introduction to criminal justice: Practice and process* (2nd ed.). Sage.

Polaschek, D., & Ward, T. (2002). The implicit theories of potential rapists: What our questionnaires tell us. *Aggression and Violent Behavior*, 7(4), 385–406.

Pollard, P. (1995). Rape reporting as a function of victim-offender relationships: A critique of the lack of effect reported by Bachman. *Criminal Justice and Behavior*, 22, 74–80.

Regehr, C., Alaggia, R., Dennis, J., Pitts, A., & Saini, M. (2013). Interventions to reduce distress in adult victims of rape and sexual violence: A systematic review. *Research on Social Work Practice*, 23(3), 257–265. https://doi.org/10.1177/1049731512474103

Rennison, C.A. (2002). Rape and sexual assault: Reporting to police and medical attention, 1992–2000 [NCJ 194530]. U.S. Department of Justice, Office of Justice Program, Bureau of Justice Statistics: www.bjs.ojp.gov/content/pub/pdf/rsarp00.pdf

Rosenberg, M.L., & Fenley, M.A. (1991). *Violence in America: A public health approach*. Oxford University Press.

Rousseau, D. (2019). The trauma of rape and the criminal justice system's response. https://sites.bu.edu/daniellerousseau/2019

Russell, D. (1975). *The politics of rape*. Stein and Day.

Schneider, M.J. (2020). *Introduction to public health* (6th ed.). Jones & Bartlett Learning.

Schram, P.J., & Tibbetts, S.G. (2014). *Introduction to criminology*. Sage.

Schwartz, M.D., & Nogrady, C.A. (1996). Fraternity membership, rape myths, and sexual aggression on a college campus. *Violence against Women*, 2(2), 148–162.

Schwendinger, J., & Schwendinger, H. (1983). *Rape and inequality*. Sage.

Seidman, I., & Pokorak, J.J. (2011). Justice responses to sexual violence. In M.P. Koss, J.W. White, & A.E. Kazdin (Eds.), *Violence against women and children* (Vol. 2, pp. 137–157). Navigating solutions. American Psychological Association. https://doi.org/10.1037/12308-007

Shields, R.T., & Feder, K.A. (2016). The public health approach to preventing sexual violence. In E.L. Jeglic & C. Calkins (Eds.), *Sexual violence: Evidence based policy and prevention* (pp. 129–144). Springer International Publishing/Springer Nature. https://doi.org/10.1007/978-3-319-44504-5_9

Siegrist, J., & Marmot, M. (2006). *Social inequalities in health*. Oxford University Press.

Siegert, R., & Ward, T. (2002). Rape and evolutionary psychology: A critique of Thornhill and Palmer's theory. *Aggression and Violent Behavior*, 7(2), 145–168.

Simpson, S. (1989). Feminist theory, crime, and justice. *Criminology*, 27, 605–632.

Smith, S.G., Chen, J., Basile, K.C., Gilbert, L.K., Merrick, M.T., Patel, N. et al. (2017). The national intimate partner and sexual violence survey (NISVS): 2010–2012 state report. Atlanta, GA: National Center for Injury Prevention and Control, Centers for Disease Control and Prevention. www.stacks.cdc.gov/view/cdc/4630

Smith, S.G., Chen, J., Lowe, A.N., & Basile, K.C. (2022). Sexual violence victimization of U.S. males: Negative health conditions associated with rape and being made to penetrate. *Journal of Interpersonal Violence*, 37(21–22), NP20953–NP20971. https://doi.org/10.1177/0886260521 1055151

Smith, S.G., Zhang, X., Basile, K.C., Merrick, M.T., Wang, J., Kresnow, M., & Chen, J. (2018). The National Intimate Partner and Sexual Violence Survey (NISVS): 2015 Data brief-updated release. National Center for Injury Prevention Control, Centers for Disease Control and Prevention. www.cdc.giv/violenceprevention/pdf/2015data-brief508.pdf

Socialworkin. (2022). *Case work practice in crisis situations: Addressing victims of rape, conflict, human trafficking, domestic abuse, and disaster situations*. Case Work Practice in Crisis Situations: Addressing Victims of Rape, Conflict, Human Trafficking, Domestic Abuse, and Disaster Situations.

Sorensen, D. (2000). Unequal protection, unequal justice. *TASH Newsletter*, 8, 27–29.

Spohn, C., & Tellis, K. (2014). *Policing & prosecuting sexual assault: Inside the criminal justice system*. Lynne Rienner Publishers.

Stemple, L., & Meyer, I.H. (2014). The sexual victimization of men in America: New data challenges old assumptions. *American Journal of Public Health*, 104(6), e19–e26.

Tharp, A.T., DeGue, S., Valle, L.A., Brookmeyer, K.A., Massetti, G.M., & Matjasko, J.L. (2013). A systematic qualitative review of risk and protective factors for sexual violence perpetration. *Trauma, Violence, & Abuse*, 14(2), 133–167. https://doi.org/10.1177/152483801 2470031

Thornhill, R. (1999). The biology of human rape. *Jurimetrics*, 39(2), 137–147.

Truman, J.L., & Morgan, R.E. (2022). Violent victimization by sexual orientation and gender identity, 2017–2020. *Statistical Brief, Bureau of Justice Statistics*, NCJ304277. https://bjs.ojp.gov/content/pub/pdf/vvsogi1720.pdf

United Nations (2021). UNODC violent crime offences. United Nations Office on Drug and Crime.

U.S. Department of Health and Human Services. (2013). Administration for children and families, administration on Children, Youth and Families, Children's Bureau. Child maltreatment survey. Exhibit 5-2 Selected Maltreatment Types by Perpetrator's Sex.

U.S. Department of Health and Human Services. (2018). Administration for children and families, administration on Children, Youth and Families, Children's Bureau. Child maltreatment survey, 2016.

U.S. Department of Justice. (2023). Criminal victimization, 2022. Office of Justice Programs, Bureau of Justice Statistics. Washington, DC.

Valenti-Hein, D., & Schwartz, L. (1995). *The sexual abuse interview for those with developmental disabilities*. James Stanfield Publishing Company.

Vera-Gray, F., McGlynn, C., Kureshi, I., & Butterby, K. (2021). Sexual violence as a sexual script in mainstream online pornography. *The British Journal of Criminology*, 61, 1243–1260.

von dem Knesebeck, O. (2015). Concepts of social epidemiology in health services research. *BMC Health Services Research*, 15(357). https://doi.org/10.1186/s12913-015-1020-z

Waechter, R. (2021). Prevention of sexual violence in America: Where do we stand? *American Journal of Public Health*, 111(3), 339–141. https://doi.org/10.2105/AJPH.2020.306120

Wallace, H. (1999). *Family violence: Legal, medical, and social perspectives* (2nd ed). Allyn and Bacon.

Wallerstein, N.B., Yen, I.H., & Syme, S. (2011). Integration of social epidemiology and community-engaged interventions to improve health equity. *American Journal of Public Health*, 101(5), 822–830.

West, C., & Johnson, K. (2013). *Sexual violence in the lives of African American women*. VAWnet. https://vawnet.org/material/sexual-violence-lives-african-american-women-risk-response-and-resilience

Westera, N.J., Kebbell, M.R., & Milne, B. (2016). Want a better criminal justice response to rape? Improve police interviews with complainants and suspects. *Violence against Women*, 22(14), 1748–1769.

Whelan, S. (2020). The criminal justice system and sexual violence. www.ecampusontario.pressbooks.pub/theballisinyourcourt/chapter/the-criminal-justice-system-and-sexual-violence/

Wilson, E., & Jiminez, D. (2023, May 23). *Victim-centered social work: Supporting survivors of child abuse and neglect, sexual assault, and crime*. Herzing University. Victim-centered social work: Supporting survivors of child abuse and neglect, sexual assault, and crime.

Wilson, M., & Webb, R. (2018). *Social work's role in responding to intimate partner violence*. Social Justice Brief. National Association of Social Workers. www.socialworkers.org/LinkClick.aspx?fileticket=WTrDbQ6CHxI%3d&portalid=0

Wong, J.Y.H., Luk, L.Y.F., Yip, T.F., Lee, T.T.L., Wai, A.K.C., Ho, J.W. (2022). Incidence of emergency department visits for sexual abuse among children in Hong Kong before and during the COVID-19 pandemic. *JAMA Network Open*, 5(10), e2236278. https://doi.org/10.1001/jamanetworkopen.2022.36278

World Health Organization (WHO). (2008). Social determinants of health. Closing the gap in a generation. Health equity though action on the social determinants of health. Geneva: World Health Organization.

World Health Organization (WHO). (2010). Preventing intimate partner and sexual violence against women: Taking action and generating evidence. *London School of Hygiene and Tropical Medicine*. Geneva, World Health Organization.

World Health Organization (WHO). (2018). Violence against women prevalence estimates. www.who.int/publications/i/item/9789240022256

World Health Organization (WHO). (2021a). Violence against women. wwww.who.int/news-room/fact-sheets/detail/violence-against-women

World Health Organization (WHO). (2021b). Devastatingly pervasive: 1 and 3 women globally experience violence: Younger women among those most at risk: WHO. Geneva/New York.

Yodanis, C.L. (2004). Gender, inequality, violence against women, and fear: A cross-national test of feminist theory against women. *Journal of Interpersonal Violence*, ttps://doi.org/10.1177/088626050426386

7

INTIMATE PARTNER VIOLENCE AND PUBLIC HEALTH

Introduction

After ten years of marriage, Amy asked Jeff for a divorce as she had several times in the past five years after enduring emotional, psychological, and physical abuse. Like before, he convinced her that a brief separation would allow them time to cool off and realize that they needed to stay together for the sake of their children and to preserve the marriage. Jeff was a devout catholic who would never entertain getting divorced. As such, they agreed to a six-month separation contingent on both attending bimonthly marital counseling sessions while the children remained with Amy. However, two months into the separation, the software company for which Jeff had been employed for 15 years downsized, and he received a pink slip notifying him of his abrupt termination. Because Jeff was no longer living in the family home, he hid being unemployed for as long as he could until his resources were depleted, because he was paying half the mortgage on the family home and leasing an apartment during the separation. Jeff felt tremendous stress and anxiety about having to inform Amy that he was fired, unable to continue paying on the mortgage, and wanted to move back into the family home. Unfortunately, he turned to alcohol to cope and to build up enough courage to confront Amy. Throughout the marriage, Jeff always had a drinking problem, which was the primary reason Amy had asked for a divorce on several occasions, since after drinking, Jeff turned belligerent, used vulgar language, and physical violence on the object of his anger. When drunk, he could not control himself. He fought Amy in private and public and in the presence of their children, who witnessed her being taken by first responders to the emergency room when Jeff got inebriated and became abusive. He would physically beat her when dinner was late. He abused her verbally when he could not account for her whereabouts. He yelled at her and fought with her when he was under pressure at work. So, after getting intoxicated, Jeff asked a friend to drive him to his family home at 9:00 p.m. to share the news about losing his job, as well as wanting to return home to be a husband and father to their children. Unfortunately, Jeff did not phone ahead, nor was Amy alone in the home. During the trial separation, she had met and fallen in love with Charles. Consequently, Jeff was met at the front door by Charles. The three got into a heated argument that ended

DOI: 10.4324/9781003373001-7

with Charles and Amy sustaining serious bodily injuries and being transported to the local hospital. Jeff was arrested, taken into custody for physical assault, and later bailed out of jail by the same friend who had driven him to his family home. Amy later filed a protective order prohibiting Jeff from coming near her. While Jeff was not allowed to return home, he stalked and harassed Amy for the next three months by driving by their home several times daily, phoning countless times each day, and mysteriously appearing at places she visited, including her job and the children's school. He also made appearances at Amy's gym and sometimes would follow her in his car as she visited friends, coworkers, and family. The ordeal with Jeff was so traumatic that Amy needed therapy to cope with the stress. Because of the health risk and economic consequences of her victimization, Amy was unable to pay for needed long-term counseling. She has also missed many days from work owing to fear, and her children missed days of school, impacting their grades. Many of her lifelong friends refused to maintain ties or allow their children to interact with hers out of fear that they would be exposed to Jeff's violence.

Intimate Partner Violence Defined

Intimate partner violence (IPV) is a public health and human rights challenge that affects millions of people globally (Patra et al., 2018). Its negative impact transcends targeted victims and reverberates through other individuals, families, communities, nations, and generations (Krug et al., 2002). IPV is also referred to as intimate partner domestic violence (IPDV). Spivak and colleagues (2014) report that IPV occurs between opposite-sex and same-sex couples. In these cases, males disproportionately direct their violence at female partners. Violence experts argue that IPV is often hidden because victims rarely report victimization or have contact with official and social services agencies. Consequently, their health problems may not be apparent until decades later (Mercy et al., 2017). IPV occurs when a perpetrator intentionally causes harm or threatens to harm a current spouse, former spouse, live-in partner, dating partner, or ongoing sexual partner (Patra et al., 2018; DeGue et al., 2012). Some experts contend that it is the pattern of controlling and coercive behavior that can be exhibited in physical, sexual, financial, verbal, emotional/psychological, cultural, spiritual, and reproductive ways against a partner (Krug et al., 2002). These experts argue that IPV involves abusive and aggressive behavior used to gain power and control over another intimate partner. While the foreknown effects are visible, other experiences that victims/survivors endure are hidden. They include being stalked, terrorized, blamed, hurt, humiliated, and intentionally isolated from social support, friends, and family. In essence, IPV also involves frightening, hurting, and manipulating persons to control them. Similarly, public health Centers for Disease Control and Prevention (CDC) officials define IPV as abuse or aggression that occurs within the context of a romantic relationship. Unlike some definitions of IPV, the CDC's definition is not limited to the spousal relationship but includes former and current spouses and dating partners (Breiding et al., 2015). To that end, it can occur even if the individuals involved are not living together when the violence or harassment occurs. According to IPV experts, this factor is what distinguishes it from IPDV. IPV often varies in terms of severity. Experts report that violence can occur only once for some victims. However, other victims can experience chronic and severe episodes of violence that could last for decades (Moorer, 2015). While the greater share of research on IPV is focused on the abuser's partner, Jewkes (2015) contends that the byproduct of

IPV also adversely impacts the silent or hidden victims, the children who are either directly or indirectly experiencing IPV. There are several types of IPV, including domestic violence, physical violence, sexual violence, emotional and psychological violence, stalking, and violence among same-sex couples (Gupta, 2023).

Nature and Extent of IPV

When measuring the extent of IPV, researchers have relied on several instruments. Critics warn that instead of refining existing instruments, new ones have emerged, complicating IPV research since different instruments (some *qualitative* and others *quantitative*) provide different results (Hamby, 2014; Waltermauer, 2005). Experts contend that this may explain the differences in IPV statistics collected from varied sources. Each year in the U.S., an estimated 10 million women and men are the victims of IPV (Huecker et al., 2023). According to the CDC, one in every four women and one in every seven men in the U.S. experience physical violence by an intimate partner in their lifetime, while one in three women and nearly one in six men will experience some form of sexual violence during their lifetime. Huecker et al. (2023) contend that one in six women and one in 19 men have been stalked during their lifetime. Moreover, the CDC provides that nearly half of all women and men have experienced psychological aggression at the hands of an intimate partner. IPV is so pervasive that the *Bureau of Justice Statistics* reports that it accounts for 15% of all violent crime. Beyond this, it is important to note that IPV is not a problem exclusive to the U.S., but rather, it is global (Patra et al., 2018). For example, in an analysis on the prevalence of IPV from 2000 to 2018 that examined 161 countries and areas, World Health Organization (WHO) at the request of the *United Nations* conducted a survey that revealed that 30% of women worldwide between the ages of 15 and 49 report being in a relationship where they were subjected to physical or sexual violence by an intimate partner or non-partner in their lifetime (World Health Organization [WHO], 2024).

IPV is a form of assaultive violence not relegated to any one group of people. It affects millions each year regardless of their marital status, sexual orientation, race/ethnicity, national origin, age, religion, education, or economic status. Bureau of Justice Statistics reported that between 2013 and 2017, an estimated 691,000 nonfatal IPV victimizations occurred each year in the U.S. Among them were some fatal incidents (Morgan & Truman, 2018). Police data reported to the Uniform Crime Reports (UCR) reveal that over 15 years, 1,400 people, mainly women, were killed in IPV situations annually by a male partner. There have been approximately 6,400 more women IPV homicides compared to men in the past decade (Cooper & Smith, 2017; Maxwell et al., 2020). Even though IPV cuts across race, class, gender, religion, and country of origin lines, some studies have isolated key factors that often increase the likelihood of IPV risk. More specifically, research points to commonalities among victims of IPV and sexual violence that include the following: lower levels of education, female, living in high poverty neighborhoods, low income (ranging from $15,000 to $24,999), harmful use of drugs and alcohol, and low level of gender equality (WHO, 2024). Regarding age, studies suggest that women ages 18–24 and 25–34, respectively, experience the highest rates of IPV. Experts contend that it can occur across the lifespan and affect people of every age, including teens to elderly couples. Research also reveals that an estimated 43% of college women who date report experiencing violence from an intimate partner, ranging from physical, sexual, verbal, or emotional abuse.

Where race/ethnicity is concerned, some studies show that historically minority women and men are disproportionately affected by IPV, especially marginalized women (Smith et al., 2017). According to a CDC *National Intimate Partner and Sexual Violence Survey*, an estimated 45.1% of Black women, and 47.5% of American Indian or Alaska Native women, and 56.6% of multicultural women, and 54% of disabled women have been the victim of IPV, rape, physical violence, or stalking at some time in their lives (Smith et al., 2017; Campbell et al., 2022). The survey also shows that an estimated 45.3% of American Indian or Alaska Native men, 38.6% of African-American men, and 39.3% of multi non-Hispanic men in the U.S. reported experiencing IPV, rape, or stalking in their lives. Where sexual identity is concerned, 43.8% of lesbian women and 61.1% of bisexual women reported being a victim of IPV, rape, or stalking at some time in their lives compared with 35% of heterosexual women. Similarly, 26% of gay men and 37.3% of bisexual men reported experiencing IPV, rape, or stalking at some point in their lives compared with 29% of heterosexual men. Moreover, a report by the *National Coalition of Anti-Violence Programs* suggests that being African-American and identifying as *LGBTQ* increases the likelihood of being subjected to physical IPV compared with non-African-Americans. Likewise, Caucasians who identify as *LGBTQ* are more likely to experience sexual violence compared to those who do not identify as Caucasian. Some research finds that IPV disproportionately affects the *LGBTQ* community because its members are invisible and face barriers when seeking protection from the legal system and social services from the healthcare systems (Messinger, 2017). Recent studies show that regardless of how one or their partner identifies, they can experience IPV (CDC, 2010).

Weapons are typically used in IPV cases, and the primary instrument of choice is a firearm (Tobin-Tyler, 2023). Where firearms are concerned, research finds that the presence of guns in IPV cases increases the likelihood of death. More specifically, research suggests that a victim of IPV is five times more likely to die when the abusive partner has access to a firearm (Tobin-Tyler, 2023). Studies show that IPV and gun violence are intersecting public health crises since over half of female homicide victims are killed either by a current or former male intimate partner (CDC, 2023). According to Wallace and colleagues (2021), firearms resulting in homicide are the leading cause of death for women during pregnancy and postpartum. There has been an increase in the number of IPV and firearm-related deaths from 2014 to 2020. Experts report that the U.S. has experienced a 58% increase that is arguably attributed to the spike in firearm sales during the COVID-19 pandemic. Some scholars report that approximately 7.5 million people purchased firearms between 2019 and 2021 (Gollan, 2021; Miller et al., 2022). More alarming is that 96% of murder–suicide victims are female. Experts argue that firearm ownership and IPV are gendered, as homicide statistics reveal that men have been more likely to purchase and use firearms compared with their female partners (Stoevers, 2019; Violence Policy Center, 2018). Firearms are not always used to kill in each case, since they are also used to cause injury, threaten, and terrorize victims and survivors. Sorenson and Schut (2016) revealed that an estimated 4.5 million women had been threatened, while one million women were either shot or shot at by an intimate partner.

Types of Intimate Partner Violence (IPV)

WHO (2010) reports that though IPV affects people of every race, ethnicity, class, age, gender, sexual identity, and sexual relationship status, it remains a gendered issue disproportionately affecting women. Because IPV is not unitary, it is important to distinguish the typologies to understand the complexities of IPV, along with its causes, correlates, and consequences (Ali et al., 2016). Research reports that types of IPV include physical violence, sexual violence, emotional abuse, psychological abuse, stalking, financial abuse, online abuse, and violence in the *LGBTQ* community (Gupta, 2023; Ricci, 2017).

Physical Violence

Physical violence occurs when an abusive partner hurts or tries to hurt by either hitting, slapping, pushing, biting, choking, strangling, throwing objects, or doing something to cause physical harm to another person's body (Patra et al., 2018). In IPV cases, abusers have also been known to hold victims down, lock them in rooms, lock them out of the home, or physically prevent them from leaving. Research suggests that there is a nexus between physical IPV and sexual violence (Ricci, 2017). Dillion and colleagues (2013) report that women with a history of IPV also experienced a range of chronic health conditions, including chronic pain, which is highly associated with IPV (Loxton et al., 2006). In a comparative study, Wuest et al. (2008) discovered that women who experienced IPV 20 months earlier still reported having high levels of debilitating pain and injuries such as swelling and painful joints. Other research studies have also reported the link between IPV and physical violence. Women with a history of IPV have reported experiencing neck pain, chronic back ache, stomach cramps, and chronic headache (Vives-Cases et al., 2011; Scheffer-Lindgren & Renck, 2008; Woods et al., 2008). In a two-year study examining an increase in HIV cases in South African women, Jewkes et al. (2010) reported that women with a history of IPV, including physical violence, faced a greater likelihood of contracting HIV compared with women who had not been abused. Similarly, in a sample of African-American women, Josephs and Abel (2009) discovered an association between the frequency of physical abuse and sexual coercion. They revealed that when women experienced violence by an abusive partner, it placed serious limitations on their decision making, free choice, and negatively impacted their ability to encourage the use of a condom during sexual relations, increasing the likelihood that they would be HIV-infected.

Sexual Violence

Sexual violence occurs when an abusive partner forces an intimate partner to engage in sexual acts without consent. The violence can be rape or sexual assault within the context of a dating relationship, marriage, or between former partners. Research shows that sexual violence includes unwanted sexual touching such as fondling and oral/anal/vaginal penetration with a penis or an object (Ricci, 2017). According to Finkelhor et al. (2015), caretakers of children and adolescents subject them to high rates of physical, sexual, and emotional victimization that are detrimental in the short and long run (Gomez, 2011). Echoing this, Lungren and Amin (2014) report that IPV and sexual violence are common among children and adolescents, changing the trajectory of their lives by aligning them to become either victims or perpetrators of IPV over their lifetime. Richards et al. (2017) also argue that child maltreatment and abuse are linked to violence within intimate partner relationships. Experts suggest a causal relationship between experiencing IPV in youth and later engaging in the behavior. Research supporting the "cycle of violence" argument postulates that IPV and sexual violence are intergenerational since children who witness violence within their family may model these behaviors in future interpersonal relationships. They also face an increased risk of being revictimized in violent relationships (Widom, 1989).

Other researchers report that IPV can occur at any time in one's lifespan. For example, it can occur from adolescence to early adulthood. However, domestic violence experts contend that IPV typically occurs in the context of marriage or cohabitation and involves physical, sexual, emotional, and acts of control. Their research also suggests that sexual violence can occur at any age and can be committed by anyone, including other children, parents, family members, teachers, peers, acquaintances, strangers, and intimate partners (Lungren & Amin, 2014). Some studies find that puberty may bring about sexual harassment or assault victimization in the home, community, or at school. Many children's first sexual experiences are the product of forced participation. Richards et al. (2017) argued that because some children experience maltreatment, often unnoticed and untreated, they face a significant risk of engaging in IPV as adults. This may explain why IPV proliferates throughout their life course. For many adolescents in the U.S. and other nations, violence becomes a recurring event throughout their relationships (Lungren & Amin, 2014).

In other parts of the world, such as Asia, marriages are arranged and take place earlier, and though dating violence is rare, IPV among the young occurs early, affecting many youths (WHO, 2010). Research conducted by Carpenter (2006) and Russell (2007) reveals that groups of male adolescents from marginalized groups, working children, homeless youths, children with mental and physical disabilities, children found in conflict-affected areas, and those who have left school are more susceptible to IPV and sexual violence victimization. In some extreme cases of IPV, abusers have been known to allow friends to join and participate in violent rapes of a spouse or intimate partner.

Emotional Abuse

Emotional abuse is aimed at hurting intimate others' feelings by undermining their self-worth. It is accomplished by criticizing them constantly or gaslighting about how they feel. This form of abuse is displayed when an abuser actively berates an intimate other publicly as well as privately, engages in name-calling, and isolates the abused from friends and family to remove and dismantle their support system or social network. It also involves preventing the victim from having a life on the outside of the abusive relationship by removing the activities they enjoy, including employment, and closely monitoring their activities (Ricci, 2017). Fuino-Estefan et al. (2016) reported that a nexus exists between IPV (especially physical and sexual abuse) exposure and poor mental health outcomes, but few studies (Sullivan et al., 2012; Mechanic et al., 2008) have focused on how emotional abuse impacts mental health. They argue that little information is available on the pathways by which emotional abuse can impact long-term depression and whether social resources are associated with its outcome (Fuico-Etefan et al., 2016). From a pilot study conducted with 156 females self-reporting depression, Fuico-Etefan et al. revealed that the effects of frequent emotional abuse itself often persist for long periods and can manifest into depression for those who experienced it several times weekly and who feared having more contact with the abuser. Other research has mirrored this finding. For example, the literature is saturated with findings supporting the notion that victims of IPV face an increased risk of experiencing depression since the rate is twice as high as what is found in the general population (Alhabib et al., 2010; Zlotnick et al., 2006). Hence, some believe that within the context of IPV relationships, emotional abuse can predict depression (Mechanic et al., 2008). Moreover, other studies conclude that psychological violence can be the most detrimental form of violence to victims' mental health (Hill et al., 2009).

Psychological Abuse

Psychological abuse in IPV is just as devastating as physical abuse since it can severely impact victims' mental and physical well-being (Pico-Alfonso, 2005; Campbell, 2002). Experts define it as the use of verbal and nonverbal communication with the intent to mentally or emotionally harm and to control the victim by instilling fear. Some studies reveal that abused women read the degree of psychological violence more than the severity of physical violence, which could bring emotional stress that lasts for an extended period (Sackett & Saunders, 1995). Wood (2000) and Weaver and Etzel (2003) report that in IPV relationships, women living with a violent and abusive partner are more likely to experience repetitive episodes of physical, psychological, and sexual violence that pose a threat to their long-term and short-term physical and mental health. Research reports a link between IPV and an increased risk of developing post-traumatic stress disorder (*PTSD*). Experts estimate that between 45% and 60% of abused women suffer from *PTSD* (Cascardi et al., 1999). The study further concluded that some women involved in abusive relationships are exposed to violence for longer and more frequently throughout their life course. As such, their high rates of *PTSD* vulnerability may be the result of cumulative and prolonged trauma exposure (Pico-Alfonso, 2005). Vitanza et al. (1995) reported that a positive correlation exists between the severity of abuse and intensity of PTSD symptomatology. Woods (2000) contends that the impact of *PTSD* is so devastating that its symptoms continue long after the abusive relationship is over. Other studies identify several mental disturbances commonly found in physically abused women, including depression, anxiety, sleeping disturbances, eating disorders, suicide ideation and attempts, and the tendency to self-medicate with substances(Campbell, 2002; Weaver & Etzel, 2003; Hegarty et al., 2004).

Stalking

In the U.S., an estimated 18.3 million women and nearly 6.5 million men report having been stalked during their lifetime (Breiding et al., 2014). Stalking occurs when an abuser makes repeated, intense unwanted contact with a partner, causing them to experience fear for their safety or the safety of someone close to them (Logan & Walker, 2017). Stalking manifests in an abuser physically showing up or following someone, phoning too frequently, sending gifts, or sending unwanted texts, emails, or social media messages. It also includes finding ways to spy (via technology-facilitated) on an intimate person or anyone as they engage in daily activities at home or work (Gupta, 2023; Ricci, 2017). This behavior is intended to annoy, frighten, harass, or harm the victim psychologically. According to the *Stalking Prevention, Awareness, and Resource Center* (n.d.), the largest category of stalking cases is linked to IPV that often escalates to behavior such as physical or sexual violence. Research revealed that many victims are stalked either by a current or past intimate partner or by someone they know (Catalano et al., 2009). Seventy-four percent of those stalked by a former intimate partner reported that the partner was violently abusive and coercive.

Eighty-one percent stalked by a current or former husband or cohabiting partner reported being physically assaulted, and 31% of women stalked by an intimate partner reported being sexually assaulted (Brewster, 2003; Tjaden & Thoennes, 1998). Chen et al. (2020) found that between 2010 and 2012, bisexual women experienced more stalking, IPV, and IPV-related impact compared with heterosexual women.

The prevalence of stalking was also recorded during the COVID-19 pandemic (Bracewell et al., 2020; Bradbury-Jones & Isham, 2020). Research finds that while a stay-at-home mandate may have been effective in protecting people from getting COVID, it increased the danger that women faced daily, given they were trapped in their homes with perpetrators of IPV. During the pandemic, scholars report that the number of calls to police nationally experienced astronomical increases (Bradbury-Jones & Isham, 2020). Bracewell et al. (2020) report that the lockdown did not prevent IPV victims from being stalked. According to Woodlock (2017), when physical stalking and IPV is not possible, perpetrators continue their behavior by being an omnipresent force resorting to using technical devices such as mobile phones, spyware, listening devices, cameras, and Global Positioning Systems (GPSs) that enable them to monitor the activities and whereabouts of their partner, former partners, or new interest (Breiding et al., 2014).

Financial Abuse

In IPV cases, financial abuse occurs when the abuser maintains control over finances and limits the other partner's ability to have equal input in determining how collective monies should be spent. Some contend it occurs when someone abuses a survivor's ability to acquire, use, or maintain resources to ensure their economic well-being and self-sufficiency (Adam et al., 2008; Johnson et al., 2022), believing this would shift the balance of power (Sanders, 2015; Gupta, 2023). Economic exploitation also occurs when one intentionally destroys a partner's financial resources by depleting them, refusing to pay debt to ruin the abused's credit, or opening lines of credit in the victim's name without permission (Stylianou, 2018). According to Postmus et al. (2012), financial abuse experienced by IPV victims is inflicted with other types of abuses, namely physical, sexual, and psychological, for an extended time. Economic abuse occurs along a continuum given in stages that reflect economic control, employment sabotage, and economic exploitation, and can continue when the relationship has ended. IPV is common: an estimated 76%–99% of survivors report that they also experienced economic abuse (Stylianou et al., 2013; Postmus et al., 2012). Littwin (2012) and Littwin (2013) contend that many IPV abusers have used the consumer credit industry to financially devastate their partner's financial history and prospects, making it almost impossible for them to leave abusive situations. While experiencing financial hardship is stressful, studies find that its effect goes beyond economics. For example, Haeseler (2013) and Fawole (2008) reported that financial abuse is also a risk factor in women's lives that increases their level of vulnerability to other aspects of violence associated with adverse health consequences, such as physical violence, sexual violence, substance abuse, *HIV*, and criminal activities. Eriksson and Ulmestig (2021) and Johnson et al. (2022) argue that financial abuse causes women to suffer poor mental and physical health, low self-esteem, and facilitates a diminished quality of life. Economic IPV is unique because it does not require close physical proximity between the abuser and victim, given that technology allows it to take place anywhere and at any time without the victim being aware (Stylianou, 2018).

Online Abuse

Online technology provides people with a wealth of easy-to-access information yet also enables abusers to do violence using email, dating apps, digital devices, tools, and services to abuse, harass, stalk, manipulate, threaten, or bully an intimate partner (Grimani et al., 2022). Burke et al. (2011) reported that approximately 65% of adults used technology to monitor a partner's activities. It is important to note that technology varies from early developments (e.g., caller identification, fax machines, calling cards, and cordless phones) to more contemporary advances (e.g., GPS and location services, cellular and wireless phones, spyware, and hidden cameras) (Al-Alosi, 2017). Studies reveal that computer-savvy IPV perpetrators use social networking sites within a community of members (e.g., victims' friends, family, and coworkers) to humiliate, manipulate, or harass a former romantic partner by revealing compromising and personal information (Brown et al., 2018; Moncur & Herron, 2018). Some contend that while many online tools are used to abuse IPV victims, the most common form is surveillance and monitoring (Brown et al., 2018). Research finds that monitoring enables perpetrators to collect information on a romantic partner that enhances their ability to exert control within the context of the relationship (Grimani et al., 2022). Tokunaga (2011) states that electronic monitoring in IPV is a surreptitious strategy used to gain access to formulate an awareness of other users' online and offline behaviors and activities. Brown et al. (2018) contend that technology-based IPV has created complications, emotional turmoil, and feelings of helplessness and hopelessness in abused victims, especially in the lives of battered women. Technology-based abuse can also be used to engage in cyberstalking. For example, Powell and Henry (2016) revealed that many victims of IPV have received unwelcome and intrusive behavior from a former partner that included repeat threats, and harassing email or other computer-mediated communication. Moncur and colleagues' (2016) research investigation reported that other online acts of abuse that victims have been exposed to include "fraping," where the former partner took control of their social media account, having their email hacked, receiving insulting communications, flooding with unwanted email, and receiving a computer virus program.

The LGBTQ Community

Most research conducted in this area has historically focused on violence perpetrated by and against heterosexuals. As such, research efforts are being made to examine the nature and extent of IPV within the LGBTQIA population. Early research established that IPV was equally as problematic in the *LGBTQ* community as it was in the heterosexual community. Some studies discovered that IPV was more pervasive in the *LGBTQ* community, but especially among those identifying as transgender. Several studies show that transgenders are more likely to experience elevated risk of violence, danger, and death compared with their cisgender *LGBTQ* peers (Decker et al., 2018; Langenderfer-Magruder et al., 2016). Members of the *LGBTQ* community in violent relationships are also more likely to experience depression and anxiety compared with their heterosexual counterparts (Edwards, 2015).

Some studies suggest that IPV victimization over the life course for LGBTQ community members surpasses those of the heterosexual community which is concerning since an estimated 26%–33% of gay men; 32%–44% of lesbian women; 37%–87% of bisexual men;

and 61%–91% of bisexual women will experience IPV victimization (Walters et al., 2013; West, 2012; Messinger, 2011). By contrast, heterosexual men and heterosexual women will experience IPV victimization over their life course at 8%–29% and 20%–35%, respectively (Goldberg & Meyer, 2013; Walters et al., 2013). Abuse experienced by *LGBTQ* members is not only experienced by adults. Reuter et al. (2017) report that IPV begins early in the lives of *LGBTQ* youth or young adults. LGBT high school students report high rates of forced sex (19% LGB and 25% transgender) compared to cisgendered students (6% LGB and 15% cisgender). LGB high school students also reported experiencing elevated rates of physical (13%) and sexual (16%) dating violence compared with their heterosexual peers at 7% and 7%, respectively. Transgender students reported facing higher rates of IPV compared with the others: physical (26%) and sexual (23%) dating violence compared to their cisgender peers at 15% and 16%, respectively (Maheux et al., 2021). Gehring and Vaske (2017) reported that adolescents experiencing IPV also face a greater risk of engaging in behaviors such as violent delinquency, binge drinking, and low academic performance compared with heterosexual adolescents.

Explaining the Roots of IPV

Health experts contend that it is important to understand the risk factors associated with IPV to reduce and prevent more cases from occurring. While IPV is a global problem causing intergenerational devastation and negative health outcomes annually, its risk factors are common among victims and perpetrators regardless of culture, socioeconomic status, and religion (Gupta, 2023). Health experts advise that risk factors should not be mistaken as causal factors but should be viewed as contributing factors increasing the likelihood of IPV occurring. Capaldi et al. (2012) provide that several risk factors often lead to IPV. Those using the ecological model to understand violence contend that the causes of IPV are complex and influenced by multiple factors operating on four levels: individual factors, relationship factors, community factors, and societal factors. Heise and Garcia-Moneno (2002) assert that these factors include engaging in aggressive or delinquent behavior as teenagers abusing alcohol or drugs, observing violence as a child, spousal conflict, the use of power and control displayed in relationships, and economic deprivation. When measuring the nature and extent of IPV, researchers in the U.S. and globally examine evidence collected in these four areas (within their social context) to better understand factors linked to the prevalence and variation of this behavior (Jewkes, 2002).

What Are the Risk Factors?

Research studies show that many factors can either increase or decrease the likelihood that one will experience being a victim of IPV or become an IPV perpetrator. For example, in a systematic review of risk factors for IPV, Capaldi and colleagues (2012) revealed two types of IPV risk factors among adults and teenagers. First, contextual characteristics of partners include demographics, neighborhood, community, and school factors. Second, developmental characteristics and behavior of partners include one's family, peers, psychological/behavioral and cognitive factors, and relationship influences and interactional patterns. Some experts even suggest that determinants are health risks related to inequalities (e.g., poverty) beyond individual control (Chung et al., 2016).

Risk factors can assist in identifying certain populations or people at a higher risk of exposure to IPV (Capaldi et al., 2012). They can also help determine if one's health risks are high or low to help people avoid negative health outcomes (Capaldi et al., 2012). Some risk factors, such as genetics or race/ethnicity, are unchangeable. However, other risk factors can be altered or changed, such as the behavior and activities one engages in (e.g., drug and alcohol use and consumption) and the relationships one may choose to enter with others (e.g., dating or marrying partner). For example, deciding to date, marry, or associate with persons who are possessive and controlling, misogynistic, drink excessively, or engage in aggressive behavior will likely place oneself at risk for IPV. Experts also postulate that the more risk factors that are present, the greater one's chances of being exposed to violence. As such, researchers contend that preventing IPV requires understanding and addressing risk factors (Capaldi et al., 2012).

Role of Inequity in IPV

Though experts point out that IPV committed against women transcends social and economic boundaries, studies report a link between wealth, inequality, and IPV (Coll et al., 2020; Raphael, 2004). These studies conclude that economic position is an important risk factor for those who experience IPV because, among lower-income populations, male abusers use violence as a resource to sabotage women from entering the labor market. This prevents them from becoming economically independent (Raphael, 2004; Kebede et al., 2022). Specifically, research shows that poverty and its stressors are present in violence occurring across socioeconomics, yet tend to proliferate among lower-class groups. This finding is well documented in the IPV literature in the U.S. as well as other countries (Coll et al., 2020; Martin et al., 1999). Yapp and Pickett (2019) reported that there is a long-standing robust relationship between income inequality and violence, including homicides, that is found globally. They also report that the economic status of women, especially in unequal societies, places women at a higher risk of IPV (Yapp & Pickett, 2019). Willie and Kershaw (2019) examined the association between gender inequality index and the prevalence of lifetime IPV among women and men at the state level, finding that women experience a lifetime prevalence of IPV ranging from 27.8% to 45.3%, while men experience a range from 18.5% to 38.6%, respectively. Liu and Olamijuwon (2024), using a sample size of 150,623 women from 24 countries in *West-Central Africa*, *East-Southern Africa*, *Middle East* and *North Africa, and South Asia*, reported that spousal resource inequality was a key factor in IPVs. Differential levels of income inequality were found to be highly associated with IPVs in lower- and middle-income countries across four regions.

In a Brazilian study, Kiss and colleagues (2012) used *WHO* interviews and other data to examine the impact of women's neighborhood socioeconomic conditions and the likelihood of experiencing IPV. Using a socioeconomical level scale, they revealed that women in the scale's middle range were significantly more likely to report IPV abuse, especially for those situations involving excessive alcohol use, controlling behavior, and multiple sexual partners. Kiss et al. recommend removing women from poverty as an effort to lower IPV rates. In a global IPV study, Coll et al. (2020) examined survey data collected between 2010 and 2017 from 46 countries. The surveys measured the prevalence and inequalities in psychological, physical, and sexual IPV among partnered women between the ages of 15 and 49. The results are consistent with other international IPV studies (Martin et al., 1999;

Strus et al., 1980; McGall & Shields, 1986), revealing that educationally, economically, and socially empowered women are more protected and report experiencing less IPV than other women. Too, data strongly suggest that younger women and those who live in rural areas experience the most IPV.

Individual Factors

Violence experts attach importance to examining IPV victims' and perpetrators' childhood history and biological factors to gain a better understanding of IPV (Renner et al., 2015). Anderson (2002) reported that emotional and behavioral disorders are risk factors for IPV perpetration. Riggs et al. (2000) revealed that males who engaged in violence toward a partner also had more depressive symptoms compared with those who did not display aggression toward a partner. Chang et al. reported an association between a history of depression and an elevated risk of physical IPV among Asian American females. Research also reports that adolescent males who have engaged in suicide attempts are more likely to commit violence against a partner in young adulthood (Kerr & Capaldi, 2011). Some studies find that low self-esteem for men increases the likelihood of committing physical IPV, especially among Latino males (Whiting et al., 2009; Kantor & Jasinski, 1998). Foran and O'Leary (2008) reported that males abusing illegal drugs and alcohol are more likely to engage in physical IPV compared with males who do not. A few studies have contradictory findings on IPV risk factors. For example, Drapkin et al. (2005) found low educational attainment as an IPV risk factor. However, Chang et al. (2009) reported that lower educational attainment decreased the likelihood of IPV perpetration, at least for Asian American women. Similarly, Caetano et al. (2000) revealed that Latina females engaged in physical IPV reported having higher levels of education compared with Latina females not engaged in IPV. Moe and Bell (2004) find that some couples with higher levels of education or employment use IPV as an ongoing process of intimidation, isolation, and control to prevent women from seeking higher aspirations. Gupta (2023) reports that aggressive behavior can be enhanced by frequent use of alcohol and drugs. Other research studies reveal that anger, hostility, use of violence to solve problems, and antisocial personality traits are linked to IPV. Poor behavioral control and impulsiveness, a history of being abusive, social isolation, economic stress, emotional insecurity, strict adherence to gender roles, the need to exercise power and control in relationships, expressing hostility to women, a favorable attitude toward violence and aggression, and a history of physical or emotional abuse as a child are linked to IPV.

Relationship Factors

Research in IPV shows a nexus exists between people who engage in IPV and their having a history of unhealthy personal relationships characterized by jealousy, possessiveness, tension, separation, and in some cases, divorce (Pichon et al., 2020). Within these relationships, the abuser may seek to dominate and control the other and is likely to engage in either physical, sexual, psychological, or emotional abuse, or a combination of these behaviors to gain power and control over the other partner (McCarthy et al., 2018). Relationship factors are indicators of the likelihood that IPV will occur and are more prevalent in families experiencing economic stressors, exacerbating relationship strains (Matjasko et al., 2013; Khalifeh et al., 2013). Those who abuse others have often been reared in unhealthy, violent, or dysfunctional family environments by parents with low educational attainment. People with childhood experiences of violence in the home are either directly or vicariously reinforced with the notion that violence is normative behavior. Consequently, children exposed to violence may engage in similar violence as adults (Jewkes, 2002). They typically have unhealthy relationships and negative interactions with their parent(s). They are often products of intergenerational violence and dysfunction, witnessing violence displayed between their parents and may have even been the target of violence at critical developmental stages in life (Fang & Corso, 2008). Experts contend that their early violent childhood experiences may have taught them to believe that violence is an acceptable dispute resolution, and that physical, psychological, and sexual violence is how people demonstrate love (Fang & Corso, 2008). The cycle of violence continues as those previously exposed to IPV repeat the behavior in intimate partner relationships as teenagers and adults (Whiting et al., 2009). They also tend to associate with others who are similarly situated and who support and reinforce risky and violent behaviors (Henneberger et al., 2013).

Community Factors

Neighborhoods characterized by high degrees of poverty, large numbers of people, low educational attainment, and a lack of economic opportunities for their residents are often besieged by crime and assaultive violence, including IPV (Post et al., 2010; McDowell & Reinhard, 2023). Research supports the notion that in socially disorganized, high poverty, and high resident mobility communities, residents do not often interact. Consequently, these community residents are prevented from exerting informal means or mechanisms of social control to eliminate IPV (Post et al., 2010). As crime and violence are displayed in these communities and witnessed by others, neighbors either are unwilling or feel powerless to intervene (McDowell & Reinhard, 2023). Other studies have discovered that in unkempt, neglected communities, the process of "broken windows" often signals to the criminal element that abandoned houses or apartments can be used to conduct illegal activities. The proliferation of firearms and dimly-lit neighborhoods invites delinquency and crime. Similarly, McDowell and Reinhard (2023) provided that concentrated disadvantages are significantly associated with IPV in neighborhoods, suggesting the need for community-wide efforts toward prevention and intervention for everyone impacted by IPV.

Societal Factors

Culture is a leading cause of IPV, especially as directed at women. Most cultures have given men the power to control the behavior and sexuality of women through religious doctrine as well as their laws (Das et al., 2015). This has featured prominently in patriarchal societies (i.e., where men dominate most social institutions, including the church, state, education, military, justice, and legal systems) as well as in other nations where women are relegated to a second-class status. In some countries, legal structures fail to recognize women's complaints of IPV if the perpetrator is a spouse. Many women are unable to leave violent and abusive relationships and return to their families or live alone (Jewkes, 2002). In some countries, females are subject to genital mutilation, men use acid to disfigure their spouse without legal consequence, or commit honor killings without legal intervention (United Nations, 2020). In some countries and cultures, women have no legal remedies allowing them to divorce or seek justice for IPV (Jewkes, 2002). A 17th-century law allowed husbands to beat their wives with impunity, but only if the stick used by men was not larger than their thumb (aka the rule of thumb law). Thus, many experts and feminist scholars conclude that globally, the culture that women find themselves in supports the violence they experience at the hands of men.

When grappling to understand the historical gaps in the IPV literature (primary focus on heterosexuals) and why less attention has been given to the variations in IPV experienced by men (Randle & Graham, 2011), feminist scholars revisit Messerschmidt's (2019) discussion of Connell's (1987) formulation of hegemonic masculinity. Partnered with emphasized femininity, it represents the highest forms of masculinity and femininity that men and women can attain in society and is also an attempt to legitimize unequal gender relations. While hegemonic masculinity and emphasized femininity are supreme, there are constructions of oppositional or subordinate forms of masculinity and femininity that can be conceptualized since masculinity and femininity can be done differently based on the settings and social structures where people find themselves. Connell (1987) viewed gender relations as being structured along with power inequities existing when emphasized femininity adapts or submits to masculine power. This suggests that hegemonic and emphasized forms are the model that matters. Within the framework of IPV studies, violence experts argue that the lion's share of research has always focused on (used samples of) heterosexual behavior and relationships, especially those displaying hegemonic masculinity and emphasized femininity to the determent of other people who do oppositional or subordinate forms of masculinity and femininity (e.g., LGBTQ members). To these experts, the lack of research attention initially devoted to other groups of IPV victims and perpetrators may be explained by how society and its culture have viewed its hierarchy of sexual identity. Many feminist scholars have argued that those who engage in oppositional forms of masculinity and femininity simply do gender differently (Messerschmidt, 2019).

Intimate Partner Violence (IPV) Is a Criminal Justice Issue

Scholars, feminists, researchers, and social workers argue that IPV has always been a criminal justice issue, but not always recognized or treated as such (Maxwell et al., 2020; Goodmark, 2017), as IPV arrests were rare, and their prosecutions were nearly unheard of (Goodmark, 2017). Before the 1980s, IPV was regarded as a private family matter. Police, courts, judiciary, and others in the criminal justice system generally took a hands-off approach to intervention (Cramer, 2004; Barney & Carney, 2011). However, due to events beginning in the late 1970s, IPV transformed into a major social problem when U.S. communities realized that IPV was a public issue requiring new systems and policies to protect women and hold abusers accountable (Maxwell et al., 2020). More specifically, the battered women's movement was instrumental in shifting IPV from being a private matter to a crime requiring official police intervention, along with criminal and civil remedies for victims in the courts and punishment for abusers (Walker, 1985; Cramer, 2004). Nationally, several lawsuits were filed by women against police departments alleging failure to enforce the laws requiring them to arrest their husbands in cases of IPV. In one egregious case, a survivor was awarded $2.3 million for damages when *Torrington, Connecticut*, police watched a woman's husband repeatedly stab and kick her without intervening (Goodmark, 2017). Sherman and Berk (1984), examining how police arrest policies in Minneapolis,

MN effected the continuation of IPV, concluded that making an arrest was effective at reducing recidivism rates in the following six months. This led to the nationwide adoption of mandatory arrest laws in cases where police officers had probable cause to believe that an assault or battery had occurred. Another important 1984 event was the *Attorney General's Task Force on Family Violence*. It issued a report listing IPV as a criminal justice matter and provided recommendations to police departments nationwide to implement policies that presume arrests were appropriate in IPV-related cases (Goodmark, 2017; Fagan, 1996). In cases where arrests were affected, some survivors were reluctant to testify in court against a partner, and many refused to move their case forward by often dropping charges (Cramer, 2004).

Criminal justice historians also point to other events occurring in the early 1970s that called attention to IPV as a crime (Walker, 1985). Women advocates and movements in cities and states throughout the country worked assiduously to bring the plight of women to the attention of the American public, protect abused women, and hold abusers accountable for their behavior. More specifically, the battered women movement was instrumental in shifting IPV from being a private matter (where police had used non-arrest alternatives such as mediation, counseling, and referrals to other agencies) to a crime requiring official police intervention, along with criminal and civil remedies for victims in the courts and punishment for abusers (Walker, 1985; Cramer, 2004, p. 168). Walker (1985) reported that by suing police departments, women obtained consent decrees that required departments to effect arrests in serious IPV cases (Phillips & Sobol, 2010). During this time, arrests were viewed as the most desired response to protect victims of domestic abuse (Walker, 1985). Despite this early effort, some still regarded IPV as a private matter with few arrests made even when police officers witnessed the abuse firsthand. In the 1980s and 1990s, communities nationwide began implementing coordinated criminal justice responses to IPV cases that included mandatory arrests, quickly becoming the norm under established legal precedent or case law (e.g., *Thurman v. City of Torrington*, 1984 and *Sherman and Berk's* domestic violence experiment). Other efforts were protective orders; aggressive prosecution strategies (e.g., no drop policies) requiring prosecutors to move forward with IPV cases even when survivors refused; monitoring court orders; court-ordered treatment for abusers; and mandatory training for justice officials on aspects of domestic violence, as well as services designed to assist the survivors and perpetrations of IPV (Maxwell et al., 2020). These responses sought coordinated efforts from criminal justice and community-based organizations that focused on the safety of victims (Davies et al., 1998). Further, the creation of the *Violence against Women Office* via the passage of the 1994 *Violence against Women Act* provides hundreds of millions of dollars to train actors (e.g., police, judges, and other criminal justice personnel) in the criminal justice system to implement criminal justice responses to IPV cases, reinforcing the need to view IPV as a crime of violence to help shape our understanding and responses to IPV (Goodmark, 2017; Cramer, 2004; Barney & Carney, 2011).

Intimate Partner Violence Is a Public Health Issue

Health officials argue that two conditions make IPV a public health issue. First is its widespread effect on the population. On average, 24 people each minute are either a victim of stalking, rape, or physical violence by an intimate partner in the U.S. (Spivak et al., 2014).

Most IPV incidents have gone unreported therefore, the actual number is unknown (Black et al., 2011). However, evidence collected by *WHO* shows that IPV affects between 15% and 71% of all women, causing them to suffer significant negative health consequences because of physical abuse, sexual abuse, emotional abuse, or a combination at least once during their lifetime (Garcia-Moreno et al., 2006). In 2010, a study revealed that 1,295 IPV-related deaths occurred, accounting for 10% of all homicides reported to the UCR that year (Federal Bureau of Investigation, 2011). Second, IPV has lasting consequences on victims' physical, emotional, and psychological health and their overall well-being. Notwithstanding the toll that it takes on families, communities, and society. Because of its global prevalence and impact, IPV is a public health crisis in every country (Kippert, 2023). Clemente-Teixeira et al. (2022) posit that globally, IPV is found in every type of family regardless of sex, age, or social dynamics between the victim and abuser. A study conducted in the U.S. reported that an estimated 37% of women and 31% of men experience sexual violence, physical violence, or stalking committed by an intimate partner during their lifetime (Smith et al., 2017).

IPV presents many negative health consequences that are difficult for victims to overcome. Health experts emphasize that if their health problems are not reported and adequately treated early, there is a risk that the violence will likely continue or manifest in a cycle of violence (Spivak et al., 2014; Clemente-Teixeira et al., 2022). Some studies reveal that IPV causes a range of concerns affecting victims' quality of life, including their physical, psychological, sexual, reproductive, relational, educational, and economic well-being (Clemente-Teixeira et al., 2022). Gilbert et al. (2023) reported that IPV victims' physical problems often include injury, chronic pain, headaches, sleeping disorders, asthma, gastrointestinal disorders, and diabetes. Women predominantly suffer physical injuries ranging from disfigurement, permanent disability, life-threatening injuries, and death (Black, 2011). Other research reveals that for women alone, an estimated two million sustain physical injuries and 1,300 are injured during IPV incidents (National Center for Injury Prevention and Control, 2003). Coker et al. (2000) reported that victims of IPV faced an elevated risk of adverse health conditions affecting the brain and nervous system, cardiovascular system, gastrointestinal system, genitourinary system, immune and endocrine system, reproductive system, and other health outcomes. Death is a rare IPV consequence but is more likely to occur in the U.S., where women are killed in IPV-related incidents at a rate of 1.2 homicides per 100,000 people (Hemenway et al., 2002).

IPV also leads to sexual and reproductive problems. Researchers report that when women are forced to engage in violent and coercive sex, they could contract *STIs (e.g., herpes, syphilis, gonorrhea, HIV/acquired immune deficiency syndrome [AIDS])* or experience unintended pregnancies. Negative health conditions may also include inflammatory pelvic disease, urinary tract infections, spontaneous and elective abortions, as well as pregnancy complications (Capitulo, 2022). Pastor-Moreno et al. (2020) found that IPV caused some women to miscarry, experience premature rupture of membranes, low birth weight, and perinatal death. Additionally, IPV can have an adverse psychological impact since it affects victims' mental health, evidenced by many reporting that during and in the aftermath of IPV, they suffered depression, post-traumatic stress disorders, and had thoughts of committing suicide. Other negative health consequences reported by victims are that many begin to abuse alcohol and drugs to cope with their situation. Finally, the ultimate consequence is that IPV can resort to homicide. Research conducted by Stockl and colleagues (2013) reports that globally, one in seven homicides is committed by an intimate partner. Black and colleagues (2002) point out that women who experience multiple forms of IPV are more likely than those who do not to develop serious health problems.

Scholars contend that IPV is a public health issue leading to substantial social and economic costs that have ripple effects impacting everyone (Walby, 2009). When women are harmed because of IPV, they often become isolated, unable to work, thereby, experiencing lost wages, becoming unable to do routine activities like taking care of an elder parent and their children, but others are also impacted, namely government, communities, and individuals (Krug et al., 2002; Walby, 2009; WHO, 2024). Peterson et al. (2018) used several IPV studies, along with the 2010–2012 *National Intimate Partner and Sexual Violence Survey* data, to determine IPV costs over the lifetime. Considering of impaired medical and mental health, lost productivity, and criminal justice activities, they revealed that IPV costs $103,767 per female and $23,414 per male victim, resulting in an estimated U.S. $3.6 trillion. Research shows that many IPV victims have healthcare needs, due to injury, requiring immediate attention such as increased visits to doctors, pharmacies, emergency rooms, and mental health providers, and may require multiple surgeries, and extended hospital stays (Krug et al., 2002). A *CDC* report estimated that in 2003, IPV in the U.S. accounted for more than 807,000 overnight hospital stays, 971,000 outpatient visits, more than 95,000 ambulance calls, and more than 486,000 emergency department visits (National Center for Injury Prevention and Control, 2003). According to Peterson et al. (2018), health officials estimate that IPV costs $2.1 trillion in medical costs, $1.3 trillion in lost productivity among victims and perpetrators, $73 billion in criminal justice activities, and $62 billion in other expenditures. Some estimate that IPV costs American taxpayers approximately $3,200 annually for associated expenses (Spivak et al., 2014).

International Comparative Statistics

Because IPV occurs in every country, it is viewed as a preventable global pandemic and a major human rights violation disproportionately affecting women and children worldwide, having lifelong health consequences (Devries et al., 2013). In 2013, the *WHO* published a review of survey data collected up to 2010. This effort used data from 81 countries and 141 studies conducted from 1990 to 2012. All studies included estimates of IPV or non-partner sexual violence or both. However, since its early attempt, *WHO* officials report that there have been substantial increases in the number of population-based surveys and studies that measure IPV worldwide (Sardinha et al., 2022). Today's data reveal that globally, the number of women and girls impacted by IPV is astronomical. To acquire a current measure of IPV worldwide, in a recent study that relied on earlier *WHO* efforts (from 2013) that measured global, regional, and country estimates of IPV (across 161 countries and areas), data from *WHO's Global Database on Prevalence of Violence Against Women (e.g., intimate-partner violence and non-partner sexual violence)*, along with additional IPV studies conducted between 2000 and 2008 that relied on a national sample of women between the age of 15 and older who either experienced physical, sexual, psychological abuse, or a combination by an intimate partner, reported that an estimated 736 million women worldwide experience IPV annually (Maheu-Giroux et al., 2022). This suggests that globally, one in four or 27% of every married/partnered woman between the ages of 15 and 49 has experienced physical, sexual, or a combination of both types of violence from an intimate in their lifetime. Moreover, one in seven or 13% of women reported experiencing it in the past year before they were surveyed (Sardinha et al., 2022).

WHO's findings also revealed that violence starts early for girls and women, since 24% revealed having experienced violence at the age of 15–19. Those ages 19–24 reported that they had experienced violence at least once since the age of 15 (Sardinha et al., 2022). Moreover, the 2011 *National Youth Risk Behavior Survey* reported that 9% of high school students revealed date-related physical violence by either a boyfriend or girlfriend. Specifically, females reported experiencing rape, physical violence, or stalking by a partner, and 22.4% had their first experience with IPV between the ages of 11 and 17 years old, 47.1% at age 18–24 years old, and 21.1% at age 25–34 years old. Of the male students who experienced rape, physical violence, or stalking by an intimate partner, 15% reported that they were between the ages of 11 and 17 years old when they had their first experience with any form of IPV. Moreover, 38.6% were between the ages of 18 and 24, and 30.6% were between the ages of 25 and 34 (CDC, 2012). Furthermore, data from the United Nations Office on Drugs and Crime (2023) also present a grim reality for women and girls by reporting that an estimated 48,800 women and girls were killed globally by an intimate partner or family member in 2024. From that number, Asia reported the highest number of victims with an estimated 18,600. This suggests that on average, more than five women or girls worldwide are killed each hour by someone known to them, typically a family member or an intimate partner. Notwithstanding, while the worldwide number of IPV victims (736 million) is disturbing, research from the WHO (2024) also provides geographical variations in the distribution of IPV prevalence. For example, recent data reveal that globally, the prevalence of lifetime IPV varies by region (Maheu-Giroux et al., 2022). According to data from the *Global Burden of Diseases, Injuries, and Risk Factors Study* that classified IPV for every partner woman between ages 15 and 49 over the lifetime for physical, sexual, or both, the highest estimated prevalence occurred in *Oceania* (49%), *Central sub-Saharan African* (44%), *Andean Latin America* (38%), and *Eastern sub-Saharan African* (38%). Moreover, the study revealed that the prevalence of lifetime physical or sexual or a combination of both for IPV was also high and exceeded the global average in *South Asia* (35%) and *North Africa* and the *Middle East* (31%), respectively (Sardinha et al., 2022). *WHO* data also showed variations in IPV in urban and rural areas. For example, prevalence is higher in *Latin American* and *Caribbean* urban areas compared with the national average of both lifetime and IPV reported in the past year. However, Sardinha et al. (2022) report the opposite pattern of higher IPV prevalence in rural areas is noted for all other regions. This was especially the case in *North Africa*, the *Middle East*, and *South Asia*. Research contends that several factors can explain the variation, such as the social, economic, and political contexts that are often impacted by inequitable gender norms, economic insecurity, social stigma, discriminatory law and practices, and other cultural factors (Maheu-Giroux et al., 2022).

Public Health and Social Work

Intersection of Public Health and Social Work

Because interpersonal violence takes different forms that "co-occur and share common risk and protective factors," it can be best understood through an integrated, intersectionality framework that considers the multiple simultaneous identities of people at risk (Decker et al., 2018, p. 65S). Experts recommend that public health carry out behavioral and structural interventions. Structural interventions include community and policy work, while behavioral interventions target individuals, groups, and families. Behavioral interventions include bystander training, school-based rape resistance training, proactive policing methods, and multi-systemic therapy, especially for reducing self-inflicted violence and suicidal behavior. These intervention and prevention measures are similar to efforts used in social work. Since social workers interact daily with persons affected by IPV, they have a responsibility to act, including in the areas of legislation, policy, and advocacy (Wilson & Webb, 2018). Social work incorporates both the victim and abuser into its IPV intervention and prevention models. When working with victims of violence, treating trauma may involve therapeutic approaches such as trauma-focused cognitive behavioral therapy (TF-CBT) (especially with youth), eye movement desensitization and reprocessing (EMDR), prolonged exposure (PE) therapy, cognitive processing therapy (CPT), dialectical behavior therapy (DBT), mindfulness-based therapies, group therapies, arts-based therapies, and holistic and body-centered therapies (Social Work Test Prep, 2023). Working with perpetrators often involves couples therapy, mind–body bridging, acceptance and commitment therapy, and restorative justice approaches (Seawright et al., 2017).

Health Disparities and Health Equities

Communities and women of color are often disproportionately affected by IPV due to the intersectionality of race, gender, status, socioeconomics, and other social constructs (Crenshaw, 2023). Living in economically distressed neighborhoods places women and men at an increased risk of IPV (Bonomi et al., 2014; Cunradi et al., 2000). Overall, many violence-related chronic diseases and mental health disorders affect African-American, Hispanic, and Asian Americans more than other ethnic or racial groups (Robert Wood Johnson Foundation, 2009; Williams, 2018).

Compared with people without violence exposure, those who experience violence are more susceptible to developing health diseases and conditions (Dube et al., 2003). For example, adults exposed to violence were found to be 2.2 times more likely to be diagnosed with ischemic heart disease, 1.9 times more likely with cancer, 2.4 times more likely with a stroke, 3.9 times more likely with chronic obstructive lung disease, and 1.6 times more likely with diabetes (Carver et al., 2008; Felitti et al., 2019). Those exposed to violence are more likely to have impaired social relationships and an increased inclination toward aggressive and/or risk-taking behaviors (Dube et al., 2003). They are also at a greater risk for substance use disorders and depression, anxiety, and suicidal behavior (Kessler et al., 2010), as well as post-traumatic stress disorder (Williams, 2018). These vulnerabilities have been linked to violence-related effects on the brain, including changes in the brain's white and gray matter (Bick & Nelson, 2016), deviations in neurotransmitter metabolism and neuroendocrine stress responses (Berens et al., 2017), ongoing inflammation (Baumeister et al., 2016), and glucose metabolic dysfunction (Maniam, 2014). Other factors active in the development of conditions and disorders include genetics, the type of violence exposure, the context of exposure (e.g., social, community, home, school), the chronicity of the exposure, and the age at which exposure began (Inslicht et al., 2006).

IPV increases generational risks of adverse pregnancy outcomes, including fetal death (Hillis et al., 2004), and postpartum depression (Fisher et al., 2012). Children of mothers who are victims of IPV have a significantly higher mortality rate than children whose mothers were not victimized (Silverman et al., 2011). Globally, research has confirmed a link between infectious diseases and violence, such as sexually transmitted diseases, and immunodeficiency viruses/AIDS (HIV/AIDS), as well as an increased risk of HIV/AIDS-related deaths (Machtinger et al., 2012). The rates of HIV/AIDS are high among women of color as IPV victims, because they are less able to demand the use of condoms (Wyatt et al., 2002) and once infected are less likely to complete antiretroviral medication regimes (Machtinger et al., 2012).

Negative Health Consequences of IPV for Men

Scant attention has been devoted to researching men as IPV victims (Scott-Storey et al., 2022). Current evidence suggests that one in seven men, or 13.9%, will experience IPV in their lifetime (Mankind Initiative, 2023). Evidence suggests that men report being victims of the same types of physical, sexual, and psychological violence as women in IPV relationships, but the methods that women use to abuse men are often different, requiring less physical aggression (Brooks et al., 2017). For example, when men report experiencing IPV physical violence, it is often described as slapping, pushing, kicking, threatening, or using a knife or object (Brook et al., 2017). Nybergh et al. (2016) reported that even when women used physical violence against male partners, the men tended to report that they were still in control of the female partner and could defuse the situation. However, Bates (2020) reported that some men revealed being afraid because of physical threats or physical violence directed at their family.

Nowinski and Bowen (2012) found that gay men were more likely to undergo similar or higher rates of physical violence than heterosexual men and they reported experiencing fear and terror owing to their gay partner's physical strength and past violence. Heterosexual men report being forced to engage in unwanted sexual acts or unprotected sexual activities with a woman inmate partner who either used threats, manipulation, pressure, or false promises (Bates, 2020). However, gay and bisexual men are more likely to report being the victims of sexual violence (Dickerson-Amaya & Coston, 2019). Furthermore, Stephenson and Finneran (2017) revealed that there is growing evidence suggesting that some men use sexual violence as a tactic on other men to transmit HIV without disclosing their HIV status. Like women, men are also subjected to psychological IPV violence. Bates (2020) reported that some men revealed being yelled at, insulted, berated, humiliated, had their sexuality questioned, experienced being controlled, monitored, and isolated from family and friends, had their competence as a father questioned, were falsely accused of child abuse, and were threatened with having their children removed. IPV is also reported to have short- and long-term negative consequences on men's health. Data, collected from the National Coalition Against Domestic Violence (n.d.), show that annually, more than 10 million men and women are physically abused by an intimate partner in the U.S. One in every 71 men has been raped in their lifetime. Moreover, an estimated 5.1 million U.S. men have been stalked by a former or current partner in their lifetime, and 6% of men were killed by a female intimate partner in a murder–suicide. Evidence taken from data collected from *the U.S. National Violence against Women Survey* from 8,001 men and 8,005 women revealed that men who are victimized by IPV report that they experience significant physical and mental health problems. This is also supported by statistics from the *National Intimate Partner and*

Sexual Violence Survey that shows one in every ten men in the U.S. experience rape, physical violence, and/or stalking by an intimate partner which has led to injury, fear, post-traumatic stress, and the use of victim services, contracting STIs, and others. Moreover, one in seven men between the ages of 18 and older in the U.S. has been the victim of serious violence by an intimate partner in their lifetime. Furthermore, 48.8% of men in IPV relationships report experiencing psychological aggression by an intimate partner in their lifetime. Men who sought help for IPV were found to be significantly suffering from poor mental health, depression, displayed symptoms of post-traumatic stress disorders (Hines & Douglas, 2015, 2018), and also demonstrated increased rates of suicide ideation (Nybergh et al., 2016). While psychological abuse was reported most often, Hines (2015) found that men in IPV relationships also sustained bruises, cuts, burns, broken bones, stabs, and gunshot wounds. There is even evidence that men also report experiencing elevated blood pressure, STIs, and asthma compared with men in the general population not in IPV relationships. Some studies find that men in relationships with other men tend to report having similar health-related IPV consequences to those of women in IPV relationships (Oliffe et al., 2014). Like their women counterparts, some men cope with the stress and trauma of IPV by turning to alcohol, drugs, substance abuse, smoking, and risky behaviors that harm their health (Nybergh et al., 2016). Comparatively, in the UK, the *Office of National Statistics* reports that 751,000 men are victims of domestic abuse annually. Of that number, an estimated 483,000 men are victims of IPV.

Criminal Justice Approaches to IPV

As early as the 1980s, collective and deliberate efforts were made to convince the public that IPV was just as serious as other types of crimes, and criminals needed to be held accountable, and victims needed to be provided services (Goodman & Epstein, 2011; Cramer, 2004). Some contend that these early efforts significantly impacted the justice system's shift from a "hands-off" to a "hands-on" approach in IPV cases. Research on IPV reveals that in the past 40 years, criminal justice practices have occurred in a threefold manner. First, the criminal justice system requires police to make an arrest in IPV cases. Prosecutors implement aggressive no drop policies (and subpoena victims as witnesses) when the state moves forward with holding batterers accountable, even when the abused refuses to press charges. Second, in the civil justice system, women activists convinced state legislatures to create and pass protection orders, empowering judges to grant IPV survivors several protections designed for their needs. Third, women activists are successful at creating public and private collaborations known as coordinated community responses, expanding the scope of the justice system's reach and response to IPV victims/survivors (Goodman & Epstein, 2011). Fagan (1996) argues that these combined efforts drastically changed the plight of victims of IPV since they, and their children, are afforded access to justice and intervention programs. As evidenced by Anderson et al. (2003), of IPV survivors in their study, 77% received assistance from public agencies, and 61% revealed being able to file a complaint with police.

Despite the achievements made to help victims of IPV, research suggests that there are obstacles often preventing the safety of victims, and many of the newly created justice reforms have given rise to unintended consequences and challenges for victims. According to Goodman and Epstein (2008), while many reforms work theoretically, they often fall short in practice for reasons such as being rigid and functioning as a one-size-fits-all without regard for context, marginalizing many women. Unintended consequences of criminal justice reform, such as mandatory arrests, have also led to women being taken into custody as part of dual arrest efforts (Hirschel & Buzawa, 2002). Women are also victims of continued violent assaults owing to ineffective monitoring of protective orders for probationer abusers (Cramer, 2004). An earlier survey on the criminal justice system's effectiveness in protecting women in IPV situations reported many limitations, given that the real problems facing women are rooted in the structured, gendered inequality found in most societies (Iovanni & Miller, 2001). While the latter is true, some violence experts contend it is more pronounced for poor women of color (Raphael, 2004).

Public Health Approaches to IPV

CDC and other health professionals criticize criminal justice approaches used to address violence (Rosenberg & Fenley, 1991). They contend that justice responses to violence prevention fall short of being more than merely punitive reactions to violence, including IPV, since they failed to address the root causes of IPV, nor were its practitioners adequately trained to address what victims and perpetrators need in IPV's aftermath. Health experts argue that what is needed in IPV cases are proactive strategies designed to reduce incidents of IPV, assist victims, perpetrators, and children with problems extending beyond the criminal justice system negative health consequences of IPV (e.g., physical, mental, and sexual problems). As such, public health approaches are needed to improve the health and well-being of everyone impacted by IPV, since a failure to do so may invariably mean that others will become victims and perpetrators of the behavior. According to Spivak et al. (2014), the role of the public health system is to use its building capacity and vast expertise by helping communities (e.g., especially impoverished ones) to develop and implement evidence-based IPV prevention strategies that identify risk factors leading to violence. To accomplish this, communities must assist public health officials in mitigating their layered risk factors that influence violence (Spivak et al., 2014). Some research suggests that communities work to replace negative norms that encourage and promote violence and replace them with positive new norms that discourage the continuation of destructive forces (Grazian & Pulcini, 2013). The Community Prevention Services Task Force (2018) reported that community efforts must also target environmental factors such as employment, education, housing, safe space, equity, and group cohesion. Moreover, by creating an infrastructure in areas known for IPV prevalence, stakeholders can work together to identify effective programs, best practices to create and implement policies to alleviate IPV incidents. Those experts who subscribe to public health, rather than criminal justice approaches, posit that by creating *primary*, *secondary*, and *tertiary* prevention strategies, successful efforts can be made to reduce IPV with widespread U.S. adoption and implementation.

Health officials at the *WHO* describe the public health approach to violence prevention as a strategy created to improve the health and safety of everyone worldwide. For example, Leight et al. (2023) conducted a systematic review on how widespread violence prevention efforts led by nongovernmental officials are beginning to target low- and middle-income countries. They contend that organizations behind these efforts employ public health strategies to alleviate the suffering that women, their families, and communities are experiencing. Chosen intervention recipients come from targeted communities and are given community mobilization and group-based training. Leight and colleagues report these efforts have been used in communities, mostly in sub-Saharan Africa to measure their impact on preventing IPV. As part of its approach, these programs educate participants by changing their attitudes and behavior associated with violence to prevent IPV. The results suggest that women who participate in these programs experience lower levels of IPV by at least 20%. The public health approach relies on the ecological framework to examine the many individual, relationship, community, and societal level risk factors increasing the likelihood that people will either become an IPV victim or perpetrator. It is designed to prevent violence on every level, including each home and community. This requires building healthy gender norms, healthy relationships, socially just institutions, changing norms, and advocating and creating protective environments (Substance Abuse and Mental Health Service Administration, 2023), especially in poor communities. The public health approach has a utilitarian focus designed to maximize benefit for the greatest number of people. The public health approach consists of four steps: (1) define the problem by collecting data that measure the extent of the problem (e.g., IPV); (2) identify the risk factors and causes of the problem (e.g., IPV). Make attempts to isolate those factors that increase or decrease the problem risk that can be modified via intervention; (3) discover what works to prevent the problem (e.g., IPV) and evaluate its effectiveness; and (4) when the intervention is proven effective, widely implement it. After implementing the intervention on the targeted risk factors, they should be monitored, and their impact assessed. Later, evaluations are needed to determine its cost-effectiveness. This helps create an evidence-based approach to be presented to policymakers, health providers, and governmental officials on the need to support sound public health policy to prevent IPV. Some studies have examined whether using public health approaches can successfully reduce IPV. Several studies reveal that the public health approach has been successfully used to prevent IPV and other types of victimization (Foshee et al., 2012). However, the most compelling data reveal that programs aimed at preventing teenage violence tend to be more effective than those targeting adults. When teens are targeted, intervention programs use a variety of people, including youths and parents. They also have components like parent-focused programs, therapeutic approaches with at-risk couples, community-based programs, and economic and policy-focused approaches. Health experts that intervention given to teens is designed to disrupt and address the negative exposure to violence they may have observed displayed by parents engaging in IPV. In a study conducted by the CDC known as *Dating Matters*, it used public health strategies to intervene in dating violence among teenagers. *Dating Matters* combined several prevention strategies that included participation from youths, their parents, educators, and other community stakeholders to help foster safe and healthy relationships for youth (Tharp, 2012). Because of its success, the CDC implemented other programs in four additional communities (Tharp, 2012).

Another IPV intervention program that targeted teen dating violence is called the *Start Strong Healthy Teen Relationship* initiative. Created in 2008, it was considered the largest private sector investment in teen dating violence prevention (Spivak et al., 2014). While relying on the social-ecological model of public health, *Start Strong* provided components such as education and targeted teens in and out of school. It also focused on educating influencers such as parents, teachers, older teens, caregivers, and other school officials. Its goal was to decrease teen IPV by increasing awareness that would translate into behavioral changes. The *Start Strong* program also enlisted other partners such as the school board to facilitate improvements to policies that promoted prevention and healthy responses to violence by using innovative social marketing and media efforts that focused on students and parents (Spivak et al., 2014). Furthermore, a research report that focused on the effect of using public health interventions to reduce dating violence among youths revealed that rates of dating violence victimizations remained between 56% and 92% lower for North Carolina teenagers who were given prevention intervention compared with those in a control group. A follow-up on its effect shows that it lasted four years (Spivak et al., 2014).

Public Health and Social Work Approaches

Public health and social work aim to engage in intervention and prevention efforts at every level of society. In addition to individual, group, and family behavioral methods of violence mediation and prevention, both professions work to bring about community modification and policy change (Decker et al., 2018). For example, public health can impact policing reform in its response to interpersonal violence and assist with empowering and mobilizing communities to become more violence-aware and safer for children. Structurally, public health strives to lower disparities connected to interpersonal violence, assists in firearm regulation change, advocates for alcohol accessibility restrictions, and promotes restorative justice options for offenders.

In 2024, one of 13 grand challenges for the social work profession was to *build healthy relationships to end violence* (Grand Challenges for Social Work, 2024). This challenge advanced the notion that broad implementation of universal and targeted violence interventions, using multilayered service delivery systems, could enhance "interpersonal relationships, reduce violence more broadly, and strengthen our mental and physical health, our families, and our communities" (p. 1). This challenge provides that over the next ten years, there can be a 10% decrease in IPV through interprofessional activities that include (p. 1)

- Identifying and facilitating prevention services for families with young children at risk of maltreatment and screening for violence exposure in health settings;
- Increasing support for evidence-based intervention and prevention programs to reduce the structural inequalities that perpetuate interpersonal violence across the lifespan;
- Harnessing healthcare resources to increase engagement, screening, brief education, and referrals from primary care providers, the expansion of home visiting, parent education, and an array of culturally relevant IPV and child abuse responses;
- Building healthy, violence-free relationships across the lifespan influencing social norms and promoting safety in the family and community;
- Increasing research funding for culturally informed evidence-based interventions that strategically address common risk and protective factor;
- Increasing the availability of parenting support (including safe-haven, birth match, and home visiting programs) for all families, and;
- Supporting the expansion of trauma-informed service delivery models that treat trauma and enhance resilience and relational health.

The challenge to build healthy relationships to end violence also requires funding for existing and new data collection, research on safe alternatives to incarceration, investments in policies and programs that strengthen relationships to reduce community risk factors associated with violence and develop programs that alleviate financial stressors.

Integrating Skills of Social Epidemiology to Address Disparities and Achieve Equity

Social epidemiology is used to describe reasons for the many social factors found in the development and growth of health problems such as disease, violence (e.g., IPV), poverty, and the risk factors linked to each (Kaplan, 2004). Simply put, social epidemiology seeks to identify certain characteristics in the environment that impact disease and health distribution by working to understand a disease's mechanisms. It relies on several concepts that include social inequalities (e.g., unequal distribution of resources), social relationships (e.g., degree of integration in social networks), social capital (e.g., features of the social structure used to engage in collective action), and work stress (e.g., job strain and work demand) to show that they improve health services research. Social epidemiologists posit that the approach has a fivefold purpose: (1) it allows them to specify the research question, (2) it clarifies methodological issues, (3) it helps them to better understand how social factors are linked to health care, (4) it allows researchers to develop and implement interventions, and (5) it addresses criticisms about health service research failure to incorporate theoretical approaches in their studies (Brazil et al., 2005). Experts argue that health disparities (e.g., a high prevalence of IPV in certain populations or communities) can be significantly reduced when social epidemiologists and community engagement intervention researchers form collaborative efforts to improve health equity (Wallenstein et al., 2011). On the one hand, epidemiologists examine risk factors in the population by analyzing the predictive power of variables, which helps to inform their interventions. On the other hand, community-engaged interventionists target the community instead of the entire population. They identify risk factors that a community sees as priorities amenable to change, such as attitudes about violence toward women and girls, and they use the community strengths to create strategies to address its risk factors (Wallenstein et al., 2011). Again, while both work to achieve health equity in the population and community, respectively, they remain separate in methodology and practice. Moreover, health experts characterize their relationship as follows: social epidemiologists tend to focus on causation and distribution of social determinants, while community-engaged interventionists rely on multiple disciplines (e.g., psychology, public health education, health promotion, health policy, and others) to focus on theories such as behavioral and social change to improve health outcome (Wallerstein et al., 2011). By partnering, social epidemiologists and community-engaged interventionists can create more effective methods to investigate health disparities since their combined efforts will allow for results to be translated into usable knowledge. Data on social determinants can aid in crafting health-enhancing policies, practices, and interventions, and benefit community-engaged researchers by informing modifications needed in their interventions, measurement of appropriate constructs, evaluating findings, and generating new theories and strategies when needed. It will allow both disciplines to apply their theories and methods to develop shared conceptual frameworks to better solve problems (Wallerstein et al., 2011; Stokols et al., 2008).

How Can IPV Be Prevented?

Because women are disproportionately the targets of IPV with historical trauma owing to structural inequalities, *WHO* and the *UN* reported that global violence against women or IPV can be prevented by using seven strategies referred to as RESPECT women (WHO, 2020). RESPECT implements interventions to keep women and teenage girls safe and empowers them by challenging culturally and societally based unequal power relationships. Those advocating for RESPECT argue that it is through its participatory process that education can lead to changes in attitudes, which can inevitably manifest in violence prevention (WHO, 2021). WHO and U.N. officials contend that nations should engage in efforts such as relationship skills strengthening, service ensured enabling environments, child and adolescent abuse prevention, and transformed attitudes, beliefs, and norms. Each strategy uses a range of interventions in low- and high-income areas. These interventions provide programs like psychological support for IPV perpetrators and survivors, economic and empowerment programs, couple counseling designed to improve communication and relationship skills, community mobilization interventions to help change unequal gender norms, and school programs that enhance safety and eliminate harsh punishment. Other efforts include changing school curriculum by removing gender stereotypes, replaced with images advocating relationships based on equality and consent, and group-based educational strategies where men and women engage in critical reflection on unequal gender power relationships (WHO, 2021).

The CDC developed *Intimate Partner Resource for Action* strategies and made them available to states and communities to implement. CDC argues that its six strategies are designed to prevent IPV, support survivors, and reduce the short- and long-term negative health consequences of IPV. Strategies include teaching safe and healthy relationship skills, engaging influential adults and peers, disrupting pathways toward partner violence, creating protective environments, strengthening economic support for women and girls, and supporting survivors by increasing their safety and minimizing harm. Experts suggest that youths should be given a social–emotional learning program and taught about healthy and safe dating, while adult couples should be provided educational programs fostering healthy relationships and sexuality. Second, engaging in processes that bring men and boys together as allies in IPV can help prevent the transmission of violence. Educating bystanders to intervene breaks social norms perpetuating violence by not allowing it to become accepted. Third, CDC officials suggest that disrupting pathways toward IPV can be an excellent tool for preventing more cases of this type. They argue that intervention should occur as early as risk factors are identified. Therefore, approaches such as early childhood home visits and preschool enrichment activities could serve as positive countermeasures. Fourth, because violence is pervasive, victims need safe spaces when the home, school, or work environment proves dangerous. Experts advocate creating safe protective environments in the school, workplace, and neighborhood. CDC officials argue that the schools should be monitored and made safe. Community safety may require changes in the physical and social environments. Fifth, CDC officials contend that efforts must be made to empower women and girls with economic and leadership opportunities. Finally, strategies that help survivors by making them safe and minimizing harm are essential for healing and recovering from victimization. This often requires victim-centered services, safe housing programs, trained first responders, patient-centered approaches, and treatment programs.

Policy Recommendations

Studies show that effectively preventing IPV requires a comprehensive prevention effort designed to target its complex nature and the host of specific risk and protective factors across individual, interpersonal, institutional, community, and societal levels (Dutton et al., 2015). However, IPV can only be properly addressed if the emphasis shifts from merely responding to treating and preventing the behavior (Spivak et al., 2014). Because of the complexity and enormity of IPV, a viable policy must also enlist the help of others by forming partnerships with officials and people within and outside of public health, criminal justice, government, education, community development, domestic violence, health care, businesses, housing, and other stakeholders (Spivak et al., 2014). A comprehensive plan of action must combine multiple strategies and approaches that focus on targeting both types of factors found at the different levels, and monitor how those factors impact people, communities, and society. Those working to prevent IPV must remember that the goal of a comprehensive plan should focus on changing attitudes, norms, environments, organizations, and behaviors that sustain and perpetuate IPV. As such, we offer the following policy recommendations: (1) use public health approaches to increase greater IPV awareness by engaging in massive educational programs; (2) teach adolescents the skillsets needed to avoid engaging in IPV and instill empathy and social–emotional learning and healthy dating practices; (3) engage influential adults and peers through family-based programs and bystander empowerment; (4) promote social norms throughout the community that are designed to protect against IPV by particularly targeting men and boys and teaching them about IPV; (5) disrupt pathways that lead to IPV by implementing strategies such as early childhood intervention, encouraging couple parenting skills and group-based training programs, and treating at-risk children, youth, and families; (6) implement strategies that address IPV risk and protective factors and examine the inequities that contribute to increased IPV risk; (7) create economic and leadership opportunities to empower those at high risk of being IPV victims(e.g., women, girls, and the *LGBTQ* community); (8) provide enhanced survivor-centered services, crisis intervention, economic support, counseling and mobilized community resources to everyone experiencing IPV; (9) create protective environments by monitoring community-level risk, implement safe workplace policies, and create safe spaces at schools; and (10) partner with law enforcement by supporting efforts to receive protective orders and implement risk assessment (Spivak et al., 2014; Leight, 2023; Niolon et al., 2017).

Summary

IPV is abuse that occurs within the context of romantic relationships. It refers to both current and former spouses and dating relationships. Research reveals that it is a preventable global problem impacting millions of people each year. While both men and women can be IPV victims, those most vulnerable include low-income women, young girls, and members of the *LGBTQ* community. Data suggest the abuse experienced by women tends to occur early in their lives and last for extended periods. The victimizations that IPV presents can have either a short- or long-term effect on its target and can also affect others who are exposed, namely children who often grow older and exhibit violence in their teenage dating relationships and later as adults. IPV has several manifestations, such as physical violence, sexual violence, emotional abuse, psychological abuse, stalking, and online abuse. Violence experts contend that it is essential to isolate and explain the causes of IPV to treat and prevent others from being either IPV victims or perpetrators. To that extent, they examine and analyze many risk factors such as the role of inequities, individual factors, relationship factors, community factors, and societal factors to determine how they influence and impact IPV. When considering how these factors influence behavior, health experts and researchers suggest they typically function in concert, rather than singularly, and while present in the environment, they are not necessarily causal. IPV is a criminal justice and public health problem, requiring a response from professionals in both systems since victims of IPV must participate in the justice process to bring offenders to justice and to seek protection orders, while those victimized by IPV experience many negative health outcomes and injuries that often have debilitating consequences. Policy experts posit that effective prevention approaches require a comprehensive plan incorporating elements of both. Recent *WHO* and *UN* statistics show that IPV is a global and humanitarian crisis that is preventable but requires public health approaches such as community mobilization or group-based training that targets women, men, or couples to change traditional, cultural, and economic attitudes and behavior about violence and women's roles in society. While many studies have examined the negative health consequences experienced by women who suffer from IPV, we also explored the health challenges that victimized men experience. As previously stated, IPV is both a criminal justice and public health problem. Therefore, we examined current and past criminal justice strategies used in response to IPV. Similarly, we examined proactive and preventive strategies used by public health officials to improve the overall well-being of victims and to prevent an increase in cases. Social epidemiologists are forming partnerships with community interventionists to create better methods for conducting research that addresses the disparities in violence and public health services, hoping to alleviate and prevent IPV. Because of the complexity and enormity of IPV, prevention efforts and public policies must be crafted to address individual, relationship, community, and societal factors perpetuating and sustaining the behavior.

Discussion Questions

1 What are some risk factors that influence IPV?
2 Explain some negative health consequences linked to IPV.
3 List and explain some criminal justice approaches used to combat IPV.
4 How can public health approaches prevent IPV?
5 What can society do to reduce the high level of violence experienced by women and young girls?
6 What is a common trait that is present in IPV cases globally?

References

Adams, A.E., Sullivan, C.M., Bybee, D., & Greeson, M.R. (2008). Development of the scale of economic abuse. *Violence against Women*, 14(5), 563–588.

Al-Alosi, H. (2017). Cyber-violence: Digital abuse in the context of domestic violence. *University of New South Wales Law Journal*, 40(4), 1573–1603.

Alhabib, S., Nur, U., & Jones, R. (2010). Domestic violence against women: Systematic review of prevalence studies. *Journal of Family Violence*, 25, 369–382. https://doi.org/10.1007/s10896-009-9298-4

Ali, P.A., Dhingra, K., & McGarry, J. (2016). A literature re view of intimate partner violence and its classifications. *Aggression and Violent Behavior*, 31, 16–25.

Anderson, K.L. (2002). Perpetrator or victim? Relationships between intimate partner violence and well-being. *Journal of Marriage and Family*, 64(4), 851–863.

Anderson, M.A., Gillig, P.M., Sitaker, M., & Mccloskey, K. (2003). Why doesn't she just leave?": A descriptive study of victim reported impediments to her safety. *Journal of Family Violence*, 18(3), 151–155.

Barner, J.R., & Carney, M.M. (2011). Interventions for intimate partner violence: A historical review. *Journal of Family Violence*, 26, 235–244.

Bates, E.A. (2020). Walking on eggshells: A qualitative examination of men's experiences of intimate partner violence. *Psychology of Men & Masculinities*, 21(3), 13–24.

Baumeister, D., Akhtar, R., Ciufolini, S., Pariante, C.M., & Mondelli, V. (2016). Childhood trauma and adulthood inflammation: A meta-analysis of peripheral C-reactive protein, interleukin-6 and tumour necrosis factor-α. *Molecular Psychiatry*, 21(5), 642–649. https://doi.org/10.1038/mp.2015.67

Berens, A.E., Jensen, S.K.G., & Nelson, C.A. (2017). Biological embedding of childhood adversity: From physiological mechanisms to clinical implications. *BMC Medicine*, 15(1), 135. Biological embedding of childhood adversity: from physiological mechanisms to clinical implications I BMC Medicine I Full Text.

Beymer, M.R., Harawa, N.T., Weiss, R.E., Shover, C.L., Toynes, B.R., Meanley, S. et al. (2017). Are partner race and intimate partner violence associated with incident and newly diagnosed HIV infection in African American men who have sex with men. *Journal of Urban Health*, 94, 666–675.

Bick, J., & Nelson, C.A. (2016). Early adverse experiences and the developing brain. *Neuropsychopharmacology (New York, N.Y.)*, 41(1), 177–196. https://doi.org/10.1038/npp.2015.252

Black, M.C. (2011). Intimate partner violence and adverse health consequences: Implications for clinicians. *Analytic Review: American Journal of Lifestyle Medicine*, https://doi.org/10.1177/1559827611410265

Black, M.C., Basile, K.C., Breiding, M.J., Smith, S.G., Walters, M.L., Merrick, M.T., Chen, J., & Stevens, M.R. (2011). *The National Intimate Partner and Sexual Violence Survey (NISVS): 2010 Summary Report*. Atlanta, GA: National Center for Injury Prevention and Control, Centers for Disease Control and Prevention.

Bonomi, A.E., Trabert, B., Anderson, M.L., Kernic, M.A., & Holt, V.L. (2014). Intimate partner violence and neighborhood income: A longitudinal analysis. *Violence against Women*, 20(1), 42–58. https://doi.org/10.1177/1077801213520580

Bracewell, K., Hargeaves, P., & Stanley, N. (2020). The consequences of the COVID-19 lockdown on stalking victimization. *Journal of Family Violence*, https://doi.org/10.1007/s10896-020-00201-0

Bradbury-Jones, C., & Isham, L. (2020). The pandemic paradox: The consequences of COVID-19 on domestic violence. *Journal of Clinical Nursing*, 29(13–14), 2047–2049. https://doi.org/10.1111/jocn.15296

Brazil, K., Ozer, E., Cloutier, M.M., Levine, R., & Stryer, D. (2005). From theory to practice: Improving the impact of health services research. *BMC Health Services Research*, 5(1), 1–5.

Breiding, M.J., Basile, K.C., Smith, S.G., Black, M.C., Mahendra, R.R. (2015). *Intimate partner violence surveillance: Uniform definitions and recommended data elements, Version 2.0*. National Center for Injury Prevention and Control, Centers for Disease Control and Prevention.

Breiding, M.J., Smith, S.G., Basile, K.C., Walters, M.L., Chen, J., & Merrick, M.T. (2014). Prevalence and characteristics of sexual violence, stalking, and intimate partner violence victimization-National Intimate Partner and Sexual Violence Survey, United States, 2011. Centers for Disease Control and Prevention. *Morbidity and Mortality Weekly Report*, 63(8), 1–17.

Brewster, M. (2003). Power and control dynamics in pre-stalking and stalking situations. *Journal of Family Violence*, 18(4), 207–217.

Brooks, C., Martin, S., Broda, L., & Poudrier, J. (2017). How many silences are there? Men's experiences of victimization in intimate partner relationships. *Journal of Interpersonal Violence*, 35(23–24), 1–24.

Brown, M.L., Reed, L.A., & Messing, J.T. (2018). Technology-based abuse: Intimate partner violence and the use of information communication technologies. In J.R. Vickery & T. Everbach (Eds.), *Mediating misogyny: Gender technology, and harassment* (pp. 209–227). Springer International Publishing.

Burke, S. C., Wallen, M., Vail-Smith, K., & Knox, D. (2011). Using technology to control intimate partners: An exploratory study of college undergraduates. *Computer in Human Behavior*, 27(3), 1162–1167. https://doi.org/10.1016/j.chb.2010.12.010

Caetano, R., Cunradi, C.B., Clark, C.L., & Schafer, J. (2000). Intimate partner violence and drinking patterns among Whites, Blacks, and Hispanic couples in the U.S. *Journal of Substance Abuse*, 11, 123–138.

Campbell, J.C. (2002). Health consequences of intimate partner violence. *Lancet*, 359, 1331–1336.

Campbell, K.A., Ford-Gilboe, M., Stanley, M., & Mackinnon, K. (2022). Intimate partner violence and women living with episodic disabilities: A scoping review protocol. *Systematic Reviews*, 11, 97–102.

Capaldi, D.M., Knoble, N.B., Short, J.W., & Kim, H.K. (2012). A systematic review of risk factors for intimate partner violence. *Partner Abuse*, 3(2), 231–280.

Capitulo, M. (2022). Aspetos medico-legais da violencia de genero e violencia domestica. In *Manual de boas praticas judiciais em materia de violencia de genero e violencia domestica: juristas*, A.P.d., Ed.: Associacao de defesa do patrimonnio de mertola.

Carpenter, C. (2006). Recognizing gender-based violence against civilian men and boys in conflict situations. *Security Dialogue*, 37, 83–103.

Carver, A., Timperio, A., & Crawford, D. (2008). Perceptions of neighborhood safety and physical activity among youth: The CLAN study. *Journal of Physical Activity & Health*, 5(3), 430–444. https://doi.org/10.1123/jpah.5.3.430

Cascardi, M., O'Leary, K.D., & Schlee, K.A. (1999). Co-occurrence and correlates of posttraumatic stress disorders and major depression in physically abused women. *Journal of Family Violence*, 14, 227–247.

Catalano, S., Smith, E., Snyder, H., & Rand, M. (2009). Female victims of violence. U.S. Department of Justice, Bureau of Justice Statistics. Office of Justice Programs. www.bjs.ojp.gov/content/pub/pdf/fvv.pdf

Centers for Disease Control (CDC) (2012). Youth risk behavior surveillance-United States, 2011. *Morbidity and Mortality Weekly Report (MMWR)*, 61(4), 1–161. www.cdc.gov/mmwr/pdf/ss/ss6 104.pd

Centers for Disease Control (CDC) and Prevention (2023). Preventing intimate partner violence. www.cdc.gov/intimate-partner-violence/prevention/index.html

Céspedes, Y.M., & Huey, S.J. (2008). Depression in Latino adolescents: A cultural discrepancy perspective. *Cultural Diversity & Ethnic Minority Psychology*, 14(2), 168–172. https://doi.org/10.1037/1099-9809.14.2.168

Chang, D.F., Shen, B., & Takeuchi, D.T. (2009). Prevalence and demographic correlates of intimate partner violence in Asian Americans. *International Journal of Law and Psychiatry*, 32, 167–175.

Chen, J., Walters, M.L., Gilbert, L.K., & Patel, N. (2020). Sexual violence, stalking, and intimate partner violence by sexual orientation, United States. *Psychology of Violence*, 10(1), 110–119.

Chung, E.K., Siegel, B.S., Garg, A., Conroy, K., Gross, R.S., Long, D.A., Lewis, G., Osman, C., Messito, M.J., Wade, R., Yin, H.S., Cox, J., & Fierman, A.H. (2016). Screening for social determinants of health among children and families living in poverty: A guide for clinicians. *Current Problems in Pediatrics and Adolescent Health Care*, 46(5), 135–153.

Clemente-Teixeira, M., Megalhaes,T., Barrocas, J., Dinis-Olivera, R.J., & Taveira-Gomes, T. (2022). Health outcomes in women victims of intimate partner violence: A 20-year-real-world study.

International Journal of Environmental Research and Public Health, 19(24), 1705. www. doi:10.3390/ijerph192417035

Coker, A.L., Smith, P.H., Bethea, L., King, M.R., & McKeown, R.F. (2000). Physical health consequences of physical and psychological intimate partner violence. *Archives of Family Medicine*, 9, 451–457.

Coker, D. (2000). Shifting power for battered women: Law, material resources, and poor women of color. *University of California Davis Law Review*, 33, 1009–1055.

Coll, C.V.N., Ewerling, F., Garcia-Moreno, C., Hellwing, F., & Barros, A.J.D. (2020). Intimate partner violence in 46 low-income and middle-income countries: An appraisal of the most vulnerable groups of women using national health surveys. *BMJ Global Health*, 5(1). https://doi.org/10.1136/bmjgh-2019-002208

Community Prevention Services Task Force (2018). Violence prevention: Primary prevention interventions to reduce perpetration of intimate partner violence and sexual violence among youth. The Community Guide. www.thecommunityguide.org/pages/about-community-prevention-services-task-force.html

Connell, R. (1987). *Gender and power*. Allen & Unwin.

Cooper, A., & Smith, E.L. (2017). *Homicide trends in the United States, 1980–2008*. Department of Justice, Bureau of Justice Statistics. NCJ 236018. www.bjs.gov/content/pub/pdf/htus8008.pdf

Cramer, E.P. (2004). Unintended consequences of constructing criminal justice as a dominant paradigm in understanding and intervening in intimate partner violence. *Women's Studies Quarterly*, 32(3/4), 164–180.

Crenshaw, K.W. (2023). Mapping the margins: Intersectionality, identity politics, and violence against women of color. In E. Taylor, D. Gillborn, & G. Ladson-Billings (Eds.), *Foundations of critical race theory in education* (3rd ed., pp. 273–307). Routledge. https://doi.org/10.4324/b23210-28

Cunradi, C.B., Caetano, R., Clark, C., & Schafer, J. (2000). Neighborhood poverty as a predictor of intimate partner violence among White, Black, and Hispanic couples in the United States: A multilevel analysis. *Annals of Epidemiology*, 10(5), 297–308. https://doi.org/10.1016/S1047-2797(00)00052-1

Das, T.K., Alam, M.F., Bhattacharyya, R., & Pervin, A. (2015). Causes and contexts of domestic violence: Tales of help-seeking married women in Sylhet, Bangladesh. *Asian Social Work and Policy Review*, 9, 163–176.

Davies, J., Lyon, E.J., & Monti-Catania, D. (1998). *Safety planning with battered women: Complex lives/difficult choices*. SAGE series on violence against women. SAGE Publisher.

Decker, M., Littleton, H.L., & Edwards, K.M. (2018). An update review of the literature on LGBTQ+ intimate partner violence. *Current Sexual Health Reports*, 10, 265–272.

Decker, M.R., Wilcox, H.C., Holliday, C.N., & Webster, D.W. (2018). An integrated public health approach to interpersonal violence and suicide prevention and response. *Public Health Reports (1974)*, 133(1S), 65S–79S. https://doi.org/10.1177/0033354918800019

DeGue, S., Simon, T.R., Basile, K.C., Yee, S.L., Lang, K., & Spivak, H. (2012). Moving forward by looking back: Reflecting on a decade of CDC's work in sexual violence prevention. *Journal of Women's Health*, 21(12), 1211–1218. https://doi.org/10.1089/jwh.2012.3973

Devries, K.M., Mak, J.Y., Garcia-Moreno, C. et al. (2013). Global health prevalence of intimate partner violence against women. *Science*, 340, 1527–1528.

Dickerson-Amaya, N., & Coston, B.M. (2019). Invisibility is not invincibility: The impact of intimate partner violence on gay, bisexual, and straight men's mental health. *American Journal of Men's Health*, 13(3), 1–12. https://journals.sagepub.com/doi/pdf/10.1177/1557988319849734

Dillion, G., Hussain, R., Loxton, D., & Rahman, S. (2013). Mental and physical health and intimate partner violence against women: A review of the literature. *International Journal of Family Medicine*, https://doi.org/10.1155/2013/313909

Drapkin, M.L., McGrady, B.S., Swingle, J.M., & Epstein, E.E. (2005). Exploring bidirectional couple violence in a clinical sample of female alcoholics. *Journal of Studies on Alcohol*, 66, 213–219.

Dube, S.R., Felitti, V.J., Dong, M., Giles, W.H., & Anda, R.F. (2003). The impact of adverse childhood experiences on health problems: Evidence from four birth cohorts dating back to 1900. *Preventive Medicine*, 37(3), 268–277. https://doi.org/10.1016/S0091-7435(03)00123-3

Dutton, M.A., James, L., Langhorne, A., & Kelley, M. (2015). Coordinated public health initiatives to address violence against women and adolescents. *Journal of Women's Health*, 24(1), 80–85.

Edwards, K.M. (2015). Incidence and outcomes of dating violence victimization among high school youth: The role of gender and sexual orientation. *Journal of Interpersonal Violence*, 33, 1–19.

Edwards, K.M., & Sylaska, K.M. (2013). The perception of intimate personal violence among LGBTQ college youth: The role of minority stress. *Journal of Youth and Adolescence*, 42, 1721–1731.

Eriksson, M., & Ulmestig, R. (2021). It's not all about money: Towards a more comprehensive understanding of financial abuse in the context of VAW. *Journal of Interpersonal Violence*, 36(3–4), NPI1625–165INP.

Fagan, J. (1996). *The criminalization of domestic violence promises and limits*. U.S. Department of Justice. National Institute of Justice. www.ncjrs.gov/pdffiles/crimdom.pdf

Fang, X., & Corso, P.S. (2008). Gender differences in the connections between violence experienced as a child and perpetration of intimate partner violence in young adulthood. *Journal of Family Violence*, 23(5), 303–313.

Fawole, O.I. (2008). Economic violence to women and girls: Is it receiving the necessary attention? *Trauma, Violence, & Abuse*, 9, 167–177.

Federal Bureau of Investigation. (2011). Crime in the United States, 2011: Expanded homicide data. Clarksburg, WV: U.S. Department of Justice, Federal Bureau of Investigation; 2012. www.fbi.gov/about-us/cjis/ucr/crime-in-the-u.s/2011/crime-in-the-u.s.-2011/offenses-known-to-law-enforcement/expanded/expanded-homicide-data

Felitti, V.J., Anda, R.F., Nordenberg, D., Williamson, D.F., Spitz, A.M., Edwards, V., Koss, M.P., & Marks, J.S. (2019). Relationship of childhood abuse and household dysfunction to many of the leading causes of death in adults: The adverse childhood experiences (ACE) study. *American Journal of Preventive Medicine*, 56(6), 774. https://doi.org/10.1016/j.amepre.2019.04.001

Finkelhor, D., Turner, H.A., Shattuck, A., & Hamby, S.L. (2015). Prevalence of childhood exposure to violence, crime, and abuse: Results from the National Survey of Children's Exposure to Violence. *JAMA Pediatrics*, 169(8), 746–754.

Fisher, J., De Mello, M.C., Patel, V., Rahman, A., Tran, T., Holton, S., & Holmes, W. (2012). Prevalence and determinants of common perinatal mental disorders in women in low- and lower-middle-income countries: A systematic review. *Bulletin of the World Health Organization*, 90(2), 139–149. https://doi.org/10.2471/blt.11.091850

Foran, H.M., & O'Leary, K.D. (2008). Alcohol and intimate partner violence: A meta-analytic review. *Clinical Psychology Review*, 28:1222–1234.

Foshee, V.A., Reyes, H.L., Ennett, S.Y., Cance, J.D., Bauman, K.E., & Bowling, J.M. (2012). Assessing the effects of families for safe dates: A family-based teen dating abuse prevention. *Journal of Adolescent Health*, 51, 349–356.

Fuino-Estefan, L., Coulter, M.L., & VandeWeerd, C. (2016). Depression in women who have left violent relationships: The unique impact of frequent emotional abuse. *Violence against Women*, 22(11), 1397–1413.

Garcia-Moreno, C., Jansen, H.A., Ellsberg, M., Heise, L., & Watts, C.H. (2006). Prevalence of intimate partner violence: Findings from the WHO multi-country study on women's health and domestic violence. *Lancet*, 368, 1260–1269.

Gehring, K.S., & Vaske, J.C. (2017). Out in the open: Consequences for intimate partner violence for victims in same sex and opposite sex relationships. *Journal of Interpersonal Violence*, 32, 669–692.

Goldberg, N.G., & Meyer, I.H. (2013). Sexual orientation disparities in history of intimate partner violence: Results from the California health interview survey, *Journal of Interpersonal Violence*, 28(5), 1109–1118. https://doi.org/10.1177/0886260512459384

Gollan, J. (2021). How the US fails to take away guns from domestic abusers: These deaths are preventable. *The Guardian*, www.theguardian.com/us-news/2021/oct/26/domestic-abuse-gun-violence-reveal

Gomez, A.M. (2011). Testing the cycle of violence hypothesis: Child abuse and adolescent dating violence as predictors of intimate partner violence in young adulthood. *Youth & Society*, 43(1), 171–192.

Goodman, L.A., & Epstein, D. (2008). *Listening to battered women: A survivor centered approach to advocacy, mental health, and justice.* American Psychological Association.

Goodman, L.A., & Epstein, D. (2011). The justice system response to domestic violence. In M.P. Koss, J.W. White, and A.E. Kazdin (Eds.), *Violence against women and children* (Vol. 2, pp. 215–235). Navigating Solutions, American Psychological Association. https://doi.org/10.1037/12308-011

Goodmark, L. (2017). *Innovative criminal justice responses to intimate partner violence.* Sage Publications.

Grand Challenges for Social Work. (2020). *Build healthy relationships to end violence.* 2020 GC Fact Sheet No. 3. BHR-One-Pager-FINAL.pdf.

Grand Challenges for Social Work. (2024). *2024 Policy recommendations for meeting the grand challenges of social work.* Policy Brief. 240701-Final-Policy-Brief-Packet_V3.pdf.

Graziano, M., & Pulcini, J. (2013). Gun violence and the role of health care: A confusing state of affairs. *American Journal of Nursing*, 113, 23–25.

Grimani, A., Gavine, A., & Moncur, W. (2022). An evidence synthesis of covert online strategies regarding intimate partner violence. *Trauma, Violence, & Abuse*, 23(2), 581–593.

Gupta, S. (2023). Understanding intimate partner violence: Relationships, toxicity, and abuse. www.verywellmind.com/intimate-partner-violence-types-signs-causes-and-impact-5324420

Haeseler, L.A. (2013). Themes of coping in the spectrum of domestic violence abuse: A review of the literature. *Journal of Evidence-Based Social Work*, 10, 25–32.

Hamby, S. (2014). Intimate partner and sexual violence research: Scientific progress, scientific challenges, and gender. *Trauma, Violence, & Abuse*, 15(3), 149–158.

Hegarty, K., Gunn, J., Chondros, P., & Small, R. (2004). Association between depression and abuse by partners of women attending general practice: Descriptive, cross-sectional survey. *British Medical Journal*, 328, 621–624.

Heise, L., & Garcia-Moreno, C. (2002). Violence by intimate partners. In E. Krug, L.L. Dahlberg, J.A. Mercy, A.B. Zwi, & R. Lozano (Eds.), *World report on violence* (pp. 87–121). World Health Organization.

Hemenway, D., Shinoda-Tagawa, T., & Miller, M. (2002). Firearm availability and female homicide victimization rates among 25 populous high-income countries. *Journal of the American Medical Women's Association*, 57, 100–104.

Henneberger, A.K., Durkee, M.I., Truong, N., Atkins, A., & Tolan, P.H. (2013). The longitudinal relationship between peer violence and popularity and delinquency in adolescent boys: Examining effects of family functioning. *Journal of Youth and Adolescence*, 42(11), 1651–1660.

Hill, T.D., Schroeder, R.D., Bradley, C., Kaplan, L.M., & Angel, R.J. (2009). The long-term health consequences of relationship violence in adulthood: An examination of low-income women from Boston, Chicago, and San Antonio. *American Journal of Public Health*, 99, 1645–1650.

Hillis, S.D., Anda, R.F., Dube, S.R., Felitti, V.J., Marchbanks, P.A., & Marks, J.S. (2004). The association between adverse childhood experiences and adolescent pregnancy, long-term psychosocial consequences, and fetal death. *Pediatrics (Evanston)*, 113(2), 320–327. https://doi.org/10.1542/peds.113.2.320

Hines, D. (2015). Overlooked victims of domestic violence: Men. *International Journal for Family Research and Policy*, 1(1), 57–79.

Hines, D.A., & Douglas, E.M. (2015). Health problems of partner violence victims: Comparing help-seeking men to a population-based sample. *American Journal of Preventive Medicine*, 48(2), 136–144.

Hines, D.A., & Douglas, E.M. (2018). Influence of intimate partner terrorism, situational couple violence, and mutual violent control on male victims. *Psychology of Men & Masculinities*, 19(4), 612–623.

Hirschel, D., & Buzawa, E. (2002). Understanding the context of dual arrest with directions for future research. *Violence against Women*, 8, 1449–1473.

Huecker, M.R., King, K.C., Jordan, G.A., & Smock, W. (2023). Domestic violence. In StatPearls. StatPearls Publishing. www.nlm.nil.gov/books/NBK499891/

Inslicht, S.S., Marmar, C.R., Neylan, T.C., Metzler, T.J., Hart, S.L., Otte, C., McCaslin, S.E., Larkin, G.L., Hyman, K.B., & Baum, A. (2006). Increased cortisol in women with intimate partner violence-related posttraumatic stress disorder. *Annals of the New York Academy of Sciences*, 1071(1), 428–429. https://doi.org/10.1196/annals.1364.035

Iovanni, L., & Miller, S.L. (2001). Criminal justice responses to domestic violence: Law enforcement and the courts. In C.M. Renzetti, J.L. Edleson, & R.K. Bergen (Eds.), *Sourcebook on Violence against Women* (pp. 303–327). Sage.

Jewkes, R.K. (2002). Intimate partner violence: Causes and prevention. *The Lancet*, 359, 1423–1429.

Jewkes, R.K. (2015). Interpersonal violence: A recent public health mandate. https://doi.org/10.1093/med/9780199661756.003.0223

Jewkes, R.K., Dunkle, K., Nduna, M., & Shai, N. (2010). Intimate partner violence, relationship power inequity, and incidence of HIV infection in young women in South Africa: A cohort study. *The Lancet*, 376(9734), 41–48.

Johnson, L., Chen, Y., Stylianou, A., & Arnold, A. (2022). Examining the impact of economic abuse on survivors of intimate partner violence: A scoping review. *BMC Public Health*, 22, 1014. https://doi.org/10.1186/s12889-022-13297-4

Josephs, L.L., & Abel, E.M. (2009). Investigating the relationship between intimate partner violence and HIV risk-propensity in Black/African American women. *Journal of Family Violence*, 24(4), 221–229.

Kantor, G.K., & Jasinski, J.L. (1998). Dynamics and risk factors in partner violence. In J. Jansinski & L. Williams (Eds.), *Partner violence: A comprehensive review of 20 years of research* (pp.1–43). Sage.

Kaplan, G.A. (2004). What's wrong with social epidemiology, and how can we make it better? *Epidemiologic Reviews*, 26, 124–135.

Kebede, S., Van Harmelen, A.L., & Roman-Urrestarau, A. (2022). Wealth inequality and intimate partner violence: An individual and ecological level analysis across 20 countries. *Journal of Interpersonal Violence*, 37, 17–18. https://doi.org/10.1177/0886205211016337

Kerr, D.C.R., & Capaldi, D.M. (2011). Young men's intimate partner violence and relationship functioning: Long-term outcomes associated with suicide attempt and aggression in adolescence. *Psychological Medicine: A Journal of Research in Psychiatry and the Allied Sciences*, 41(2), 759–769.

Kessler, R.C., McLaughlin, K.A., Green, J.G., Gruber, M.J., Sampson, N.A., Zaslavsky, A.M., Aguilar-Gaxiola, S., Alhamzawi, A.O., Alonso, J., Angermeyer, M., Benjet, C., Bromet, E., Chatterji, S., de Girolamo, G., Demyttenaere, K., Fayyad, J., Florescu, S., Gal, G., Gureje, O., ... Williams, D.R. (2010). Childhood adversities and adult psychopathology in the WHO world mental health surveys. *British Journal of Psychiatry*, 197(5), 378–385. https://doi.org/10.1192/bjp.bp.110.080499

Khalifeh, H., Hargreaves, J., Howard, L.M., & Birdthistle, I. (2013). Intimate partner violence and socioeconomic deprivation in England: Findings from a national cross-sectional survey. *American Journal of Public Health*, 103(3), 462–472.

Kippert, A. (2023). Why domestic violence is a public health crisis: Intimate partner violence isn't just harming the primary victims; its negatively affecting our entire population. www.domesticshelters.org/articles/ending-domestic-violence/why-domestic-violence-is-a-public-health-crisis

Kiss, L., Schraiber, L.B., Heise, L., Zimmerman, C., Gouveia, N., & Watts, C. (2012). Gender-based violence and socioeconomic inequalities: Does living in more deprived neighborhoods increase women's risk of intimate partner violence? *Social Science & Medicine*, 74, 1172–1179.

Krug, E.G., Dahlberg, L.L., Mercy, J.A. et al., (2002). *World report on violence and health*. World Health Organization.

Langenderfer-Magruder, L., Whitfield, D.L., Walls, N.E., Kattari, S.K., & Ramos, D. (2016). Experiences of intimate partner violence and subsequent police reporting among lesbian, gay, bisexual, transgender, and queer adults in Colorado: Comparing rates of cisgender and transgender victimization. *Journal of Interpersonal Violence*, 31(5), 855–871.

Leight, J., Cullen, C., Ranganathan, M., & Yakubovich, A. (2023). Effectiveness of community mobilization and group-based interventions for preventing intimate partner violence against women in low-and -middle-income countries: A systematic review and meta-analysis. *Journal of Global Health*, https://doi.org/10.7189/jogh13:04115

Littwin, A. (2012). Coerced debt: The role of consumer credit in domestic violence. *California Law Review*, 100, 951–1026.

Littwin, A. (2013). Escaping battered credit: A proposal for repairing credit reports damaged by domestic violence. *University of Pennsylvania Law Review*, 161, 363–429.

Liu, C., & Olamijuwon, E. (2024). The link between intimate partner violence and spousal resource inequality in lower-and middle-income countries. *Social Science & Medicine*, 345, https://doi.org/10.1016/j.socscimed.2024.116688

Logan, T.K., & Walker, R. (2017). Stalking: A multidimensional framework for assessment and safety planning. *Trauma, Violence, & Abuse*, 18(2), 200–222. https://doi.org/10.1177/1524838015603210

Loxton, D., Scholield, M., Hussain, R., & Mishra, G. (2006). History of domestic violence and physical health in midlife. *Violence against Women*, 12(8), 715–731.

Lundgren, R., & Amin, A. (2014). Addressing intimate partner violence and sexual violence among adolescents: emerging evidence of effectiveness. *Journal of Adolescent Health*, 56(1), S42–S50. https://doi.org/10.1016/j.jadohealth.2014.08.012

Machtinger, E.L., Wilson, T.C., Haberer, J.E., & Weiss, D.S. (2012). Psychological trauma and PTSD in HIV-positive women: A meta-analysis. *AIDS and Behavior*, 16(8), 2091–2100. https://doi.org/10.1007/s10461-011-0127-4

Maheu-Giroux, M., Sardinha, L., Stockl, H., Meyer, S.R., Godin, A., Alexander, M., & Garcia-Moreno, C. (2022). A framework to model global, regional, and national estimates of intimate partner violence. *BMC Medical Research Methodology*, 22, 159. www.doi:10.1186/s12874-022-01634-5

Maheux, A.J., Zhou, Y., Thoma, B.C., Salk, R.H., & Choukas-Bradley, S. (2021). Examining sexual behavior among U.S. transgender adolescents. *The Journal of Sex Research*, 58(8), 1050–1060.

Maniam, J., Antoniadis, C., & Morris, M.J. (2014). Early-life stress, HPA axis adaptation, and mechanisms contributing to later health outcomes. *Frontiers in Endocrinology (Lausanne)*, 5, 73–73. https://doi.org/10.3389/fendo.2014.00073

Mankind Initiative. (2023). Statistics on male victims of domestic violence. Office for National Statistics. www.mankind.org.uk/statistics/statistics-on-male-victims-of-domestic-abuse/#

Martin, S.L., Tsui, A.O., Maitra, K, & Marinshaw, R. (1999). Domestic violence in Northern India. *American Journal of Epidemiology*, 150, 417–426.

Matjasko, J.L., Niolon, P.H., & Valle, L.A. (2013). The role of economic factors and economic support in preventing and escaping from intimate partner violence. *Journal of Policy Analysis and Management*, 32(1), 122–128.

Maxwell, C.D., Sullivan, T.P., Backes, B.L., & Kaufman, J.S. (2020). New approaches to policing high-risk intimate partner victims and offenders. *NIJ Journal*, 282. https://nij.ojp.gov/topics/articles/new-approaches-policing-high-risk-intimate-partner-victims-and-offenders

McCarthy, K.J., Mehta, R., & Haberland, N.A. (2018). Gender, power, and violence: A systematic review of measures and their association with male perpetrators of IPV. *PLOS One*, 13(11), e0207091.

McCauley, H.L., Silverman, J.G., Decker, M.R., Agenor, M., Borrero, S., Tancredi, D.J., et al. (2015). Sexual and reproductive health indicators and intimate partner violence victimization among female family planning clinic patients who have sex with women and men. *Journal of Women's Health*, 24, 621–629.

McDowell, M., & Reinhard, D. (2023). Community characteristics and the geographic distribution of intimate partner violence: A partial test of social disorganization theory. *Journal of Interpersonal Violence*, 38(1), 1494–1516.

McGill, G.J., & Shield, N.M. (1986). Social and structural factors in family violence. In M. Lystad (Ed.), *Violence in the home: Interdisciplinary perspectives* (pp. 98–123). Brunner/Mazel.

Mechanic, M.B., Weaver, T.L., & Resick, P.A. (2008). Mental health consequences of intimate partner abuse: A multidimensional assessment of four different forms of abuse. *Violence against Women*, 14, 634–654.

Mercy, J. A., Hillis, S.D., Burtchart, A., Bellis, M.A., Ward, C.L., Fang, X., & Rosenberg, M.L. (2017). Interpersonal violence: Global impact and path to prevention. In C.N., Mock, R. Nugent, O. Kobusingye, & K. R. Smith (Eds.), Injury prevention and environmental health (3rd ed.). The Work. www.ncbi.nlm.nih.gov/books/NBK525218/pdf/Bookshelf_NBK525218.pdf

Messerschmidt, J.W. (2019). The salience of "hegemonic masculinity." *Men and Masculinities*, 22(1), 85–91.

Messinger, A.M. (2011). Invisible victims: Same-sex IPV in the national violence against women survey. *Journal of Interpersonal Violence*, 26(11), 2228–2243. doi:10.1177/0886260510383023

Messinger, A.M. (2017). *Introduction: Making the invisible visible, in LGBTQ intimate partner violence*. University of California.

Miller, M., Zhang, W., & Azrael, D. (2022). Firearm purchasing during the COVID-19 pandemic: Results from the 2021 national firearms survey. *Annals of Internal Medicine*, 175(2), 219–225.

Moe, A.M., & Bell, M.P. (2004). Abject economics: The effects of battering and violence on women's work and employability. *Violence against Women*, 10, 29–55.

Moncur, W., & Herron, D. (2018). How to digitally disentangle after a breakup-some new rules. The Conversation. www.theconversation.com/how-to-digitally-disentangle-after-a-break-up-some-new-rules-90592

Moncur, W., & Orzech, K.M., & Neville, F.G. (2016). Fraping, social norms and online representations of self. *Computers in Human Behavior*, 63, 125–131.

Moorer, O. (2015). Intimate partner violence vs. domestic violence: Eliminating racism empowering women YWCA. Spokane, Washington. www.ywcaspokane.org/what-is-intimate-partner-domestic-violence/

Morgan, R.E., & Truman, J. L. (2018). Criminal Victimization, 2017, Washington, DC: U.S. Department of Justice, Bureau of Justice statistics. NCJ 252472. www.bjs.gov/content/pub/pdf/cv17.pdf

National Center for Injury Prevention and Control. (2003). *Costs of intimate partner violence against women in the United States*. Department of Health and Human Services. Centers for Disease Control and Prevention. www.ncdsv.org/uploads/1/4/2/2/142238266/cdc_costsofipvagainstwomenintheus_2003.pdf

National Coalition Against Domestic Violence. (n.d.). Statistics. www.thehotline.org/stakeholders/domestic-violence-statistics

Niolon, P.H., Kearns, M., Dills, J., Rambo, K., Irving, S., Armstead, T.L., & Gilbert, L. (2017). *Preventing intimate partner violence across the lifespan: A technical package of programs, policies, and practices*. Center of Disease Control and Prevention. www.cdc.gov/violenceprevention/pdf/ipv-technicalpackages.pdf

Nowinski, S.N., & Bowen, E. (2012). Partner violence against heterosexual and gay men: Prevalence and correlates. *Aggression & Violent Behavior*, 17(1), 36–52.

Nybergh, L., Enander, V., & Krantz, G. (2016). Theoretical considerations on men's experiences of intimate partner violence: An interview-based study. *Journal of Family Violence*, 31(2), 191–202.

Oliffe, J.L., Han, C., Maria, E.S., Lohan, M., Howard, T., Stewart, D.E., & MacMillan, H. (2014). Gay men and intimate partner violence: A gender analysis. *Sociology of Health & Illness*, 36(4), 564–579.

Pastor-Moreno, G., Ruiz-Perez, I., Henares-Montiel, J., Escriba-Aguir, V., Higueras-Callejon, C., & Ricco-Cabello, I. (2020). Intimate partner violence and perinatal health: A systematic review. *BJOG: An International Journal of Obstetrics and Gynecology*, 127(5), 537–547.

Patra, P., Prakash, J., Patra, B., & Khanna, P. (2018). Intimate partner violence: Wounds are deeper. *Indian Journal of Psychiatry*, 60(4), 494–498.

Peterson, C., Kearns, M.C., McIntosh, W.L., Estefan, L.F., Nicolaidis, C., McCollister, K.E., Gordon, A., & Florence, C. (2018). Lifetime economic burden of intimate partner violence among U.S. adults. *American Journal of Preventive Medicine*, 55(4), 433–444.

Phillips, S.W., & Sobol, J.J. (2010). Twenty years of mandatory arrest: Police decision making in the face of legal requirements. *Criminal Justice Policy Review*, 21(1), 98–118. https://doi.org/10.1177/0887403408322962

Pichon, M., Treves-Kagan, S., Stern, E., Kyegombe, N., Stockl, H., & Buller, A.M. (2020). A mixed methods systematic review: Infidelity, romantic jealousy, and intimate partner violence against women. *International Journal of Environmental Research and Public Health*, 17(16), 5682. https://doi.org/10.3390/ijerph17165682

Pico-Alfonso, M.A. (2005). Psychological intimate partner violence: The major predictor of posttraumatic stress disorder in abused women. *Neuroscience and Biobehavioral Reviews*, 29, 181–193.

Post, L.A., Klevens, J., Maxwell, C.D., Shelley, G.A., & Ingram, E. (2010). An examination of whether coordinated community responses affect intimate personal violence. *Journal of Interpersonal Violence*, 25(1), 75–93.

Postmus, J.L., Plummer, S.B., McMahon, S., Murshid, N.S., & Sung, K.M. (2012). Understanding economic abuse in the lives of survivors. *Journal of Interpersonal Violence*, 27, 411–430.

Powell, A., & Henry, N. (2016). Policing technology-facilitated sexual violence against adult victims: Police and service sector perspectives. *Policing and Society*, 28(3), 291–307. www.tandfonline.com/doi/full/10.1080/10439463.2016.1154964

Randle, A.A., & Graham, C.A. (2011). A review of the evidence on the effects of intimate partner violence on men. *Psychology of Men & Masculinities*, 12(2), 97–111.

Raphael, J. (2004). Rethinking criminal justice responses to intimate partner violence. *Violence against Women*, 10(11), 1354–1366.

Renner, L.M., Whitney, S.D., & Vasquez, M. (2015). Individual and interpersonal risk factors for physical intimate partner violence perpetration by biological sex and ethnicity. *Violence and Victims*, 30(1), 97–119. http://dx.doi.org/10.1891/0886-6708.VV-D-13-00123

Reuter, T.R., Newcomb, M.E., Whitton, S.W., & Mustanski, B. (2017). Intimate partner violence victimization in LGBT young adults: Demographic differences and association with health behavior. *Psychology of Violence*, 7(1), 101–109.

Ricci, S. S. (2017). Violence against women: A global perspective. *Women's Health Open Journal*, 3(1), e1–e2.

Richards, T.N., Skubak-Tillyer, M., & Wright, E.M. (2017). Intimate partner violence and the overlap of perpetration and victimization: Considering the influence of physical, sexual and emotional abuse in childhood. *Child Abuse & Neglect*, 67, 240–248.

Riggs, D., Caulfield, M., & Street, A. (2000). Risk factors associated with perpetration and victimization. *Journal of Clinical Psychology*, 56(10), 1289–1316.

Robert Wood Johnson Foundation. (2009). *Race and socioeconomic factors affect opportunities for better health*. Issue Brief 5: Race and Socioeconomic Factors. The Robert Wood Johnson Foundation Commission to Build a Healthier America. Issue Brief 5 April 09 – Race and Socioeconomic Factors.pdf.

Rosenberg, M.L., & Fenley, M.A. (1991). *Violence in America: A public health approach*. Oxford University Press.

Russell, W. (2007). Sexual violence against violence men and boys. *Forced Migration Review*, 27, 22–23.

Sackett, L.A., & Saunders, D.G. (1994). The impact of different forms of psychological abuse on battered women. *Violence and Victims*, 14, 105–117.

Sanders, C.K. (2015). Economic abuse in the lives of women abused by an intimate partner: A qualitative study. *Violence against Women*, 21, 3–29.

Sardinha, L., Maheu-Giroux, M., Stockl, H., Meyer, S.R., & Garcia-Moneno, C. (2022). Global, regional, and national prevalence estimates of physical or sexual, or both, intimate partner violence against women in 2018. *Lancet*, 399(10327), 803–813. https://doi.org/10.1016/S0140-6736(21)02664-7

Scheffer-Lindgren, M., & Renck, B. (2008). It is still deep-seated, the fear: Psychological stress reactions as consequences of intimate partner violence. *Journal of Psychiatric and Mental Health Nursing*, 15(3), 219–228.

Scott-Storey, K., O'Donnell, S.O., Ford-Giboe, M., Varcoe, C., Wathen, N., Malcolm, J., & Vincent, C. (2022). What about the men? A Critical review of men's experiences of intimate partner violence. *Trauma, Violence, & Abuse*, 24(2), 858–872.

Seawright, J., Whitaker, B., Droubay, B., & Butters, R. (2017). *Treatment for perpetrators of domestic violence: A review of the literature*. Utah Criminal Justice Center, University of Utah. Background and Introduction.

Sherman, L.W., & Berk, R.A. (1984). The specific deterrent effects of arrest for domestic assault. *American Sociological Review*, 49, 261–272.

Silverman, J.G., Decker, M.R., Cheng, D.M., Wirth, K., Saggurti, N., McCauley, H. L., Falb, K.L., Donta, B., & Raj, A. (2011). Gender-based disparities in infant and child mortality based on maternal exposure to spousal violence: The heavy burden borne by Indian girls. *Archives of Pediatrics & Adolescent Medicine*, 165(1), 22–27. https://doi.org/10.1001/archpediatrics.2010.261

Smith, S.G., Chen, K.C., Basile, L.K., Gilbert, M.T., Merrick, N., Patel, M., Walling, & Jain, A. (2017). The National Intimate Partner and Sexual Violence Survey (NISVS): 2010–2012 State Report, National Center for Injury Prevention and Control, Centers for Disease Control and Prevention. www.c:/Users/Owners/Downloads/cdc_46305_DSi%20(3).pdf

Social Work Test Prep (SWTP). (2023). Blog: *The impact of stress, trauma, and violence*. www.socialworktestprep.com/blog/2023/october/13/the-impact-of-stress-trauma-and-violence/

Sorenson, S.A., & Schut, R.A. (2016). Nonfatal gun use in intimate partner violence: A systematic review of the literature. *Trauma, Violence and Abuse*, 19(4), 431–442.

Spencer, C.M., Mendez, M., & Stith, S.M. (2019). The role of income inequality on factors associated with male physical intimate partner violence perpetration: A meta-analysis. *Aggression and Violent Behavior*, 48, 116–123.

Spivak, H.R., Jenkins, E.L., Van Audenhove, K., Lee, D., Kelly, M., & Iskander, J. (2014). CDC grand rounds: A public health approach to prevention of intimate partner violence. *Morbidity and Mortality Weekly Report*, 63(02) 38–41.

Stalking Prevention, Awareness, and Resource Center (n.d.). *Stalking & intimate partner violence: Fact sheet*. Washington, DC: stalkingawareness.org.

Stephenson, R., & Finneran, C. (2017). Minority stress and intimate partner violence among gay and bisexual men in Atlanta. *American Journal of Men's Health*, 11(4), 952–961.

Stockl, H., Devries, K., Rotstein, A., Abrahams, N., Campbell, J., Watts, C., & Moreno, C.G. (2013). The global prevalence of intimate partner violence. *Lancet*, 382(9895), 859–865. www.doi.10.1016/S0140-6736(13)61030-2

Stoever, J.K. (2019). Firearms and domestic violence fatalities: Preventable deaths. *Family Law Quarterly*, 53(3), 183–212.

Stokols, D., Hall, K.L., Taylor, B.K., & Moser, R.P. (2008). The science of team science: Overview of the field and introduction to the supplement. *American Journal of Preventive Medicine*, 35(2 Suppl), S77–S89.

Straus, M.A., Gelles, R.J., & Steinmetz, S.K. (1980). *Behind closed doors: Violence in the American family*. New York: Anchor Press.

Stylianou, A.M. (2018). Economic abuse within intimate partner violence: A review of the literature. *Violence and Victims*, 33, 3–22.

Stylianou, A.M., Postmus, J.L., & McMahon, S. (2013). Measuring abuse behaviors: Is economic abuse a unique form of abuse? *Journal of Interpersonal Violence*, 28(16), 186–204.

Substance Abuse and Mental Health Service Administration (2023). Mental health: Get the facts. www.samhsa.gov/mental-health/what-is-mental-health/facts

Sullivan, T.P., McPartland, T.S., Armeli, S., Jaquier, V., & Tennen, H. (2012). Is it the exception or the rule? Daily co-occurrence of physical, sexual, and psychological partner violence on a 90-day study of substance-using, community women. *Psychology of Violence*, 2, 154–164.

Tharp, T. (2012). Dating matters: The next generation of teen dating violence prevention. *Prevention Science*, 13, 398–401.

Tjaden, P., & Thoennes, N. (1998). *Stalking in America: Findings from the national violence against women survey* (NCJ#169592). Washington, DC: National Institute of Justice Centers for Disease Control and Prevention.

Tobin-Tler, E. (2023). Intimate partner violence, Firearm injuries and homicides: A health justice approach to two intersecting public health crises. *Journal of Law, Medicine & Ethics*, 51, 64–76.

Tokunaga, R.S. (2011). Social networking site or social surveillance site? Understanding the use of interpersonal electronic surveillance in romantic relationships. *Computers in Human Behavior*, 27(2), 705–713.

United Nations (2020). Achieve gender equality and empower all women and girls. Department of economic and Social Affairs. Statistics Division.

United Nations Office on Drugs and Crime (2023). Gender-related killings of women and girls (femicide/feminicide): Global estimate of female intimate partner/family-related homicides in 2022. Ending Violence Against Women Section, United Nations Entity for Gender Equality and the Empowerment of Women (UN Women).

Violence Policy Center (2018). *American roulette: Murder-suicide in the United States* (6th ed.). Washington, DC. www.vpc.org/studies/amroul2018.pdf

Vitanza, S., Vogel, L.C., & Marshall, L.L. (1995). Distress and symptoms of posttraumatic stress disorder in abused women. *Violence and Victims*, 10, 23–34.

Vives-Cases, C., Ruiz-Cantero, T., Aguir-Escriba, V., & Miralles, J. (2011). The effect of intimate partner violence and other forms of violence against women on health. *Journal of Public Health*, 33(1), 15–21.

Walby, S. (2009). The cost of domestic violence: Up-date 2009. Lancaster University. www.openaccess.city.ac.uk/id/eprint/21695

Walker, S. (1985). *Sense and nonsense about crime: A policy guide*. Monterey, CA: Brooks/ Cole Publishing.

Wallace, M., Gillispie-Bell, V., & Cruz, K. (2021). Homicide during pregnancy and the postpartum period in the United States, 2018–2019. *Obstetrics and Gynecology*, 138, 762–769.

Wallerstein, N. (1992). Powerlessness, empowerment, and health: Implications for health promotion programs. *American Journal of Health Promotion*, 6(3), 197–205.

Wallerstein, N.B., Yen, I.H., & Syme, S.L. (2011). Integration of social epidemiology and community-engaged interventions to improve health equity. *American Journal of Public Health*, 101(5), 822–830.

Waltermauer, E. (2005). Measuring intimate partner violence (IPV): You may only get what you ask for. *Journal of Interpersonal Violence*, 20(4), 501–506.

Walters, M.L., Breiding, M.J., & Chen, J. (2013). The national intimate partner and sexual violence survey: 2010 findings on victimization by sexual orientation. www.cdc.gov/violenceprevention/pdf/nisvs_sofindings.pdf

Weaver, T.L., & Etzel, J.C. (2003). Smoking patterns, symptoms of PTSD and depression: Preliminary findings from a sample of severely battered women. *Addictive Behaviors*, 28, 1665–1679.

West, C.M. (2012). Partner abuse in ethnic minority and gay, lesbian, bisexual, and transgender populations. *Partner Abuse*, 3(3), 336–357.

Whiting, J.B., Simmons, L.A., Havens, J.R., Smith, D.B., & Oka, M. (2009). Intergenerational transmission of violence: The influence of self-appraisals, mental disorders, and substance abuse. *Journal of Family Violence*, 24(8), 639–648.

WHO (2010). Preventing intimate partner violence and sexual violence against women: Taking action and generating evidence. WHO. www.who.int/publications/i/item/preventing-intimate-partner-and-sexual-violence-against-women-taking-action-and-generating-evidence

WHO (2020). RESPECT-seven strategies to prevent violence against women. www.who.int/publications/i/item/WHO-RHR-19.11

WHO (2024). *Violence against women*. World Health Organization. www.who.int/news-room/fact-sheets/detail/violence-against-women

Widom, C.S. (1989). Child abuse, neglect, and violent criminal behavior. *Criminology*, 27(2), 251–271.

Williams, D. R. (2018). Stress and the mental health of populations of color: Advancing our understanding of race-related stressors. *Journal of Health and Social Behavior*, 59(4), 466–485. https://doi.org/10.1177/0022146518814251

Willie, T.C., & Kershaw, T.S. (2019). An ecological analysis of gender inequality and intimate partner violence in the United States. *Preventive Medicine*, 118, 257–263.

Wilson, M., & Webb, R. (2018). *Social justice brief: Social work's role in responding to intimate partner violence*. Social Justice Brief. National Association of Social Workers. Washington, DC: Intimate Partner Violence – Social Justice Brief.

Woodlock, D. (2017). The abuse of technology in domestic violence and stalking. *Violence against Women*, 23(5), 584–602. https://doi.org/10.1177/1077801216646277

Woods, S.J. (2000). Prevalence and patterns of posttraumatic stress disorder in abused women and post abused women. *Issues in Mental Health Nursing*, 21, 309–324.

Woods, S.J., Hall, R.J., Campbell, J.C., & Angott, D.M. (2008). Physical health and posttraumatic stress disorder symptoms in women experiencing intimate partner violence. *Journal of Midwifery and Women's Health*, 53(6), 538–546.

Wuest, J., Merritt-Gray, M., Ford-Gilboe, M., Lent, B., Varcoe, C., & Campbell, J.C. (2008). Chronic pain in women survivors of intimate partner violence. *Journal of Pain*, 9(11), 1049–1057.

Wyatt, G.E., Myers, H.F., Williams, J.K., Kitchen, C.R., Loeb, T., Carmona, J.V., Wyatt, L.E., Chin, D., & Presley, N. (2002). Does a history of trauma contribute to HIV risk for women of color? Implications for prevention and policy. *American Journal of Public Health (1971)*, 92(4), 660–665. https://doi.org/10.2105/AJPH.92.4.660

Yapp, E., & Pickett, K.E. (2019). Greater income inequality is associated with higher rates of intimate partner violence in Latin America. *Public Health*, 175, 87–89.

Zlotnick, C., Johnson, D.M., & Kohn, R. (2006). Intimate partner violence and long-term psychological functioning in a national sample of American women. *Journal of Interpersonal Violence*, 21, 262–275.

8

ELDERLY ABUSE AND PUBLIC HEALTH

Introduction

Jane had not seen her friend Harry, 87, at Mass for weeks. This was not like her friend since Harry went to Mass almost every Sunday. Jane stopped by Harry's house. Harry answered the door and Jane was shocked. Her friend had lost weight, looked terrible, and had obviously been crying. Jane noticed what appeared to be bruising on his face and arms. Harry told Jane in a hushed voice that since his daughter had moved in, she would not let him go to church, the senior center, or even out of the house. Harry said that his daughter was now controlling everything including his money and what he ate. Before Jane could say anything, Harry's daughter started yelling in a threatening manner and calling him demeaning names. Harry quickly closed the door (*adapted from* United States Department of Justice, n.d.b, 18).

Elderly Abuse (EA) Defined

Elder abuse (EA) is defined as the intentional harming of an older person (i.e., 60 years old or older), usually by a trusted caregiver (United States Centers for Disease Control and Prevention [CDC], 2024a; World Health Organization [WHO], 2024a). Abuse can be a single event or many events over time and be perpetrated in the home or community/institutional settings. WHO (2024a) considers this as a type of violence that causes victims to lose dignity and respect. While the abuser is typically a known person, the elderly can also fall victim to fake organizations or persons pretending to represent organizations, otherwise known as *scamming*, that is perpetrated via mail, phone, and the internet (Weissberger et al., 2020). *Agism,* or rather the stereotyping of, discriminating against, or showing prejudice against older persons, is one of the most pervasive sources of injustice, giving rise to biased actions and attitudes at all levels of society with harmful consequences including injury, morbidity, social isolation, and marginalization (National Center on Elder Abuse [NCAE], 2021).

DOI: 10.4324/9781003373001-8

Nature and Extent of EA

It is estimated that 1 in every 10 older Americans was reportedly abused (Rosay & Mulford, 2017), with numbers rising to 1 in 5 elders during the COVID-19 pandemic (Chang & Levy, 2021). While these numbers seem high, it is believed that only 1 in 24 cases of EA are ever reported (Storey, 2020). In addition, only about 1 in 57.5 cases of elder neglect are reported for services (Lachs & Berman, 2011). For the U.S., using data from 8,419 studies, the 2022 median prevalence rates are reported by type of EA: 6% physical abuse, 9% sexual abuse, 5% psychological abuse, 5% financial abuse, and 5% neglect (WHO, 2022). Many elders experience poly-victimization, or rather, being the victim of more than one type of abuse. The exact number of victims is difficult to establish because of the reluctance to seek help for nonfatal injuries or because they get care from providers who fail to report (CDC, 2024a). Failed reporting, the decision not to self-report, or the inability to report can lead to death. For example, between the years of 2002 and 2016, more than 19,000 elders were murdered (Logan et al., 2019). Research has shown the mortality rate of EA victims to be three times the rate of non-victims (Dong, 2005). Moreover, with the *baby boomer* cohort graying, over 70 million people are projected to be 65 and older by 2030, increasing to over 90 million by 2060 (Vespa et al., 2020). Simultaneously, the population of those over 85 is estimated to double by 2035 and triple by 2060.

Types of EA

Physical Abuse

Elder physical abuse includes the "illness, injury, functional impairment, or death" of an older person by intentional means (CDC, 2024a, p. 2). It can include slapping, burning, cutting, bruising (Bhagat & Htwe, 2018), hitting or pushing (CDC, 2024a), restraining, or threatening with a weapon (Burnes et al., 2019a), and the breaking of bones, causing internal injuries and damage to organs, poisoning, asphyxiating, using medications inappropriately, physically restraining, force-feeding, and stomping (Hall et al., 2016). Burnes and colleagues (2019a) found that victims of physical abuse were more likely to seek help than victims of other single abuse types, likely because of the danger of physical abuse and the possibility of death.

Sexual Abuse

Elder sex abuse is defined as forced or unwanted sexual interaction that may include forced penetration or non-physical sexual harassment (CDC, 2024a, p. 2). It may also be pornography, molestation, and undressing (Burnes et al., 2018). There is also unwanted touching while undressed or through clothing, "intrusive, and/or painful procedures in caring for genitals or rectal area," and voyeurism (Hall et al., 2016, p. 32). Because of medical and physical issues that may result in communication problems, confusion, or memory loss, elders may not be able to report the abuse (Nursing Home Abuse Center, 2024). Signs of sexual abuse include pelvic injuries, difficult walking or sitting, bleeding from and/or irritation of the anus or vagina, panic attaches, post-traumatic stress symptoms, agitation, engagement in inappropriate behaviors, and suicide attempts. Both men and women nursing home residents are sexually abused by staff and other residents each year (Malmedal et al., 2015).

Economic Abuse and Financial Exploitation

Elder economic abuse, sometimes referred to as financial abuse, includes the unauthorized and illegal use of "money, benefits, property, or assets" of an older person for the benefit of someone else (CDC, 2024a, p. 2). This may also occur in the form of theft of items, unauthorized credit card use, the forging of the victim's signature on checks, and forcing elders to sign inheritance and power of attorney forms (Hall et al., 2016). DeLiema and colleagues (2018) found that victims of fraud suffered three times the losses than victims of financial exploitation. Rogers and colleagues (2023) found that financial abuse was the second most reported single type of abuse (43%, n = 255), preceded only by poly-victimization (53%, n = 257). Weissberger and colleagues (2020), in an analysis of 818 calls to the National Center on Elder Abuse (NCEA) resource line, found that calls about financial abuse were predominant. Having high levels of social support was found to be a buffer against financial exploitation (Beach et al., 2010) and fraud (DeLiema et al., 2018).

Psychological Abuse

Elderly psychological abuse, including emotional abuse, can be verbal or nonverbal actions that incite fear or distress for the older person, such as threats, humiliation, forms of harassment (CDC, 2024a, p. 2), and infantilizing (Hall et al., 2016). It may also include scolding, coercion, and ignoring the elder (Burnes et al., 2019a). Emotional abuse may also be in the form of intentionally isolating the elder through intentional seclusion, withholding assistive devices such as wheelchairs, or even locking the elder away (Hall et al., 2016). Victims of emotional abuse were found to have relatively low levels of help-seeking behavior potentially because this type of abuse is more socially accepted and tolerated (Burnes et al., 2019a).

Neglect and Abandonment

Elder neglect is likely the most unreported form of abuse (Lachs & Berman, 2011). Neglect can include a range of activities, but ultimately, it includes action or inaction where an older person's needs go unmet (CDC, 2024a). These actions may allow elders to go without food, shelter, health care and medications, heat and cooling, and hygienic care. Inaction on behalf of older adults, including omission of vaccinations, can lead to the occurrence of preventable diseases such as "pneumococcal diseases, influenza, and tetanus" (Hall et al., 2016, p. 29). Elders may be left unattended and lying in bed for days with no communication ability and no one checking in. At times, neglect may be that elders are left in unsanitary and unsafe conditions such as the "proper disposal of urine, feces, and other bodily waste," and infestations of rodents and roaches (Hall et al., 2016, p. 34). There may also be elder *self-neglect* where, because of mental or physical disability, they cannot perform self-care routines, have difficulty managing their finances, and rely on others to obtain the necessary medical care, medications, and food (Older Americans Act Amendments, 2006).

Poly-Victimization

Many abused elders can be categorized as experiencing poly-victimization or being the victim of more than one type of abuse. Poly-victimization is considered a more severe form of EA (Hamby et al., 2016), and this may be the reason that victims of poly-victimization are four times more likely to seek help than elders experiencing only one type of abuse (Burnes et al., 2019a). Rogers and colleagues (2023) found a 43% (n = 257) prevalence rate of poly-victimization involving two, three, and four different subtypes of abuse: financial paired with psychological abuse was reported at 21%, followed most closely by financial abuse and neglect (6%), financial abuse, psychological abuse, and neglect (5%), and psychological abuse and neglect (4%). However, Williams and colleagues (2020) found that, for 101 study participants, the most prevalent forms of poly-victimization involved emotional abuse (72.3%), neglect (57.6%), and physical abuse (43.7%). These poly-abuse victims also reported past-year sexual abuse and neglect. In contrast to both studies, Weissberger and colleagues (2020) found that the most predominant poly-abuse types reported to the NCEA (n = 818 calls) involved physical abuse and at least one additional form of abuse. Data also revealed that family members were the most accused group of perpetrators for poly-victimization, highlighting the role that caregiver stressors likely played in these cases (Weissberger et al., 2020) or associated with caregiver problems (Amstadter et al., 2011; Anme et al., 2004; Conrad et al., 2019; Fulmer, 2013).

Explaining the Roots of EA

Lachs and Pillemer (2015) estimate that EA, both community and institutional, has existed throughout time, although it was not described in the medical literature until sometime in the 1970s. Originally, EA, otherwise known as *granny-battering*, was defined solely in terms of the physical abuse of older persons (Burston, 1975) and was portrayed as the consequence of stressors found in multi-generational homes. Today, we may refer to this as caregiver *burnout* or rather, "physical, emotional, and/or mental exhaustion" leading to negative caregiver attitudes (American Medical Association, 2018, p. 4). In 1980, a series of articles was published by a social worker, wherein he reported on the agist attitudes and denials of professionals about the abuse they were witnessing and prompted him to publish alert signs of EA (Eastman, 1980). More specifically, Eastman expanded the existing perspective and definition of EA to include physical abuse, neglect, financial exploitation, and finally, sexual abuse (Eastman & Sutton, 1982). In 1982, a correlation was found between caring for an elder with dementia and caregiver morale: the greater the dementia, the lower the morale (Gilhooly, 1982). Bergmann and colleagues (1984) researched caregiver and victim relationship dynamics, resulting in the descriptions of three relationship patterns likely to foster abuse:

- a *mother–daughter [mother–son/father–son] syndrome* in which a daughter is dependent on a dominant mother who ages and becomes frailer, putting more demands on the daughter,
- a *fallen tyrant* who, once was dominant in the family, because of frailty now exerts power through manipulation, and
- *power reversal*, wherein a typically compliant elder exploits the power that comes from needing care.

By 1984, Eastman had again revised the definition of EA to include the systematic nature of the abuse and that the abuse was inflicted by a caregiver (Eastman, 1984). However, by 1989, questions arose about the nature of caregiving, about caregivers who did not abuse, about other caregiver or relationship factors that increased the likelihood of abuse, and whether there were different explanations for different types of EA (McCreadie, 1991). Research into both caregiving and EA, in domestic and institutional settings, continued and led to inquiries about the needs of older persons (Stevenson, 1989).

Legal and protective initiatives began as well ranging from the establishment of the National Council on Aging in 1950, American Society on Aging in 1954, Adult Protectives Services in 1979, the establishment of the NCEA in the 1980s, and key legislation (i.e., the Elder Justice Act [EJA] in 2010 and the Elder Abuse Prevention and Prosecution Act [EAPPA] in 2017) (American Bar Association, 2019). Further, the Commission on Law and Aging (COLA) has contributed by assisting organizations with understanding and handling EA through various actions including the development or production of the following: *Elder Abuse in the State Courts – Three Curricula for Judges and Court Staff* (1997), *Legal Issues Related to Elder Abuse: A Pocket Guide for Law Enforcement*, and the *nationally recognized annual state guardianship legislative update*. The U.S. Department of Justice (DOJ) created the Elder Justice Initiative (EJI) providing public information, training, and other resources on EA (United States Department of Justice, n.d.a). While the topic of aging has become prominent, largely because of the baby-boomer phenomenon, there is still research to be conducted for understanding the full scope and prevalence of EA and prevention methodology.

What Are the Risk Factors

Risk factors are characteristics of a person or their surroundings that increase the likelihood of encountering something unfavorable, such as violence or illness. There are a host of factors placing older persons at risk for harm: individual, relationship, environmental, and community. Moreover, risk factors for EA have been categorized as either *static* or *dynamic* (Andrews & Bonta, 2010): static factors are those that tend to go unchanged such as the abuser's past criminal or violent behavior, while dynamic factors include those that interventions may be able to change or mediate, such as abuser substance use, anxiety, or depression (Douglas & Skeem, 2005). Some forms of EA are multifactorial and the more risk factors one has, the higher the likelihood of abuse. For example, many risk factors have been linked to physical, emotional, and psychological abuse such as functional impairment, daily living activity impairment, poor social support, low socioeconomic status, and poor health (Beach et al., 2010; Burnes et al., 2015).

Role of Inequity in EA

Studies tracking the levels of EA with social inequities are either limited or missing from the literature. More prevalent are studies that correlate health *status* and the likelihood of abuse. However, there are a few studies that attempt to examine social determinants of health as they correlate with elder victimization. One such study compared the socioeconomic statuses (SES) of seven cities in seven European countries to the rates of different subtypes of EA. Fraga and colleagues (2014) found that across these seven countries, the rate of reported abuse as correlated with SES, varied by type of abuse. For example, Italy had the lowest rates of reported psychological EA (10.4%) and Sweden, the highest (29.7%). When examining the study populations, comprised persons 60–84 years of age, Italy's participants had lower levels of university education, but Sweden had fewer old-age social benefits. Athens, Greece, with the lowest level of tertiary education, had the highest combined rates of physical, psychological, and sexual abuse. Although findings are mixed, many have found relationships between the level of income and abuse overall such as Naughton and colleagues (2012), who demonstrated that in Ireland, persons with lower SES were twice as likely to experience EA of any kind. A study by Sinha and colleagues (2021) demonstrated similar findings in India: the poorest elders had the least ability to protect themselves from abuse.

Lower income has been identified as a variable in elder mistreatment (Burnes et al., 2015; Burnes et al., 2017) and in studies examining elder poly-victimization. In a cohort of 1,017 Medicaid recipients, Buri and colleagues (2006) found an overall self-reported abuse rate of 20.9%: "15.8% reported experiencing one type of abuse, 4.0% reported experiencing two types of abuse, and 1.0% reported experiencing three types of abuse" (p. 569). In addition to finances, other characteristics of this population included the following: low social support, aloneness, and increased emergency room visits. DeLiema and colleagues (2012) discovered high rates of poly-victimization in a population of older, low-income Latino elders.

Williams and colleagues (2020) studied the rate of victimization, along with the correlation of social factors, in a three-group comparison: one who experienced no abuse, one who experienced a single type of abuse, and a poly-victimization group. The final sample consisted of 2,300 (39.8%) males and 3,477 (60.2%) females with a mean age of 71.46 years (SD = 8.08). Eighty-four percent (n = 4,876) identified as Caucasian, 6.7% (n = 386) as African-American, 4.3% (n = 245) as Hispanic, 2.3% (n = 132), and the rest as American Indian or Alaskan Native, Asian, and Pacific Islanders. Lower income was strongly related to both the single-type abuse and poly-abuse groups (n = 297) (56.8 %) and n = 50 (65.8%), respectively. While having poor health and identifying as a racial minority were significant in both groups, these factors were most prominent in the polyvictim population: 50% of the polyvictim group reported poor health, and 25.5% identified as a racial minority, including Hispanic.

In a systematic review of EA, Wei and Balser (2024) identified risk and protective factors for EA among racial minorities. Dependency on caregivers, and therefore intensifying caregiver stress, increased the risk of EA for African-Americans (Enguidanos et al., 2014), Hispanic Americans (Enguidanos et al., 2014), and Native Americans (Brown, 1989). Other common factors were found to be isolation from services and family, higher levels of functional impairment, mental health and health problems, and substance use by the perpetrator, family, and/or community (Wei and Balser, 2024). Either witnessing trauma and/or being a victim of trauma also increased the risk of violence. For African-American older women, perpetrator trauma was linked to having experienced family violence as a child or having witnessed violence (Paranjape et al., 2009). Overall, risk factors mirrored those found in studies not focused on race or culture with some variations and exceptions. Some studies examining socio-cultural factors in EA have determined that ethnicity can be a protective factor. Cultural Hispanic values, such as valuing family closeness and a responsibility to care of older relatives, may provide protection for the elderly (Montoya,

1997). Respect for elders found in the African-American (Paranjape et al., 2009) and Indian cultures (Nagpaul, 1997) may also act as buffers against abuse.

Individual Factors

Individual factors that increase the likelihood that an older person may suffer abuse include mental illness and stress (Johannesen & LoGuidice, 2013), past trauma (Acierno et al., 2010), a history of or current substance abuse, physical diagnoses (and/or disability), poor coping skills, social isolation, and childhood exposure to violence (Storey, 2020). Having dementia, poor social support, social isolation, and poor health have been linked to becoming a victim of EA (DeLiema, 2018). Rogers and colleagues (2023) found that elders with a dementia diagnosis, and therefore requiring more care, were more vulnerable to financial abuse than those without a diagnosis. Older persons who experienced depression and low levels of family cohesion were also found to be at a higher risk of mistreatment (Gao et al., 2019). Surprisingly, age as a factor to abuse vulnerability applies to the younger-old population who are more likely to live with spouses or adult children compared with the oldest-old living in long-term care facilities (Lauman et al., 2008). Low income and lower levels of education also increase the likelihood of being a victim (Burnes et al., 2017; Williams et al., 2020).

Gender

There has been little research about differences in the occurrence of abuse by gender. However, some speculated that women are likely to be victimized more because of their longer life expectancy (Roberto & Hoyt, 2021). Friedman and colleagues (2017) studied 259 cases of elder physical abuse and found factors that placed elders at risk of revictimization: being female, widowed, being diagnosed with dementia, and being returned to the home where the abuse occurred. Evans and colleagues (2017) found that older women were disproportionately diagnosed with EA during emergency room visits. Gender was also a factor identified by Rogers and colleagues, with women being abused at a prevalence of 71% (n = 424 victims). In a study of 2,713 older Chinese Americans, females were shown to have a higher risk of caregiver neglect (Dong & Wang, 2017). They speculated that this occurs because of the traditional expectation that women care for the family but may not be shown the same regard when needing care. Some studies show, however, that compared with female elderly, there has been a higher likelihood that older men will be nonfatally injured and that non-Hispanic American Indian/Alaskan Natives and Hispanic or Latino persons (not age specific) will be victims of homicide (Logan et al., 2019). For male elderly, firearm deaths increased between the years of 2014 and 2017: contexts included "familial or intimate partner problems, robbery or burglary, argument, and illness-related [including mercy-killing]" (Shawon et al., 2021, p. 1).

Relationship Factors

Relationship factors are characteristics and qualities of an older person's relationships with family, intimate partners, acquaintances and friends, caregivers, healthcare providers, neighbors, and others. There are relationship risk factors common to EA: emotional and financial dependence on an older person and little to no social support (Johannesen & LoGuidice, 2013), a history of family conflict (Wang et al., 2015), and the inability to establish meaningful relationships (Storey, 2020). Beyond these lies a complicated web of risk factors, taking into consideration relationship status, that makes it more likely that someone will abuse an elder.

Rosay and Mulford (2017) distinguish between intimate and non-intimate partner abusers. Whereas intimate partners can include current and past romantic others, non-intimate partners can include family, friends, coworkers, or additional persons that the victim has known for years (Oasis against Violence, 2021). They found that elders were more often physically and psychologically abused by *both* intimate and non-intimate partners (72.6% psychological abuse and 77.7% physical abuse, respectively) compared with only intimate partners (22.2% and 27.4%, respectively) and only non-intimate partners (57.1% and 34.8%, respectively). This indicates that elders are more likely to be emotionally abused by someone other than a partner or spouse. Rogers and colleagues (2023), in a study of 299 elders with dementia and 299 without dementia, found that the abuser was most often an adult child (59%), followed by a spouse or partner (12%). They also found that elders with dementia exhibited more depression and cognitive risk factors, including cognitive decline. Study findings from Weissberger and colleagues (2020) also support family members as being the greatest identified group of perpetrators across all abuse types, suggesting that an elder's risk of abuse increases with the number of family members in the household.

Caregiver Relationships

Caregivers with poor health and medical problems, disabilities, and functional problems (Anme et al., 2004), and difficulties with activities of daily living (Fulmer et al., 2005) are more likely to display perpetrator behavior. Mental illness is a major factor in EA, especially depression (with the rate of mental illness among caregivers found to be between 25% and 35%) (Amstadter et al., 2011). One of the most prominent factors of EA is caregiver substance abuse (Conrad et al., 2019). Other related factors include abuser dependence on the victim for housing and/or finances (Roberto, 2016), problems coping with stress (Johansson, 2018), having been the victim or observer of abuse (Jackson & Hafemeister, 2011), experiencing social isolation, and feeling as though they are not receiving enough social support for proving care (Lachs & Pillemer, 2015). Relationship factors can act as barriers to elders' self-reporting abuse and seeking assistance. The situation of being dependent on a perpetrator for care can dissuade a victim from acknowledging the seriousness of abuse (Burnes et al., 2017). This dependence can even lead to a tit-for-tat situation where the victim allows the abuse in exchange for benefits such as food, physical assistance, medication assistance, and not being placed in a facility (Enguidanos et al., 2014).

Community Factors

Institutions and Facilities

Community risk factors are present in both institutional and non-institutional settings. Nursing homes and other long-term care communities can be either safe or dangerous for vulnerable elders who rely on care. Many facilities have staffing issues such as staff shortages and untrained or under-trained workers, and burnout from stressful environmental conditions (Yon et al., 2019). In 2021, 94% of nursing home providers and 81% of assisted living providers described critical staffing shortages (American Health Care Association and National Center for Assisted Living, 2021). According to the NCEA (2012), the main types of abuse in nursing homes are as follows: physical abuse (29%), resident-to-resident abuse (22%), gross neglect (14%), financial abuse (7%), and sexual abuse (7%). In samples of nursing home staff, it was revealed that 40% (Hawes, 2003) and even 50% (NCEA, 2012) admitted to having abused or mistreated residents. Even if residents are taken to emergency rooms for treatment, many physicians and nurses may not be trained in diagnosing elder victimization (Patel et al., 2021). Duffy and colleagues (2024) carried out a multi-country review of EA occurring in care facilities, such as nursing homes. Common characteristics were found that placed elders in residential care at increased risk for abuse: advanced age and few to no visitors (Mysyuk et al., 2016; Wang et al., 2018), marital status, cognitive decline or dementia, and physical disability (Borda & Yarnoz, 2015), incontinence (Cohen et al., 2010), mental health issues (Wang et al., 2018), and communication problems (Teaster et al., 2007). Behaving in a hostile or aggressive manner and complaining often were also resident traits that increased worker frustration and, therefore, created a higher risk for abuse.

Ruralness

Rural America comprises approximately 97% of the nation's land and, as of July 2017, 19% of rural America was 65 years old and older (United States Department of Justice, n.d.c). Zhang and colleagues (2022) found that approximately 33%, or 3 of 10, older rural persons experience abuse and/or neglect. This is significantly higher than the 10% global estimate reported by Ho and colleagues (2017). Elders in rural areas face unique challenges that increase their risk of abuse such as geographical isolation, inadequate transportation, barriers to reporting, and availability of support services (Warren & Blundell, 2019; Yunus, 2021) as well as the lack of nutritious food (food desert) and adequate broadband (National Sheriff's Association, 2018). It was found that rural elders are at an elevated risk for abuse due to individual and community factors including "less education, limited occupations, lower income, poorer health, higher rates of cognitive impairment and social isolation" (National Sheriff's Association, 2018, p. 25). Even after an elder is identified as a victim, necessary community assistance such as "social services, health care services, mental health services, victim services, aging in place services, opioid treatment, and/or civil and criminal justice services" are very often hard to access if they exist (p. 25). Shortages in social services likely equate to a shortage in adult protective services workers. This is critical in rural areas hard-hit by the opioid epidemic. Roberto and colleagues (2022) found that the U.S. Appalachian area demonstrated a high rate of elder exploitation among older women, citing that the cases examined were "complex, with family loyalties and interdependences influencing how the cases played out" (p. 50). For example, in cases where an elder's medication was stolen by a relative the victim may not have reported any negative side-effects from missing doses, seen as a likely strategy for protecting the perpetrator. As a result, many if not most allegations of exploitation or neglect may go unsubstantiated. Rural law enforcement, although eager to help, often faces impediments to rendering aid: lack of training in identifying and reporting

EA, expansive areas to cover, little time to participate in agency meetings, a lack of language interpreters, and a shortage of funding (National Sheriff's Association, 2018).

EA Is a Criminal Justice Issue

The criminal justice system is an invaluable means of protection from abuse for the elderly. It communicates to the offender that the act is a crime and that he/she will be apprehended for its commission. Krienert and colleagues (2009) suggest that prior to 1990, EA was not considered a criminal justice issue. However, it was a shift in philosophical conceptualization that began to view the abuser of elders as closely aligned with family violence. Family violence was already a criminal justice issue. Therefore, the inclusion of elderly abuse related to family violence was logical given that most individuals who abused the elderly were their family members.

Elderly individuals are protected under criminal and civil law. Acts of EA violate criminal law, but these acts vary by state, with some acts constituting violations of civil law. Some possible crimes of elderly abuse are as follows in most states: (1) elderly physical abuse can constitute assault, aggravated assault, attempted murder, battery, domestic violence, kidnapping, and murder; (2) elderly sexual abuse can constitute assault, aggravated assault, battery, domestic violence, rape, sexual assault, sexual battery, and human trafficking; (3) psychological abuse of the elderly can constitute EA, harassment, and hate crimes; (4) elderly abandonment can constitute EA, manslaughter, murder, neglect, negligent, or involuntary homicide; (5) neglect can constitute EA, manslaughter, and murder; (6) financial exploitation can constitute EA, embezzlement, false instrument, financial exploitation, forgery, fraud (e.g., credit card, tax, or Medicaid), identity theft, larceny, money laundering, theft, and trafficking (Stiegel, 2014). Laws enacted in all states within the U.S. have established systems of reporting and investigating elderly abuse through adult protective services.

Police officers, bank tellers, and health providers are required by law to report cases of elderly abuse (U.S. Government Accountability Office, 2011). Abuse statutes vary by state concerning types of abuse, definitions of abuse, requirements for reporting, procedures for investigation, and remedies. For example, some state statutes exclude psychological abuse, sexual abuse, and abandonment; some states cover older adults who live in the community and others cover abuse that occurs within institutions. Some states regard elderly abuse as a criminal offense and others as a civil matter (American Bar Association Commission on Law and Aging, 2005).

Jackson (2015) argues that the criminal justice conceptualization of elderly abuse as a crime started the elder justice movement in the U.S. The DOJ became involved in EA in 2002, and the phrase EA was replaced with elder justice further supplanting elder abuse as a crime. The EJA was passed in 2010 as part of the Patient Protection and Affordable Care Act (ACA, P.L. 111–148, as amended). The Act was intended to provide a coordinated federal response to EA by emphasizing various public health and social service approaches to prevent, detect, and treat abuse. The Act is also Congress' first attempt at comprehensive legislation to address abuse, neglect, and exploitation of the elderly at the federal level (Colello, 2020). The DOJ established the EJI to support and coordinate the department's efforts to combat EA, neglect, and financial fraud and scams that target the nation's seniors. Specifically, the EJI, due to Americans living longer and to the baby boomers becoming seniors, has developed several resources to assist local, state, federal, and tribal law enforcement officers in responding to crimes of EA and financial exploitation.

EA Is a Public Health Issue

Elder abuse is a global public health issue in light of the growing older generation in key countries (Teaster & Hall, 2018). Worldwide, 1 in 6 persons will be aged 60 and older by 2030, numbering 1.4 billion (WHO, 2024b). In fact, World Health Organization (WHO) estimates that by 2050, this number will double to over 2 billion, nearly 22% of the global population, with nearly two-thirds of the world's citizens residing in low- and middle-income countries. In addition to medical and psychological/emotional conditions associated with aging, there are also "geriatric syndromes" (p. 6), which are diagnosed when there are multiple complex health conditions present. The quality of life and opportunities that aging brings to the older person and their family is, to a large degree, dependent on the older persons' health. Societal ageism, however, has marked much of the older generation as frail, dependent, and as a burden. This stigmatization strongly affects how older persons are cared for by family and the community, how they are treated and discriminated against, and how policy does or does not address their many needs. Too many times, the consequence of ageism is EA.

EA is considered a public health problem because of the types of response needed to address its detection, intervention, and prevention (Teaster & Hall, 2018). Between 2021 and 2036, the rise in demand for additional U.S. healthcare workforce was projected as follows: allied health care, 23%; behavioral health personnel, 62%; long-term care workers, 38%; and primary care, 14%. In total, the expected demand increase for health care is 11%, while the supply is projected at –1% by 2036 (Department of Health and Human Services, 2024). Currently, the public healthcare workforce, including geriatric specialists, is experiencing a severe shortage, especially in rural areas. In 2020, there were approximately 52.4 million older persons and roughly 8,220 full-time geriatricians, or rather, doctors who have additional training in treating older adults (American Geriatrics Society, 2025). By 2030, the demand for this specialty will increase by 50%, but the supply of geriatricians will have decreased (Gurwitz, 2023), with rural America feeling the brunt of the shortage. As the older population grows and outnumbers the healthcare system's capacity, EA is likely to grow and continue to go unnoticed.

EA also has costs attached. Older adults who are victims of financial abuse incur losses totaling over $28 billion each year (Gunther, 2023). These losses often include retirement savings which can place the victim into a state of dependency on family members. It is estimated that 70% of Alzheimer's care is provided by family members either in direct aid or by the provision of medications, food, housing, and other support (Alzheimer's Association, 2025). Subtypes of abuse, such as physical and sexual abuse or neglect, can lead to costly consequences such as admissions to long-term stay facilities and subsequent hospital admissions, resulting in expenditures that total billions of dollars of Medicare and Medicaid costs (Office of Inspector General, 2014). It was also found that EA victims are less likely to see a primary care provider and more likely to present in emergency rooms—nearly three times that of non-mistreated elders—another costly consequence that typically does not lead to an identification of abuse (Platts-Mills et al., 2014; Rosen et al., 2023).

International Comparative Statistics

EA continues to grow as a global public health concern. In a global study analysis of EA prevalence, Ho and colleagues (2017) found that third-party caregiver studies (e.g., nursing facilities and extended stay facilities) reported EA at a rate of three times that of community-based studies relying on self-report. This difference in reporting is thought to be linked to fear of the abused elder about reporting a family or intimate partner caregiver. Ho and colleagues also found a 10% difference in EA reporting between western and non-western countries, likely due to cultural and family structure differences. As with other prevalence studies, women are abused at a higher rate globally than men: 17% and 10.9%, respectively (p. 49). For 2022, the subtype of EA most reported in the U.S was sexual abuse, followed by physical abuse. However, globally, it was found that emotional abuse was the most prevalent (71.5%) followed by physical abuse with sexual abuse as the least reported (p. 49).

It was also reported that abuse was more often related to child and spouse caregiving and caregivers who lived in the home with the elder. This was believed to be related to caregiver emotional health and burnout. Abuse was negatively associated with older persons, with good support, who were able to age at home longer and delay community placements.

WHO (2022) reports EA median prevalence rates at the county and global WHO region level. The region highest for physical abuse and financial abuse is the African region at 15% and 13%, respectively. The region highest for sexual abuse is the Americas at 6%. Moreover, four regions are noted for their prevalence of psychological abuse: the Western Pacific region (China) at 21%, the African region (Nigeria) at 11%, the European region (Czechia, Croatia, Italy, Spain, Portugal, the Netherlands, the U.K., and Ireland) at 10%, and the South-East Asia Region at 11%. The Eastern Mediterranean Region, including Israel and Egypt, has the highest prevalence of elder neglect at 42%.

Public Health and Social Work

Intersection of Public Health and Social Work

Public health and social work intersect at critical junctions when it comes to EA. Social workers act alongside public health workers, intersecting with elder victims in nearly every venue where elders interact, reside, and receive care. At times, they work as a member of a unit or team, such as in social service agencies (e.g., with adult protection or with securing benefits), public health departments, long-term care facilities, and hospitals. At other times, they cross paths with elders at senior centers, elder daycare, food banks, psychiatric and healthcare outpatient clinics, during in-home care visits, and substance use disorder programs. Social workers act as advocates on behalf of elder victims for identifying, investigating, intervening with, and preventing EA (National Indigenous Elder Justice Initiative, 2023). They also advocate on behalf of family or other unpaid caregivers, seeking to ensure that they have access to resources that meet their needs (National Association of Social Workers [NASW], 2010). As mentioned previously, caregiver stress and burnout have been recognized as a key factor for the occurrence of EA (Amstadter et al., 2011; Anme et al., 2004; Conrad et al., 2019; Fulmer et al., 2005; Weissberger et al., 2020). By making sure that caretakers have adequate support and wellness resources, it is intended that caregivers' burden is reduced, thereby decreasing the prevalence of abuse. Moreover, community health workers, likewise, promote wellness, implement programs, and advocate for those, such as the elderly and their caregivers, who have limited access to services (Bureau of Labor Statistics, n.d.). They work alongside social workers, nurses, and substance use and behavioral health counselors to help promote healthy living, coordinate care for individuals and communities, provide coaching and support and home visits, as well as provide basic health screenings. Through collaborative efforts, they are more likely to see opportunities for intervention on EA.

Social workers, like public health workers, act to create and champion policy and programs targeting healthy aging and the protection of vulnerable populations. For example, NASW also has worked, as a member of the Nursing Home Reform Coalition, to improve nursing home quality through better staffing and transparency (Herman, 2024). The NASW also established the NASW Standards for Social Work Services in Long-Term Care Facilities to "address the use of long-term services and supports by people across the lifespan in both facility and home- and community-based settings" (Herman, 2024, 14). In addition, the profession of social work has access to a wide selection of resources through NASW such as elder care continuing education, a community of elder care workers via the *aging specialty practice section*, and practice perspective publications (e.g., elder justice and racial justice). The care of elders and abuse prevention are interwoven throughout the NASW's *2021 Blueprint of Federal Social Policy Priorities* where they emphasize 21 topics including the improvement of access to mental and behavioral health and social care services, the building of healthy relationships to end violence, eradication of social isolation, and advancement of long and productive lives. In this plan, NASW called for action, including but not limited to, the reauthorization of the EJA, increased funding for adult protective services and long-term care ombudsman programs, the strengthening of Medicare outreach and enrollment, improvement of long-term care patient-to-staff ratio and increased staff qualifications, the development of an equitable social insurance system, and the passage of the Improving Access to Mental Health Act (NASW, 2021).

Health Disparities and Health Equities

Ageism, or rather age discrimination, is a key factor in health disparities associated with older persons and EA (WHO, 2024b). For instance, ageism is linked to an increased risk of mortality, lower cognitive functioning, and recovering more slowly when ill (Burnes et al., 2019b). It is also associated with higher rates of depression, emotional distress and anxiety, isolation, and a lower perceived quality of life (Ermer et al., 2020). Levy and colleagues (2020) found that several of the most common health issues among older persons can be attributed to ageism. In fact, they estimated that a 10% reduction in ageism could result in 1.7 million fewer cases of health conditions. It is not only the ageist attitude held by society that is damaging, but the ageist self-perceptions held by older persons are just as toxic. Self-perceived negative images have been associated with low self-confidence (Voss et al., 2018), can increase stress, interfere with cognition, increase the risk of Alzheimer's (Chang et al., 2020), and cause other deleterious brain changes (Levy et al., 2020). While ageism is damaging for all older persons, Perron (2018) found that the experience of ageism was higher among African-Americans (77%), compared with Latinos (61%) and Whites (59%), respectively.

While ageism and other present-day factors (e.g., climate change, rising food costs, healthcare inaccessibility, and lack of affordable housing) play a significant part in the determinants of health for older persons, one's historical experiences are perhaps the most significant factor in determining health in older age. This is known as the *life course perspective* and is critical to understanding health outcomes of socioeconomically disadvantaged and racial and ethnic minority populations (Jones et al., 2019). For example, childhood exposure to environmental hazards and violence, malnourishment, homelessness, and/or parental behaviors due to poverty, behavioral health, or substance abuse, especially during critical periods of development, can be formative for later life (Zeanah et al., 2011). These health disparities, and their impact over the life course, increase an older person's vulnerability to victimization of all abuse subtypes (WHO, 2002). According to the National Institute on Aging (n.d.), factors that create and/or maintain health disparities for older persons include the following:

- Environmental factors such as income, education, occupation, retirement, and wealth (e.g., savings, property, and stocks),
- Social factors, including social or structural discrimination such as ageism and racism,
- Cultural factors such as food preferences, coping mechanisms, and attitudes toward lifestyle factors (e.g., alcohol consumption, drug use, and exercise),
- Behavioral factors including life outlook and sense of personal control (optimism and internal loci versus pessimism and external loci), and
- Biological factors which may be genetic or epigenetic, such as factors shaping stress response systems (Jones et al., 2019).

EA itself is viewed as a determinant of health from being identified as a form of interpersonal violence. Being older, low-income, and a member of a minority group increases the likelihood of mistreatment and abuse (Burnes et al., 2015).

Negative Health Consequences of EA

EA can have long-lasting consequences on its victims. In addition to premature mortality (Yunus et al., 2019), it has also been shown to cause serious health conditions and poor mental health including depression, anxiety, and post-traumatic stress symptoms (Acierno et al., 2017; Yunus et al., 2019). Those with dementia are particularly vulnerable to negative effects, as the abuse compounds already existing issues. Medication non-adherence was attributed to first, caregiver neglect and second, dementia (Grocki & Huffman, 2007). Medical consequences of EA were found to include cardiovascular disease, chronic obstructive pulmonary disease, peptic ulcers, digestive disorders, metabolic diseases, acute inflammation, tumors, and injuries (Fang et al., 2018). When elders are subjected to extreme heat or cold temperatures, because of neglect or abuse, injuries or even death may occur (Hall et al., 2016). Immediate and chronic pain from physical abuse can range from "mild discomfort or dull distress to acute, often unbearable, agony," as well as having difficulties with or being unable to perform activities or daily living, work, or recreation (Hall et al., 2016, p. 31).

Suicide

The 2022 suicide rate in the U.S. was highest for persons ages 75 and older (Curtin et al., 2023). From 49,449 confirmed suicides, there were 10,443 among those persons aged 65 and older. They were primarily male (CDC, 2024b). When compared to 2021, the rate of suicide for this age group (65+) rose by 8.1%. Furthermore, there are many factors influencing the decision to commit suicide such as isolation, loss of independence forcing reliance on others, chronic illness, and cognitive impairment (National Council on Aging [NCOA], 2025)—all of which have been reviewed in this chapter as being factors associated with EA. An elder's decision to end their life by assisted suicide may also be influenced by abuse in the forms of neglect (Wand et al., 2018). Neglect, as discussed earlier, produces harm and distress, at times through undue influence that arises through relational dynamics. Van Orden and colleagues (2010) found a correlation between the factors of an older person's sense of burdensomeness and isolation as they pertain to the decision to commit suicide. Caregivers or other family members can influence the decision to commit suicide through abusive actions including how they speak to or about the elder. For example, persons may speak at or in earshot of the elder about what an inconvenience being a carer is, or about how much better their lives would be if not burdened with caring. They may also complain about the finances involved in being a caregiver. These actions and attitudes can intensify the older person's internalized sense of burdensomeness, loneliness, and depression. Suicide in elders, with and without a history of abuse, has been associated with depression. In a study of older Koreans, Lee and Atteraya (2019) found positive associations between suicide ideation, depression, poverty, and past abuse in comparison to those who did not experience these factors. Alexopulous and colleagues (1999) found that the severity of depression was the predominant determinant of suicidal behavior and that elders with severe depression, a history of suicide attempts, and poor social support were at the highest risk of committing suicide.

Criminal Justice Approaches

The "aging" of America has wide-ranging implications for virtually every aspect of our society, including the criminal justice system. The criminal justice system will be confronted with more elderly victims and the offenders who abuse them. In response to the elderly, law enforcement officers have initiated several programs which are designed to improve their response to them, particularly those who are abused or at risk of abuse. The DOJ established the Elder Abuse Protection Act of 2021, which provides statutory authority for the EJI, which coordinates criminal enforcement and public engagement efforts to combat EA, neglect, and financial fraud and scams that target elders (Elder Abuse Protection Act of 2021).

The Act requires EJI to establish through local, state, federal, and tribal law enforcement offices a national elder fraud telephone hotline, promote civil legal aid to victims of elder fraud and EA, and make resources available online in English and Spanish. Moreover, the DOJ provides law enforcement officers with training, toolkits, and resources to assist in their mission to combat EA and financial exploitation. These resources include the following: (1) EAGLE (Elder Abuse Guide for Law Enforcement) which is a web module to support law enforcement in EA and financial exploitation cases; (2) SAFTA (Senior Abuse Financial Training and Accounting), a downloadable toolkit to assist financial exploitation investigations and prosecution; (3) providing informative videos, such as financial abuse by a stranger, physical abuse, and understanding EA to assist in identifying and understanding EA; (4) working collaboratively with other professionals to build strong working relationships;

(5) providing documents and websites specifically for law enforcement involved in EA and financial exploitation cases; and, (6) a curated list of elder justice webinars for law enforcement officers.

EJI also provides information for local, state, and federal prosecutors who handle EA, neglect, and financial exploitation cases. For prosecutors who are new to the field training, videos and resources are provided to help successfully prosecute cases; it also provides federal and state EA statutes, and research that prosecutors will need to handle elderly abuse cases. Victim specialists also work with prosecutors, law enforcement, and other staff members to ensure that EA victims are treated with respect, know their rights, and understand their role within the criminal justice system. They help victims navigate the criminal justice system by providing support, assessing a victim's needs, developing a safety plan, connecting victims to resources, and identifying gaps in service. EJI also provides several community outreach resources such as presentations, flyers, and videos to encourage older adults to get involved in preventing financial exploitation (United States Department of Justice, 2025). Through the DOJ and EJI, the criminal justice system meets the needs of the elderly.

Public Health Approaches

EA has been recognized as a public issue only since 2001, when, at the National Policy Summit on Elder Abuse, ten recommendations for a coordinated federal response to EA were made and a proposal of a national EA agenda was put forth (Aravanis, 2002). A response has been for public health to coordinate its ten essential public health services with other response frameworks used in both violence prevention and public health (Irving & Hall, 2018). We offer a summary of how these ten services could be used in the prevention of EA. First, *monitoring is required to identify and solve community health problems*. Even though there are reporting mechanisms used by official sources, such as the police, there are many more occurrences that go unreported. According to Connolly and Trilling (2014), there are an estimated 23 unreported instances of EA for everyone that is registered. Public health can enhance surveillance by training community-level workers to recognize and report EA. Public health officials can also spearhead efforts to increase reporting by working with other frontline personnel to learn about and share how EA is defined and counted, to identify challenges of distinguishing EA surveillance from other types of violence and to establish agreements about data sharing and combining resources for "collecting, analyzing, and applying EA data" (Irving & Hall, 2018).

Second, public health services are needed to *diagnose and investigate community health hazards and problems*. This is where public health can continue to help practitioners, "better elucidate co-occurring factors, risk factors, and protective factors" (Irving & Hall, 2018, p. 27). This knowledge is crucial in helping researchers understand the dynamics between factors such as characteristics of perpetrators and victims, relationship factors, and societal influence. Public health can assist in monitoring the increase or decrease of EA and to improve the effectiveness of risk assessment, identification of cases, and abuse investigations. Third, an essential public health function is to *inform, educate, and empower people about health issues* such as EA. Educating the public not only raises the potential for more case identification but it also gives the public resources and information for creating policy, programs, and awareness campaigns (Irving & Hall, 2018). Health education about EA can be used to tailor intervention and prevention efforts for specific community populations. In other words, knowledge is power and having awareness of EA may empower individuals to collectively combat EA.

Fourth, collective action is needed to *mobilize community partnerships to identify and solve health problems*. Irving and Hall (2018) suggest that the engagement of community-based stakeholders may assist in increasing "cultural relevance of the solutions while also increasing the awareness of cultural issues among the public health practitioners" (p. 31). Additionally, it may be that community partnerships will be able to create sustainable efforts. Fifth, public health approaches can develop policies and plans *"that support individual and community health efforts"*(p. 32). While individual agency and program policies are helpful, policies at the local, state, federal, and global levels are necessary to ensure that proper attention is given to EA and that interest in and action to prevent EA is properly established and maintained. Irving and Hall (2018) suggest that public health can assist in proving "contextual evidence, experiential evidence, and the best available research evidence" (p. 33) needed to evaluate EA policy and practices. Sixth, an essential public health function is *enforcing laws and regulations that protect health and ensure safety*. Public health law exists when policy is not enough to maintain public health due to a lack of voluntary compliance to policy (Martin, 2008). Public health law services to elucidate the importance of public health policy and it uses precise language to explain the government's position on an issue. Laws passed during the COVID-19 pandemic are instructive. For mandatory reporting of EA, laws vary by state. As such, the effectiveness of these laws is something that public health could assist with achieving as well as working with long-term care ombudsmen to more heavily oversee long-term care facilities (Irving & Hall, 2018).

Seventh, public health links *people to needed personal health services and assuring the provision of health care when otherwise unavailable*. This function was discussed earlier as a service that community health workers and social workers often provided. These services may include primary prevention activities and programs to reduce risks for EA, secondary prevention or intervention services, and lastly are those services needed to address the physical, emotional, and psychological effects of EA victimization (Irving & Hall, 2018). Some critical issues are the availability and accessibility of these services which are challenging in any environment but especially in rural areas.

Eighth, the prime concern of essential service is to *assure a competent public and personal healthcare workforce*. As demonstrated earlier, there is and will continue to be an overall healthcare workforce shortage as the number of older persons continues to rise. Specifically, Gurwitz (2023) predicted that by 2030, the demand for geriatricians would increase by 50%, but the supply decreases. Irving and Hall (2018) purport that public health can assist in the development of a competent workforce by identifying specific training needs, creating academic partnerships, and creating opportunities for the development of EA-focused training for individuals, teams, units, and organizations. Ninth, public health agencies must evaluate *the effectiveness, accessibility, and quality of personal and population-based health services*. "Process, outcome, and impact evaluation" (Irving & Hall, 2018, p. 38) are necessary for improving current efforts, establishing lessons learned, and determining future public health and collaborative actions. While evaluation of current efforts leads to impactful changes, research should always be ongoing. Tenth, public health must continue to *conduct research to obtain new insights and innovative solutions to health problems*. As Irving and Hall (2018) point out, effective prevention policy is impossible without accurate, up-to-date, and culturally relevant data. Public health can contribute by researching risk factors to examine the diverse populations of older adults, to clarify if some risk factors are more critical than others, and how combinations of risk factors increase the likelihood of EA. As stated above, research can sway policy, determine funding for prevention and intervention measures (availability and accessibility), and influence the amount of effort put toward EA innovation and prevention.

Public Health and Social Work Approaches

In an earlier chapter section, *Intersection of Public Health and Social Work*, some roles of social workers in the prevention of elder suicide were mentioned, such as advocacy on behalf of elders and their caregivers for getting the intervention and resources they need to both intervene with and prevent circumstances leading to abuse. The role social workers play in policy reforms was also mentioned. However, the scope of their EA efforts goes further. For example, some social workers are employed by local *Area Agency on Aging* (AAA) organizations where they act as case managers, program managers, or agency directors (Herman, 2022). While nearly all AAAs offer at least one EA prevention service, they typically provide seven different programs. Furthermore, social workers are often employed as a long-term care ombudsman with the following responsibilities:

- Identifying, investigating, and resolving complaints made by or on behalf of residents;
- Providing information to residents about long-term services and supports;
- Ensuring that residents have regular and timely access to ombudsman services;
- Representing the interests of residents before governmental agencies and seeking administrative, legal, and other remedies to protect residents; and
- Analyzing, commenting on, and recommending changes in laws and regulations that pertain to the health, safety, welfare, and rights of residents (Administration for Community Living [ACL], 2020a, para. 3).

Social workers may also act on behalf of elders as court investigators and eldercaring coordinators. As a court investigator, the social worker ensures that potential legal guardians for elders are suitable and make recommendations to a judge for guardian assignment (Herman, 2022). Eldercaring coordination is a court-ordered dispute resolution process for resolving high-stress family conflicts that could lead to elder mistreatment (Association for Conflict Resolution & Florida Chapter of the Association of Family and Conciliation Courts, n.d.). They are members of *EAe multidisciplinary teams* that focus on complex cases of "elder abuse, neglect, and exploitation" (p. 9). These social workers may also work for crime victim assistance programs, such as the Elder Abuse Prevention and Elimination Services, and participate in *abuse in later life programs*. Additionally, social workers are trained to develop and implement community education and public awareness campaigns, and they are involved in *elder justice coalitions*. Social workers are vital to elder prevention across the service continuum "including in health, housing, mental health, and substance use programs" (p. 19).

Integrating Skills of Social Epidemiology to Address Disparities and Achieve Equity

Social epidemiology is a field of epidemiology that "aim[s] to identify social characteristics that affect the pattern of disease and health distribution in a society and to understand its mechanisms" (von dem Knesebeck, 2015, p. 1 of 4). It is concerned with larger systems, such as social structures, institutions, and relationships, and the impact of these systems on well-being (Berkman et al., 2014). In other words, social epidemiology is concerned with "describing and intervening on social conditions that either promote or harm health" (Kawachi, 2002, p. 1739). Therefore, social epidemiology has a unique way of examining health inequities. For example, the higher mortality rates of disenfranchised groups of people have, by some, been viewed as an outcome of those groups' inactivity in the political process (Kawachi & Subramanian, 2018). However, Rodriguez and colleagues (2015) examined mortality from a different perspective by focusing on the effect of the inequalities in mortality (a pattern of disease) on electoral participation (social institution). Another example is the connection between income distribution (a social structure) and population health (pattern of disease or health distribution). Though some researchers have posited that the connection between lower income and poor health is poverty, social epidemiologists have posited that the connection is income distribution and that a more equal distribution of income and wealth will result in improved population health (Brodish & Hakes, 2016).

When thinking about EA and the myriad of factors that facilitate the abuse, the social epidemiology perspective can help address disparities. Take, for example, the relationship between low income and lower levels of education and the increased likelihood of being an EA victim (Burnes et al., 2017; Williams et al., 2020). As with the previous example examining health and income (Brodish & Hakes, 2016), poverty could be attributed as the factor leading to EA. However, by applying the social epistemological lens, it can be argued that a redistribution of income could potentially reduce the amount of EA. Looking at health disparities from a different (i.e., social epidemiology) perspective can lead to the creation and implementation of more effective interventions that are focused on legitimate root causes.

How Can EA Be Prevented

Preventing EA is multi-pronged. One of the most measurable ways to prevent EA is to focus prevention efforts on targeted risk factors for change or management (Douglas et al., 2013). For example, intimate partner violence has been researched to a higher degree leading to risk assessment instruments to be used in practitioner offices for assessing and managing future intimate partner violence (Nicholls et al., 2013). Routine screenings for use in detecting abuse or violence have been suggested by the National Advisory Committee on Rural Health and Human Services (2015). Care providers and other agencies encountering elders can find violence screening tools and protocols at violence prevention websites by the American Family Physician (www.uspreventiveservicestaskforce.org/) and NCEA Research to Practice: Elder Abuse Screening Tools for Healthcare Professionals (usc.edu).

Given that only 15% of EA victims seek help (Burnes et al., 2019a), more research is needed to develop easily accessible help-seeking mechanisms either through emergency services, healthcare providers, or other pathways. It was found that help-seeking was the lowest among those who were dependent on their abuser. Burnes and colleagues also found that victims who had knowledge about and knew police were more likely to seek assistance, suggesting that community policing may be an effective abuse deterrent.

Educational programs for elders that define the seriousness of any abuse should be readily available. These programs should also educate elders about what happens when they make a report: many elders are afraid that their perpetrator will be jailed when often this is not the case, especially with less dangerous forms of abuse such as emotional abuse or mistreatment prevention efforts, therefore, should follow a "client-centered harm reduction model" (Burnes et al., 2019a, p. 895). Given the complex relationship that most often exists between perpetrator and victim, it may be helpful to teach both parties problem-solving skills, especially since most perpetrators are family members (O'Donnell et al., 2014). It has also been suggested that specific types of intervention and prevention be developed for the distinct subtypes of abuse, rather than, depending on a single method of addressing EA as a problem in general (Jackson, 2016). Goergen and Beaulieu (2010) proposed that interventions be devised in terms of perpetrator intent to harm and if the abuse carries over situationally. As an example, if there is an incident where the abuser did not intend to harm the elder and the context is limited to one situation, then intervention would be much different than if there was an intent to do harm and the abuse was carried out across multiple contexts.

Caregiver protective factors are also important in curbing EA. Fang and colleagues (2018) cited the significance of emotion-focused and solution-focused coping and the perception of familism. While solution-focused techniques work to eliminate sources of stress, emotion-focused techniques focus on negative emotion regulation (Kristofferzon et al., 2018). Familism is a sense that the care of one's family supersedes that of one's own (Steidel & Contreras, 2003). Additionally, it has been discovered that preparing caregivers for their role is beneficial since it allows them to foresee potential stressors and learn coping skills ahead of time (Hancock et al., 2022). Wei and colleagues (2024) discovered that it was critical to tailor caregiver educational programs for those caring for elders diagnosed with dementia.

Policy Recommendations

Comprehensive policy guidelines and protocols for addressing EA are crucial (Wei et al., 2024). In 2015, policy priorities for EA were established to enhance a public health response (Board on Global Health et al., 2014). As the number of elders increases, and the incidence of EA becomes greater, these priorities remain relevant today. One priority is to develop a policy that views EA as a public health issue. Even while there are efforts to confront and combat EA, those efforts are few when compared to those targeting child abuse and domestic violence. In other words, while EA is an issue connected with "law enforcement, prosecution, social services, and financial issues" (p. 4), it is also one connected with uncountable consequences for "individuals, families, and society" (p. 4) and, therefore, should be treated according to the public health model that addresses data collection, surveillance, and sound methods for determining effective intervention. Improved surveillance not only locally but globally for monitoring and tracking EA is essential for informing prevention policy (Alias, 2023). Relatedly, the workforce shortage for addressing EA is a significant barrier to adequate prevention and intervention. It is imperative to train an adequate workforce for identifying, tackling, and preventing EA, as well as training professionals who are interested in EA research (Board on Global Health et al., 2014). This workforce should include not only geriatricians, but physicians, nurses, other health professionals, community workers, social workers, law enforcement—those who encounter older persons regularly (Wei et al., 2024). Wei and colleagues also advocate for specialized training in recognizing and responding to EA elderly abuse victims who are diagnosed with dementia.

Another proposed policy priority is research, especially in five areas: intervention, defining success, prevention, data collection, and cost (Board on Global Health et al., 2013). Research on *intervention* is necessary to reveal which actions are effective and with which populations. While EA agencies have their own *definitions of intervention success*, it is still unknown to those who are most impacted by EA what is considered successful, so there is much work to be done in identifying success from a victim/survivor perspective. Examining *prevention* strategies is imperative for ensuring that measures, such as EA awareness campaigns, are effective. Because of the barriers for accurate reporting of EA, *data collection* and surveillance methods need to be enhanced for accuracy. Research that assesses the economic burden of EA is also required to calculate its effect on healthcare costs and "economic losses for employers, businesses, families, and individuals" (p. 14). Demonstrating the financial impact of EA can be an incentive to lawmakers to take policy action and can also highlight areas for intervention that may have been unnoticed.

Other priority policy recommendations include translating what we learn into practice, such as addressing inadequate provider training and outdated tools that assist in making decisions for intervention and reporting, establishing funding for EA research, building infrastructure that maintains consistent and appropriate policy attention to EA, developing a political constituency, and promoting innovation such as multidisciplinary teams and forensic geriatricians (Board on Global Health et al., 2014). Among many more policy recommendations are those that promote rights for EA victims to seek appropriate compensation from their perpetrators and those that add more protections for elders residing in long-term care facilities—more protections not only against staff abuse but abuse from other residents (Elderabuse.org, 2019).

Summary

EA is a long-standing societal problem that is projected to worsen as the older population grows. Compounding the geriatric population's increase is a shortage of an adequately trained healthcare workforce, both in credentialing and number. Relatedly, are the added stressors placed on caregivers, both family and institutional, that increase the likelihood of EA, especially in rural areas which are lacking resources and where there is added social isolation. Many other factors increase the likelihood of EA occurring. Caregiver factors such as substance abuse, dependency on the elder for shelter and income, mental health diagnoses, and poor coping skills. Victim characteristics are involved as well such as being diagnosed with dementia, having several physical illnesses, being socially isolated, and being part of a family with low cohesion or closeness. Inequities play a significant part in the occurrence and persistence of EA. Low income has been associated with EA (single and poly-victimization) because of the stressors that financial strain places on families. Other factors associated with low-income communities synergize to create a storm of influences such as climate change, rising food costs, healthcare inaccessibility, and lack of safe and affordable housing. However, a more significant inequity is found to be one's persona, typically traumatic, experiences occurring over the *lifespan*: childhood exposures to violence, lead, abuse, caregiver mental illness, and substance use, etc. In other words, trauma experienced early on can lay a pathway leading to further trauma and debilitating inequities in the future. The consequences of EA are vast and varied ranging from elder neglect to mistreatment, to abuse, suicide, and even death or murder. The most common forms of EA are physical abuse, psychological abuse, financial abuse, and sexual abuse. There are subtypes of each of these and they all occur to varying degrees. Prolonged trauma, depression and hopelessness, worsening health and frailty, economic ruin, shame, and loss of dignity are all examples of EA outcomes. The fields of social work and public health are very active in responding to and preventing EA. Both social workers and community health workers become established in communities seeking to assist caregivers, to spread awareness of EA and the causes of EA such as ageism, and to investigate reports of EA through programs such as adult protective services. Social work is active politically, supporting policy and law for the prevention and intervention of EA. Public health supports epidemiological measures to surveil, prevent, and intervene in EA through the support of major public health policy and action measures. Health care, along with law enforcement, and other public service entities can be and/or are being trained in the recognition and reporting of EA—very similar to the efforts that have occurred with child abuse. According to WHO's studies on the prevalence of EA, a global prevention effort is imperative. Since EA is both a personal and societal experience, it can only be addressed through comprehensive measures that enforce and enable accountability. It is a multisystemic problem requiring creativity and innovation, increased person-power, resources, and advocacy for producing an effective response.

Discussion Questions

1 Considering identified risk factors for EA, what are some community-based prevention measures you would recommend for implementation?
2 How can the criminal justice system and social workers effectively collaborate to address EA while ensuring that the autonomy and dignity of the elder are respected?
3 Considering that elder abuse manifests differently across geographics and cultures, what culturally sensitive approaches should be employed in the prevention and intervention of EA in diverse populations?
4 What are the advantages and limitations of addressing EA through a public health lens? Social work lens?
5 How can current policies, such as the Elder Justice Act or the Older Americans Act, be strengthened to better address EA?
6 What additional policy measures could be introduced to further protect older adults?

References

Acierno, R., Hernandez-Tajeda, M.A., Amstadter, A.B., Resnick, H.S., Steve, K., Muzzy, W., & Kilpatrick, D.G. (2010). Prevalence and correlates of emotional, physical, sexual, and financial abuse and potential neglect in the United States: The national elder mistreatment study. *American Journal of Public Health*, 100, 292–297. https://doi.org/10.2105/AJPH.2009.163089
Acierno, R., Hernandez-Tejada, M.A., Anetzberger, G.J., Loew, D., & Muzzy, W. (2017, August–October). The national elder mistreatment study: An 8-year longitudinal study of outcomes.

Journal of Elder Abuse & Neglect, 29(4), 254–269. https://doi.org/10.1080/08946566.2017.1365 031. PMID: 28837418.

Administration for Community Living (ACL). (2020a). *Longterm care ombudsman program*. U.S. Department of Health and Human Services. https://acl.gov/programs/Protecting-Rights-and-Pre venting-Abuse/Long-term-Care-Ombudsman-Program

Alexopoulos, G.S., Bruce, M.L., Hull, J., Sirey, J.A., & Kakuma, T. (1999). Clinical determinants of suicidal ideation and behavior in geriatric depression. *Archives of General Psychiatry*, 56(11), 1048–1053. https://doi.org/10.1001/archpsyc.56.11.1048

Alias, A.N., Mokti, K., Ibrahim, M.Y., Saupin, S., & Madrim, M.F. (2023). Elderly abuse and neglect on population health: Literature review and interventions from selected countries. *Korean Journal of Family Medicine*, 44(6), 311–318. https://doi.org/10.4082/kjfm.23.0046

Alzheimer's Association. (2025). Caregiving. www.alz.org/alzheimers-dementia/facts-figures#:~:text= Of%20the%20total%20lifetime%20cost,long%2Dterm%20care%20expenses%20or

American Bar Association. (2019). Elder abuse then and now: 1979–2019. *American Bar Association Journal*, 41(2), 174–176. Elder Abuse Then and Now (1979–2019) (americanbar.org).

American Bar Association Commission on Law and Aging. (2005). Information about laws related to elder abuse. Newark, DE: National Center on Elder Abuse.

American Geriatrics Society. (2025. *State of the geriatrician workforce*: Geriatrics workforce by the numbers. www.americangeriatrics.org/geriatrics-profession/about-geriatrics/geriatrics-workforce-numbers

American Health Care Association and National Center for Assisted Living. (2021, June 23). *Survey: 94 percent of nursing homes face staffing shortages. Press Release*. Survey: 94% of US nursing homes experiencing staff shortage amid pandemic.

American Medical Association. (2018). *Caring for the caregiver: A guide for physicians*. www. ama-assn.org/sites/ama-assn.org/files/corp/media-browser/public/public-health/caregiver-burnout-guide.pdf

Amstadter, A.B., Cisler, J.M., McCauley, J.L., Hernandez, M.A., Muzzy, W., & Acierno, R. (2011). Do incident and perpetrator characteristics of elder mistreatment differ by gender of the victim? Results from the national elder mistreatment study. *Journal of Elder Abuse & Neglect*, 23(1), 43–57. https://doi.org/10.1080/08946566.2011.534707

Andrews, D.A., & Bonta, J. (2010). *The psychology of criminal conduct* (5th ed.). Matthew Bender.

Anme, T. (2004). A study of elder abuse and risk factors in Japanese families: Focused on the social affiliation model. *Geriatrics & Gerontology International*, 4(s1), S262–S263. https://doi.org/ 10.1111/j.1447-0594.2004.00221.x

Aravanis, S.C. (2002). A profile of the national policy summit on elder abuse: Perspective and advice on replication. *Journal of Elder Abuse & Neglect*, 14(4), 55–69. https://doi.org/10.1300/J084v1 4n04_06

Association for Conflict Resolution & Florida Chapter of the Association of Family and Conciliation Courts. (n.d.). What is eldercaring coordination? Retrieved April 5, 2021, from www.eldercaringc oordination.com/description

Beach, S.R., Schulz, R., Castle, N.G., & Rosen, J. (2010). Financial exploitation and psychological mistreatment among older adults: Differences between African Americans and non-African Americans in a population-based survey. *The Gerontologist*, 50(6), 744–757. https://doi.org/ 10.1093/geront/gnq053

Bergmann, K., Manchee, V., & Woods, R.T. (1984). Effect of family relationships on psychogeriatric patients. *Journal of the Royal Society of Medicine*, 77, 91–95. https://doi.org/10.1177/0141076 88407701008

Berkman, L. F., Kawachi, I., & Glymour, M. M. (Eds.). (2014). *Social epidemiology* (2nd ed.). Oxford University Press.

Bhagat, V., & Htwe, K. (2018). A literature review of findings in physical and emotional abuse in elderly. *Research Journal of Pharmacy and Technology*, 11(10), 4731–4738. https://doi.org/ 10.5958/0974-360X.2018.00862.4

Board on Global Health, Institute of Medicine, National Research Council, & Forum on Global Violence Prevention. (2014). II.2 seven policy priorities for an enhanced public health response to elder abuse--marie-therese connolly and ariel trilling. In R.M. Taylor (Ed.), *Elder abuse and its prevention* (pp. 59–66). National Academies Press.

Borda, N.F., & Yarnoz, A.Z. (2015). Perceptions of abuse in nursing home care relationships in Uruguay. *Journal of Transcultural Nursing*, 26(2), 164–170. https://doi.org/10.1177/104365961 4526458

Brodish, P.H., & Hakes, J.K. (2016). Quantifying the individual-level association between income and mortality risk in the United States using the national longitudinal mortality study. *Social Science & Medicine*, 170, 180–187. https://doi.org/10.1016/j.socscimed.2016.10.026

Brown, A.S. (1989). A survey on elder abuse at one Native American tribe. *Journal of Elder Abuse & Neglect*, 1(2), 1738. https://doi.org/10.1300/J084v01n02_03

Bureau of Labor Statistics. (n.d.). U.S. department of labor, occupational outlook handbook: community health workers. www.bls.gov/ooh/community-and-social-service/community-health-workers.htm

Buri, H., Daly, J.M., Hartz, A.J., & Jogerst, G.J. (2006). Factors associated with self-reported elder mistreatment in Iowa's frailest elders. *Research on Aging*, 28(5), 562–581. https://doi.org/10.1177/0164027506289722

Burnes, D., Acierno, R., & Hernandez-Tejada, M. (2019a). Help-seeking among victims of elder abuse: Findings from the national elder mistreatment study. *The Journals of Gerontology. Series B, Psychological Sciences and Social Sciences*, 74(5), 891–896. https://doi.org/10.1093/geronb/gby122

Burnes, D., Lachs, M.S., & Pillemer, K. (2018). Addressing the measurement challenge in elder abuse interventions: need for a severity framework. *Journal of Elder Abuse & Neglect*, 30(5), 402–407. https://doi.org/10.1080/08946566.2018.1510354

Burnes, D., Pillemer, K., Caccamise, P.L., Mason, A., Henderson, C.R., Berman, J., Cook, A.M., Shukoff, D., Brownell, P., Powell, M., Salamone, A., & Lachs, M.S. (2015). Prevalence of and risk factors for elder abuse and neglect in the community: A Population-based study. *Journal of the American Geriatrics Society (JAGS)*, 63(9), 1906–1912. https://doi.org/10.1111/jgs.13601

Burnes, D., Pillemer, K., & Lachs, M.S. (2017). Elder abuse severity: A critical but understudied dimension of victimization for clinicians and researchers. *The Gerontologist*, 57(4), 745–756. https://doi.org/10.1093/geront/gnv688

Burnes, D., Sheppard, C., Henderson Jr., C.R., Wassel, M., Cope, R., Barber, C., & Pillemer, K. (2019b). Interventions to reduce ageism against older adults: A systematic review and meta-analysis. *American Journal of Public Health*, 109(8), e1–e9, 40. https://doi.org/10.2105/AJPH.2019.305123

Burston, G.R. (1975). Do your elderly patients live in fear of being battered? *British Medical Journal*, 3, 592. https://doi.org/10.1136/bmj.3.5983.592-a

Chang, E., & Levy, B. (2021). High prevalence of elder abuse during the COVID-19 pandemic: Risk and resilience factors. *American Journal of Geriatric Psychiatry*, 29(11), 1152–1159. https://doi.org/10.1016/j.jagp.2021.01.007. https://pubmed.ncbi.nlm.nih.gov/33518464/

Chang, E.S., Kannoth, S., Levy, S., Wang, S.Y., Lee, J.E., & Levy, B.R. (2020). Global reach of ageism on older persons' health: A systematic review. *PloS One*, 15(1), e0220857. https://doi.org/10.1371/journal.pone.0220857

Cohen, M., Halevy-Levin, S., Gagin, R., Priltuzky, D., & Friedman, G. (2010). Elder abuse in long-term care residences and the risk indicators. *Ageing and Society*, 30(6), 1027–1040. https://doi.org/10.1017/S0144686X10000188

Colello, K. (2020). The Elder Justice Act: Background and issues for Congress. *Congressional Research Services*, R43707. https://sgp.fas.org/crs/misc/R43707.pdf

Connolly, M.T., & Trilling, A. (2014). Seven policy priorities for an enhanced public health response to elder abuse. In *Forum on global violence prevention*; Board on Global Health; Institute of Medicine; National Research Council. Elder Abuse and Its Prevention: Workshop Summary. Washington, DC: National Academies Press (US); PMID: 24624478. www.ncbi.nlm.nih.gov/books/NBK208578/

Conrad, K.J, Liu, P.J., & Iris, M. (2019). Examining the role of substance abuse in elder mistreatment: Results from mistreatment investigations. *Journal of Interpersonal Violence*, 34(2), 366–391. https://doi.org/10.1177/0886260516640782

Curtain, S., Garnett, M., & Ahmad, F. (2023, November). *Provisional estimates of suicide by Demographic Characteristics: United States, 2022*. Vital Statistics Rapid Release; no 34. November 2023. https://doi.org/10.15620/cdc:133702

DeLiema, M. (2018). Elder fraud and financial exploitation: Application of routine activity theory. *The Gerontologist*, 58, 706–718. https://doi.org/10.1093/geront/gnw258

DeLiema, M., Gassoumis, Z.D., Homeier, D.C., & Wilber, K.H. (2012). Determining prevalence and correlates of elder abuse using promotores: Low income immigrant Latinos report high rates of abuse and neglect. *Journal of the American Geriatrics Society*, 60, 1333–1339.

Dong, X. (2005). Medical implications of elder abuse and neglect. *Clinics in Geriatric Medicine*, 21, 293–313. www.geriatric.theclinics.com/action/showPdf?pii=S0749-0690%2804%2900125-9

Dong, X., & Wang, B. (2017). Incidence of elder abuse in a U.S. Chinese population: Findings from the longitudinal cohort PINE study. *Journals of Gerontology Series A: Biological Sciences & Medical Sciences*, 72, S95–S101. https://doi.org/10.1093/gerona/glx005

Douglas, K.S., Hart, S.D., Groscup, J.L., & Litwack, T.R. (2013). Assessing violence risk. In I.B. Weiner & R.K. Otto (Eds.), *Handbook of forensic psychology* (4th ed., pp. 403–460). John Wiley & Sons.

Douglas, K.S., & Skeem, J.L. (2005). Violence risk assessment: Getting specific about being dynamic. *Psychology, Public Policy, and Law*, 11, 347–383. https://doi.org/10.1037/1076-8971.11.3.347

Duffy, A., Connolly, M., & Browne, F. (2024). Older people's experiences of elder abuse in residential care settings: A scoping review. *Journal of Advanced Nursing*, 80(6), 2214–2227. https://doi.org/10.1111/jan.15992

Eastman, M. (1980). Granny-battering: An unrecognised problem. *Community Care*, 310, 12–14.

Eastman, M. (1984). *Old age abuse*. Age Concern England.

Eastman, M., & Sutton, M. (1982). Granny battering. *Geriatric Medicine*, 12, 11–15.

Elder Abuse Protection Act of 2021, H.R. 2922, 117th Cong. (2021). www.congress.gov/bill/117th-congress/house-bill/2922

Elderabuse.org. (2019). Elder abuse policy and advocacy. Elder Abuse Policy and Advocacy – elderabuse.org.

Enguidanos, S., DeLiema, M., Aguilar, I., Lambrinos, J., & Wilber, K. (2014). Multicultural voices: Attitudes of older adults in the United States about elder mistreatment. *Aging and Society*, 34, 877–903. https://doi.org/10.1017/S0144686X12001389

Ermer, A.E., York, K., & Mauro, K. (2020). Addressing ageism using intergenerational performing arts interventions. *Gerontology & Geriatrics Education*, 42(3), 1–315. https://doi.org/10.1080/02701960.2020.1737046

Evans, C.S., Hunold, K.M., Rosen, T., & Platts-Mills, T.F. (2017). Diagnosis of elder abuse in U.S. emergency departments. *Journal of the American Geriatrics Society*, 65, 91–97. https://doi.org/10.1111/jgs.14480

Fang, B., Yan, E., Chan, K.L., & Ip, P. (2018). Elder abuse and its medical outcomes in older Chinese people with cognitive and physical impairments. *International Journal of Geriatric Psychiatry*, 33(8), 1038–1047. https://doi.org/10.1002/gps.4890

Fraga, S., Lindert, J., Barros, H., Torres-González, F., Ioannidi-Kapolou, E., Melchiorre, M.G., Stankunas, M., & Soares, J.F. (2014). Elder abuse and socioeconomic inequalities: A multilevel study in 7 European countries. *Preventive Medicine*, 61, 42–47. https://doi.org/10.1016/j.ypmed.2014.01.008

Friedman, L.S., Avila, S., Rizvi, T., Partida, R., & Friedman, D. (2017). Physical abuse of elderly adults: Victim characteristics and determinants of revictimization. *Journal of the American Geriatrics Society*, 65, 1420–1426. https://doi.org/10.1111/jgs.14794

Fulmer, T. (2013). Elder abuse and neglect assessment. *Journal of Gerontological Nursing*, 29(6), 4–5. https://doi.org/10.3928/0098-9134-20030601-04

Fulmer, T., Paveza, G. J., VandeWeerd, C., Guadagno, L., Fairchild, S., Norman, R., Abraham, I., & Bolton-Blatt, M. (2005). Neglect assessment in urban emergency departments and confirmation by an expert clinical team. *The Journals of Gerontology: Series A*, 60(8), 1002–1006.

Gao, X., Sun, F., Marsiglia, F.F., & Dong, X. (2019). Elder mistreatment among older Chinese Americans: The role of family cohesion. *International Journal of Aging & Human Development*, 88, 266–285. https://doi.org/10.1177/0091415018773499

Gilhooly, M. (1982). Social aspects of senile dementia. In R. Taylor & A. Gilmore (Eds.), *Current trends in British Gerontology*. Gower.

Goergen, T., & Beaulieu, M. (2010). Criminological theory and elder abuse research—Fruitful relationship or worlds apart? *Ageing International*, 35, 185–201. https://doi.org/10.1007/s12126-010-9063-2

Grocki, J.H., & Huffman, K.K. (2007). Medication adherence among older adults. *Journal of Evidence-Based Social Work*, 4(1–2), 97–120. www.tandfonline.com/doi/epdf/10.1300/J394v0 4n01_07?needAccess=true

Gunther, J. (2023). *The scope of elder financial exploitation: What it costs victims*. AARP Public Policy Institute. https://doi.org/10.26419/ppi.00194.001

Gurwitz, J.H. (2023). The paradoxical decline of geriatric medicine as a profession. *JAMA*, 330(8), 693–694. https://doi.org/10.1001/jama.2023.11110

Hall, J., Karch, D., & Crosby, A. (2016). Elder abuse surveillance: Uniform definitions and recommended core data elements. CDC, National Center for Injury Prevention and Control, Division of Violence Prevention. Elder Abuse Surveillance: Uniform Definitions and Recommended Data Elements (cdc.gov).

Hamby, S., Smith, A., Mitchell, K., & Turner, H. (2016). Polyvictimization and resilience portfolios: Trends in violence research that can enhance the understanding and prevention of elder abuse. *Journal of Elder Abuse & Neglect*, 28, 217–234. https://doi.org/10.1080/08946 566.2016.1232182

Hancock, D.W., Czaja, S., & Schulz, R. (2022). The role of preparedness for caregiving on the relationship between caregiver distress and potentially harmful behaviors. *American Journal of Alzheimer's Disease & Other Dementias*, 37, 1–7. https://doi.org/10.1177/15333175221141552

Hawes, C. (2003). Elder abuse in residential long-term care settings: What is known and what information is needed? In R.J. Bonnie & R.B. Wallace (Eds.), *National research council (US) panel to review risk and prevalence of elder abuse and neglect*. Elder Mistreatment: Abuse, Neglect, and Exploitation in an Aging America. National Academies Press (US). 14. Available from: www.ncbi. nlm.nih.gov/books/NBK98786/

Herman, C. (2024, May). *Older Americans month 2024: What is NASW doing to support social work with older adults?* Tips and tools for social workers. www.socialworkers.org/Practice/Tips-and-Tools-for-Social-Workers/Older-Americans-Month-2024

Herman, C. (with Anetzberger, G.J., Brandl, B., & Breckman, R). (2022, May). Social work roles in elder abuse prevention and response: A report by the National Association of Social Workers. National Association of Social Workers. https://bit.ly/NASW-SW-ElderJustice-2022

Ho, C.S.H., Wong, S.Y., Chiu, M.M., & Ho, R.C.M. (2017). Global prevalence of elder abuse: A meta-analysis and meta-regression. *East Asian Archives of Psychiatry*, 27(2), 43–55. www.proqu est.com/scholarly-journals/global-prevalence-elder-abuse-meta-analysis/docview/2792053609/se-2

Irving, S., & Hall, J. (2018). Elder abuse and the core function of public health: Using the 10 Essential public health services as a framework for addressing elder abuse. In P. Teaster & J. Hall (Eds.), *Elder abuse and the public's health* (pp. 19–44). Springer Publishing Company.

Jackson, S.L. (2015). The shifting conceptualization of elder abuse in the United States: From social services to criminal justice, and beyond. International Psychogeriatrics. *International Psychogeriatric Association* (2016), 28(1), 1–8. https://doi.org/10.1017/S1041610215001271

Jackson, S.L. (2016). All elder abuse perpetrators are not alike: The heterogeneity of elder abuse perpetrators and implications for intervention. *International Journal of Offender Therapy and Comparative Criminology*, 60(3), 265–285. https://doi.org/10.1177/0306624X14554063

Jackson, S.L., & Hafemeister, T.L. (2011). Risk factors associated with elder abuse: The importance of differentiating by type of elder maltreatment. *Violence and Victims*, 26, 738–757. https://doi.org/10.1891/0886-6708.26.6.738

Johannesen, M., & LoGuidice, D. (2013). Elder abuse: A systematic review of risk factors in community-dwelling elders. *Age and Ageing*, 42(3), 292–298. https://doi.org/10.1093/ageing/afs195

Johansson, A. (2018). Risk markers associated with caregiver elder abuse: A meta-analytic study (Doctoral dissertation). Loma Linda University.

Jones, N.L., Gilman, S.E., Cheng, T.L., Drury, S.S., Hill, C.V., & Geronimus, A.T. (2019). Life course approaches to the causes of health disparities. *American Journal of Public Health*, 109(S1), S48–S55. https://doi.org/10.2105/AJPH.2018.304738

Kawachi, I. (2002). Social epidemiology? *Social Science and Medicine*, 54(12), 1739–1741. https://doi.org/10.1016/S0277-9536(01)00144-7

Kawachi, I., & Subramanian, S.V. (2018). Social epidemiology for the 21st century. *Social Science & Medicine*, 196, 240–245. https://doi.org/10.1016/j.socscimed.2017.10.034

Krienert, J.L., Walsh, J.A., & Turner, M. (2009). Elderly in America: A descriptive study of elder abuse examining national incident-based reporting system (NIBRS) data, 2000–2005. *Journal of Elder Abuse & Neglect*, 21, 325–345. https://doi.org/10.1080/08946560903005042

Kristofferzon, M.L., Engström, M., & Nilsson, A. (2018). Coping mediates the relationship between sense of coherence and mental quality of life in patients with chronic illness: A cross-sectional study. *Quality of Life Research*, 27(7), 1855–1863. https://doi.org/10.1007/s11136-018-1845-0

Lachs, M.S., & Berman, J. (2011). *Under the radar: New York state elder abuse prevalence study*. Lifespan of Greater Rochester, Weill Cornell Medical Center of Cornell University, and NY City Department for the Aging. (nyc.gov).

Lachs, M.S., & Pillemer, K. (2015). Elder abuse. *The New England Journal of Medicine*, 373, 1947–1956. Elder Abuse (nejm.org).

Laumann, E.O., Leitsch, S.A., & Waite, L.J. (2008). Elder mistreatment in the United States: prevalence estimates from a nationally representative study. *The journals of gerontology. Series B, Psychological sciences and social sciences*, 63(4), S248–S254. https://doi.org/10.1093/geronb/63.4.S248

Lee, S.-Y., & Atteraya, M.S. (2019). Depression, poverty, and abuse experience in suicide ideation among older Koreans. *The International Journal of Aging and Human Development*, 88(1), 46–59. https://doi.org/10.1177/0091415018768256

Levy, B.R., Slade, M.D., Chang, E.S., Kannoth, S., & Wang, S.Y. (2020). Ageism amplifies cost and prevalence of health conditions. *The Gerontologist*, 60(1), 174–181. https://doi.org/10.1093/geront/gny131

Logan, J.E., Haileyesus, T., Ertl, A., Rostad, W.L., & Herbst, J.H. (2019). Nonfatal assaults and homicides among adults aged ≥60 years—United States, 2002–2016. *MMWR. Morbidity and Mortality Weekly Report*, 68(13), 297–302. https://doi.org/10.15585/mmwr.mm6813a1

Malmedal, W., Iversen, M.H., & Kilvik, A. (2015). Sexual abuse of older nursing home residents: A literature review. *Nursing Research and Practice*, 2015(2015), 1–7. https://doi.org/10.1155/2015/902515

Martin, R. (2008). Law, and public health policy. *International Encyclopedia of Public Health*, 30–38. https://doi.org/10.1016/B978-012373960-5.00236-7. Epub 2008 Aug 26. PMCID: PMC7150113.

McCreadie, C. (1991). *Elder abuse: An exploratory study*. Age Concern. Institute of Gerontology, King's College.

Montoya, V. (1997). Understanding and combating elder abuse in hispanic communities. *Journal of Elder Abuse & Neglect*, 9(2), 5–17. https://doi.org/10.1300/J084v09n02_02

Mysyuk, Y., Westendorp, R.G.J., & Lindenberg, J. (2016). How older persons explain why they became victims of abuse. *Age and Ageing*, 45(5), 695–702. https://doi.org/10.1093/ageing/afw1

Nagpaul, K. (1997). Elder abuse among Asian Indians: Traditional versus modern perspectives. *Journal of Elder Abuse & Neglect*, 9(2), 77–92. https://doi.org/10.1300/J084v09n02_07

National Advisory Committee on Rural Health and Human Services. (2015, March). Intimate partner violence in rural America: Policy Brief. Microsoft Word – IPV Brief (Final).docx (hrsa.gov).

National Association of Social Workers (NASW). (2010. NASW standards for social work practice with family caregivers of older adults: Standard 7, Advocacy. www.socialworkers.org/Practice/NASW-Practice-Standards-Guidelines/NASW-Standards-for-Social-Work-Practice-with-Family-Caregivers-of-Older-Adults#:~:text=Social%20workers%20shall%20advocate%20for,to%20meet%20their%20biopsychosocial%20needs

National Association of Social Workers (NASW). (2021, January 28). NASW releases its 2021 blueprint of federal social policy priorities [News release]. NASW releases its 2021 Blueprint of Federal Social Policy Priorities.

National Center on Elder Abuse (NCAE). (2012). *Abuse of residents of long-term care facilities* [Research brief]. National Center on Elder Abuse. www.centeronelderabuse.org/docs/ResearchBrief_LongTermCare_508web.pdf

National Center on Elder Abuse (NCAE). (2021). *Ageism.* NCEA Research Brief: Ageism (acl.gov).

National Council on Aging (NCOA). (2025). Depression & anxiety: *Suicide and older adults: What you should know.* www.ncoa.org/article/suicide-and-older-adults-what-you-should-know/

National Indigenous Elder Justice Initiative. (2023). Tribal elder protection team: Social Worker. https://iasquared.org/wp-content/uploads/2023/09/tribal-ept-social-worker.pdf

National Institutes on Aging. (n.d.). *The national institute on aging: strategic directions for research, 2020-2025. Goal F: Understand health disparities related to aging and develop strategies to improve the health status of older adults in diverse populations.* Health Disparities and Aging | NIA (nih.gov).

National Sheriff's Association. (2018). *Elder abuse: The rural response.* A law enforcement handbook. Elder Justice Initiative, US Department of Justice. www.justice.gov/elderjustice/law-enforcement-1

Naughton, C., Drennan, J., Lyons, I., Lafferty, A., Treacy, M., Phelan, A., O'Loughlin, A., & Delaney, L. (2012). Elder abuse and neglect in Ireland: results from a national prevalence survey. *Age Ageing*, 41, 98–103. http://refhub.elsevier.com/S0091-7435(14)00025-5/rf0060

Nicholls, T.L., Pritchard, M.M., Reeves, K.A., & Hilterman, E. (2013). Risk assessment in intimate partner violence: A systematic review of contemporary approaches. *Partner Abuse*, 4, 76–168. https://doi.org/10.1891/1946-6560.4.1.76

Nursing Home Abuse Center. (2024). *Sexual abuse: Sexual abuse of the elderly. Sexual abuse of the Elderly – Signs of sexual elder abuse (nursinghomeabusecenter.com).*

Oasis against Violence. (2021, October 01). Non-intimate partner violence. Non-Intimate Partner Violence (oasisagainstviolence.org).

O'Donnell, D., Treacy, M.P., Fealy, G., Lyons, I., & Lafferty, A. (2014). The case manage-ment approach to protecting older people from abuse and mistreatment: Lessons from the Irish experience. *British Journal of Social Work.* Advance online publication. https://doi.org/10.1093/bjsw/bcu027

Office of Inspector General. (2014). Adverse events in skilled nursing facilities: National incidence among medicare beneficiaries. (OEI-06-11-00370.) Washington, DC: Department of Health and Human Services. Adverse Events in Skilled Nursing Facilities: National Incidence among Medicare Beneficiaries (OEI-06-11-00370; 02/14).

Older Americans Act Amendments of 2006, Pub. L. No. 109-365, 120 Stat. 2522 (2006). www.govinfo.gov/content/pkg/PLAW-109publ365/pdf/PLAW-109publ365.pdf

Paranjape, A., Corbie-Smith, G., Thompson, N., & Kaslow, N.J. (2009). When older African American women are affected by violence in the home: A qualitative investigation of risk and protective factors. *Violence against Women*, 15(8), 977–990. https://doi.org/10.1177/1077801209335490

Patel, K., Bunachita, S., Chiu, H., Suresh, P., Patel, U.K. (2021). Elder abuse: A comprehensive overview and physician-associated challenges. *Cureus*, 13(4), e14375. https://doi.org/10.7759/cureus.14375

Perron, R. (2018). The value of experience: Age discrimination against older workers persists. *AARP Research*, 10. https://doi.org/10.26419/res.00177.002

Platts-Mills, T.F., Barrio, K., Isenberg, E.E., & Glickman, L. (2014). Emergency physician identification of a cluster of elder abuse in nursing home residents. *Annals of Emergency Medicine*, 64, 99–100. https://doi.org/10.1016/j.annemergmed.2014.03.023

Roberto, K.A. (2016). The complexities of elder abuse. *American Psychologist*, 71, 302–311.

Roberto, K.A., & Hoyt, E. (2021). Abuse of older women in the United States: A review of empirical research, 2017–2019. *Aggression and Violent Behavior*, 57, 101487. https://doi.org/10.1016/j.avb.2020.101487

Roberto, K.A., McCann, B.R., Teaster, P.B., & Hoyt, E. (2022). Elder abuse and the opioid epidemic: Evidence from APS cases in central Appalachia. *Journal of Rural Mental Health*, 46(1), 50–62. https://doi.org/10.1037/rmh0000181

Rodriguez, J.M., Geronimus, A.T., Bound, J., & Dorling, D. (2015). Black lives matter: differential mortality and the racial composition of the U.S. electorate, 1970-2004. *Social Science & Medicine*, 136–137, 93–199, https://doi.org/10.1016/j.socscimed.2015.04.014

Rogers, M.M., Storey, J.E., & Galloway, S. (2023). Elder mistreatment and dementia: A comparison of people with and without dementia across the prevalence of abuse. *Journal of Applied Gerontology*, 42(5), 909–918. https://doi.org/10.1177/07334648221145844

Rosay, A.B., & Mulford, C.F. (2017). Prevalence estimates and correlates of elder abuse in the United States: The national intimate partner and sexual violence survey. *Journal of Elder Abuse & Neglect*, 252390. U.S. Department of Justice: Office of Justice Programs. https://nij.ojp.gov/library/publications/prevalence-estimates-and-correlates-elder-abuse-united-states-national-0

Rosen, T., Zhang, H., Wen, K., Clark, S., Elman, A., Jeng, P., Baek, D., Zhang, Y., Gassoumis, Z., Fettig, N., Pillemer, K., Lachs, M., & Bao, Y. (2023). Emergency department and hospital utilization among older adults before and after identification of elder mistreatment. *JAMA Network Open*, 6(2), e2255853. https://doi.org/10.1001/jamanetworkopen.2022.55853

Shawon, R.A., Adhia, A., DeCou, C., & Rowhani-Rahbar, A. (2021). Characteristics and patterns of older adult homicides in the United States. *Injury Epidemiology*, 8(1), 1–11. https://doi.org/10.1186/s40621-021-00299-w

Sinha, D., Mishra, P.S., Srivastava, S., & Kumar, P. (2021). Socio-economic inequality in the prevalence of violence against older adults – findings from India. *BMC Geriatrics*, 21(1), 322–322. https://doi.org/10.1186/s12877-021-02234-6

Steidel, A.G.L., & Contreras, J.M. (2003). A new familism scale for use with Latino populations. *Hispanic Journal of Behavioral Sciences*, 25(3), 312–330. https://doi.org/10.1177/0739986303256912

Stevenson, O. (1989). *Age and vulnerability*. Age Concern England.

Stiegel, L.A. (2014). *Legal issues related to elder abuse a pocket guide for law enforcement commission on law and aging*. American Bar Association Commission on Law. ABA-ElderAbuseGuide.pdf

Storey, J.E. (2020). Risk factors for elder abuse and neglect: A review of the literature. *Aggression and Violent Behavior*, 50. https://doi.org/10.1016/j.avb.2019.101339

Teaster, P.B., & Hall, J.E. (Eds.). (2018). *Elder abuse and the public's health*. Springer.

Teaster, P.B., Ramsey-Klawsnik, H., Mendiondo, M.S., Abner, E., Cecil, K., & Tooms, M. (2007). From behind the shadows: A profile of the sexual abuse of older men residing in nursing homes. *Journal of Elder Abuse and Neglect*, 19(1–2), 29–45. https://doi.org/10.1300/J084v19n01_03

United States Centers for Disease Control and Prevention (CDC). (2024a, November 2). *About abuse of older persons: What is Older person abuse?* www.cdc.gov/elder-abuse/about/index.html

United States Centers for Disease Control and Prevention (CDC). (2024b, March 26). Suicide data and statistics | Suicide Prevention | CDC. www.cdc.gov/suicide/facts/data.html

United States Department of Justice. (n.d.a). *Elder justice initiative*. Elder Justice Initiative (EJI) | Elder Justice Initiative (EJI).

United States Department of Justice. (n.d.b). *Elder justice initiative: Abuse stories*. www.justice.gov/elderjustice/abuse-stories#Physical%20Abuse%20Stories

United States Department of Justice. (n.d.c). *Elder abuse statistics: Rural statistics*. www.justice.gov/elderjustice/rural-and-tribal-resources

United States Department of Justice. (2025, June 16). Justice department highlights enforcement efforts protecting older Americans from transnational fraud schemes in recognition of 2025 world elder abuse awareness day. www.justice.gov/opa/pr/justice-department-highlights-enforcement-efforts-protecting-older-americans-transnational#:~:text=News-,Justice%20Department%20Hig
hlights%20Enforcement%20Efforts%20Protecting%20Older%20Americans%20From%20Tr
ansnational,2025%20World%20Elder%20Abuse%20Awareness

United States Government Accountability Office. (2011). *Elder justice. Report of the chairman, special committee on aging, U.S. Senate.* GAO-11-208. Author.

U.S. Department of Health and Human Services. (2024). *Health care workforce: Key issues, challenges, and the path forward.* Office of the Assistant Secretary for Planning and Evaluation. https://aspe.hhs.gov/sites/default/files/documents/82c3ee75ef9c2a49fa6304b3812a4855/aspe-workforce.pdf

Van Orden, K.A., Witte, T.K., Cukrowicz, K.C., Braithwaite, S.R., Selby, E.A., & Joiner, T.E. (2010). The interpersonal theory of suicide. *Psychological Review*, 117(2), 575–600. https://doi.org/10.1037/a0018697

Vespa, J., Medina, L., & Armstrong, D. (2020). *Demographic turning points for the United States: Population projections for 2020 to 2060.* Current Population Reports, P25–1144. U.S. Census Bureau, Washington, DC. www.census.gov/content/dam/Census/library/publications/2020/demo/p25-1144.pdf

von dem Knesebeck, O. (2015). Concepts of social epidemiology in health services research. *BMC Health Services Research*, 15(1), 35357. https://doi.org/10.1186/s12913-015-1020-z

Voss, P., Bodner, E., & Rothermund, K. (2018). Ageism: The relationship between age stereotypes and age discrimination. In L. Ayalon & C. Tesch-Römer (Eds.), *Contemporary perspectives on ageism.* Springer International Publishing AG. https://doi.org/10.1007/978-3-319-73820-8_2

Wand, A., Peisah, C., Draper, B., & Brodaty, H. (2018). The nexus between elder abuse, suicide and assisted dying: The importance of relational autonomy and undue influence. *Macquarie Law Journal*, 18(6), 79–92. https://20.austlii.edu.au/cgi-bin/viewdoc/au/journals/MqLawJl/2018/6.html#fn24

Wang, F., Meng, L.I.R., Zhang, Q., Li, L., Nogueira, B.O.C.L., Ng, C.H., Ungvari, G.S., Hou, C.-L., Liu, L., Zhao, W., Jia, F.-J., & Xiang, Y.T. (2018). Elder abuse and its impact on quality of life in nursing homes in China. *Archives of Gerontology and Geriatrics*, 78, 155–159. https://doi.org/10.1016/j.archger.2018.06.011

Wang, X.M., Brisbin, S., Loo, T., & Straus, S. (2015). Elder abuse: An approach to identification, assessment and intervention. *CMAJ Canadian Medical Association Journal*, 187(8), 575–581. https://doi.org/10.1503/cmaj.141329

Warren, A., & Blundell, B. (2019). Addressing elder abuse in rural and remote communities: Social policy, prevention and responses. *Journal of Elder Abuse & Neglect*, 31(4–5), 424–436. https://doi.org/10.1080/08946566.2019.1663333

Wei, W., & Balser, S. (2024). *A systematic review: Risk and protective factors of elder abuse for community-dwelling racial minorities.* Sage. https://doi.org/10.1177/15248380221140123

Wei, W., Balser, S., Nguyen, A.W., & Qin, W. (2024). Elder abuse in older adults with dementia: Protective factors and adverse effects. *Trauma, Violence & Abuse*, 25(5), 3827–3842. https://doi.org/10.1177/15248380241265379

Weissberger, G.H., Goodman, M.C., Mosqueda, L., Schoen, J., Nguyen, A.L., Wilber, K.H., Gassoumis, Z.D., Nguyen, C.P., & Han, S.D. (2020). Elder abuse characteristics based on calls to the national center on elder abuse resource line. *Journal of Applied Gerontology*, 39(10), 1078–1087. https://doi.org/10.1177/0733464819865685

Williams, J.L., Racette, E.H., Hernandez-Tejada, M.A., & Acierno, R. (2020). Prevalence of elder polyvictimization in the United States: Data from the national elder mistreatment study. *Journal of Interpersonal Violence*, 35(21–22), 4517–4532. https://doi.org/10.1177/0886260517715604

World Health Organization (WHO). (2002). World report on violence and health. Geneva, Switzerland: WHO. www.who.int/publications/i/item/9241545615

World Health Organization (WHO). (2022). *Studies of abuse of older people prevalence.* Interactive global map by country and type of abuse using 214 studies. https://apps.who.int/violence-info/abuse-of-older-people

World Health Organization (WHO). (2024a, June 15). *Abuse of older people: Overview* [Fact sheet]. www.who.int/news-room/fact-sheets/detail/abuse-of-older-people

World Health Organization (WHO). (2024b). *Ageing and health.* Ageing and health (who.int).

Yon, Y., Ramiro-Gonzalez, M., Mikton, C.R., Huber, M., & Sethi, D. (2019). The prevalence of elder abuse in institutional settings: A systematic review and meta-analysis. *European Journal of Public Health*, 29(1), 58–67. https://doi.org/10.1093/eurpub/cky093

Yunus, R.M. (2021). The under-reporting of elder abuse and neglect: a Malaysian perspective. *Journal of Elder Abuse & Neglect*, 33(2), 145–150. https://doi.org/10.1080/08946566.2021.1919271

Yunus, R.M., Hairi, N.N., & Yuen, C.W. (2019). Consequences of elder abuse and neglect: A systematic review of observational studies. *Trauma, Violence, & Abuse*, 20(2), 197–213. https://doi.org/10.1177/1524838017692798

Zeanah, C.H., Gunnar, M.R., McCall, R.B., Kreppner, J.M., & Fox, N.A. (2011). VI. Sensitive periods. *Monographs of the Society for Research in Child Development*, 76(4), 147–162. https://doi.org/10.1111/j.1540-5834.2011.00631.x

Zhang, L.P., Du, Y.G., Dou, H.Y., & Liu, J. (2022). The prevalence of elder abuse and neglect in rural areas: A systematic review and meta-analysis. *European Geriatric Medicine*, 13(3), 585–596. https://doi.org/10.1007/s41999-022-00628-2

9

SUICIDE AND PUBLIC HEALTH

Introduction

A 30-year-old Black male, Tyrone, was brought from his place of employment by a personnel representative. Tyrone had been thinking of suicide "all the time" because he "can't cope." He said that he had a knot in his stomach; that his sleep and appetite were down (sleeps only 3 hours per night); and that he planned either to shoot himself, jump off a bridge, or drive recklessly off a ravine. He told about constant fighting with his wife, leading to a recent breakup (there is a long history of mutual verbal/physical abuse). His medical record also shows a history of serious suicide attempts, preceded by a divorce, wherein he jumped off a ledge and fractured both legs. He has been in a state of grieving because the attempt was not successful. There is a history of chemical dependency with two courses of treatment and there appears to be no current problem with alcohol or drugs. The patient is tearful, shaking, frightened, hopeless, and at a high risk for impulsive acting out. He states that life isn't worthwhile. He has also mentioned that he has been questioning his gender identity, an ongoing inner battle since early childhood, causing constant turmoil. He was raised in the church as a young boy and often worries about the forgiveness of "sin." "I don't know what to do!" he shouts, "I just want to die!" (*adapted from* Patterson, 1981, p. 24).

Suicide Defined

The National Institute of Mental Health (n. d.) defines *suicide* as "death caused by self-directed injurious behavior with the intent to die as a result of the behavior" (p. 1). A suicide attempt is a "non-fatal, self-directed, potentially injurious behavior with intent to die as a result of the behavior" (¶ 1), and suicidal ideation refers to "thinking about, considering, or planning suicide." Ideation may also encompass details of the suicide act, such as "when, where, and how," and the impact of one's suicide on others (Hawton & Fortune, 2008). Goodfellow and others (2019) found that most definitions of suicide have four consistent features allowing for the exploration of the meaning of suicide across countries and

DOI: 10.4324/9781003373001-9

cultures: "agency (self-or other-inflicted), knowledge of the potential fatal outcome, intent (to die, or other), and outcome (death, injury, or other)" (p. 490).

Nature and Extent of Suicide

Extent

Suicide is a leading cause of death in the U.S., but it is more prominent among some age groups. For all age groups and races combined, in 2021, it was the 11th leading cause of death. Suicide was the second cause of death among those 10–14 years old (n = 598) and 25–34 years old (n = 8,862), the third cause of death for those 15–24 (n = 6,528), the fifth cause of death for those 35–44 (n = 7,862), the seventh cause of death for those 45–54 (n = 7,400), and the ninth cause of death for those ages 55–64 (National Institute of Mental Health, n. d.). However, for Hispanics, the order of cause of death differed: suicide was the fourth cause of death among ages 10–14, the eighth cause of death for those 45–54, and was not listed as a leading cause of death for persons ages 55 and older. Between 2000 and 2021, there were steady increases in the suicide rate overall, but with some gender differences. In 2021, the suicide rate for males was four times that of females (22.8 per 100,000 and 5.7 per 100,000, respectively) and was highest for males ages 75 and older (42.2 per 100,000) (Centers for Disease Control and Prevention [CDC], n.d.b). For that same year, female suicides were highest for the age group 45–64 (8.2 per 100,000).

Nature

In 2021, the prominent methods of suicide for females were firearms (34.5%), suffocation (28.4%), and poisoning (27.8%). For males, the primary methods were firearms (59.8%) and suffocation (25.1%). In 2022, for ages 10–14, 51.9% of suicides were committed by suffocation, followed by firearms (35.5%), poisoning (8.5%), and falls (2.4%) (CDC, n.d.c). Suffocation was prominent for females (62.1%), whereas a firearm (47.2%) was dominant for males, followed by suffocation (45.5%). For those aged 15–24, the leading method of suicide was a firearm (53.7%), followed by suffocation (28%), poisoning (9.4%), and falls (3.3%) (CDC, n.d.d).

Suicide Ideation and Attempts

Ideation may be indicative of future suicide attempts and completions (Castle et al., 2011; Deykin & Buka, 1994). In 2022, the prevalence of suicidal ideation was 4.8%, or rather, over 12 million adults (Reinert et al., 2022). Ideation was highest among males and females ages 18–25 (13.6%) and for persons identifying as two or more races (9.3%–11%), followed by American Indian/Alaskan Native (7.0%), Black (5.5%), White (5.2%), Hispanic (4.6%), and Asian (3.4%) (Substance Abuse and Mental Health Services Administration [SAMHSA], 2022). The numbers were highest for ages 18–25. *Suicide attempt* trends demonstrated Blacks had a rate of 0.9% and Whites, along with Hispanics, a rate of 0.6%—showing lower rates of attempts compared to ideation for these three groups (SAMHSA, 2022). Richesson and Hoenig (2021) reported that the age group with the highest percentage of attempts was 18–25 (1.9%), followed by ages 26–49 (0.4%), and ages 50+ (0.1%).

Types of Suicide

LGBTQIA Adults

The prevalence of LGBTQIA suicides is difficult to calculate. Currently, there is no U.S. agency collecting sexual orientation and/or gender identity decedent information, and transgender decedents are misgendered on death certificates and other documents (Clark & Blosnich, 2024; Haas et al., 2019). The most accurate LGBT suicide numbers are for those who self-report having prior suicide attempts, ideation, and plans. The Trevor Project (2023) reported that 1.4 million U.S. LGB adults, ages 18–25, had suicidal thoughts in the past year. In 2020, approximately 81% of U.S. transgender adults reported suicide ideation, 42% reported prior attempts, and 56% demonstrated nonfatal self-injurious behaviors (Krueger et al., 2020). Among the 10.4% of transgender decedents recorded in the National Violent Death Reporting System (NVDRS) from 2003 to 2014, 67.7% were documented as male-to-female, 10.8% female-to-male, and 21.5% were in the process of transitioning or their self-identified gender was unknown (Lyons et al., 2019, p. 3). Moreover, Ramchand and others (2021b), by analyzing 2015–2019 data from the National Survey on Drug Use and Health, found that suicide risk for LGB adults was three to six times higher than for heterosexual adults, even when considering age, race, and ethnicity. They discovered that between 12% and 17% of gay and bisexual men had suicidal ideation in the past 12 months, 5% had a plan, and roughly 2% attempted. The survey also showed that between 11% and 20% of lesbian and bisexual women experienced suicidal thoughts in the past 12 months, 7% had a plan, and approximately 3% attempted. LGBTQIA community subgroup differences were found among 41,412 college students (Horwitz et al., 2020). "Among sexual minorities, those identifying as pansexual, bisexual, queer, or mostly gay/ lesbian had greater odds of endorsing 2+ suicide risk factors relative to students identifying as mostly heterosexual, gay/lesbian, [or] asexual" (p. 1). Pansexual students had higher odds compared with bisexual students for reporting two or more suicide risk factors.

Circumstances surrounding LGBTQIA suicides include mental health or substance use disorders and intimate partner or family relationship problems (Lyons et al, 2019; Patten et al., 2022), stigma and discrimination (Moagi, 2021), income and employment status (Hanley, 2021), and minority stress caused by added, chronic stress experienced over a lifetime from stigmatization and discrimination due to "social processes, institutions, and structures" (Meyer, 2003, p. 4) beyond the individual's control. Survey data from 445 asexual study participants revealed that this subgroup reports higher levels of depression compared with non-asexual persons (Lech et al., 2024). Forty-two percent of asexual participants were aged 18–25 years and 36.4% ages 26–35, while 44% identified as female, and 33% as queer.

Approximately 1.7% of the population identify as *intersex*, characterized by "differences in sex traits or reproductive anatomy" (Interact, n.d.). As with those identifying as asexual, there has been little research devoted to their mental health, including suicidal behavior. The mental health of intersex people is usually embedded in the analysis of other LGBTQIA-focused studies that demonstrate the elevated risks for suicide ideation, attempts, and nonfatal self-injuries, such as that of Marchi et al. (2022). Australian research revealed in a sample of 46 intersex participants ages 18–67, 87% (n = 40) had experienced suicidal thoughts, 52.6% (n = 20) attempted suicide, and 81% (n = 31) had, at some time, been diagnosed with depression (Amos et al., 2023). These results mirror a national health study of 198 intersex adults ages 18 and older, where 61% had been diagnosed with a depressive disorder, 62.6% with an anxiety disorder, and 81% with PTSD. Only 14.3% indicated that they had never considered suicide, while 25.4% had suicidal thoughts, 28.6% had a plan, 10.1% attempted but did not want to die, and 21.7% attempted and hoped to die (Rosenwohl-Mack et al., 2020).

Adolescents
According to the National Youth Risk Behavior Survey (NYRBS) (CDC, 2024e), mental health for high schoolers has worsened since 2013 with key areas most affected including the number of students experiencing persistent feelings of sadness/hopelessness (four of ten students), who seriously considered suicide (two of ten), and made a plan and attempted suicide (one in ten). Female and LGBTQ students had the highest numbers for suicidal thoughts and behaviors. American Indians/Alaskan Natives (AI/AN) youth (male and female) had the highest percentage of students having persistent feelings of sadness/hopelessness (45%), followed by Hispanic students (42%), multiracial students (41%), Black students (40%), and White students (39%). Of all genders and ethnicities, LGBTQ students scored more than twice the rate of cisgendered and heterosexual students at 65% versus 31%, respectively. Of students attempting suicide during the last 12 months, at the time of the survey, the majority were female (13%), Native Hawaiian/Pacific Islander (NH/PI) (15%), and LGBTQ (20%).

Between 2007 and 2021, suicide rates for youth ages 10–24 increased by 62%, jumping from 6.8% to 11.0 % per 100,000 (Curtain & Garnett, 2023). In 2020, approximately 3 million U.S. adolescents, ages 12–17, had serious thoughts about suicide, 1.3 million made a plan, and 629,000 attempted suicide (Richesson & Hoenig, 2021). In 2020, there were 6,643 completed suicides for persons ages 10–24 (CDC, n.d.c, n.d.d). According to Reinert and others (2022), 16% of youth reported experiencing at least one major depressive episode, and more than 2.7 youth experienced severe major depression. However, 60% of youth with major depression did not receive treatment, and more than 1.2 million youth having private insurance did not have coverage for mental health services.

Factors related to childhood and adolescent suicide that transcend ethnicity include adverse childhood experiences (ACEs) (Bowen et al., 2022; Camacho & Henderson, 2022); lack of parent or caregiver support (King et al., 2018); parental incarceration (Quinn et al., 2022); community violence (Lambert et al., 2022); school bullying (Benbenishty et al., 2018); social determinants of health leading to hopelessness, or despair (Shanahan & Copeland, 2021); social media (Macrynikola et al., 2021), including cyberbullying (Romanelli et al., 2022); substance use (Rizk et al., 2021); and access to lethal means, such as firearms (Morris-Perez et al., 2023). Research demonstrated that youth with access to firearms had 1.52 times greater odds of experiencing suicide ideation and 1.61 times higher odds of prior suicide attempts (Kemal et al., 2023). Other factors include connectedness at school, unstable housing, racism in school, and experiencing unfair discipline at school (CDC, 2024c).

Black Youth
In 2018, suicide became the second leading cause of death for Black youth ages 10–14 and the third cause of death for Black youth aged 15–19 (Bridge et al., 2018). Black male high school students reported suicide attempts requiring medical attention more than White male students (Gaylor et al., 2023). Research reveals, Black youth engage in and

complete treatment for depression at lower rates than White youth, and outpatient mental health treatment less than White youth, even after a suicide attempt (Fontanella et al., 2020; Gordan, 2020). These disparities, in addition to suicide rates, may reflect that Black youth lack access to mental health services and/or Black youth distrust those in the helping professions.

Hispanic Youth

From 2010 to 2019, the rate of suicide for Hispanic youth ages 11 years and younger increased by 92.3%, making suicide the seventh leading cause of death for Latino children (Price & Khubchandani, 2022). Specifically, suicide was greater for males (59.6%) and for those ages 10–12 years (94.9%). Research suggests that suicides could be linked to inequities for this population owing to a lack of access to care, unmet mental health needs, and low socioeconomics. Hispanics were found to use mental health services at a significantly lower rate than non-Hispanics, possibly due to shame and stigma linked to having a diagnosis, fear of deportation, and religious concerns (Caplan, 2019).

LGBTQ Youth

According to the 2023 NYRBS, transgender and questioning students had the highest rates of poor mental health (42.6% and 53.7%, respectively) when compared to their cisgender counterparts (CDC, 2024c). The Trevor Project (2023) reported that 46% of transgender and non-binary youth ages 13–24, compared to 30% of cisgender youth, considered suicide during 2023. In addition, 14% of transgender and non-binary youth, compared to 7% of cisgender youth, attempted suicide. This disparity was consistent when examining CDC data (Suarez et al., 2024) for serious consideration of attempting suicide in the last 12 months, making a suicide plan in the last 12 months, attempting suicide in the previous 12 months, and having a suicide attempt medically treated in the last 12 months. Of those 14% LGBTQ youth attempting suicide, only 11% were White compared with youth of color: 22% Indigenous, 18% Middle Eastern/Northern African, 17% multiracial, 16% Black, 15% Latinx, and 10% Asian American or Pacific Islander (The Trevor Project, 2023).

Conversion therapy, considered as a form of victimization, is a treatment aimed at converting an LGB person's sexual orientation, played a significant role in suicide ideation and attempts. For 2023, 27% of U.S. LGBTQ youth who were exposed to conversion therapy attempted suicide, and 27% of those threatened with conversion therapy committed suicide (The Trevor Project, 2023). Other forms of victimization, linked to gender identity and/or sexual orientation that are associated with increased suicide attempts and abuse happen in schools: verbal harassment, restrictions in dressing according to gender identity of choice, disciplinary sanctions for fighting back against bullies, unwanted sexual contact, and physical attacks. Failure to have gender-affirming spaces at school or home accounted for 16% and 18% of LGBTQ suicide attempts in 2023 (The Trevor Project, 2023). Of the 81% of LGBTQ youth who wanted mental health treatment, only 44% were able to access care. Barriers to care included fear of talking about mental health issues (47%), not wanting to get parental consent (41%), fear of not being taken seriously (40%), and cost (38%) (The Trevor Project, 2023).

Military

During 2022, 6,407 veteran suicides were equally 17.6 per day—271 females and 6,136 males making suicide the 12th leading cause of death for veterans, but the second leading cause of death for those younger than age 45 (United States Department of Veteran Affairs [USDVA], 2024b). Suicide was highest for veterans between the ages of 18 and 34, followed by those ages 35–54. Approximately 73% of these suicides involved a firearm, followed by suffocation, and poisoning. The rate of suicide was higher (50.4%) among those who had recently used Veteran's Health Administration (VHA) care than those who did not (49.6%). Research suggests there are several reasons why these veterans have a higher suicide risk: lower annual income (USDVA, 2024b), poorer self-reported health status (Agha et al., 2000), increased chronic medical diagnoses (Dursa et al., 2016), self-reported disability due to physical or mental health conditions (Nelson, 2007), greater depression and anxiety (Fink et al., 2022), greater reporting of trauma, lifetime psychopathology, and current suicidality (Meffert et al., 2019).

The average number of veteran suicides per day rose between 2001 and 2022, from 16.5% to 17.6%, respectively (USDVA, 2024b). The rates of suicide for veterans 12 months following their separation from active duty fluctuated between 2010 (34.8%) and 2021 (46.2%) (USDVA, 2024b). Among military branches, between 2010 and 2021, Marine veterans had the highest rate of suicide, followed by the Army, Navy, and Air Force. Of diagnoses given to decedents 12 months before active military separation, the rates were highest for suicidal ideation and substance use disorder, followed by "mental health" (p. 16). Suicide for veterans with the diagnoses of "other psychoses" reached the rate of 207.1 per 100,000, surpassing bipolar disorder (125.4) and schizophrenia (92.6) (USDVA, 2024a, p. 18). The 2022 rate of veteran suicide for those diagnosed with a sedative use disorder was found to be 236.7 per 100,000, an increase of 29.2% from 2021.

Other veteran suicide risk factors include homelessness, military sexual trauma (MST), and being involved in justice programs (USDVA, 2024a). Homelessness among veterans was found as a factor among decedents at a rate (per 100,000) ranging from approximately 80 (2014) to 79 (2022), with a spike above 100 occurring sometime in mid-2021. Between 2009 and 2022, for both males and females, the rates of suicide were higher among veterans experiencing MST. The rates of veteran suicide decedents, for both genders, were approximately 75% higher among those who disclosed MST than those who did not. The rate of suicides for female veterans who reported MST fell 18% from 2021 to 2022 (for those who recently utilized VHA services). However, for male veterans who recently used VHA and disclosed MST, the suicide rate rose by 37.5% from 2021 to 2022.

Active military suicide rates are also considerable. In 2022, the rate, per 100,000, was 25.1% or 331 decedents, highest for the Marine Corps (34.9%), followed by the Army (28.9%), Navy (20.6%), and Air Force (19.7%), a gradual increase from 2011 (United States Department of Defense [USDOD], 2023). Of these decedents, 93.1% were male and 6.9% female, 71.6% White, 15.4% Black, 5.4% Asian, and 1.2% AI/AN. Most were in the age group of 20–24 years (40.8%), followed by 25–29 years (22.1%), 30–34 years (15.4%), and 35–39 years (11.5%), similar to veteran statistics. While only 7.3% of decedents were commissioned officers, 90.9% were enlisted (E1–E4: 46.2% and E5–E9: 44.7%, respectively). As with veteran suicides, the primary method was a firearm, followed by hanging. Investigations revealed that mental health (45%), intimate relationship problems (42%), work problems (26%), administrative or legal concerns (26%), and financial strain (10%) were life stressors known to have been experienced by decedents pre-suicide. Mental health issues included substance use disorder, depression, anxiety, trauma or stress-related disorders, and sleep disorders (USDOD, 2023)—another similarity to veteran suicides. Data from 2022 also showed that there were 64 reservist suicides and 97 National Guard suicides. While there were many completed suicides, there were also 1,278 attempted suicides that involved the use of poison.

While military suicides typically refer to military personnel decedents, less attention is given to military family member suicides. In 2022, 114 spouses and 54 dependents ended their lives, involving active duty, reserve, and National Guard families (USDOD, 2023). Of spousal decedents, 52% were female, and 84% were younger than 40 years. Nearly 50% of spousal decedents were active duty or veterans. Of dependent decedents, 30% were female and 69% were younger than 18 years old. As with most military suicides, the primary method of death was a firearm.

Elder Suicides

The 2022 suicide rate in the U.S. was highest (23%) for persons aged 85 and older, those aged 75–84 (20.3%), 45–54 (19.2%), and 25–34 (19%) (CDC, 2025). From the 49,449 confirmed suicides in 2022, there were over 8,000 aged 65+, primarily male decedents (National Center for Health Statistics, 2024). Elder suicide may go unnoticed as death among the elderly is common. The human lifespan in many countries has increased significantly and doubled in some (Crimmins, 2015). According to Bell and Miller (2005), life expectancy at ages 65 and 85 increased nearly 50% over the past 100 years. However, a longer lifespan does not equate to a healthier or happier life. Gimeno and colleagues (2024) found that while years of living have increased in America and other high-income countries, younger cohorts have reported more self-reported doctor-diagnosed chronic diseases, such as diabetes, high cholesterol, and moderate disability. There have also been demonstrated increases in multimorbidity (Bishop et al., 2022) as well as cancer, hypertension, and lung and heart disease in the U.S. (Beltrán-Sánchez et al., 2016; Payne, 2022).

Research finds that there are many factors linked to unhealthy longevity that often influence the decision to commit suicide. They include isolation, loss of independence, reliance on others, loss of dignity, cognitive impairment, decreased quality of life, lower sense of meaning and life purpose, and perceived diminished personal value and self-esteem (Fässberg et al., 2016). Functional impairment is common, as is loneliness, pain, and the development of depression. Loneliness may be thought of as the absence of reciprocal relationships or disconnection, often resulting from family dysfunction and/or abuse (Joiner, 2005; Van Orden et al., 2010). Alexopoulos and colleagues (1999) found that the severity of depression was the predominant determinant of suicidal behavior and that elders with severe depression, a history of suicide attempts, and poor social support were at the highest risk of suicide.

Explaining the Roots of Suicide

According to Mueller and colleagues (2021), Emile Durkheim's *Suicide: A Study in Sociology (2005)*, first published in 1858, provides two major principles about suicide: suicide rates are a function of the structure of social relationships, and social relationships are varied by "level of integration and [moral] regulation" (p. 2). Durkheim wrote that "[Suicide] must necessarily depend upon social causes and be in itself a collective phenomenon" (Durkheim, 2005, p. 97), believing that social types of suicide should be classified by the social conditions that caused the suicide. Social integration refers to the closeness of collective relationships providing people with life purpose and meaning (Mueller et al., 2021). Durkheim (2005) wrote about two kinds of external individual conditions that may lead to suicide: external circumstances, such as events and situations in one's life—which Durkheim did not consider the determining cause of suicide, and "the moral constitution of society [which] establishes the contingent of voluntary deaths," further described as "a definite amount of energy, impelling men to self-destruction . . . a prolongation of a social condition which they express externally" (p. 263). This condition, he purported, is responsible for suicide rates in any society and, therefore, explains the variations found globally. In short, although someone might be quick to blame an individual's emotional state or financial status for self-destruction, the real reason, believed by Durkheim, was the consistent state of the social environment in which one's relationships were embedded. According to Mueller and colleagues (2021), those without collective belonging would not have the protection from suicides resulting from isolation.

Klonsky and May (2015) offer a different theory—the *Three-Step Theory (3ST)* in which there is a progression from suicide ideation to following through with the act. Step One hypothesizes that *ideation* occurs due to the compounding effects of psychological pain (or any pain) and hopelessness, against which connectedness is a protective factor from *ideation escalation* (Step Two). Step Three is the progression from ideation escalation to attempts "as facilitated by dispositional, acquired, and practical contributors to the capacity to attempt suicide" (p. 114). Does the person have the necessary wherewithal to complete an attempt? Klonsky and May (2015) build upon Thomas Joiner's *The Interpersonal Theory of Suicide* wherein high capacity brings high potentially lethal self-harm: fearlessness—not being afraid of pain—is required to follow through with ideation, along with a sense of burdensomeness on others and feeling "hopelessly alienated" (Joiner, 2010).

What are the Risk Factors

Role of Inequity in Suicide

Many forms of inequity contribute to the occurrence of suicide among disadvantaged populations: insufficient insurance coverage to pay for mental health treatment, stigma of being diagnosed and/or receiving help, systemic racism (e.g., implicit, explicit, short- or long term, and generational), and linguistic and cultural barriers and biases occurring in interactions between patients and providers (SAMHSA, 2024). Consequently, there are long wait times for receiving services, a decreased quality of care, limited community treatment options, and a mistrust of medical institutions that result in the avoidance of pursuing help. Inequity can be found among any demographic of people. However, for this discussion, we will focus on Black/African-American, and Indian/Alaskan Native peoples due to their higher rates of suicide compared with other populations.

Black and African-American Youth and Adults

The suicide rate of Blacks and African-Americans has remained lower than non-Hispanic Whites: 50% lower in 2020 (CDC, 2022). However, the rate has been climbing steadily. Castle and colleagues (2011) found that Black male suicide was likely connected to suicide and death ideation (SDI), especially when there was also severe depression (Garlow, 2008). However, it was discovered that SDI could occur in the absence of depression (Joo et al., 2016) while still associated with emotional distress (Ribeiro et al., 2018). Kogen and colleagues (2024) found, depression aside, that childhood adversities, including racial discrimination, characterized by both deprivation and threat, were linked to self-reporting of SDI in a study relying on a sample of 504 Black men with a mean age of 20 years. A national study found that participants who had experienced childhood adversities were three times more likely to consider suicide than those without adversities (Thompson et al., 2019).

Black men and women in the U.S. are disproportionately exposed to childhood adversities (Dumornay et al., 2023) encompassing abuse and neglect, community violence, substance use, family disengagement, and incarceration (Felitti et al., 1998) as well as adulthood adversities such as continuous, multidimensional, and contextual discrimination in many areas of life (e.g., housing, finances, employment, policing, and education) that can be generational (Bernard et al., 2021). Black young women, particularly between the ages of 15–24 and 25–34, are disproportionately affected by the national suicide upswing that occurred between 2018 and 2020 (Joseph et al., 2023; Price & Khubchandani, 2019; Ramchand et al., 2021a). While specific drivers of these suicides are still under investigation, systematic racial discrimination (Polanco-Roman et al., 2019), an increase in youth cyberbullying (Arnon et al., 2022), neighborhood factors (e.g., domestic violence, community violence, and poverty) that lead to poor mental health with limited access to services (Lacey et al., 2015; Goodwill & Yasui, 2022), workplace discrimination (Parker et al., 2022), and maternal health stressors (Ertel et al., 2012) have been cited as possible suicide factors. Research also suggests that Black youth engage in and complete treatment for depression at lower rates and receive outpatient mental health treatment less than White youth, even after a suicide attempt (Gordan, 2020). These disparities, in addition to suicide rates, may be, in part, due to a lack of access to mental health services.

American Indians and Alaskan Natives (AI/AN) Youth and Adults

Non-Hispanic AI/AN, when compared to the U.S. general population (GP), have a higher rate of suicide. Suicide was the second leading cause of death for these populations in 2022 for ages 10–34 (CDC, n.d.b). In 2021, the suicide rate for AI/AN young females, between ages 10 and 14, was over five times that for non-Hispanic females of the same age group (CDC, n.d.c). In 2020, the AI/NA suicide rate was 23.9% compared to the U.S. overall rate of 13.5%, despite AI/NA persons composing only 1.3% of the U.S. population (CDC, 2020). The rate for AI/AN suicide between 2011 and 2020 was highest for those between ages 25 and 34 (38.2%) followed by ages 15–24 (34.5%), 35–44 (29%), and 45–54 (20.7%) (CDC, 2020). AI/NA suicide rates for males over the same period were 33.6% and 10.3% for females compared to the U.S. overall numbers of 22.9% and 6.2%, respectively (CDC, 2020). The prevalence rate for AI/NA high school youth reporting injurious suicide attempts in 2023 was 5.2%, who seriously considered suicide was 24.5%, and who made a plan to attempt suicide was 25.7%—all higher than for any other race (CDC, n.d.a).

Stone and colleagues (2022) published results on AI/NA suicides from the 2015–2020 state-based NVDRS surveillance system. This study reported on 3,397 AI/NA suicides. Causal factors included relationship problems or loss, other life stressors, crises or anticipated crises, and mental health or substance use treatment. While specific drivers of these suicides are still being investigated, a significant factor was violence. When compared with non-Hispanic White women, violence rates for AI/NA women were significantly higher. Using data from the National Intimate Partner and Sexual Violence Survey (NISVS) (U.S. Department of Health and Human Services [U.S.DHSS], 2016), Rosay (2016) found that AI/AN:

> women are 1.2 times as likely as non-Hispanic White-only women to have experienced violence in their lifetime, 1.7 times as likely to have experienced violence in the past year, . . . more likely to have experienced stalking and physical violence by an intimate partner, as well as psychological aggression by an intimate partner.

Relying on the same NISVS data, Rosay (2016) discovered that AI/NA men were:

> 1.3 times as likely as non-Hispanic White-only men to have experienced lifetime violence in their lifetime, . . . 1.4 times as likely to have experienced physical violence by an intimate partner, and 1.4 times as likely to have experienced psychological aggression by an intimate partner.

Largely, the perpetrators of this violence have been non-AI/NA for both female (97%) and male (90%) victims (National Institute of Justice, n.d.). This could mean that the violence against AI/NA persons is largely racially motivated and a form of overt discrimination. AI/AN peoples have historically been the victims of genocide, forced displacement, and colonization, in addition to racism leading to generational trauma (Edwards & Kelton, 2020). Generational adversity can lead to what is known as epigenesis, or rather, genetic changes that leave individuals more susceptible to generational occurrences of adverse health, stress, disease, and mortality (Lehrner & Yehuda, 2018).

Individual Factors

Many individual risk factors have been linked to suicidal behaviors, although it is rare that only a single factor is considered causative. Some factors include an individual's past suicide attempts, serious illness or chronic pain, a history of criminality or legal issues, job loss or financial struggles, impulsivity or aggressive predispositions, and prior victimization or perpetration (CDC, 2024a). The more common factors include substance use, a history of mental illness (such as depression), a sense of hopelessness (CDC, 2024a), and ACEs (Camacho & Henderson, 2022).

Adverse Childhood Experiences

ACEs can be a pivotal factor in suicidal behavior for youth and adults. ACEs are traumatic events occurring in childhood that are associated with negative health outcomes throughout the lifespan and are prevalent in the lives of underserved and underprivileged populations—those most likely to live through frequent or prolonged stressful experiences (Bowen et al., 2022). These events are not in isolation but are considered *intersectional* with other risk factors involving politics, geographics, economics, social factors, and intergenerational inequities and trauma (Camacho & Henderson, 2022). Some events that are considered traumatic include emotional, physical, and sexual abuse, physical neglect, witnessing violence against your mother, growing up in a household where someone is using alcohol and other drugs and/or is mentally ill, losing a parent due to separation or divorce, and growing up with someone who is incarcerated (University of Rochester Medical Center [URMC], 2014). A seminal study on ACEs was conducted by Permanente using a survey distributed to approximately 27,000 patients (Felitti et al., 1998). The results revealed that nearly 63% of patients who completed the survey had experienced at least one traumatic event, while more than 20% had experienced three or more events (URMC, 2014). It was concluded that exposure to one adverse event equated to an 80% likelihood of experiencing another (Felleti et al., 1998). The study showed that the more traumatic incidents one encountered, the greater their risk for experiencing one or more of the following: "alcoholism and alcohol abuse, chronic obstructive pulmonary disease, depression, fetal death, poor health quality of life, illicit drug use, ischemic heart disease, liver disease, risk of intimate partner violence, *and suicide* among others" (p. 2).

Substance Abuse and Mental Health

In the U.S. GP, 50 million people reported having a mental health condition in 2022. Of that number, 55% did not receive treatment due to cost or lack of access (Reinert et al., 2022). The prevalence was highest for ages 18–25 (30.6%), followed by ages 26–49 (25.3%), and 50+ (14.5%) (Richesson & Hoenig, 2021). According to NVDRS data, approximately 46% of suicide decedents had a known mental health diagnosis (USDHSS, 2016). Global studies have found correlations between mental illness and suicide risk. For example, higher rates of suicide were linked to bipolar disorder in Denmark and Sweden (Hoyer et al., 2000; Osby et al., 2001). Elevated rates of suicide were found among patients diagnosed with schizophrenia in England (Hunt et al., 2006). In a Finland study of 137,112 persons diagnosed with bipolar disorder and schizophrenia, 1,475 committed suicide within one year of their first episode featuring psychosis (Sariaslan et al., 2023). Bertolote and colleagues (2004) examined suicides that occurred in Europe and North America. They found that when suicidal decedent deaths from a psychiatric inpatient hospital population (HP) and the GP were combined, 30.2% of the decedents were diagnosed with a mood disorder (20.8 HP versus 44.5–34.3 GP), 17.6% with a substance use disorder (9.8 HP versus 19.2–23.0 GP), 14.1 schizophrenia (19.9 HP versus 7.5–11.2 GP), personality disorders 13% (15.2 HP versus 3.2–13.1 GP), and organic mental disorder 6.3% (15.0 HP versus 2.1–.9 GP). The diagnoses most prevalent with the HP group were schizophrenia, personality, and organic mental disorders, while mood disorders and substance-related disorders were most prevalent in the GP group. In another comparative investigation, a Korean study, by Song and colleagues (2020), examined 40,692 non-suicidal GP deaths and 597 suicidal deaths. The suicides had occurred among persons who were psychiatric outpatient users, had been hospitalized in a psychiatric ward, or had received a psychiatric consultation. The study found the rate of suicide for psychiatric patients to be 5.13 times higher than in the GP. Among those 597 suicidal deaths, 187 patients were diagnosed with severe mental illness (psychotic disorder), 138 with depressive disorder, 71 with organic mental disorder, 68 with bipolar disorder, 39 with anxiety disorder, and 20 with substance use disorder. Substance use is linked to violence in general and should not exclude violence toward self or suicide. According to the U.S. NVDRS data (USDHSS, 2016), AI/NA suicide decedents were more likely than non-AI/NA decedents to have a substance use problem, with higher odds of alcohol, amphetamine, or marijuana use. However, other, non-AI/NA suicide decedents were more likely to have had problems with "opioids, benzodiazepines, cocaine, antidepressants, antipsychotics, or barbiturates" (Stephensen, 2022). Emerson and colleagues (2017), using 2012–2013 U.S. National Epidemiologic Survey on Alcohol and Related Conditions-III data, found PTSD and alcohol use disorder were present in 9.5% of AI/NA men suicide decedents and 3.1% of non-Hispanic White men decedents, and in 4.3% of AI/NA women decedents compared to 1.8% of non-Hispanic White women decedents (Emerson et al., 2017). Reinert and colleagues (2022) found that while 15% of adults were diagnosed with a substance use disorder, 93.5% did not receive treatment.

The combination of alcohol use and any mental health disorder can lead to injury and/ or death. According to the NVDRS (USDHSS, 2016), the rate of AI/NA suicide decedents with reported alcohol use was 31.4%, alcohol used in hours before death, 30.8%, and *any* current mental health diagnosis, 41.5% including depression (29.4%), bipolar disorder (5%), and PTSD (3.1%). Of 1,431 AI/NA decedents, 19.4% were currently involved in mental health or substance use disorder treatment, and 29.5% had a history of treatment (USDHSS, 2016).

Relationship Factors

According to the CDC (2024a), relationship factors that can be a risk for suicide include bullying, a family member's history of suicide, loss of relationships, conflictual or violent relationships, and social isolation. Stanley and colleagues (2023) report that a precursor to adult suicide may be intimate partner problems (IPP) according to their analysis of information reported in the NVDRS database showing suicide statistics from 2003 to 2020 (CDC, 2021b). They determined that specific circumstances increased the likelihood of IPP-related suicides: interpersonal violence perpetration and victimization, arguments, financial problems, job problems, and family problems (p. 385) as well as "depressed mood, history of suicidal thoughts, history of suicide attempts, and alcohol problems" (p. 388). Significant for IPP decedents, when compared with non-IPP decedents, were the life stressors of "perpetration of interpersonal violence . . ., arguments . . ., interpersonal violence victimization . . ., and financial problems" (p. 388). It was also discovered that alcohol use, compared to drug use, played a prominent role in IPP-suicides. Similar to ACEs, the more types of relationship violence one encounters, the greater the risk of an IPP-related suicide (Wilkins et al., 2015).

Till and colleagues (2017) found that both relationship status and satisfaction were suicide risk factors. Their study concluded that "suicidal ideation, hopelessness, and depression were highest among singles" than others who were in "happy, romantic" relationships (p. 12). *The Interpersonal Theory of Suicide* (Joiner, 2005 Van Orden et al., 2010) may account for this, proposing that persons experiencing low belongingness are at an increased risk for suicide. Till and colleagues discovered three types of relationships: "relationships with solutions to conflicts, relationships without solutions to conflicts, and relationships without conflicts" (p. 12). In addition to single persons, those in a relationship with problems, and finding no solutions, were also observed to have higher levels of suicidality, hopelessness, and depression. Unresolved issues were noted as leading to more inter-couple conflict and increased dissatisfaction, potentially resulting in a heightened risk of self-harm or suicide.

Community Factors

According to the CDC (2024a), community risk factors for suicide include limited access to health care, community suicide clusters, acculturation stress, community violence, generational/historical trauma, and pervasive discrimination. Several of these factors have been discussed in other chapters; however, community suicide clusters and acculturation stress are new to the discussion.

Suicide Clusters

Suicide clusters have occurred among varied populations including psychiatric inpatients (Haw, 1994; Taiminen et al., 1992), adolescents and young adults (Annor et al., 2018; Jacobs et al., 2021), students at school (Askland et al., 2003; Swedo et al., 2021), prisoners (Cox & Skegg, 1993; Hawton et al., 2014), and AI/NA communities (SAMHSA, 2017). Cluster suicides are either *point* clusters occurring "in a community/county or an institution such as a school, university, or psychiatric inpatient setting" (Ballesteros et al., 2024, p. 1) or *mass* clusters pertaining to a high number of suicides geographically spread but occurring during a specific time. Suicide clusters are most common among male adolescents or young adults with a history of self-harm and mental illness (Haw et al., 2013; Niedzwiedz et al., 2014). Research suggests factors such as suicide contagion (Lake & Gould, 2014), associated with a suicide decedent (Haw et al., 2013), and media reporting of suicides (Sinyor et al., 2018) could be linked to suicide clusters. Cerel and colleagues (2016) found that depression and anxiety were higher among those previously exposed to suicide and that they were more likely than non-exposed individuals (9% versus 5%) to reveal suicidal ideation. The odds for experiencing depression, anxiety, and PTSD were higher for those who described themselves as close to the suicide decedent.

Acculturative Stress

Acculturative stress, related to adapting to the beliefs, practices, values, and lifestyle of a dominant culture, has been linked to suicide (Berry, 1998). Acculturative stress entails racial discrimination felt by the acculturating person, changes and conflict within family dynamics, problems with forming new relationships, and a low sense of belonging (Fuertes & Westbrook, 1996; Mena et al., 1987). Acculturative stress has been linked to anxiety, depression, and suicidal ideation, especially among Latino, Black/African-American, and Asian populations (Walker et al., 2008). In a study with 969 ethnically diverse young adults (ages 18–25), data analysis demonstrated that familial acculturative stress was linked with two times the odds of predicting a past suicide attempt: over two times higher odds with Asian participants, four times higher odds for Black participants, more than three times higher odds with non-U.S.-born White participants, and more than three times higher odds for Latino participants (Gomez et al., 2011). Perceived discrimination was a critical factor, being associated with more than five times higher odds of a suicide attempt, especially for White U.S.-born and Latino participants. Polanco-Roman and Miranda (2013) performed a similar study, adding the dimension of hopelessness, predicted by higher measures of acculturative stress and discrimination. An increased risk of suicidal ideation was linked to higher levels of both depression and hopelessness for emerging adults from Asian, White, Latino, and Black populations.

Stigma

In some communities, the stigma surrounding suicide can prevent those needing help from seeking and receiving it. Monteith and colleagues (2020) discovered that the stigma in a rural community likely led to a lack of community awareness and resources to prevent veteran suicides. Some participants stated, "It goes back to 'we know about it, we just don't want to talk about it'" (p. 373). In a study using 3,269 adult participants, suicide stigma was found to be correlated with a lower likelihood of getting professional help, but a higher likelihood of reaching out to friends or family (Oexle et al., 2022). Conversely, the normalization of suicide was linked to a reduced likelihood of seeking help and thereby increased odds of suicidality. Suicide-related stigma was also shown to be associated with increased grief suicidality, and decreased personal growth (Oexle et al., 2018a). Oexle and colleagues (2018b) also found that stigma exists for those who have previously attempted suicide, thereby increasing their risk for suicide completion.

Criminal Justice Issue

Suicide under common law was a felony punishable by forfeiture in the U.S. States removed the common law punishment because it was impossible to punish the deceased. The U.S. criminal justice system regards euthanasia as well as attempted suicide as crimes prohibited by the federal government in all 50 states based on general homicide laws (Giorgi, 2024). The only country allowing the act of assisted dying performed by someone other than a physician is Switzerland (MacLeod et al., 2012). Elsewhere, any assisted death is regarded as a criminal offense and is prosecutable through legal means. For example, in the U.K., all forms of assisted dying are illegal and considered under criminal law as manslaughter or murder (Emanuel et al., 2016). Studies (Fazel et al., 2017; Snowden et al., 2017) reveal that most suicide victims had prior justice system involvement. Suicide is one of the leading causes of mortality among prisoners, accounting for approximately 30% of all prison deaths (Favril et al., 2019; Kaur et al., 2019). In 2015, suicide was the leading cause of death and made up more than one-third of all prisoner deaths (Noonan et al., 2015). Prison amplifies health disparities that are present in the community (Dolan et al., 2016), causing increased risk of inmate suicide.

Snowden and colleagues (2017) assert that veterans are at an increased risk for justice system involvement: nearly one in three veterans report having been arrested and booked into jail, relative to only one in five non-veterans. An investigation by Holliday and colleagues (2021) revealed that justice-involved veterans were nearly twice as likely to attempt suicide as non-veterans without justice involvement. These researchers further report that contact with the criminal justice system can create disruptions in health care for those who are transitioning between the community and incarceration. Research has shown that veterans who have been involved with the criminal justice system may experience PTSD, traumatic brain injury, depression, and substance abuse disorders, which all intensify suicidal risk (Holliday et al., 2023; Blodgett et al., 2015; Taylor et al., 2020). Many individuals who are processed by the criminal justice system have increased suicide risk, have used drugs or alcohol to alleviate stress, and may have had previous contact with psychiatric services (Webb et al., 2011).

There are an increasing number of law enforcement officers in the U.S. who commit suicide or are at risk of suicide. President Biden issued "Executive Order 14074" which included provisions preventing suicide among law enforcement officers. This Order recognized the importance of officers'/psychological health to public safety. Law enforcement work can lead to chronic stress, fatigue, compassion fatigue, burnout, and depression that causes negative physical, mental, interpersonal, and behavioral outcomes, including substance use and misuse (Lambert et al., 2022; Bosman & Henning, 2022). Officers' access to lethal weapons and lack of access to mental health services can lead to suicide and endanger public safety. For those involved in the criminal justice system, through incarceration or law enforcement employment, the thought of suicide is likely the result of living or working in stressful situations without preventative measures for suicide risk.

Public Health Issue

Suicide is a public health issue affecting individuals, families, and communities (American Public Health Association (APHA), 2021). For a problem to be considered a public health concern, four conditions are considered: (1) the problem is linked to high mortality, morbidity, loss of quality of life, and high costs; (2) the prevalence of the problem is the result of and/or creates disparities for populations already overburdened by disadvantages; (3) public health strategies must be observed as helpful to reducing the problem; and (4) prevention strategies are not extensively in place (Saaddine et al., 2003; Schoolwerth et al., 2006). Suicide meets all of these requirements. In 2022, suicide mortality in the U.S. reached beyond 49,000, a 30% increase over the last 20 years (CDC, 2025). In 2022, 13.2 million thought about suicide, 3.8 million planned to commit suicide, and 1.6 million made a nonfatal attempt.

Suicide is also financially costly. Suicide and nonfatal self-harm injuries totaled $510 billion annually from 2015 to 2020 with the following totals: "cost of lost life years ($484B), fatal and nonfatal injuries ($13B), injury morbidity reduced quality of life ($10B), and work loss due to nonfatal injuries ($3B)" (Peterson et al., 2024, p. 130). *Severity* is another public health characteristic when measuring burden of disease. While this measurement can be difficult to calculate, suicide presents a clear burden of disease when viewing its toll on the vulnerable and disadvantaged, such as AI/AN persons (CDC, n.d.b), the LGBTQIA community (James et al., 2016), and young Black males (CDC, n.d.d).

Suicide cannot be remedied through the individual efforts of medical and psychological providers disconnected from larger, well-funded, monitored, and data-driven efforts tailored to specific populations. Initiatives should be evidence-based public health strategies (A Comprehensive Approach to Suicide Prevention within a Public Health Framework, 2021). Approaches should be widespread and inclusive of geographies, neighborhoods and communities, schools and universities, hospitals and clinics, and places of work and leisure to ensure accessibility of education and other prevention efforts, intervention, and postvention programs—creating "an umbrella of impacts that cover entire populations" (Armitage, 2022). Approaching suicide from a public health perspective is not a novel idea, but it is still in its formative stage, which is where repositories of information, such as the Suicide Prevention Resource Center, play a significant role by providing suicide information, prevention strategies, training, a best practices registry, an online library, and up-to-date news.

Public health matters also tend to be *communicable*, like diseases (Armitage, 2022). For example, suicide can be *transmissible* as in generational, via genetic biomarkers and mediated by the environment (Joaquim et al., 2021; O'Reilly et al., 2020), parent behaviors (O'Reilly et al., 2020), and other domains such as social relations, physical domain and risk of suicide, and the psychological domain (Joaquim et al., 2021). Armitage also cites the role of health systems by acknowledging that subpar systems—those not accessible, efficient, safe, quality, acceptable, or affordable—are part of the continuance, if not the development, of a public health issue.

International Comparative Statistics

Worldwide, approximately 703,000 people commit suicide annually (World Health Organization (WHO), 2021). Worldwide, suicide was the fourth leading cause of death in persons between the ages of 15 and 29 for males and females (WHO, 2021). Reasons for suicide are complex, and yet, there are many reoccurring factors historically: most suicides occur among men (WHO, 2021), previously attempting suicide is the strongest predictor of dying by suicide (WHO, 2025), and someone with depression is 20 times more likely to complete suicide than someone without a depression diagnosis (Ferrari et al., 2014). Nearly 73% of suicides occurred in high-income countries in 2021, followed by middle-income countries, upper-middle, and lower-income (WHO, 2024). While 20 countries do not consider suicide a legal offense, many that follow Sharia law do and can impose small fines up to life in prison on those who make suicidal attempts (Marisha & Weisstub, 2016).

Internationally, in 2021, suicide rates per 100,000 persons varied widely, with Greenland having the greatest rate at 59.62 for all genders (86.96 males versus 29.4 females) and Palestine, the lowest at 0.78 (1.24 males versus 0.31 females) (World Population View, 2024). In the top five countries with the highest rates, in addition to Greenland, were Guyana (31.26), Lithuania (27.9), South Korea (25.81), and Russia (24.1). The lowest five countries, in addition to Palestine, included Syria (0.89), Lebanon (0.94), Egypt (1.012), and Oman (1.04). Rates of countries between the two polars include, but are not limited to, the U.S. (15.25), Canada (12.51), Denmark (11.27), DR Congo (8.12), and Italy (6.14).

In South Korea in 2023, suicide was the fourth leading cause of death, preceded by cerebrovascular disease, pneumonia, heart disease, and cancer (Statistica, n.d.). The suicide rate for Korean females has been on the rise since 2018. By 2021, it was at a rate of 16.2 per 100,000 persons (Statistics Korea, 2022). Korea is an anomaly because the increasing rates have been especially true for women in their 20s and 30s and elderly women aged 70 and older (Jang et al., 2023). Common methods of suicide, from 2019 to 2021, were hanging (46.9%), falling (24.5%), and carbon monoxide (8.0%). It is believed that a primary factor in female suicides has been the expectations and demands of dual roles: domestic caretaker and workforce employee, where they may face workplace discrimination (The Economist, 2023). Other prejudices, adding to existing stress, can include sexist beauty standards, misogyny, and sexual abuse. For elderly women, age has a positive correlation with suicide, along with economic instability, more so than educational attainment (Kim et al., 2020).

Public Health and Social Work

Intersection of Public Health and Social Work

Social workers, alongside public health personnel, are critical players in screening for, preventing, and responding to suicide. They comprise the largest group of mental health professionals in the U.S. (American Board of Clinical Social Work, 2022). In surveys of U.S. mental health and non-mental health social workers, approximately 50%–98% had engaged with persons who reported fatal and/or nonfatal suicide behavior (Sanders et al., 2008). Social workers connect with clients diagnosed with several mental health disorders, making suicide intervention training necessary. Research demonstrates that there is a high prevalence of mental illness—as high as 90%—among decedents (Mann et al., 2005). To treat disorders and prevent suicide, licensed clinical social workers (LCSWs) use a range of psychotherapies, including cognitive behavioral therapy (CBT) (Lazar, 2014), psychodynamic treatment, interpersonal psychotherapy, social skills training, and problem-solving therapy (Cuijpers et al., 2008) with persons diagnosed with mood and anxiety disorders. Clients with a diagnosis of PTSD can be treated with cognitive processing therapy, prolonged exposure therapies, and trauma-focused CBT (Rubin et al., 2013). Motivational enhancement therapy (Lenz et al., 2016), motivational interviewing (Smedslund et al., 2011), group therapy (Lazar, 2014), and CBT are likely therapies for substance use disorders, and dialectical behavioral therapy (DBT) for those diagnosed with borderline personality disorder (Linehan et al., 2015). Additionally, social workers perform family therapy with at-risk persons and their caregivers, providing education, resources, and support. These skills are also used when working with someone imminently suicidal, providing suicide risk assessment, emergency services referral, crisis intervention (Rose & Molina, 2017), safety planning (Stanley & Brown, 2012), and psychotherapy (Méndez-Bustos et al., 2019).

Social workers are skilled in suicide prevention with larger groups identified as high risk or at risk for suicide behaviors, such as the military (Milligan & Kelber, 2024), unemployed, homeless, justice-involved, LGBTQIA youth, and immigrants (Levine & Sher, 2020), utilizing their knowledge in case management activities per need. Services are likely to include finding assistance for dealing with relationships, money, or housing issues, locating support groups and services outside of medical systems, or providing high-level services such as intensive outpatient case management (ICM). ICM is characterized by smaller caseloads, long-term follow-up, and frequent contact with patients. Social workers also offer postvention services for the bereaved. Postvention services can also be in the form of critical incident stress management debriefing for groups of first responders (Bell, 1995), medical professionals (Spitzer & Neely, 1992), and in schools (Miller, 2003).

Health Disparities and Health Equities

Health disparities in suicide impact many groups, including those with poor access to suicide prevention programs and services, and current and past societal disadvantage or limited autonomy (Honchhauser et al., 2020). Suicide—preceded only by homicide and accidents—was found to be the third leading cause of death for Black and African-American males between ages 10 and 24 (CDC, n.d.d). LGBTQIA youth and adults experience higher rates of suicide ideation and attempts compared with non-LGBTQIA youth and adults (James et al., 2016). Data reveal that the rate of suicide for all youth, but especially females between the ages of 15 and 19, has increased (CDC, n.d.d). Non-Hispanic AI/NA persons (CDC, n.d.b) and veterans also have higher rates of suicide. Data show that adults with disabilities were twice as likely as non-disabled persons to have suicidal ideation, planning, and attempts (Marlow et al., 2021). Other suicide disparities of note include males working in specific professions (e.g., mining, quarrying, and oil and gas extraction, and construction), those with less than a high school diploma, persons living in rural areas, middle-aged adults, male non-Hispanic Whites, non-Hispanic Black females ages 10–24, multiracial persons ages 25–44, and older people ages 70 and over (U.S. DHHS, 2024). Social determinants of health that influence suicide disparities involve racism, "economic hardship, poverty, limited affordable [and safe] housing, lack of educational opportunities, and barriers to physical and mental healthcare access, among others" (CDC, 2024b). A common thread that links these groups is historical marginalization—acts of discrimination that impact the lives of people in a manner that increases their risk of suicide (Saunders & Panchal, 2023).

Negative Health Consequences of Suicide Ideation

Most research literature about suicide pertains to those who have had suicide ideation, made suicide attempts, and have completed suicide. Scant research is written about the consequences of suicide experienced by those who are witnesses to the act and/or those who are close friends, family, and coworkers of decedents. For each suicide, it has been estimated that between 6 (Shneidman et al., 1970) and 135 (Cerel et al., 2014) persons are affected. Using the conservative number of six persons and multiplying that by 703,000 suicides (WHO, 2021), approximately 4,218,000 persons are impacted annually.

Survivors have reported health and psychological consequences. The extent to which they are affected is often contingent on their attachment to or familiarity with the decedent (Cerel et al., 2014). Suicide bereavement may include negative mental health outcomes such as depression and suicidal ideation (Levi-Belz & Gilo, 2020; Maple et al., 2017), psychiatric hospitalization and suicide attempts (Pitman et al., 2014; Pitman et al., 2016), and diagnosed PTSD (Spillane et al., 2018). When compared to survivors of sudden natural death decedents, young adult suicide survivors demonstrated a higher likelihood of future suicide attempts (Pitman et al., 2016). Some literature reports that negative mental effects suffered by survivors can be prolonged for years. Guilt and shame (Sveen & Walby, 2008), sadness, relief, numbness, and blame (Spillane et al., 2018) are also documented psychological effects. Psychosomatic symptoms of bereavement were discovered to include physical pain, severe abdominal pain, trouble breathing, chest pain, loss of appetite, low energy levels, nightmares, memory loss, intrusive images, and an inability to sleep (Spillane et al., 2018). Through qualitative survivor interviews, Spillane et al. (2018) found that some survivors tried to cope with suicide through alcohol use and overeating. Formal and informal supports were discovered important to a survivor's coping and healing (Levi-Belz, 2019; Spillane et al., 2018). If the decedent was actively receiving or had previously received treatment, a patient suicide can be a traumatic experience, often requiring the treating psychiatrist or therapist to seek professional peer support and/or care (Pisnoli & Van der Hallen, 2022; Tamworth et al., 2022).

Criminal Justice Approaches

The Suicide Prevention Resource Center (2020) has established procedures for those employed in the criminal justice system who play a vital role in preventing suicide among those they serve. Useful strategies include providing suicide prevention training to personnel, establishing protocols for physical safety in all facilities, and responding to suicidal crises. Correctional officers work with inmates daily and are often the first responders when suicides or attempted suicides occur. Inmates can become suicidal at any point during incarceration. Therefore, prevention methods should start at the point of arrest and continue throughout incarceration. Arrest and conviction, as well as confinement in the prison environment, may increase the inmates' risk of suicide. In addition to staying alert and taking all threats and attempts of suicide seriously, the Suicide Prevention Resource Center (2020) recommends that the correctional and criminal justice system use the following approaches:

- Talk with inmates and encourage them to express their feelings.
- Ask if the inmate is thinking about suicide and do not disregard the immediate threat.
- Remove lethal means from an inmate who appears to be suicidal or threatens suicide.
- Contact designated mental health professional.
- Keep the inmate in a supervised environment until seen by a mental health professional.
- If an inmate is suicidal, he or she should be placed in a suicide-resistant cell under suicide precautions and checked every 10–15 minutes or continuously.

Executive Order 14074 directed the Department of Justice, in coordination with the Department of Health and Human Services to present evidence-informed recommendations regarding the prevention of death by suicide of law enforcement officers, including methods to encourage submission of data to the Law Enforcement Suicide Data Collection (LESDC) Program, in a manner that respects the privacy interest of officers and is consistent with applicable law. As such, some evidence-based approaches include (Department of Justice, 2023) the following:

1 Utilizing Public Policy to Advance Efforts

- Investing in intervention, and postvention programs to reduce risk factors for and build protective factors against suicide;
- Creating and implementing strategic plans and action plans, in partnership with the workforce, to advance psychological health and well-being.

2 Improving Data Collection Efforts

- Supporting agencies to employ data-driven approaches to identify the impact and performance of agency efforts.

3 Strengthening Coordination and Information Sharing

- Institutionalizing information sharing, and collaboration between entities that support suicide prevention programs, conduct research on suicide/suicide prevention, and collect and analyze data on deaths by suicide and attempted suicide.

4 Supporting Standards for Routine Mental Wellness Visits

- Exploring standards for and utilization of routine individual mental wellness visits.

5 Supporting Education and Training that Increases Knowledge and Provides Skills

- Prioritizing evidence-based education and training as preventative measures throughout one's career—into retirement—and evidence-based training for agency personnel to develop skills to protect against the effects of stressful experiences and exposure to trauma;

- Developing resources, conducting outreach, and providing education to mental health professionals who serve/will serve law enforcement (and other public safety) agency personnel.

6 Strengthening Communication

- Having easy access to current information and resources on evidence-based prevention, intervention, and postvention programs that reduce risk factors for and build protective factors against suicide.

The criminal justice system should be equipped with mental health clinicians who can draw on their skill sets to educate the community, those confined, and the workforce about mental illness and suicide warning signs and prevention. This may result in systematic improvements in wellness and suicide prevention.

Public Health Approaches

The CDC funds the *Comprehensive Suicide Prevention Program* (CSP), which aims to reduce suicide disparities (i.e., suicide and suicide attempts) by 10% in identified populations and to reach a national suicide reduction of 20% by 2025. Annually, the CDC invests $21 million, with monies allocated to selected state departments of health programming that implement and evaluate a wide-ranging public health suicide prevention approach (CDC, 2024e). The CSP program has five key components:

1 Strong leadership to convene and connect multisectoral partnerships;
2 Data to (1) identify disproportionately affected populations with increased risk of suicide, (2) understand contributors to suicide and suicidal behaviors, and (3) track trends in suicide deaths and suicidal behavior;
3 Identification and assessment of gaps in existing programs in the jurisdiction;
4 Implementation and evaluation of complementary strategies with the best available evidence from the Suicide Prevention Resource for Action; and
5 Development, implementation, and evaluation of a communication and dissemination plan to communicate trends, progress, successes, and lessons learned to partners.

After recognizing the large suicide disparity for AI/NA people, the CDC funded the Tribal Suicide Prevention Program through a *Strengthening Public Health Systems and Services in Indian Country* cooperative agreement. As of 2024, the CDC has invested $51.3 million. The program is intended to assist tribal organizations to enhance community protective factors, identify those at risk and link them to services, strengthen crisis identification and postvention services, prevent cluster suicides, and build capacity and infrastructure for developing local suicide surveillance (CDC, 2024d).

The APHA issued a policy on a comprehensive approach to suicide prevention within a public health framework (APHA, 2021) based on evidence-based strategies. This approach uses prevention, intervention, treatment, and postvention efforts for a comprehensive strategy. According to APHA, this has five requirements: (1) accurate and timely suicide-related data; (2) more money for suicide research, programs, and program evaluation; (3) addressing contextual factors to reduce suicide especially in those populations that have been historically underserved and that demonstrate suicide and health disparities; (4) making suicide attempt methods less accessible and other prevention policies that can be employed at the population level; and (5) developing suicide-related services. There is community-based suicide prevention that emphasizes collaborative suicide prevention partnerships, a suicide aware workplace culture, and research-informed suicide prevention community activities using communication science (U.S. DHHS, 2024). Other community prevention elements include a shared vision, leaders, strategic planning, readiness, strategic communication campaigns, and sustainability (EDC.ORG, 2025). Additional communities, such as the military, have specific programs tailored to address the needs of their members such as enhancing the quality of life, addressing stigma related to receiving services, improving the delivery of mental health care, promoting a culture of lethal means safety in a crisis, and continuing evaluation of suicide prevention efforts (USDOD, 2023).

Public Health and Social Work Approaches

In an earlier chapter section, *Intersection of Public Health and Social Work*, it was established that social workers interact with persons at risk for suicide in several ways including the use of psychotherapies (Cuijpers et al., 2008; Lazar, 2014; Rubin et al., 2013), motivational interviewing (Smedslund et al., 2011), group therapy (Lazar, 2014), and case management (Milligan & Kelber, 2024). They perform suicide risk assessment, emergency services referral, crisis intervention (Rose & Molina, 2017), safety planning (Stanley & Brown, 2012), and psychotherapy (Méndez-Bustos et al., 2019). Additionally, they often teach safe gun storage practices and advocate for temporary transfer of gun ownership or storage during stressful periods (Abrams et al., 2022). Social workers and nurses provide family intervention, in the form of suicide prevention education, to caretakers of persons diagnosed with mental illness and/or who are at risk for suicide (Sun et al., 2013).

To improve their skills and intervention proficiency, it has been suggested that the social work profession pay special attention to demographic patterns and trends in suicide, especially concerning preventive measures for older youth and young adults (Joe & Niedermeier, 2008). In addition, it is recommended that social workers make risk assessment and management readily available to those undergoing current stressors such as divorce, moving into nursing homes, being incarcerated, and experiencing long periods of unemployment. While LCSWs do preventive work with clients, the importance of religious and spiritual support needs to be considered, particularly for women.

Integrating Skills of Social Epidemiology to Address Disparities and Achieve Equity

Social epidemiology focuses on "social-structural factors" and their effects on health and "assumes that the distribution of advantages and disadvantages in a society reflects the distribution of health and disease" (Honjo, 2004, p. 193). Social structures that affect health include "social class, gender, race and ethnicity, discrimination, social network, social capital, income distribution, and social policy" (p. 194). Altering any one of these structures could change a disparity and bring about more equality.

The suicide literature is replete with information about social connectedness and suicide. Cero and colleagues (2024) used knowledge from Durkheim (2005) and recent research about social connectedness as the foundation of their study on social networks as a suicide prevention. The Trevor Project (2023) reported on LGBTQIA adolescent mental health survey results. Accordingly, LGBTQIA youth and young adults do not feel a sense of belongingness or support in their homes, communities, or schools. Therefore, disconnectedness results in health disparities (e.g., higher rates of mental and physical illness, self-injurious behaviors, suicide ideation, and attempts). Research also shows that social connectedness, including "caring, support, and quality of communication," is a proven, significant protective factor against suicide (Wasserman et al., 2021, p. 8).

Social network is formed by choice, and network members influence one another (Christakis & Fowler, 2013). When members' influence is negative, a suicide cluster could occur. However, clusters are rare (Ballesteros et al., 2024) and most people are not suicidal. In 2022, 49.5 million died by suicide compared to the total 2022 U.S. population of 333,287,557 (United States Census Bureau, 2022). According to Cero and colleagues (2024), this is important because healthy people are likely to have healthy connections even after an unhealthy person enters the group. A healthy network could increase the health of an at-risk person. This phenomenon can be utilized in an epidemiological approach to positively shift a social network to impact one at-risk person or even an at-risk cluster. In short, an area of intervention for suicide, according to epidemiology, should be the social networks of those at risk for suicide. In keeping with an epidemiological framework, another area of structural change to decrease LGBTQIA suicide would be social policy, such as in schools or federal policy. For example, transsexual and non-binary youth who report having access to gender-neutral bathrooms at school disclose fewer suicide attempts than those who did not (The Trevor Project, 2023). Haas and colleagues (2011) stated, "The well-established association between mental disorders and suicide attempts in at least some LGBT subgroups points to the need to include advocacy for policy change as a component of a comprehensive plan for LGBT suicide prevention" (pp. 39–40).

How Suicides Can Be Prevented

In addition to the suicide prevention efforts already discussed, SAMHSA sponsors many suicide prevention initiatives as a focus in its strategic plan (SAMHSA, 2024b). They fund programs that provide prevention, early intervention, crisis support, treatment, recovery, and postvention for youth and adults. Examples include mobile crisis response units, college campus programs, community-based programs for state and tribal behavioral health, a national suicide prevention resource center (SPRC), a Black youth suicide prevention initiative, the *zero suicide* framework model for multi-setting suicide prevention (lead, train, identify, engage, treat, transition, and improve), and the 988 suicide and crisis 24/7 lifeline phone service.

School suicide prevention programs can differ across states and school systems. For some schools, services have been provided by one mental health agency, and others may provide services through counselors and social workers. They might offer case management, crisis intervention, family therapy, group counseling, individual therapy, substance use group counseling, and substance use counseling. There are several websites with free prevention programming, such as the Rural Health Information Hub (School-Based Programming for

Suicide Prevention—RHIhub Toolkit), Student Mental Health Resource Directory (OC-School-Based-Prevention-Campaign.pdf), and the Sandy Hook award-winning prevention curriculum, *Say Something* for grades K–12 (Home | Sandy Hook Promise Learning Center).

Globally, the International Association for Suicide Prevention (IASP) has developed an effective forum, proactively creating strong collaborations and promoting evidence-based prevention programs. They offer crisis support, they maintain a free helpline that operates in over 50 countries, they publish *The Journal of Crisis Intervention and Suicide Prevention*, and they produce the *Reach-In, Reach Out* podcast. These resources can be found on the website, IASP.

Policy Recommendation

The agencies and programs involved in suicide prevention nationally and globally offer several policy recommendations. For example, WHO (2023) issued a policy brief on decriminalizing suicide and suicide attempts, arguing that such criminalization represents a significant barrier to the 2030 30% reduction of suicide mortality goal. This reduction is a target stated in the United Nations Sustainable Development Goals and the WHO Global Mental Health Action Plan. At least 23 countries still consider suicide and suicide attempts illegal under civil and criminal law (International Association for Suicide Prevention, 2020). It was also recommended that these countries "develop a comprehensive national suicide prevention strategy, establish rights-oriented, community-based mental health services, and reform or develop new mental health-related laws, policies and strategic plans that promote the rights of persons with mental health conditions" (p. 8).

The Biden/Harris Administration produced the new 2024 National Strategy for Suicide Prevention (U.S. DHHS, 2024) to assist in creating a more comprehensive and coordinated suicide prevention strategy for U.S. communities. While most of the actions outlined in the national strategy are achievable through collaborations and partnerships, there are several that demand policy advocacy such as the development and utilization of comprehensive community-based suicide prevention strategies and initiatives, the reduction of access to lethal means among people at risk of suicide, the integration of suicide prevention into the culture of the workplace and into other community settings, the implementation of effective suicide prevention services as a core component of health care, and the creation of an equitable and diverse suicide prevention workforce. The national strategy also includes federal government actions requiring policy work such as the provision of adequate funding for a mobile crisis locator for 988 crisis centers and the sustained support for decedent survivors.

As for youth, Ackerman and Horowitz (2022) offer policy recommendations that target specific young adults. These recommendations include the implementation of universal, culturally sensitive, and sustainable suicide prevention in schools, the development of suicide risk screening and assessment approaches to use with children beginning in elementary school, the utilization of evidence-based suicide interventions by healthcare settings, the inclusion of "minority-specific" resources (p. 103) in suicide prevention and postvention services, and the assurance of "state-level licensing requirements that require continuing education in suicide" (p. 104).

Summary

Suicide is a global concern, encompassing suicidal ideation, suicide plans, suicide attempts, and suicide completions. Suicide is a public health problem affecting individuals, families, and communities. One suicide can affect countless others, ranging from relatives to friends, to coworkers, neighbors, and others that a decedent interacted with. Most importantly, suicide is preventable. Some populations carry a disparate burden of suicide inequity, such as military active duty and veterans, LGBTQIA youth, young Black males and men, in addition to Black women and girls, AI/NA persons, and the elderly aged 85 and older. Why is this? Research provides information to help understand these suicide disparities: individual and systemic discrimination, isolation and loneliness, trauma experienced as children and as adults, the influence of alcohol and other substances, relationship issues, mental illness, the inability to access help, stigma associated with getting help, and other factors. These influences add to other social, economic, genetic, geographical, and psychological factors, such as chronic illness, community violence, rural inaccessibility to services, the sense of burdensomeness, the feeling of disconnectedness, acculturative stress, and access to lethal means of self-harm. While many therapists and mental health workers engage with persons exhibiting suicidal behaviors, the problem exists at a much larger scope, too big to be dealt with person by person. Meeting the characteristics of what constitutes a public health issue, suicide can only be approached effectively using the tools and practices of public health, much as with the COVID pandemic or other contagious diseases. Supported by private and public funding, governed by state, federal, and global policy, and positioned in every community, suicide prevention and postvention services and efforts require the awareness, education, and commitment of everyone. Just as no one is immune to suicide risk, everyone is needed in efforts to decrease or even eliminate suicide. These efforts, as recommended, should begin in elementary schools, healthcare practices, hospitals, clinics, dental offices, community agencies and programs, long-term care, departments of social services, and other government organizations, and at home.

Discussion Questions

1 What is one group of people that is shown to experience suicide disparity and what are three factors involved in creating that disparity?
2 What are at least two prevention or intervention strategies that could be used to decrease suicide among that group?
3 What could you do in your community to help strengthen the effort to decrease suicide?
4 What special skill sets do social workers use to prevent suicides?
5 How can suicide clusters be confronted in efforts to prevent suicide?
6 Why are some people more at risk to committing suicide compared with others?

References

Abrams, L.S., Dettlaff, A.J., & Risley-Curtiss, C. (2022). social workers and safe gun storage: Bridging the divide to promote child safety. *Families in Society*, 103(2), 263–277. https://doi.org/10.1177/10443894221081577.

Ackerman, J.P., & Horowitz, L.M. (2022). *Youth suicide prevention and intervention: Best practices and policy implications* (p. 169). Springer Nature.

Agha, Z., Lofgren, R.P., VanRuiswyk, J.V., & Layde, P.M. (2000). Are patients at veterans affairs medical centers sicker? A comparative analysis of health status and medical resource use. *Archives of Internal Medicine*, 160(21), 3252–3257. https://doi.org/10.1001/archinte.160.21.3252

Alexopoulos, G.S., Bruce, M.L., Hull, J., Sirey, J.A., & Kakuma, T. (1999). Clinical determinants of suicidal ideation and behavior in geriatric depression. *Archives of General Psychiatry*, 56(11), 1048–1053. https://doi.org/10.1001/archpsyc.56.11.1048

American Board of Clinical Social Work. (2022, November 28). What is clinical social work? www.abcsw.org/what-is-clinical-social-work

American Public Health Association (APHA). (2021, October 25). A comprehensive approach to suicide prevention within a public health framework [Policy brief]. Policy 20213. www.apha.org/policies-and-advocacy/public-health-policy-statements/policy-database/2022/01/07/a-comprehensive-approach-to-suicide-prevention-within-a-public-health-framework

Amos, N., Hart, B., Hill, A.O., Melendez-Torres, G.J., McNair, R., Carman, M., Lyons, A., & Bourne, A. (2023). Health intervention experiences and associated mental health outcomes in a sample of LGBTQ people with intersex variations in Australia. *Culture, Health & Sexuality*, 25(7), 833–846. https://doi.org/10.1080/13691058.2022.2102677

Annor, F.B., Zwald, M.L., Wilkinson, A., Friedrichs, M., Fondario, A., Dunn, A., Nakashima, A., Gilbert, L.K., & Ivey-Stephenson, A.Z. (2018). Characteristics of and precipitating circumstances surrounding suicide among persons aged 10–17 years — Utah, 2011–2015. *MMWR. Morbidity and Mortality Weekly Report*, 67(11), 329–332. https://doi.org/10.15585/mmwr.mm6711a4

Armitage, R. (2022, February). *Suicide prevention: Current landscape*. College of Policing. https://assets.college.police.uk/s3fs-public/2022-02/Suicide-prevention-current-landscape.pdf.

Arnon, S., Klomek, A., Visoki, E., Moore. T.M., Argabright, S.T., DiDomenico, G.E., Benton, T.D., & Barzilay, R. (2022). Association of cyberbullying experiences and perpetration with suicidality in early adolescence. *JAMA Network Open*, 5(6), e2218746. https://doi.org/10.1001/jamanetworkopen.2022.18746

Askland, K.D., Sonnenfeld, N., & Crosby, A. (2003). A public health response to a cluster of suicidal behaviors: Clinical psychiatry, prevention, and community health. *Journal of Psychiatric Practice*, 9, 219–27. https://doi.org/10.1097/00131746-200305000-00005

Ballesteros, M.F., Ivey-Stephenson, A.Z., Trinh, E., & Stone, D.M. (2024). Background and rationale—CDC guidance for communities assessing, investigating, and responding to suicide clusters, United States. *MMWR Supplements*, 73(Suppl-2), 1–7. http://dx.doi.org/10.15585/mmwr.su7302a1

Bell, J.L. (1995). Traumatic event debriefing: Service delivery designs and the role of social work. *Social Work*, 40(1), 36–43. https://doi.org/10.1093/sw/40.1.36

Bell, F.C., & Miller, M.L. (2005). *Life tables for the United States social security area 1900–2100*. Social Security Administration, Office of the Chief Actuary, SSA Pub. No. 11-11536.

Beltrán-Sánchez, H., Jiménez, M.P., & Subramanian, S.V. (2016). Assessing morbidity compression in two cohorts from the health and retirement study. *Journal of Epidemiology and Community Health*, 70(10), 1011–1016. https://doi.org/10.1136/jech-2015-206722

Benbenishty, R., Astor, R.A., & Roziner, I. (2018). A school-based multilevel study of adolescent suicide ideation in California high schools. *Journal of Pediatrics*, 196, 251–257. https://doi.org/10.1016/j.jpeds.2017.12.070

Bernard, D.L., Calhoun, C.D., Banks, D.E., Halliday, C.A., Hughes-Halbert, C., & Danielson, C.K. (2021). Making the "C-ACE" for a culturally-informed adverse childhood experiences framework to understand the pervasive mental health impact of racism on Black youth. *Journal of Child & Adolescent Trauma*, 14(2), 233–247. https://doi.org/10.1007/s40653-020-00319-9

Berry, J.W. (1998). Acculturative stress. In P. Organista, K. Chun, & G. Marin (Eds.), *Readings in ethnic psychology* (pp. 117–122). Routledge.

Bertolote, J.M., Fleischmann, A., De Leo, D., & Wasserman, D. (2004). Psychiatric diagnoses and suicide: Revisiting the evidence. *Crisis*, 25(4), 147–55. https://doi.org/10.1027/0227-5910.25.4.147

Bishop, N.J., Haas, S.A., & Quiñones, A.R. (2022). Cohort trends in the burden of multiple chronic conditions among aging U.S. adults. *The Journals of Gerontology, Series B: Psychological Sciences and Social Sciences*, 77(10), 1867–1879. https://doi.org/10.1093/geronb/gbac070

Blodgett, J.C., Avoundjian, T., Finlay, A.K., Rosenthal, J., Asch, S.M., Maisel, N.C., & Midboe, A.M. (2015). Prevalence of mental health disorders among justice-involved veterans. *Epidemiologic Reviews*, 37(1), 163–176. https://doi.org/10.1093/epirev/mxu003

Bosma, L. J., & Henning, S. L. (2022). Compassion fatigue among officers. Retrieved from FBI, Law Enforcement Bulletin (LEB): https://leb.fbi.gov/articles/featured-articles/compassion-fatigue-among-officers

Bowen, F.R., Lewandowski, L.A., Snethen, J.A., Childs, G., Outlaw, F.H., Greenberg, C.S., Burke, P.J., Sloand, E., Gary, F., & DeSocio, J. (2022). A schema of toxic stress informed by racism, transgenerational stress, and disadvantage. *Journal of Pediatric Health Care*, 36(2), 79–89. https://doi.org/10.1016/j.pedhc.2021.08.005

Bridge, J.A., Horowitz, L.M., Fontanella, C.A., Sheftall, A.H., Greenhouse, J.B., Kelleher, K.J., & Campo, J.V. (2018). Age-related racial disparity in suicide rates among U.S. youths between 2001 and 2015. *JAMA Pediatrics*, 172(7), 697–699. https://doi.org/10.1001/jamapediatrics.2018.0399

Camacho, S., & Clark Henderson, S. (2022). The social determinants of adverse childhood experiences: An intersectional analysis of place, access to resources, and compounding effects. *International Journal of Environmental Research and Public Health*, 19(17), 10670. https://doi.org/10.3390/ijerph191710670

Caplan, S. (2019). Intersection of cultural and religious beliefs about mental health: Latinos in the faith-based setting. *Hispanic Health Care International*, 17(1), 4–10. https://doi.org/10.1177/1540415319828265

Castle, K., Conner, K., Kaukeinen, K., & Tu, X. (2011). Perceived racism, discrimination, and acculturation in suicidal ideation and suicide attempts among Black young adults. *Suicide and Life-Threatening Behavior*, 41(3), 342–351. https://doi.org/10.1111/j.1943-278X.2011.00033.x

Centers for Disease Control and Prevention (CDC). (n.d.a). 1991-2023 high school youth risk behavior survey data. Available at www.cdc.gov/yrbs/

Centers for Disease Control and Prevention (CDC). (n.d.b). *Leading causes of death: Suicide for ages 10-34, United States 2022, All Sexes, All Races.* Web-based Injury Statistics Query and Reporting System (WISQARS). Atlanta, GA: National Centers for Injury Prevention and Control, Centers for Disease Control and Prevention. www.cdc.gov/injury/wisqars/index.html

Centers for Disease Control and Prevention (CDC). (n.d.c). *Leading causes of death: Suicide for ages 10-14, United States 2022, All Sexes, All Races.* Web-based Injury Statistics Query and Reporting System (WISQARS). Atlanta, GA: National Centers for Injury Prevention and Control, Centers for Disease Control and Prevention. www.cdc.gov/injury/wisqars/index.html

Centers for Disease Control and Prevention (CDC). (n.d.d). *Leading cause of death: Suicide for ages 15-24, United States, 2022, All Sexes, All Races.* Web-based Injury Statistics Query and Reporting System (WISQARS). Atlanta, GA: National Centers for Injury Prevention and Control, Centers for Disease Control and Prevention. www.cdc.gov/injury/wisqars/index.html

Centers for Disease Control and Prevention (CDC). (2020). About underlying cause of death, *1999–2020: Wide ranging online data for epidemiological research (WONDER), multiple cause of death files* [Data file]. National Center for Health Statistics. http://wonder.cdc.gov/ucd-icd10.html

Centers for Disease Control and Prevention (CDC). (2021a). CDC WONDER: About underlying cause of death, 1999–2020. Atlanta, GA: US Department of Health and Human Services, CDC; 2021. https://wonder.cdc.gov/ucd-icd10.html

Centers for Disease Control and Prevention (CDC). (2021b). National center for injury prevention and control. Web Based Injury Statistics Query and Reporting System (WISQARS). National Violent Death Reporting System. Violent Deaths Report.

Centers for Disease Control and Prevention (CDC). (2022). Suicide prevention resource for action: A compilation of the best available evidence. Atlanta, GA: National Center for Injury Prevention and

Control, Centers for Disease Control and Prevention. www.cdc.gov/suicide/pdf/preventionresou rce.pdf

Centers for Disease Control and Prevention (CDC). (2024a, April 25). *Risk and protective factors for suicide*. Risk and Protective Factors for Suicide I Suicide Prevention I CDC.

Centers for Disease Control and Prevention (CDC). (2024b, May 16). Suicide Prevention: Health disparities in suicide. Health Disparities in Suicide I Suicide Prevention I CDC.

Centers for Disease Control and Prevention (CDC). (2024c, August 06). *Youth risk behavior survey data summary & trends report: 2013–2023*. U.S. Department of Health and Human Services; 2024. www.cdc.gov/yrbs/dstr/index.html

Centers for Disease Control and Prevention (CDC). (2024d, August 28). *Suicide prevention: Tribal suicide prevention*. www.cdc.gov/suicide/programs/tribal.html

Centers for Disease Control and Prevention (CDC). (2024e, September 10). *Suicide prevention: Comprehensive suicide prevention*. Comprehensive Suicide Prevention I Suicide Prevention I CDC.

Centers for Disease Control and Prevention (CDC). (2025, March 26). *Suicide data and statistics* [Data brief]. www.cdc.gov/suicide/facts/data.html

Cerel, J., Maple, M., van de Venne, J., Moore, M., Flaherty, C., & Brown, M. (2016). Exposure to suicide in the community: Prevalence and correlates in one U.S. state. *Public Health Reports (1974)*, 131(1), 100–107. https://doi.org/10.1177/003335491613100116

Cerel, J. McIntosh, J., Neimeyer, R., Myfanwy, M., & Marshall, D. (2014). The continuum of "Survivorship": Definitional issues in the aftermath of suicide. *Suicide and Life-Threatening Behavior*, 44(6), 591–600. https://doi.org/10.1111/sltb.12093

Cero, I., De Choudhury, M., & Wyman, P.A. (2024). Social network structure as a suicide prevention target. *Social Psychiatry and Psychiatric Epidemiology*, 59, 555–564. https://doi.org/10.1007/s00 127-023-02521-0

Christakis, N.A., & Fowler, J.H. (2013). Social contagion theory: Examining dynamic social networks and human behavior. *Statistics in Medicine*, 32, 556–577. https://doi.org/10.1002/sim.5408

Clark, K.A., & Blosnich, J.R. (2024). Limitations of sexual orientation and gender identity information as reported in the National Violent Death Reporting System. *LGBT Health*, 11(3), 173–177. https://doi.org/10.1089/lgbt.2022.0297

Cox, B., & Skegg, K. (1993). Contagious suicide in prisons and police cells. *Journal of Epidemiology and Community Health*, 47, 69–72. https://doi.org/10.1136/jech.47.1.69

Crimmins, E.M. (2015). Lifespan and healthspan: Past, present, and promise. *The Gerontologist*, 55(6), 901–911. https://doi.org/10.1093/geront/gnv130

Curtin, S.C., & Garnett, M.F. (2023, June). *Suicide and homicide death rates among youth and young adults aged 10–24: United States, 2001–2021*. NCHS Data Brief, Centers for Disease Control and Prevention (CDC). www.cdc.gov/nchs/data/databriefs/db471.pdf

Cuijpers, P., van Straten, A., Andersson, G., & van Oppen, P. (2008). Psychotherapy for depression in adults: A meta-analysis of comparative outcome studies. *Journal of Consulting and Clinical Psychology*, 76(6), 909–922. https://doi.org/10.1037/a0013075

Deykin, E.Y., & Buka, S.L. (1994). Suicidal ideation and attempts among chemically dependent adolescents. *American Journal of Public Health*, 84(4), 634–639. https://doi.org/10.2105/AJPH.84.4.634

Dolan, K., Wirtz, A.L., Moazen, B., Ndeffo-Mbah, M., Galvani, A., Kinner, S.A., Courtney, R., McKee, M., Amon, J.J., Maher, L., Hellard, M., Beyrer, C., Altice, F.L. (2016). Global burden of HIV, viral hepatitis, and tuberculosis in prisoners and detainees. *Lancet*, 388(10049), 1089–1102. https://doi.org/10.1016/S0140-6736(16)30466-4

Dumornay, N.M., Lebois, L.A.M., Ressler, K.J., & Harnett, N.G. (2023). Racial disparities in adversity during childhood and the false appearance of race-related differences in brain structure. *The American Journal of Psychiatry*, 180(2), 127–138. https://doi.org/10.1176/appi.ajp.21090961

Durkheim, E. (2005). *Suicide, a study in sociology* (2nd ed.). Free Press. https://doi.org/10.4324/9780203994320

Dursa, E.K., Barth, S.K., Bossarte, R.M., & Schneiderman, A.I. (2016). Demographic, military, and health characteristics of VA health care users and nonusers who served in or during operation enduring freedom or operation Iraqi freedom, 2009–2011. *Public Health Reports*, 131(6), 839–843. https://doi.org/10.1177/0033354916676279

EDC.ORG. (2025). *Community-led suicide prevention*. Community-Led Suicide Prevention.

Edwards, T.S., & Kelton, P. (2020). Germs, genocides, and America's indigenous peoples. *Journal of American History*, 107(1), 52–76. https://doi.org/10.1093/jahist/jaaa008

Emanuel, E.J., Onwuteaka-Philipsen, B.D., Urwin, J.W., & Cohen, J. (2016). Attitudes and practices of euthanasia and physician-assisted suicide in the United States, Canada, and Europe. *JAMA*, 316(1), 79–90. https://doi.org/10.1001/jama.2016.8499

Emerson, M.A., Moore, R.S., & Caetano, R. (2017). Association between lifetime posttraumatic stress disorder and past year alcohol use disorder among American Indians/Alaska Natives and non-Hispanic Whites. *Alcoholism: Clinical and Experimental Research*, 41(3), 576–584. https://doi.org/10.1111/acer.13322

Ertel, K.A., James-Todd, T., Kleinman, K., Krieger, N., Gillman, M., Wright, R., & Rich-Edwards, J. (2012). Racial discrimination, response to unfair treatment, and depressive symptoms among pregnant Black and African American women in the United States. *Annals of Epidemiology*, 22(12), 840–846. https://doi.org/10.1016/j.annepidem.2012.10.001

Fässberg, M.M., Cheung, G., Canetto, S.S., Erlangsen, A., Lapierre, S., Lindner, R., Draper, B., Gallo, J., Wong, C., Wu, J., Duberstein, P., & Wærn, M. (2016). A systematic review of physical illness, functional disability, and suicidal behaviour among older adults. *Aging & Mental Health*, 20(2), 166–194. https://doi.org/10.1080/13607863.2015.1083945

Favril, L., Wittouck, C., Audenaert, K., & Vander Laenen, F. (2019). A 17-year national study of prison suicides in Belgium. *Crisis*, 40(1), 42–53. https://doi.org/10.1027/0227-5910/a000531

Fazel, S., Ramesh, T., & Hawton, K. (2017). Suicide in prisons: An international study of prevalence and contributory factors. *Lancet Psychiatry*, 4, 946–952.

Felitti, V.J., Anda, R.F., Nordenberg, D., Williamson, D.F., Spitz, A.M., Edwards, V., Koss, M.P., & Marks, J.S. (1998). Relationship of childhood abuse and household dysfunction to many of the leading causes of death in adults. The Adverse Childhood Experiences (ACE) Study. *American Journal of Preventive Medicine*, 14(4), 245–258. https://doi.org/10.1016/S0749-3797(98)00017-8

Ferrari, A.J., Norman, R.E., Freedman, G., Baxter, A.J., Pirkis, J.E., Harris, M.G., Page, A., Carnahan, E., Degenhardt, L., Vos, T., & Whiteford, H.A. (2014). The burden attributable to mental and substance use disorders as risk factors for suicide: findings from the Global Burden of Disease Study 2010. *PLoS One*, 9(4), e91936. https://doi.org/10.1371/journal.pone.0091936

Fink, D.S., Stohl, M., Mannes, Z.L., Shmulewitz, D., Wall, M., Gutkind, S., Olfson, M., Gradus, J., Keyhani, S., Maynard, C., Keyes, K.M., Sherman, S., Martins, S., Saxon, A.J., & Hasin, D.S. (2022). Comparing mental and physical health of U.S. veterans by VA healthcare use: Implications for generalizability of research in the VA electronic health records. *BMC Health Services Research*, 22, Article number 1500. https://doi.org/10.1186/s12913-022-08899-y

Fontanella, C.A., Warner, L.A., Steelesmith, D.L., Brock, G., Bridge, J.A., & Campo, J.V. (2020). Association of timely outpatient mental health services for youths after psychiatric hospitalization with risk of death by suicide. *JAMA Network Open*, 3(8), e2012887. https://doi.org/10.1001/jamanetworkopen.2020.12887

Fuertes, J.N., & Westbrook, F.D. (1996). Using the Social, Attitudinal, Familial, and Environmental (S.A.F.E.) Acculturation Stress Scale to assess the adjustment needs of Hispanic college students. *Measurement and Evaluation in Counseling and Development*, 29, 67–76.

Garlow, S.J., Rosenberg, J., Moore, J.D., Haas, A.P., Koestner, B., Hendin, H., & Nemeroff, C.B. (2008). Depression, desperation, and suicidal ideation in college students: Results from the American foundation for suicide prevention college screening project at Emory University. *Depression and Anxiety*, 25(6), 482–488. https://doi.org/10.1002/da.20321

Gaylor, E.M., Krause, K.H., Welder, L.E., Cooper, A.C., Ashley, C., Mack, K.A., Crosby, A.E., Trinh, E., Ivey-Stephenson, A.Z., & Whittle, L. (2023). Suicidal thoughts and behaviors among high school students–youth risk behavior survey, United States, 2021. *MMWR Supplements*, 72(1), 45–54. https://doi.org/10.15585/mmwr.su7201a6

Gimeno, L., Goisis, A., Dowd, J.B., & Ploubidis, G.B. (2024). Cohort differences in physical health and disability in the United States and Europe. *The Journals of Gerontology. Series B, Psychological Sciences and Social Sciences*, 79(8). gbae113. https://doi.org/10.1093/geronb/gbae113

Giorgi, A. (2024). *Euthanasia: Understanding the quality factors and legality*. Verywell Health. www.verywellhealth.com/euthanasia-8701113

Gomez, J., Miranda, R., & Polanco, L. (2011). Acculturative stress, perceived discrimination, and vulnerability to suicide attempts among emerging adults. *Journal of Youth and Adolescence*, 40(11), 1465–1476. https://doi.org/10.1007/s10964-011-9688-9

Goodfellow, B., Kõlves, K., Leo, D., & Franz, C. P. (2019). Contemporary definitions of suicidal behavior: A systematic literature review. *Suicide & Life-Threatening Behavior*, 49(2), 488–504. https://doi.org/10.1111/sltb.12457

Goodwill, J.R., & Yasui, M. (2022). Mental health service utilization, school experiences, and religious involvement among a national sample of Black adolescents who attempted suicide: Examining within and cross-race group differences. *Child and Adolescent Social Work Journal*, 41, 545–560. https://doi.org/10.1007/s10560-022-00888-8

Gordan, J. (2020). *Addressing the crisis of Black youth suicide*. National Institute of Mental Health, Director's Messages. Addressing the Crisis of Black Youth Suicide – National Institute of Mental Health (NIMH).

Haney, J.L. (2021). Suicidality risk among adult sexual minorities: Results from a cross-sectional population-based survey. *Journal of Gay & Lesbian Social Services*, 33(2), 250–271. https://doi.org/10.1080/10538720.2021.1875946

Haas, A.P., Eliason, M., Mays, V.M., Mathy, R.M., Cochran, S.D., D'Augelli, A.R., Silverman, M.M., Fisher, P.W., Hughes, T., Rosario, M., Russell, S.T., Malley, E., Reed, J., Litts, D.A., Haller, E., Sell, R.L., Remafedi, G., Bradford, J., Beautrais, A. L., …, & Clayton, P.J. (2011). Suicide and suicide risk in lesbian, gay, bisexual, and transgender populations: Review and recommendations. *Journal of Homosexuality*, 58(1), 10–51. https://doi.org/10.1080/00918369.2011.534038

Haas, A.P., Lane, A.D., Blosnich, J.R., Butcher, B.A., & Mortali, M.G. (2019). Collecting sexual orientation and gender identity information at death. *American Journal of Public Health (1971)*, 109(2), 255–259. https://doi.org/10.2105/AJPH.2018.304829

Haw, C.M. (1994). A cluster of suicides at a London psychiatric unit. *Suicide and Life-Threatening Behavior*, 24, 256–266. PMID: 7825198 https://doi.org/10.1111/j.1943-278X.1994.tb00750.x

Haw, C., Hawton, K., Niedzwiedz, C., & Platt S. (2013). Suicide clusters: A review of risk factors and mechanisms. *Suicide and Life-Threatening Behavior*, 43, 97–108. https://doi.org/10.1111/j.1943-278X.2012.00130.x

Hawton, K., & Fortune, S. (2008). Suicidal behavior and deliberate self-harm. In *Rutter's child and adolescent psychiatry* (pp. 648–669). https://doi.org/10.1002/9781444300895

Hawton, K., Linsell, L., Adeniji, T., Sariaslan, A., & Fazel, S. (2014, March 29). Self-harm in prisons in England and Wales: an epidemiological study of prevalence, risk factors, clustering, and subsequent suicide. *Lancet*, 383(9923), 1147–1154. https://doi.org/10.1016/S0140-6736(13)62118-2

Hochhauser, S., Rao, S., England-Kennedy, E., & Roy, S. (2020). Why social justice matters: A context for suicide prevention efforts. *International Journal for Equity in Health*, 19(1), 1–8. https://doi.org/10.1186/s12939-020-01173-9

Holliday, R., Forster, J.E., Desai, A., Miller, C., Monteith, L.L., Schneiderman, A.I., & Hoffmire, C.A. (2021). Association of lifetime homelessness and justice involvement with psychiatric symptoms, suicidal ideation, and suicide attempt among post-9/11 veterans. *Journal of Psychiatric Research*, 144, 455–461. https://doi.org/10.1016/j.jpsychires.2021.11.007

Holliday, R., Kinney, A.R., Smith, A.A., Forster, J.E., Stimmel, M.A., Clark, S.C., Liu, S., Monteith, L.L., & Brenner, L.A. (2023). Suicide risk among veterans using VHA justice-involved services: A latent class analysis. *BMC Psychiatry*, 23(1), 235. https://doi.org/10.1186/s12888-023-04725-9

Honjo, K. (2004). Social epidemiology: Definition, history, and research examples. *Environmental Health and Preventive Medicine*, 9(5), 193–199. https://doi.org/10.1007/BF02898100

Horwitz, A.G., Berona, J., Busby, D.R., Eisenberg, D., Zheng, K., Pistorello, J., Albucher, R., Coryell, W., Favorite, T., Walloch, J.C., & King, C.A. (2020). Variation in suicide risk among subgroups of sexual and gender minority college students. *Suicide and Life-Threatening Behavior*, 50(5). https://doi.org/10.1111/sltb.12637

Hoyer, E.H., Mortensen, P.B., & Olesen, A.V. (2000). Mortality and causes of death in a total national sample of patients with affective disorders admitted for the first time between 1973 and 1993. *British Journal of Psychiatry*, 176, 76–82. https://doi.org/10.1192/bjp.176.1.76

Hunt, I.M., Kapur, N., Windfuhr, K., Robinson, J., Bickley, H., Flynn, S., Parsons, R., Burns, J., Shaw, J., & Appleby, L. (2006). Suicide in schizophrenia: Findings from a national clinical survey. *Journal of Psychiatric Practice*, 12(3), 139–147. https://doi.org/10.1097/00131746-200605000-00002

Interact . (2021, January 26). Frequently asked questions. Interact: Advocates for intersex youth. https://interactadvocates.org/faq/

International Association for Suicide Prevention. (2020). The decriminalisation of attempted suicide: Policy position statement. Washington (DC): International Association for Suicide Prevention. www.iasp.info/wp-content/uploads/IASP-Decriminalisation-Policy-Position-Statement-GA.pdf

Jacobs, R., Grobler, C., & Strumpher, J. (2021). Identifying a probable suicide cluster in an acute care psychiatric hospital in the Eastern Cape, South Africa. *South African Journal of Psychiatry*, 19(27), 1646. https://doi.org/10.4102/sajpsychiatry.v27i0.1646

James, S., Herman, J., Rankin, S., Keisling, M., Mottet, L., & Anafi, M. (2016). *The report of the 2015 U.S. transgender survey* (p. 302). The National Center for Transgender Equality. USTS-Full-Report-Dec17.pdf

Jang, H., Lee, S., Park, S., Kang, B., & Choi, H. (2023). Analysis of suicide statistics and trends between 2011 and 2021 among Korean women. *Korean Journal of Women Health Nursing*, 29(4), 348–356. https://doi.org/10.4069/kjwhn.2023.12.14.1

Joaquim, R.M., Guatimosim, R.F., da Silva Araújo, R.J., Nardi, A.E., Veras, A.B., & de Medeiros Alves, V. (2021). Vulnerability biomarkers for mental illness and suicide risk: Regards for the development of pharmacological and psychological therapies. *Current Research in Behavioral Sciences*, 2, 100050. https://doi.org/10.1016/j.crbeha.2021.100050.

Joe, S., & Niedermeier, D. (2008). Preventing suicide: A neglected social work research agenda. *British Journal of Social Work*, 38(3), 507–530. https://doi.org/10.1093/bjsw/bcl353

Joiner, T. (2005). *Why people die by suicide*. Harvard University Press.

Joiner, T. (2010, April 28). NPR: Mental health. Deconstructing 'Myths about Suicide' interview. Talk of the Nation. www.npr.org/2010/04/28/126365907/deconstructing-myths-about-suicide

Joo, J., Hwang, S., & Gallo, J.J. (2016). Death ideation and suicidal ideation in a community sample who do not meet criteria for major depression. *Crisis: The Journal of Crisis Intervention and Suicide Prevention*, 37(2), 161–165. https://doi.org/10.1027/0227-5910/a000365

Joseph, V.A., Martínez-Alés, G., Olfson, M., Shaman, J., Gould, M.S., Gimbrone, C., & Keyes, K.M. (2023). Trends in suicide among Black women in the United States, 1999-2020. *The American Journal of Psychiatry*, 180(12), 914–917. https://doi.org/10.1176/appi.ajp.20230254

Kaur, J., Manders, B., & Windsor-Shellard, B. (2019, July 25). Drug-related deaths and suicide in prison custody in England and Wales: 2008 to 2016. *Office for National Statistics. Drug-related deaths and suicide in prison custody in England and Wales*

Kemal, S., Krass, P., Brogan, L., Min, J., Quarshie, W.O., & Fein, J.A. (2023). Identifying suicide risk in adolescents with firearm access: Screening in the emergency department. *Academic Pediatrics*, 23(1), 165–171. https://doi.org/10.1016/j.acap.2022.05.011

Kim, J.W., Jung, H.Y., Won, D.Y., Shin, Y.S., Noh, J.H., & Kang, T.I. (2020). Landscape of elderly suicide in South Korea: Its trend according to age, gender, and educational attainment. *OMEGA – Journal of Death and Dying*, 82(2), 214–229. https://doi.org/10.1177/0030222818807845

King, K.A., Vidourek, R.A., Yockey, R.A., & Merianos, A.L. (2018). Impact of parenting behaviors on adolescent suicide based on age of adolescent. *Journal of Child and Family Studies*, 27(12), 4083–4090. https://doi.org/10.1007/s10826-018-1220-3

Klonsky, D., & May, A. (2015). The three-step theory (3ST): A new theory of suicide rooted in the "Ideation-to-action" framework. *International Journal of Cognitive Therapy*, 8(2). https://doi.org/10.1521/ijct.2015.8.2.114

Kogan, S.M., Reck, A.J., Curtis, M.G., & Oshri, A. (2024). Childhood adversity and racial discrimination forecast suicidal and death ideation among emerging adult Black men: A longitudinal analysis. *Cultural Diversity & Ethnic Minority Psychology*. https://doi.org/10.1037/cdp0000641

Krueger, E.A., Divsalar, S., Luhur, W., Choi, S.K., & Meyer, I.H. (2020). *TransPop – U.S. transgender population health survey (methodology and technical notes)*. Los Angeles, CA: The Williams Institute. Retrieved from: www.transpop.org/s/TransPop-Survey-Methods-v18-FINAL-copy.pdf

Lacey, K.K., Parnell, R., Mouzon, D.M., Matusko, N., Head, D., Abelson, J.M., & Jackson, J.S. (2015). The mental health of US black women: The roles of social context and severe intimate partner violence. *BMJ Open*, 5(10), e008415. https://doi.org/10.1136/bmjopen-2015-008415

Lake, A.M., & Gould, M.S. (2014). Suicide clusters and suicide contagion. In S. Koslow, P. Ruiz, & C. Nemeroff (Eds.), *A concise guide to understanding suicide: Epidemiology, pathophysiology and prevention* (pp. 52–61). Cambridge University Press.

Lambert, S.F., Boyd, R.C., & Ialongo, N.S. (2022). Protective factors for suicidal ideation among Black adolescents indirectly exposed to community violence. *Suicide and Life-Threatening Behavior*, 52(3), 478–489. https://doi.org/10.1111/sltb.12839

Lazar, S.G. (2014) The cost-effectiveness of psychotherapy for the major psychiatric diagnoses. *Psychodynamic Psychiatry*, 42(3), 423–457. https://doi.org/10.1521/pdps.2014.42.3.423

Lech, S., Köppe, M., Berger, M., Alonso-Perez, E., Gellert, P., Herrmann, W., & Buspavanich, P. (2024). Depressive symptoms among individuals identifying as asexual: A cross-sectional study. *Scientific Reports*, 14(1), 16120–16127. https://doi.org/10.1038/s41598-024-66900-6

Lehrner, A., & Yehuda, R. (2018). Cultural trauma and epigenetic inheritance. *Development and Psychopathology*, 30(5), 1763–1777. https://doi.org/10.1017/S0954579418001153

Lenz, A.S., Rosenbaum, L., & Sheperis, D. (2016). Meta-analysis of randomized controlled trials of motivational enhancement therapy for reducing substance use. *Journal of Addictions & Offender Counseling*, 37(2), 66–86. https://doi.org/10.1002/jaoc.12017

Levi-Belz, Y. (2019). With a little help from my friends: A follow-up study on the contribution of interpersonal characteristics to posttraumatic growth among suicide-loss survivors. *Psychological Trauma: Theory, Research, Practice, and Policy*, 11, 895–904. https://doi.org/10.1037/tra0000456

Levi-Belz Y., & Gilo T. (2020). Emotional distress among suicide survivors: The moderating role of self-forgiveness. *Frontiers in Psychiatry*, 11, 341. https://doi.org/10.3389/fpsyt.2020.00341

Levine, J., & Sher, L. (2020). How to increase the role of social workers in suicide preventive interventions. *Acta Neuropsychiatrica*, 32, 186–195. https://doi.org/10.1017/neu.2020.11

Linehan, M.M., Korslund, K.E., Harned, M.S., Gallop, R.J., Lungu, A., Neacsiu, A.D., McDavid, J., Comtois, K.A., & Murray-Gregory, A.M. (2015). Dialectical behavior therapy for high suicide risk in individuals with borderline personality disorder: A randomized clinical trial and component analysis. *JAMA Psychiatry (Chicago, IL.)*, 72(5), 475–482. https://doi.org/10.1001/jamapsychiatry.2014.3039

Lyons, B.H., Walters, M.L., Jack, S.P.D., Petrosky, E., Blair, J.M., & Ivey-Stephenson, A.Z. (2019). Suicides among lesbian and gay male individuals: Findings from the national violent death reporting system. *American Journal of Preventive Medicine*, 56(4), 512–521. https://doi.org/10.1016/j.amepre.2018.11.012

Macleod, R.D., Wilson, D.M., & Malpas, P. (2012). Assisted or hastened death: The healthcare practitioner's dilemma. *Global Journal of Health Sciences*, 4, 87–98.

Macrynikola, N., Auad, E., Manjivar, J., & Miranda, R. (2021). Does social media use confer suicide risk? A systematic review of the evidence. *Computers in Human Behavior Reports*, 3(100094). https://doi.org/10.1016/j.chbr.2021.100094

Mann, J.J., Apter, A., Bertolote, J., Beautrais, A., Currier, D., Haas, A., Hegerl, U., Lonnqvist, J., Malone, K., Marusic, A., Mehlum, L., Patton, G., Phillips, M., Rutz, W., Rihmer, Z., Schmidtke, A., Shaffer, D., Silverman, M., Takahashi, Y., ..., & Hendin, H. (2005). Suicide prevention strategies: A systematic review. *JAMA: The Journal of the American Medical Association*, 294(16), 2064–2074. https://doi.org/10.1001/jama.294.16.2064

Maple, M., Cerel, J., Sanford, R., Pearce, T., & Jordan, J. (2017). Is exposure to suicide beyond kin associated with risk for suicidal behavior? A systematic review of the evidence. *Suicide and Life-Threatening Behavior: Volume*, 47, 461–474. https://doi.org/10.1111/sltb.12308

Marchi, M., Arcolin, E., Fiore, G., Travascio, A., Uberti, D., Amaddeo, F., Converti, M., Fiorillo, A., Mirandola, M., Pinna, F., Ventriglio, A., Galeazzi, G.M., & Italian Working Group on LGBTIQ Mental Health. (2022). Self-harm and suicidality among LGBTIQ people: A systematic review and meta-analysis. *International Review of Psychiatry (Abingdon, England)*, 34(3–4), 240–256. https://doi.org/10.1080/09540261.2022.2053070

Marlow, N.M., Xie, Z., Tanner, R., Jo, A., & Kirby, A.V. (2021). Association between disability and suicide-related outcomes among US adults. *American Journal of Preventive Medicine*, 61(6), 852–862. https://doi.org/10.1016/j.amepre.2021.05.035

Meffert, B.N., Morabito, D.M., Sawicki, D.A., Hausman, C., Southwick, S.M., Pietrzak, R.H., & Heinz, A.J. (2019). US veterans who do and do not utilize veterans affairs health care services. *The Primary Care Companion for CNS Disorders*, 21(1). https://doi.org/10.4088/pcc.18m02350

Mena, F.J., Padilla, A.M., & Maldonado, M. (1987). Acculturative stress and specific coping strategies among immigrant and later generation college students. *Hispanic Journal of Behavioral Sciences*, 9, 207–225.

Méndez-Bustos, P., Calati, R., Rubio-Ramírez, F., Olié, E., Courtet, P., & Lopez-Castroman, J. (2019). Effectiveness of psychotherapy on suicidal risk: A systematic review of observational studies. *Frontiers in Psychology*, 10, 277–277. https://doi.org/10.3389/fpsyg.2019.00277

Meyer, I.H. (2015). Resilience in the study of minority stress and health of sexual and gender minorities. *Psychology of Sexual Orientation and Gender Diversity*, 2(3), 209–213. https://doi.org/10.1037/sgd0000132

Miller, J. (2003). Critical incident debriefing and social work: Expanding the frame. *Journal of Social Service Research*, 30(2), 7–25. https://doi.org/10.1300/J079v30n02_02

Milligan, T., & Kelber, M. (2024). The role of case management in suicide prevention. Health.mil: The official website of the Military Health System. https://health.mil/Military-Health-Topics/Centers-of-Excellence/Psychological-Health-Center-of-Excellence/Clinicians-Corner-Blog/The-Role-of-Case-Management-in-Suicide-Prevention

Mishara, B.L., & Weisstub, D.N. (2016). The legal status of suicide: A global review. *International Journal of Law and Psychiatry*, 1(44), 54–74. https://doi.org/10.1016/j.ijlp.2015.08.032

Moagi, M.M., Van Der Wath, A.E., Jiyane, P.M., & Rikhotso, R.S. (2021). Mental health challenges of lesbian, gay, bisexual and transgender people: An integrated literature review. *Health SA Gesondheid*, 26(1), a1487. https://doi.org/10.4102/hsag.v26i0.1487

Monteith, L., Smith, N., Holliday, R., Dorsey Holliman, B., LoFaro, C., & Mohatt, N. (2020). We're afraid to say suicide. *The Journal of Nervous and Mental Disease*, 208(5), 371–376. https://doi.org/10.1097/NMD.0000000000001139

Morris-Perez, P., Abenavoli, R., Benzekri, A., Rosenbach-Jordan, S., & Boccieri, R.G. (2023). Preventing adolescent suicide: Recommendations for policymakers, practitioners, program developers, and researchers. *Social Policy Report*, 36(2–3), 1–32. https://doi.org/10.1002/sop2.30

Mueller, A.S., Abrutyn, S., Pescosolido, B., & Diefendorf, S. (2021). The social roots of suicide: Theorizing how the external social world matters to suicide and suicide prevention. *Frontiers in Psychology*, 12, 621569. https://doi.org/10.3389/fpsyg.2021.621569

National Center for Health Statistics. (2024). Mortality multiple cause-of-death. U.S. Department of Health & Human Services, CDC, National Vital Statistics System. Public-use data file documentation: Mortality multiple cause-of-death.

National Institute of Justice. (n.d.). *Figure 1: Estimates of lifetime interracial and intraracial violence.* Office of Justice Programs: Washington, DC. https://nij.ojp.gov/media/image/19456

National Institute of Mental Health. (n. d.). Mental health information: *Suicide.* www.nimh.nih.gov/health/statistics/suicide

Nelson, K.M., Starkebaum, G.A., & Reiber, G.E. (2007). Veterans using and uninsured veterans not using veterans affairs (VA) health care. *Public Health Reports*, 122(1), 934–100. https://doi.org/10.1177/003335490712200113

Niedzwiedz, C., Haw, C., Hawton, K., & Platt, S. (2014). The definition and epidemiology of clusters of suicidal behavior: a systematic review. *Suicide and Life-Threatening Behavior*, 44, 569–581. https://doi.org/10.1111/sltb.12091

Noonan, M., Hohloff, H., & Ginder, S. (2015). Mortality in local jails and state prisons, 2000-2013 statistical tables. *Bureau of Justice Statistics.* www.bjs.gov/index.cfm?ty=pbdetail&iid=5341

Oexle, N., Feigelman, W., & Sheehan, L. (2018a). Perceived suicide stigma, secrecy about suicide loss and mental health outcomes. *Death Studies*, 44(4), 248–255. https://doi.org/10.1080/07481187.2018.1539052

Oexle, N., Herrmann, K., Staiger, T., Sheehan, L., Rüsch, N., & Krumm, S. (2018b). Stigma and suicidality among suicide attempt survivors: A qualitative study. *Death Studies*, 43(6), 381–388. https://doi.org/10.1080/07481187.2018.1474286

Oexle, N., Valacchi, D., Grübel, P., Becker, T., & Rüsch, N. (2022). Two sides of the same coin? The association between suicide stigma and suicide normalisation. *Epidemiology and Psychiatric Sciences*, 31, e78, 1–7. https://doi.org/10.1017/S2045796022000610

Ösby, U., Brandt, L., Correia, N., Ekbom, A., & Sparén, P. (2001). Excess mortality in bipolar and unipolar disorder in Sweden. *Archives of General Psychiatry*, 58(9), 844. https://doi.org/10.1001/archpsyc.58.9.844

Parker, J.S., Haskins, N., Clemons, A., McClure, E., & Washington, J. (2022). Early career Black women in school-based mental health fields: Understanding their experiences of workplace discrimination. *Journal of School Psychology*, 92, 49–65. https://doi.org/10.1016/j.jsp.2022.02.004

Patten, M., Carmichael, H., Moore, A., & Velopulos, C. (2022). Circumstances of suicide among lesbian, gay, bisexual and transgender individuals. *The Journal of Surgical Research*, 270, 522–529. https://doi.org/10.1016/j.jss.2021.08.029

Patterson, C.W. (1981). Suicide. In basic psychopathology: A programmed text. Suicide risk: Case studies and vignettes. Case 7, Syracuse University: School of Education. Suicide Risk: Case Studies and Vignettes | Syracuse University School of Education.

Payne, C.F. (2022). Expansion, compression, neither, both? Divergent patterns in healthy, disability-free, and morbidity-free life expectancy across U.S. birth cohorts, 1998–2016. *Demography*, 59, 949–973. https://doi.org/10.1215/00703370-9938662

Peterson, C., Haileyesus, T., & Stone, D.M. (2024). Economic cost of U.S. suicide and nonfatal self-harm. *American Journal of Preventive Medicine*, 67(1), 129–133. https://doi.org/10.1016/j.amepre.2024.03.002

Pisnoli, I., & Van der Hallen, R. (2022). Attitudes toward suicide and the impact of client suicide: A structural equation modeling approach. *International Journal of Environmental Research and Public Health*, 19, 5481. https://doi.org/10.3390/ijerph19095481

Pitman, A., Osborn, D., King, M., & Erlangsen, A. (2014). Effects of suicide bereavement on mental health and suicide risk. *The Lancet Psychiatry*, 1(1), 86–94. https://doi.org/10.1016/S2215-0366(14)70224-X

Pitman, A.L., Osborn, D.P.J., Rantell, K., & King, M.B. (2016). Bereavement by suicide as a risk factor for suicide attempt: A cross-sectional national UK-wide study of 3432 young bereaved adults. *BMJ Open*, 6(1), e009948. https://doi.org/10.1136/bmjopen-2015-009948

Price, J.H., & Khubchandani, J. (2019). The changing characteristics of African-American adolescent suicides, 2001–2017. *Journal of Community Health*, 44(4), 756–763. https://doi.org/10.1007/s10900-019-00678-x

Polanco-Roman, L., & Miranda, R. (2013). Culturally related stress, hopelessness, and vulnerability to depressive symptoms and suicidal ideation in emerging adulthood. *Behavior Therapy*, 44(1), 75–87. https://doi.org/10.1016/j.beth.2012.07.002

Polanco-Roman, L., Anglin, D.M., Miranda, R., & Jeglic, E.L. (2019). Racial/ethnic discrimination and suicidal ideation in emerging adults: The role of traumatic stress and depressive symptoms varies by gender not race/ethnicity. *Journal of Youth and Adolescence*, 48(10), 2023–2037. https://doi.org/10.1007/s10964-019-01097-w

Quinn, C.R., Beer, O.W.J., Boyd, D.T., Tirmazi, T., Nebbitt, V., & Joe, S. (2022). An assessment of the role of parental incarceration and substance misuse in suicidal planning of African American youth and young adults. *Journal of Racial and Ethnic Health Disparities*, 9(3), 1062–1074. https://doi.org/10.1007/s40615-021-01045-0

Ramchand, R., Gordon, J.A., & Pearson, J. L. (2021a). Trends in suicide rates by race and ethnicity in the United States. *JAMA Network Open*, 4(5), e2111563. https://doi.org/10.1001/jamanetworkopen.2021.11563

Ramchand, R., Schuler, M.S., Schoenbaum, M., Colpe, L., & Ayer, L. (2021b). Suicidality among sexual minority adults: Gender, age, and race/ethnicity differences. *American Journal of Preventive Medicine*. https://doi.org/10.1016/j.amepre.2021.07.012

Ribeiro, J.D., Huang, X., Fox, K.R., & Franklin, J.C. (2018). Depression and hopelessness as risk factors for suicide ideation, attempts and death: Meta-analysis of longitudinal studies. *The British Journal of Psychiatry*, 212(5), 279–286. https://doi.org/10.1192/bjp.2018.27

Richesson, D., & Hoenig, J. (2021). *Key substance use and mental health indicators in the United States: Results from the 2020 national survey on drug use and health*. Substance Abuse and Mental Health Services Administration (SAMHSA), U.S. Department of Health and Human Services (HHS). www.samhsa.gov/data/sites/default/files/reports/rpt35325/NSDUHFFRPDFWHTMLFiles2020/2020NSDUHFFR1PDFW102121.pdf

Reinert, M., Fritze, D., & Nguyen, T. (2022, October). *"The state of mental health in America 2023."* Mental Health America, Alexandria VA. https://mhanational.org/sites/default/files/2023-State-of-Mental-Health-in-America-Report.pdf

Rizk, M.M., Herzog, S., Dugad, S., & Stanley, B. (2021). Suicide risk and addiction: The impact of alcohol and opioid use disorders. *Current Addiction Reports*, 8(2), 194–207. https://doi.org/10.1007/s40429-021-00361-z

Romanelli, M., Sheftall, A.H., Irsheid, S.B., Lindsey, M.A., & Grogan, T.M. (2022). Factors associated with distinct patterns of suicidal thoughts, suicide plans, and suicide attempts among US adolescents. *Prevention Science*, 23(1), 73–84. https://doi.org/10.1007/s11121-021-01295-8

Rose, R., & Molina, N. (2017). Interventions. In I. Galynker (Ed.), *The suicidal crisis: Clinical guide to the assessment of imminent suicide risk* (pp. 1–8). Oxford University Press.

Rosenwohl-Mack, A., Tamar-Mattis, S., Baratz, A.B., Dalke, K.B., Ittelson, A., Zieselman, K., & Flatt, J.D. (2020). A national study on the physical and mental health of intersex adults in the U.S. *PLoS One*, 15(10), e0240088. https://doi.org/10.1371/journal.pone.0240088

Rosay, A. (2016, June 01). Violence against American Indian and Alaska Native men and women: An NIJ-funded study shows that American Indian and Alaska Native women and men suffer violence at alarmingly high rates. *National Institute of Justice Journal*, 277, 1–50. National Institute of Justice. Office of Justice Programs. Washington, DC. www.ojp.gov/pdffiles1/nij/249821.pdf

Rubin, A., Weiss, E.L. & Coll, J.E. (2013). *Handbook of military social work*. Wiley & Sons.

Saaddine, J.B., Narayan, K.M., & Vinicor, F. (2003). Vision loss: A public health problem? *Ophthalmology*, 110, 253–254. www.aaojournal.org/action/showPdf?pii=S0161-6420%2802%2901839-0

Sanders, S., Jacobson, J.M., & Ting, L. (2008). Preparing for the inevitable: Training social workers to cope with client suicide. *Journal of Teaching in Social Work*, 28(1–2), 1–18. https://doi.org/10.1080/08841230802178821

Sariaslan, A., Fanshawe, T., Pitkänen, J., Cipriani, A., Martikainen, P., & Fazel, S. (2023). Predicting suicide risk in 137,112 people with severe mental illness in Finland: External validation of the oxford mental illness and suicide tool (OxMIS). *Translational Psychiatry*, 13(1), 126–126. https://doi.org/10.1038/s41398-023-02422-5

Saunders, H., & Panchal, N. (2023). A look at the latest suicide data and change over the last decade. KFF. A Look at the Latest Suicide Data and Change Over the Last Decade | KFF Schoolwerth, A.C., Engelgau, M.M., Hostetter, T.H., Rufo, K.H., Chianchiano, D., McClellan, W.M., Warnock, D.G., & Vinicor, F. (2006). Chronic kidney disease: A public health problem that needs a public health action plan. *Preventing Chronic Disease*, 3(2), A57. PMCID: PMC1563984 PMID: 16539798.

Shanahan, L., & Copeland, W.E. (2021). Psychiatry and deaths of despair. *JAMA Psychiatry*, 78(7), 695–696. https://doi.org/10.1001/jamapsychiatry.2021.0256

Shneidman, E., Farberow, N., & Litman, R. (1970). *The psychology of suicide*. Science House.

Sinyor, M., Schaffer, A., Nishikawa, Y., Redelmeier, Donald, A., Niederkrotenthaler, T., Sareen, J., Levitt, A.J., Kiss, A., & Pirkis, J. (2018). The association between suicide deaths and putatively harmful and protective factors in media reports. *Canadian Medical Association Journal (CMAJ)*, 190(30), E900–E907. https://doi.org/10.1503/cmaj.170698

Smedslund, G., Berg, R.C., Hammerstrøm, K.T., Steiro, A., Leiknes, K.A., Dahl, H.M., & Karlsen, K. (2011). Motivational interviewing for substance abuse. *Cochrane Database of Systematic Reviews*, 2011(5), CD008063. https://doi.org/10.1002/14651858.CD008063.pub2

Snowden, D.L., Oh, S., Salas-Wright, C.P., Vaughn, M.G., & King, E. (2017). Military service and crime: New evidence. *Social Psychiatry & Psychiatric Epidemiology*, 52(5), 605–615. http://doi.org/10.1007/s00127-017-1342-8

Song, Y., Rhee, S.J., Lee, H., Kim, M.J., Shin, D., & Ahn, Y.M. (2020). Comparison of suicide risk by mental illness: A retrospective review of 14-year electronic medical records. *Journal of Korean Medical Science*, 35(47), e402. https://doi.org/10.3346/jkms.2020.35.e402

Spillane, A., Matvienko-Sikar, K., Larkin, C., Corcoran, P., & Arensman, E. (2018). What are the physical and psychological health effects of suicide bereavement on family members? an observational and interview mixed-methods study in Ireland. *BMJ Open*, 8(1), e019472. https://doi.org/10.1136/bmjopen-2017-019472

Spitzer, W.J., & Neely, K. (1992). Critical incident stress: The role of hospital-based social work in developing a statewide intervention system for first-responders delivering emergency services. *Social Work in Health Care*, 18(1), 39–58. https://doi.org/10.1300/j010v18n01_03. PMID: 1298101.

Stanley, A.R., Aguilar, T., Holland, K.M., & Orpinas, P. (2023). Precipitating circumstances associated with intimate partner problem–related suicides. *American Journal of Preventive Medicine*, 65(3), 385–394. https://doi.org/10.1016/j.amepre.2023.03.011

Stanley, B., & Brown, G.K. (2012). Safety planning intervention: A brief intervention to mitigate suicide risk. *Cognitive and Behavioral Practice*, 19(2), 256–264. https://doi.org/10.1016/j.cbpra.2011.01.001

Statistica. (n.d.). Number of deaths in South Korea in 2023, by cause of death (per 100,000 inhabitants). South Korea: death rate by cause of death 2023 | Statista.

Statistics Korea. (2022, September 27). *Causes of death statistics in 2021*. https://kostat.go.kr/boardDownload.es?bid=11773&list_no=421206&seq=1

Stephenson, J. (2022). High suicide rates among American Indian or Alaska Native persons surging even higher. *JAMA Health Forum*, 3(9), e224179. https://doi.org/10.1001/jamahealthforum.2022.4179

Stone, D.M., Jones, S.E., & McGuire, L.C. (2022). Suicides Among American Indian or Alaska Native Persons — National Violent Death Reporting System, United States, 2015–2020. *Morbidity and Mortality Weekly Report (MMWR)*, 71(37), 1177–1183. http://dx.doi.org/10.15585/mmwr.mm7137a1

Suarez, N.A., Trujillo, L., McKinnon, I.I., Mack, K.A., Lyons, B., Robin, L., Carman-McClanahan, M., Pampati, S., Cezair, K.L.R., & Ethier, K.A.(2024). Disparities in school connectedness, unstable housing, experiences of violence, mental health, and suicidal thoughts and behaviors among transgender and cisgender high school students–youth risk behavior survey, united states, 2023.

Morbidity and Mortality Weekly Report. Supplement, 73(4), 50–58. https://doi.org/10.15585/mmwr.su7304a6

Substance Abuse and Mental Health Services Administration (SAMHSA). (2017). Suicide clusters within American Indian and Alaska Native communities: A review of the literature and recommendations. Rockville, MD. US Department of Health and Human Services, Center for Mental Health Services. https://store.samhsa.gov/sites/default/files/d7/priv/sma17-5050.pdf

Substance Abuse and Mental Health Services Administration (SAMHSA). (2024a). *Suicide prevention strategies for underserved youth*. Publication No. PEP24-06-005. Substance Abuse and Mental Health Services Administration. Suicide Prevention Strategies for Underserved Youth

Substance Abuse and Mental Health Services Administration (SAMHSA). (2024b). SAMHSA's suicide prevention initiatives. Suicide prevention initiatives | SAMHSA.

Substance Abuse and Mental Health Services Administration (SAMHSA). (2022). *2022 national survey on drug use and health*. Substance Abuse and Mental Health Services Administration. 2022 NSDUH Detailed Tables | CBHSQ Data

Suicide Prevention Resource Center. (2020). The role of adult correctional officers in preventing suicide. Supported by a grant from the U.S. Department of Health and Human Services, Substance Abuse and Mental Health Services Administration (SAMHSA) under Grant No. 5U79SM059945.

Suicide Prevention Resource Center. (2023). Barriers and opportunities for suicide prevention among correctional officers: An issue brief for clinicians. https://sprc.org/wp-content/uploads/Correctional-Officers-Brief.pdf

Sun, F.K., Long, A., & Hsieh, P.C. (2013). Short-term effects of a suicide education intervention for family caregivers of people who are suicidal. *Journal of Clinical Nursing*, 22(19-20), 2824–2834. https://doi.org/10.1111/jocn.12351.

Sveen, C.A., & Walby, F.A. (2008). Suicide survivors' mental health and grief reactions: A systematic review of controlled studies. *Suicide and Life-Threatening Behavior*, 38(1), 13–29. https://doi.org/10.1521/suli.2008.38.1.13

Swedo, E.A., Beauregard, J.L., de Fijter, S., Werhan, L., Norris, K., Montgomery, M.P., Rose, E.B., David-Ferdon, C., Massetti, G.M., Hillis, S.D., & Sumner, S.A. (2021). Associations between social media and suicidal behaviors during a youth suicide cluster in Ohio. *Journal of Adolescent Health*, 68(2), 308–316. https://doi.org/10.1016/j.jadohealth.2020.05.049

Taiminen, T., Salmenperä, T., & Lehtinen, K. (1992). A suicide epidemic in a psychiatric hospital. *Suicide and Life-Threatening Behavior*, 22(3), 350–363.

Tamworth, M., Killaspy, H., Billings, J., & Gibbons R. (2022). Psychiatrists' experience of a peer support group for reflecting on patient suicide and homicide: A qualitative study. *International Journal of Environmental Research and Public Health*, 19, 14507. https://doi.org/10.3390/ijerph192114507

Taylor, E.N., Timko, C., Nash, A., Owens, M.D., Harris, A.H.S., & Finlay, A.K. (2020). Posttraumatic stress disorder and justice involvement among military veterans: A systematic review and meta-analysis. *Journal of Traumatic Stress*, 33(5), 804–812. https://doi.org/10.1002/jts.22526

The Economist. (2023). South Korea's suicide rate fell for years. Women are driving it up again. *The Economist*. www.proquest.com/docview/2817788571?OpenUrlRefId=info:xri/sid:summon&accountid=10639&sourcetype=Magazines

The Trevor Project. (2023). 2023 U.S. national survey on the mental health of LGBTQ young people. The Trevor Project: 2023 U.S. National Survey on the Mental Health of LGBTQ Young People.

Thompson, M.P., Kingree, J.B., & Lamis, D. (2019). Associations of adverse childhood experiences and suicidal behaviors in adulthood in a U.S. nationally representative sample. *Child: Care, Health and Development*, 45(1), 121–128. https://doi.org/10.1111/cch.12617

Till, B., Tran, U.S., & Niederkrotenthaler, T. (2017). Relationship satisfaction and risk factors for suicide. *Crisis: The Journal of Crisis Intervention and Suicide Prevention*, 38(1), 7–16. https://doi.org/10.1027/0227-5910/a000407

United States Census Bureau. (2022). Annual estimates of the resident population for the United States, regions, states, District of Columbia, and Puerto Rico: April 1, 2020 to July 1, 2022. Table. Accessed from 2022 National and State Population Estimates Press Kit.

United States Department of Defense (USDOD). (2023, October 26). *Annual report on suicide in the Military CY 2022*. Defense Suicide Prevention Office. www.dspo.mil/Portals/113/Documents/ARSM_CY22.pdf

United States Department of Health and Human Services (U.S. DHHS). (2016). Centers for disease control and prevention. National Center for Injury Prevention and Control. National Intimate Partner and Sexual Violence Survey (NISVS): General Population Survey Raw Data, 2010. Inter-university Consortium for Political and Social Research [distributor], 2016-06-09. https://doi.org/10.3886/ICPSR34305.v1

United States Department of Health and Human Services (U.S. DHHS). (2024, April). *National strategy for suicide prevention*. Washington, DC: HHS. 2024 National Strategy for Suicide Prevention.

United States Department of Justice. (2023, August). *Recommendations regarding the prevention of death by suicide of law enforcement*. www.justice.gov/d9/2023-09/ecats_2023-201340_sec._4c_report.pdf

United States Department of Veteran Affairs (USDVA). (2024a). *National veteran suicide prevention annual report, part 1 of 2: In-depth reviews*. 2024 National Veteran Suicide Prevention Annual Report. 2024 National Veteran Suicide Prevention Annual Report

United States Department of Veteran Affairs (USDVA). (2024b). *National veteran suicide prevention annual report, part 2 of 2: Report findings*. 2024 National Veteran Suicide Prevention Annual Report.

University of Rochester Medical Center (URMC). (2014). *The adverse childhood experiences study*. The Adverse Childhood Experiences Study.

Van Orden, K.A., Witte, T.K., Cukrowicz, K.C., Braithwaite, S.R., Selby, E.A., Joiner, T.E., Jr. (2010). The interpersonal theory of suicide. *Psychological Review*, 117(2), 575–600. https://doi.org/10.1037/a0018697

Walker, R.L., Wingate, L.R., Obasi, E.M., & Joiner, T.E., Jr. (2008). An empirical investigation of acculturative stress and ethnic identity as moderators for depression and suicidal ideation in college students. *Cultural Diversity & Ethnic Minority Psychology*, 14(1), 75–82. https://doi.org/10.1037/1099-9809.14.1.75

Wasserman, D., Carli, V., Iosue, M., Javed, A., & Herrman, H. (2021). Suicide prevention in childhood and adolescence: A narrative review of current knowledge on risk and protective factors and effectiveness of interventions. *Asia-Pacific Psychiatry*, 13, e12452. https://doi.org/10.1111/appy.12452

Webb, R.T., Qin, P., Stevens, H., Mortensen, P.B., Appleby, L., & Shaw, J. (2011). National study of suicide in all people with a criminal justice history. *Archives Of General Psychiatry*, , 68(6), 591–599. https://doi.org/10.1001/archgenpsychiatry.2011.7

Wilkins, N., Hertz, M., Kuehl, T., & Klevens, J. (2015). 0040 Connecting the dots: Understanding and addressing the links between multiple forms of violence. *Injury Prevention*, 21(Suppl 1), A2. https://doi.org/10.1136/injuryprev-2015-041602.4

World Health Organization (WHO). (2021). *Suicide worldwide in 2019: Global health estimates*. Geneva. License: CC BY-NC-SA 3.0 IGO. 9789240026643-eng.pdf.

World Health Organization (WHO). (2023, September 12). WHO *launches new resources on prevention and decriminalization of suicide* [Department update]. www.who.int/news/item/12-09-2023-who-launches-new-resources-on-prevention-and-decriminalization-of-suicide

World Health Organization (WHO). (2025, March 25). *Suicide* [Fact sheet]. www.who.int/news-room/fact-sheets/detail/suicide

World Population View. (2024). *Suicide rate by country 2024*. Suicide rate by country 2024.

10

POLICE VIOLENCE AND PUBLIC HEALTH

Introduction

Sharmane, a 21-year-old African-American transgender woman was well known and liked by residents of her housing project where she had been born and reared. Most remember her as having a wonderful and bright personality. Members of the local *LGBQT* community which she was a part of were saddened to hear about her untimely death at the hands of local police. According to eyewitness accounts, police were dispatched to Sharmane's home to prevent her from harming herself or her grandmother whom she lived with. The police department and its officers were not strangers to Sharmane or the community since it was accustomed to receiving routine calls from concerned neighbors for several issues ranging from intimate partner violence (IPV), and drug sales, to a host of other matters including Sharmane when she would go off her meds and experience a psychotic break. Community residents explained that while these matters were always annoying, they were afraid to call for police assistance given that many police shootings of unarmed Black men were occurring nationwide, and they did not want it to happen in their community. Moreover, they expressed being reluctant to ask the police for help because they were aware of the historical tensions and distrust between police and African-American community, especially, its attitudes and perceptions toward young unemployed men and those who identify as *LGBTQ*, but they never imaged that requesting help would end in tragedy. Because it was a typical occurrence, the community knew Sharmane was not dangerous, everyone simply wanted Sharmane's loud outboasts to defuse so they could have peace and quiet. However, this time, when first responders arrived at the scene, the exchange between police officers and Sharmane escalated. As police approached Sharmane's grandmother's apartment, they immediately noticed that Sharmane was burnishing a knife. Officers on the scene reported that when they ordered her to drop the weapon, she appeared incoherent and aloof to the extent that the officer in charge quickly informed the other officers to let him handle the situation since he was aware of Sharmane's mental health status. After being held at a standstill for an hour, a newly assigned officer rushed and tackled Sharmane to the ground and she reacted by stabbing him. When this occurred, one police officer shot Sharmane

DOI: 10.4324/9781003373001-10

several times in her chest and another officer slammed her thin body to the ground. The officers quickly placed her in handcuffs and turned her face down toward the ground. They left her alone as they went to check on the officer who was stabbed. Sharmane cried out for help and said that she was holding the knife because she was raped before officers arrived at the scene. After 30 minutes passed, one officer returned to check on Sharmane and noticed she was unresponsive. Despite this, no attempts were made by any officer to resuscitate her. Police waited another hour before calling for emergency assistance. She subsequently bled to death from the gunshot wounds. In response, Sharmane's family filed a wrongful death lawsuit that alleged the local police department engaged in brutality by using excessive force to apprehend Sharmane when arriving at the scene. The police countered by stating that its action was predicated on its perception that she posed a threat to the safety of police officers, herself, and community residents. The family also alleged that the officers were not properly trained to respond to persons exhibiting mental health signs. In the wake of community outcry, several protests were staged at the police department, city hall, and Sharmane's community by members of the public *including Black Lives Matter*, the *MeToo Movement*, and others who denounced police violence (PV).

Police Violence Defined

Criminal justice experts posit that what most people know as police brutality is referred to as PV (Cuncic, 2023). While the use of violence is a core aspect of policing since it must be used in law enforcement (in isolated cases), it is not meant to be the norm (Bittner, 1970). In fact, police officers are empowered by state and federal constitutional authority to engage in the use of force under specific circumstances, or when it is legally proscribed such as when an officer's life or someone else is under immediate threat of death. del Carmen (1991) argues that there are two types of force used in police work: nondeadly force and deadly force. Accordingly, when nondeadly force is used, a suspect is not likely to sustain serious bodily harm or death. When deadly force is used in policing, it is the level of force that would lead a reasonable officer at the scene to assume that a suspect will face a high risk of serious bodily injury or death (del Carmen, 1991). This suggests there are constitutional restrictions placed on police behavior, namely what is considered reasonable behavior within the meaning of state and federal constitutions. It also begs the question, how is PV defined? Some police experts define PV as the use of overwhelming force against persons or suspects to accomplish a law enforcement objective (Alder et al., 1994). Other police scholars view it as any use of unnecessary physical force by police that causes injuries to citizens (Champion, 2005). Because PV is not simply an American problem, *WHO* reports that PV is a global concern that has several manifestations that include beatings, racial abuse, unlawful killings, torture, or indiscriminate use of riot control agents at protests. *WHO* also reports that PV is a global health issue that can result in human rights violations (Deivanayagam et al., 2021).

Nature and Extent of Police Violence

Experts argue that it is very difficult to calculate the total amount of PV that is committed each year in the U.S. considering that most behavior goes underreported, especially acts of beatings, injuries related to shootings, and other violent acts of suppression. Despite this admission, some reports revealed that between 1980 and 2018, an estimated 30,000 people were killed and 52,000 were treated in emergency departments for injuries sustained in exchanges with U.S. police officers (*The Lancet*, 2021a; Miller et al., 2017). What most scholars and researchers agree on is that it is relatively easy to determine the number of homicides that police engage in each year since these data are collected by certain agencies, repository, *the Washington Post*, and databases (Lett et al., 2020). Despite this, some justice experts contend that there is a lack of definitive official data that stores national estimates of the prevalence of police use of force resulting in death (Schindler & Kittredge, 2020). Most statistics indicate that police commit an estimated 1,000 fatal shootings annually (Ludwig, 2023). However, in 2023, police accounted for 1,232 shooting deaths (*The Guardian*, 2024). While this number is outrageous to most citizens, justice officials believe, it is a low estimation given that many violent encounters between civilians and police go unheeded, unacknowledged, and uncounted (*The Lancet*, 2021; *The Guardian, 2024*). What is more alarming about police homicides in the U.S. is that *Black, Indigenous, and People of Color* (BIPOC) are disproportionately the victims of these killings (Nix & Shjarback, 2021; Lett et al., 2020). Research reveals that while Black people make up only 13% of the U.S. population, they account for 25% of fatal police shootings (Nix & Shjarback, 2021). In 2023, there were 425 Whites, 229 Blacks, 133 Hispanics, 29 Others, and 344 unknowns killed by police. Currently, statistics show that 159 Whites, 98 Blacks, 71 Hispanics, 13 Others, and 128 unknowns have been killed by police (Statista, 2024). These statistics paint a grim picture of the racial disparity that exists in PV in the U.S. According to police experts, Blacks account for more than 1 in 4 or 25% of the people killed by police followed by Hispanics and Native Americans, while Asian/Pacific Islanders and Whites are underrepresented among those killed in police shootings given their population proportions. These findings suggest that racially minoritized communities are more likely to suffer police brutality which significantly increases their mortality rates and dramatically increases their chances of experiencing other physical and psychological problems (Alang et al., 2023).

Concerned about the disproportionality of police killings experienced by Blacks, Hispanics, and Indigenous populations compared with Whites, a recent comprehensive study examined the extent of underreporting of deaths caused by PV in the U.S. The study relied on data from the *National Vital Statistics System* (NVSS) that were taken from 1980 to 2018 along with three non-governmental databases on PV: *Fatal Encounters* from 2005 to 2019, *Mapping Police Violence* from 2013 to 2019, and *The Counted* from 2015 to 2016. The study revealed that the NVSS underreported deaths caused by PV by 55.5%. This represented 17,100 out of 30,800 deaths committed from 1980 to 2018. Data also show that the proportions of underreported deaths were highest among non-Hispanic Black men since 59.5% were misclassified, followed by non-Hispanic White persons at 56.1%. Hispanic persons of any race were misclassified by 50% and non-Hispanic persons of other races were misclassified by 32.6%. The results also revealed that underreporting varied by state (GBD, 2021). Similarly, officials at the CDC argue that national crime data that provide estimates of homicides by police have been flawed for decades since more than half of police killings kept by agencies and stored in databases are often mislabeled as either generic homicides or suicides (*The Guardian*, 2023). Moreover, the GBD study showed that the death rate for non-Hispanic Blacks was higher than for non-Hispanic Whites for every year included in the study. From 2010 to 2019, morality rates for non-Hispanic Blacks increased in 42 states compared with non-Hispanic Whites. The researchers stated the findings in the study highlight the need for evidence-based strategies to address systematic racism and discrimination in policy as well as personal implicit biases in the U.S. and the likelihood that they impact reporting police killings to the NVSS. The conclusion drawn from the study is that most datasets on police use of deadly force severely underestimate the rate of police use of deadly force (GBD, 2021). At the same time, these statistics reveal a system that has tolerated police use of violence and fatal policy practices that are unfair and applied unequally across race and ethnicity leading some experts to conclude that this exists because the use of fatal violence against people of color is deeply entrenched in the U.S. culture and structure (Serchen et al., 2020; *The Lancet*, 2021). Moreover, Harris and Cortes (2022) described PV as stemming from structural racism which provides institutional practices, laws, and policies that sustain racial and ethnic inequalities.

With respect to race/ethnicity, Black men and boys experience the highest amount of inequity in mortality rates from PV since they are killed at a rate of 2.5 times higher than their White counterparts over the life course (Edward et al., 2019; Ludwig, 2023). Research shows that people of color face a greater likelihood of being killed by police compared with other groups and while the risk peaks when they are young adults, it persists throughout the life course (Edward et al., 2019). Age is an important factor in police shootings that result in death. According to the *Washington Post*, police killings are a leading cause of death for young men in the U.S., but especially for Black men (Schindler & Kittredge, 2020). The *Washington Post* further reports that in 2017, Black emerging adults (those under 24), were killed by police at a rate of death that was tripled that of their White counterparts (Schindler & Kittredge, 2020). Other studies also reveal the risk of death is more pronounced for young Black men between the ages of 25 and 29 years old since they are killed by police at a rate between 2.8 and 4.1 per 100,000. Comparatively, other racial/ethnic groups in the same age category are killed by police as follows: American Indian and Alaska Native men are killed by the police at a rate of 1.5 and 2.8 per 100,000. Asian/Pacific Islander men are killed by police at a rate of 0.3 and 0.6 per 100,000, respectively. Moreover, Latinx men are killed by police at a rate of 1.4 and 2.2 per 10,000 while White men are killed by police at a rate of 0.9 and 1.4 per 100,000 (Edward et al., 2019). In a longitudinal study conducted by Lett and colleagues (2020), that examined the rate of fatal police shootings of *Black Indigenous People of Color* (BIPOC), researchers relied on 5,367 fatal police shootings reported by the *Washington Post* from 2015 to May 2020. The study excluded 627 cases from the analysis because race was marked as either unknown or other. As such, the study relied on 4,470 deaths. Data revealed that there were White (51%), Blacks (26.7), Hispanic (18.8%), Asian (2%), and Native American (1.6%). The median age was 34, but varied across groups with young Black victim's average age being 30, while the median age for Whites was 38 (Edward et al., 2019). Despite this, statistics collected from *The Counted Project*, show that Blacks were nine times more likely to be killed by police in 2015 compared to any other racial or ethnic group (*The Guardian*, 2017; *American Psychiatric Association*, 2018).

Some investigations have isolated the reasons why police encounters resulted in death. In 2023, 139 killings (11%) were attributed to claims of an officer seeing a weapon, 107 killings (90%) started as a traffic violation that escalated into death, 100 killings (8%) were owing to either a mental health or welfare check, 79 killings (6%) were in response to a domestic violence call, 73 killings (6%) were not provided with an excuse, 265 killings (22%) involved an alleged non-violent offense, and 469 killings (38%) were claimed to be precipitated by a violent or serious crime (*The Guardian*, 2024). Data also show that minorities are often killed while fleeing from law enforcement. More specifically, from 2013 to 2023, an estimated 39% of Blacks who were killed by police were in the process of either driving or running away. Moreover, 35% of Latinx were killed by police while fleeing, and 30% of Native Americans were killed while fleeing compared with 29% of Whites and 22% of Asian Americans killed, respectively (*The Guardian*, 2024).

Types of Police Violence

In the past few years, research and television broadcasts have presented findings and images of police nationwide inflicting acts of violence against U.S. citizens who were merely exercising their *First Amendment* right to engage in peaceful protests to express their grievances against the government. Some of these protests were about *racial justice, police violence against Blacks, COVID-19, labor movements, LGBTQ rights, political candidates, White nationalisms*, and others (Kajeepeta & Johnson, 2023). Constitutional scholars contend that the *First Amendment* is viewed as part of the cornerstone of American democracy (Kajeepeta & Johnson, 2023; del Carmen, 1991). Despite engaging in peaceful protests, reports reveal that for some protests, police used militarized crackdown responses against unarmed citizens by inflicting violence against them that has varied in severity ranging from the use of excessive or lethal force that has resulted in deaths, countless unprovoked beatings, use of tear gas during the *COVID-19* pandemic, indiscriminate use of rubber bullets, pepper spray, driving police vehicles into crowds of protesters, indiscriminate use of riot control agents at protests, to the untimely deaths of those viewed as a threat to the state (*Amnesty International*, 2020; Barker et al., 2021). Critics observe that there have been striking disparities in police responses at racial justice demonstrations compared with others. For example, police are more likely to be present (57.3%) and demonstrate a willingness to escalate violence by dispatching riot police, state police, and in some cases, the national guard as reinforcements compared with the aforesaid protests (18.4%) that are categorized as unrelated to racial justice (Kejeepeta & Johnson, 2023).

Police Violence against Black Male Protesters

In the aftermath of the police killing of *George Floyd*, hundreds of cities around the nation were the sites of protests, demonstrations, as well as widespread failures in American policing (Schindler & Kittredge, 2020). Some experts estimate that tens of millions of Americans, along with people around the world staged protests over the killings of Blacks by police including the deaths of *Breonna Taylor and George Floyd* (Kajeepeta & Johnson, 2023). Reports from *Demonstration and Political Violence in America* (2020) suggested that during this time, there were more protests that any other period in American history because there were over 7,000 public demonstrations for racial justice in more than 2,400 locations in the U.S. (Buchanan et al., 2021). Nationwide reports revealed that police used batons to beat, sprayed tear gas, and shot projectiles into crowds of protesters at *BLM* demonstrations as a method of crowd control. While most protests were peaceful, police responded by engaging in aggressive behavior since by all accounts, they escalated, rather than, de-escalated encounters with protesters. Studies report that officers were ill-prepared, lacked adequate planning, and were ill-trained to respond to random protests. As such, they acted reactively instead of proactively (Barker et al., 2021).

Chaudhary and Richardson (2022) and Schindler and Kittredge (2020) reported that *BLM* protests of racialized PV were met by repressive violence from state authorities (e.g., riot police, state police, national guard, and others) along with far-right-wing civilian militia groups that have increased the devastating effects of racism and PV. They contend that during the summer of 2020, many states throughout the nation engaged in widespread incidents of mistreatment of *BLM* demonstrators that were captured on the local news and posted in social media outlets. They also postulated that there are no organized data clearinghouses on state violence against citizens, or the over 19,000 police agencies required by law to report officer-related shootings or violence to any federal databases. Therefore, it is impossible to truly measure the extent of damage that police inflicted on demonstrators. However, in the absence of official data, the *Armed Conflict Location and Event Data* project (ACLED), an independent nonprofit data collaborative, has been used by some experts and is considered a reliable data source to track protest-related PV in the U.S. during the summer of 2020. In describing the political violence, it found that 9% of *BLM* demonstrations experienced some type of state intervention such as physical force or other compared with 4% of right-wing demonstrations and 3% of all demonstrations. Moreover, police disproportionately targeted *BLM* protestors even though 94% of their demonstrations were non-violent compared with 86% of right-wing protests. ACLED also noted that state interventions used against *BLM* members were more violent compared with interventions used against right-wing demonstrators. For example, 51% of *BLM* protestors were met with physical force such as chemical irritants such as tear gas, robbery bullets, pepper balls, bean bag rounds, and beat with batons compared with 33% of right-wing demonstrators and 26% of other types of demonstration. Some of the injuries that *BLM* protestors sustained ranged from chronic respiratory disorder to permanent vision loss, globe ruptures to amputations to traumatic brain injuries, to death (Chaudhary & Richardson, 2022). ACLED reported that the presence of *BLM* demonstrations has been countered by demonstrations from far-right civilian militia groups holding a range of interrelated ideological beliefs such as *proTrump, Republican, proPolice, Stop-the-Steal*, and others that variously synergized with militarized policing strategies to stifle dissent from *BLM* demonstrators (Chaudhary & Richardson, 2022).

Police Violence against Black Males

The idea of police committing violence against Black men in America is nothing new, but rather, it has deep roots that have created historical trauma for many racial and ethnic minorities (Bryant-Davis et al., 2017). History is replete with examples of police murdering unarmed Black men that date to the inception of modern policing when it started out as slave patrols (Kappeler, 2014). Kratcoski and Cebulak (2000) reported that early colonizers appointed constables to police and kill Indigenous peoples to take ownership of their land. Similarly, Hinton and Cook (2021) revealed that during the antebellum South, White men of every station were hired by landowners to capture, whip, arrest, rape, shoot, harass, and lynch enslaved and freed Blacks. Scholars contend that while PV has always been part of the American fabric, it was during the mid-1960s and 1970s that nationwide protests over police brutality against Black men started to emerge. Unfortunately, instead of those efforts helping to reduce PV, history shows that they exacerbated police brutality and caused further strain in police–community relations (Kajeepeta & Johnson, 2023; Davenport et al., 2011). In an effort to address nationwide turmoil generated by protests against police brutality, the *Kerner Commission* identified biased policing practices and militarized law enforcement, as major causes of civil unrest, along with other forms of systemic racial inequities such as voter suppression, housing discrimination, and the mass incarceration of minorities (Kajeepeta & Johnson, 2023).

Despite three national commissions that addressed police brutality against Black protestors and riots, the practice continues, and the system remains unchanged (Kahn et al., 2021). Today, police respond to Black demonstrations against fatal PV and racial inequities by escalating it when intervening with counterproductive militarized responses (Jahn & Schwartz, 2024). Many law enforcement experts argue that, rather than, implementing crowd control management tactics to defuse tense situations, during recent protests led by *BLM* and others, police escalated matters by employing widespread use of militarized policing tactics that relied on riot gear, pepper spray, releasing clouds of tear gas, and rubber bullets (Barker et al., 2021; Schwartz, 2020). These experts postulate that militarized policing and its war-like approach prepares officers for riot control and often come with riot gear, advanced weaponry, night vision goggles, and tripod-mounted rifles typically used by snipers. This aggressive approach places law enforcement officers in the mindset that conflict with protesters and others is imminent. Therefore, they do not see citizens exercising their *First Amendment* right to engage in peaceful protest, but rather, they view everyone (e.g., protesters, bystanders, photojournalists, reporters, medics, and camera crews) in their way as combatants who are enemies of the State (Gottbrath & Strickland, 2020; Kraska & Kappeler, 1995). While it is unsurprising to hear about confrontations that Black men have with police since many are routinely stopped and subjected to a frisk or a pat-down, some think it unusual for violence to be used against Black men by off-duty police. A recent study that examined data taken from *Mapping Police Violence* assessing off-duty police killings of citizens from 2013 to 2021 found that nearly 40% of the victims were Black men, while Whites and Latinx men ranked second and third at a rate of 25.2% and 11.2%, respectively.

Police Violence against Women

Violence experts and public health professionals argue that most studies about police use of violence against marginalized communities (e.g., Blacks, immigrants, people of color, Indigenous, lesbians, gays, transgenders, bisexuals, disabled people) have historically focused on brutality disproportionately committed against Black men, and what has been a neglected area of research is violence that women have sustained from their encounters with police, especially since Black women are 1.4 times more likely to be killed by police compared with White women (Edward et al., 2019). They are also more likely than their counterparts to either experience, witness, or worry about a family member facing police brutality (Alang et al., 2017; Harris & Cortes, 2022; *The Lancet*, 2021). Feminist scholars contend that Black women have experienced similar levels of violence as others in the Black community dating as far back as slavery. They experienced systematic rapes, beatings, lynchings, denial of reproductive autonomy, theft of their children, and other unspeakable forms of state-sanctioned behavior, in the U.S., but they are not the only women who experience violence at the hands of police. Feminists posit that Black women and other women of color, including nonconforming people of color are harmed by police, yet their violent encounters go undocumented as though these women were invisible (Ritchie, 2017; Ritchie, 2016). Black women and other women experience racial disparities in the number of stops and frisks compared to their White counterparts (Crenshaw & Ritchie, 2014). Within the context of routine traffic stops by police, Quinn (2015) and Sullum (2015) reported that many Black women are subjected to degrading and unlawful experiences such as unprovoked physical violence, along with strip searches conducted on the side of the road under the pretext of drug searches (Zennie & Grieg, 2013).

Studies show that Black women have been killed in police custody (Edwards, 2015). Consider the example of Sandra Bland who was killed in police custody, along with Alesia Thomas, who was kicked to death by a policeman after being placed in a squad car. The death of Natasha McKenna is also instructive in this regard since after being placed in custody at a jail, several guards used 50,000 volts of electricity from their tasers to shock her while she was chained to a chair (Jackman & Jouvenal, 2015). Furthermore, the *War on Drugs* fought in minority communities during the 1980s and 1990s is replete with examples of state-sanctioned violence the police perpetrated against Black women. During this time, Black women were routinely subjected to racial profiling, and strip searches that often extended to body cavity searches that were conducted in public places such as airports, jails, and street corners. Research reveals that sometimes, these encounters ended in death. The cases of Frankie Perkins and Theresa Henderson are examples in this regard since they were both choked to death after police profiled them as drug carriers and later argued that their deaths occurred as they attempted to retrieve drug evidence that the decease women swallowed (Crenshaw & Ritchie, 2014).

Another study reported that Black women and women of color experience a disproportionate amount of sexual harassment and assault from police compared to White women. In a New York study conducted in 2014, researchers found that two in every five (40%) young women reported being sexually harassed by an NYPD police officer. This finding was similar to a report from transgender women in New Orleans who experienced routine sexual harassment and extortion from police officers. In their study, Stinson and colleagues (2014) discovered that many women including young women of color, homeless and low-income women, lesbian and transgender women, and other women connected to vice crimes (e.g., drug and sex trades) were routinely targeted by police for sexual favors (Kraska & Kappeler, 1995). Nembhard and colleagues (2022) also reported that women of color disproportionately experience sexual violence perpetrated by police. Feminists contend that the violence police commit against women has been marginalized from the public and what it understands about police brutality and the threat it poses to the safety of women. They argue that police have been committing different types of violence against women since its inception. However, women's stories have been suppressed from becoming part of mainstream narratives by misogynistic men who protect violent men (Blain, 2020).

Police Violence against LGBTQIA

Members of the *LGBTQ+* also have a history of violence and discrimination from the law enforcement community dating by to the 1940s, 1950s, and 1960s when efforts were made to purge the nation of people engaging in homosexuality from government service and other areas of the American experience. Mallory and colleagues (2015) report that members of the *LGBTQ+* community continue to face profiling, discrimination, and harassment by police officers. Other research is more specific about what members of the community experience from law enforcement officers. Data from a 2014 national survey revealed the experiences people identifying as members of the *LGBTQ+* community had with police. The survey found that 73% of respondents reported experiencing personal contact with police in the past five years and 21% indicated that their interaction was hostile, 14% reported being verbally assaulted by police, 3% indicated that they were sexually harassed, while 2% reported they were physically assaulted. The survey revealed that most abuse was reported by respondents of color and transgender and gender nonconforming respondents (Lambda Legal, 2014). In their study that examined 220 low-income Latina transgender women in Los Angeles, they found that two-thirds of the respondents reported being verbally abused by police, 21% reported they received physical abuse, and 24% indicated that they were sexually abused by police (Woods et al., 2013).

Studies on PV against the *LGBTQ+* community find that the behavior remains constant and stems from institutionalized racism, homophobia, and transphobia that is anchored in the criminal justice system, especially regarding how it normalizes discrimination by the way it handles hate crime in general, but particularly, how it treats the victimizations experienced by *LGBTQ+* people. Research shows that their victimization is not always taken seriously, is underestimated, and processed unprofessionally as well as with indifference. Crimes and victimizations committed against *LGBTQ+* people are also not taken as seriously as those reported by non-*LGBTQ+* people (Drey et al., 2020; Nadal et al., 2012). Besides being seriously victimized by people in their own neighborhoods and elsewhere, Tucker and colleagues (2019) and Nadal and colleagues (2012), report that *LGBTQ+* victims experience patterns of police discriminatory and unlawful practices that include microaggression and verbal abuse, sexual misconduct, and physical violence. Where microaggression is concerned, it occurs when police oversexualize *LGBTQ+* people by using language such as "*faggot*" and "*dyke*" as derogatory terms and by assuming that homosexuality is either morally wrong or a psychological disorder (Platt & Lenzen, 2013). Furthermore, it occurs when police use language to objectify or subordinate women, use sexist comments, and misgender those who are gender nonconforming (Nadal et al., 2012). Moreover, Wolff and Cokely (2007) reveal that verbal abuse by police often escalates into physical violence that includes police engaging in inappropriately touching, beating, and using coercive methods to restrain *LGBTQ+* people. Based on reports from the *International Association of Chiefs of Police* (2011), when *LGBTQ+* people are sexually harassed, it is referred to as police sexual misconduct that includes actions used to intimidate victims. Statistics suggest that they are overwhelmingly young, lesbian, bisexual, transgender, and gender nonconforming people (Serpe & Nadal, 2017; *Amnesty International*, 2005). While *LGBTQ+* people experience more PV than cisgender persons (*American Civil Liberties Union*, 2024), those among them who receive the worst treatment are Black transgender persons since research shows that they are more likely to experience routine unwanted detention and gender searches by police officers who often require them to strip publicly to check and confirm their sex. They are also three times more likely to experience physical abuse, violence, and arrest (30.7%) compared with cisgender persons (*Amnesty International*, 2005; *National Coalition of Anti-Violence Programs*, 2012; *American Civil Liberties Union*, 2024). Braunstein (2017) posits that there are five types of police sexual misconduct that *LGBTQ+* people are subjected to that include being threatened with sexual assault, illegal strip searches, exhortation of sexual favors, coercive sexual conduct, and rape. Fileborn (2019) contends that *LGBTQ+* people are the victims of discriminatory police practices that lead to profiling based solely on gender identity and sexual orientation. Because of their negative experiences with police, research reveals that 71% of *LGBTQ+* people report that they are less likely to call police for help compared with 87% of non-LGBTQ people who indicated they would be inclined to call police for help (*American Civil Liberties Union*, 2024).

Police Violence against the Media/Reporters/Medics

A class action lawsuit filed by members of the press in Minneapolis, Minnesota alleged that local and state police violated their *First Amendment* right to freedom of the press. Journalists contend that while covering social protests, police officers made them targets of arrests, intimidation, assaults, and excessive force even when they identified themselves as members of the press (Gottbraith & Strickland, 2020; Hauss & Nelson, 2020). Reports contend that after the death of *George Floyd*, police across the country deliberately inflicted brutality against protesters as well as members of the press (e.g., photojournalists, reporters, camera crews) and medics. Medics at the scene of protests reported that while attempting to aid those who sustained injuries from being beaten, pepper sprayed, or shot with rubber bullets, they, too, were attacked by police officers who escalated, rather than, defused volatile situations. In another report, lawsuits have been filed by the *American Civil Liberties Union Foundation of Oregon* against the *Department of Homeland Security*, *U.S. Marshalls Service*, and the *City of Portland* by volunteer street medics who allege they were the victims of state-sponsored violence. The lawsuit states that local police and federal agents violated their *First* and *Fourth Amendment* rights when they opened fire indiscriminately into crowds using rubber bullets, tear gas, pepper spray, batons, and flash-bangs. The plaintiffs in the case contend that they were brutally attacked and sustained injuries by state and federal agents as they attempted to administer medical aid, services, and treatment to injured protesters and innocent bystanders. Additionally, *Human Rights Watch* (2020) reported that nationwide estimates of at least 300 incidents of violent confrontations between police and members of the press have occurred in 33 states including more than 49 arrests, 192 assaults, and 42 incidents of newsroom equipment damage. However, two weeks after nationwide protests erupted over Floyd's murder, the *U.S. Free Freedom Tracker* found that there were over 400 documented incidents of press freedom violations committed by law enforcement agents ranging from harassment and indiscriminate arrests, equipment damage, projectiles fired at press workers, attacks on reporters, journalists, and camera crews, to being shot with rubber bullets and sprayed with tear gas.

Explaining the Roots of Police Violence

Experts contend that to prevent PV from occurring, they must first understand the underlying factors that cause it to occur (Cuncic, 2023). Of note, some police experts and scholars argue that brutality exists in American policing for multiple reasons including its history of originating out of the institution of slavery and structural racism, which conspired to legally sanction control over Blacks. Racism was exacerbated by the economic fears of Whites. As such, slave patrols were instruments created to ensure that Whites would be protected from those fears. Some experts believe that racism has always fueled American policing. While some may wonder whether this argument is passed, recently, accounts of police brutality by Abramson and Denenberg (2024) support that contention since they posit that racism not only exists in American policing, but it is a common cause of police brutality which enables police officers to inflict violence on people based solely on race, ethnicity, gender, religion, sexual orientation, or social origins. Similarly, officials at *Amnesty International* (2020) report that sometimes while making arrests and being fueled by racism, police have killed and injured many people. Racism and other types of discrimination influence many law enforcement practices and how people are processed by the justice system (*Amnesty International*, 2020). This is demonstrated by who gets targeted by police for excessive or lethal force. The literature is replete with studies and reports that suggest police target certain segments of the population compared with how Whites are treated by police and processed in the justice system. Other forms of targeting include selective law enforcement practices based on a lack of evidence where police officers effect *stops, frisks, searches, and arrests,* of people fitting the profile of drug couriers (*Amnesty International*, 2020).

PV is also linked to its institutional culture. Experts argue that the nature of police culture is unique compared with other groups and organizations since it emphasizes traits such as group solidarity, loyalty, and bravado. Officers are taught that they can only trust and depend on each other for protection against what they will encounter in the line of duty. Skolnick and Fyfe (1993) revealed that the cultural world of policing, especially its socialization of officers accepting the attitudes of viewing their role as soldiers in a war on crime and drugs and the insularity and authoritarianism of some police administrations. Consequently, officers began to internalize that their behavior is beyond accountability since they routinely witness entrenched impunity (*Amnesty International*, 2020). These traits are taught and instilled in officers in their respective training academies where officers are nurtured to develop a sense of *esprit de corps* that bonds them (Bionidi, 2000). They are also reminded of the group's values, attitudes, and practices. According to some police experts, most practices they receive are racist and anti-Black (Abramson & Denenberg, 2024). As such, what police are taught in the training academies is reinforced when they are paired with a veteran partner. Unfortunately, it is the culture of solidarity or the "thin blue line" that insulates and protects corrupt officers who engage in violence and brutality from being disciplined and removed from police service (Bionidi, 2000). They are protected by the silence of fellow officers who believe that police must protect each other to the detriment of seeing justice served when they fail to assist in having violent officers reprimanded for engaging in brutality or discriminatory practices such as racial profiling. This has led some policing experts to conclude that the lack of moral courage from good police who fear being labeled a traitor for reporting bad officers are complicit in furthering and perpetuating future aggressive behavior that could cause death to some civilians since the culture supports PV and predispose them to look the way while facilitating a deadly cycle of violence (Rahr, 2023; Chicago Citizen, 1997; *Amnesty International*, 2020).

Other reports reveal that police officers who engage in brutality may suffer from poor mental health. A study conducted in 2019 that surveyed police officers who self-reported participating in abusive practices revealed that they also reported having higher levels of *PTSD* symptoms. This finding has led some experts to believe that police officers who experience stressors and trauma from work may also be more likely compared with other police officers to respond to incidents with aggressive behavior. Experts contend that this may also explain why these officers tend to overreact by using excessive force or lethal violence when the situation does not demand such action. This finding is similar to a report given by police brutality expert, James J. Fyfe who argued that PV occurs when police officers are placed in overwhelmingly high stressful situations without having a realistic expectation of success. According to Fyfe (1991), we require too much from police officers since they are viewed as soldiers who are fighting an unwinnable war on crime and disorder which are symptoms of broader social problems. Yet, we ask these soldiers who are only trained for six months at an academy to address larger societal problems that they are not adequately prepared or trained to do. To assist, we armed them with militarized weapons and asked them to do the impossible. Fyfe believes that the standards that society has set for police officers are too high and add stress that they are unable to control. Likewise, another cause of police brutality that is not fully accepted by most people is that some police officers, especially those who engage in unprovoked aggressive behavior toward civilians may suffer from antisocial personality disorder *(APD)* which is believed to be more common among some officers compared with people in the general population.

What Are the Risk Factors?

Research on PV reveals that while anyone in the U.S. can experience police brutality, there are consistent patterns that have emerged that paint a picture of those who are disproportionately its victims, people from communities of color, especially young Black males (Goff & Rau, 2020). According to the results from a *Harvard University* study conducted in 2020 that examined nearly 5,400 police fatalities from 2013 to 2017, Blacks were three times more likely to be killed by police compared with their White counterparts. In another study conducted at *Rutgers University* in 2019, researchers concluded that one of the leading causes of death for Black young men in the U.S. is police since Blacks are 2.5 times more likely to be killed by police compared to Whites. Researchers at *Boston University* reported the presence of a relationship between fatal police shootings and living in segregated neighborhoods (e.g., Black compared to White) as a predictor of police killings (Dunn, 2020). As previously mentioned, throughout American history, there has not been a shortage of examples of police killing young Black men. However, during the past several years, the world community witnessed the danger that Blacks faced at the hands of police in riot gear as mass protests erupted throughout the U.S. in response to calls for justice and an end to police murdering unarmed Black men (Dunn, 2020). This has led many scholars, practitioners, and experts to conclude that race and ethnicity are risk factors that are supported in the literature, but it is not the only risk factor. Recent research investigations report that there is a nexus between police shootings and gun ownership. More specifically, a 2019 study found that fatal police shootings are 40% more likely to occur in states with higher rates of gun ownership (Dunn, 2020).

In their research, Stoddard and colleagues (2024), relied on data collected from the *Chicago Police Department* from 2010 to 2018 in cooperation with the *University of Chicago's Crime Lab* and the *Illinois Attorney General's Office*. The study asked, what are the risk factors that predict police misconduct? The study revealed that when police officers have accumulated patterns of prior behavior (either minor or serious), rather than, a single violent action, their behavior is likely to escalate into egregious behavior such as PV. Stated differently, a history of problem behavior is more predictive than a single act of misconduct (Stoddard et al., 2024). To isolate risk factors in police shootings, Ridgeway

(2015) examined police data taken from the *New York City Police Department* of a sample of 291 officers who were involved in shootings that were adjudicated between 2004 and 2006. Data from this two-year timeframe revealed that veteran police officers pose a lower risk of being involved in shootings, Black officers were three times more likely compared with White officers to engage in shootings, officers who accumulate negative reports in their files were three times more likely to shoot others, and officers who made many misdemeanor arrests were four times less likely to engage in shootings (Ridgeway, 2015). An important study conducted by Goff and Rau (2020) found those risk factors that contribute to racially disparate and aggressive police behavior occur under two conditions. First, when officers experience emotional and physical threats (perceived or real) directed at their self-concept or police collectively. Second, when officers consistently interact with segments of society they view as disgusting (e.g., drug addicts, sex workers, homeless, mentally ill) largely influenced by cultural stereotypes that dehumanize people, they see themselves as being at risk of the consequences of exposure from being required to interact with these elements. As such, they are more likely to use excessive force. Despite these findings, experts argue that the most significant risk factors are those that examine the role of inequity in PV, individual factors in PV, relationship factors in PV, community factors in PV, as well as societal factors in PV.

Role of Inequity in Police Violence

The notion that inequality in society can be linked to police repression and violence is not a new one. As early as the 1960s, many critical scholars, social control theorists, sociologists, and radical criminologists, especially conflict theorists argued that the state exercises a monopoly on violence that is sanctioned and supported by people who benefit from the existing arrangement (Jacob & Britt, 1979; Beirne & Messerschmidt, 1991). Similarly, Parks (1970) argues that the main purpose of police is to protect existing unequal relationships in society by protecting the interests of the dominant class from redistributive violence. Likewise, Blauner (1972) held that the racial aspect of the conflict argument is that police are not neutral agents, but rather, they are used to control subordinate groups by being a physical presence in their communities. As such, powerful groups are more inclined to deploy social agents (e.g., police and military) to maintain the status quo to the detriment of poor and powerless groups. In a national study, Jacob and Britt (1979) measured the number of killings committed by police officers, income inequality, urbanization, and southern locations. The results revealed that disparities in social class and race, along with increasing crime in rapidly growing cities were linked to more police presence and killings. Jacob and Britt (1979) found support for police officers nationwide increasingly invoking the use of lethal force against rapidly growing populations composed of poor Blacks when they are perceived as a threat to the White majority. Carmichael and Kent's (2014) study also supports the racial threat and income inequality argument. They report that when there is an increase in racial composition and economic inequality in cities, it has the effect of creating a racial threat that leads to substantial shifts and mobilizations in the sizes of police departments placed in those areas to control inhabitants. In a recent study, Feldman (2020) measured the association between social class and racial inequalities and their impact on police killings, he matched 6,451 police killings that were committed in the last five years to the census tract data (e.g., neighborhoods where the fatal shootings occurred). The results revealed that socioeconomics played a major role in policing killings. According to these data, the highest-poverty areas experienced police killings at a rate of 6.4 per million, while the lowest-poverty areas experienced police killings at a rate of 1.8 per million. Feldman's study concluded that class differences make up more than 100% of the differences between White and Latinx killings committed by police, and class differences account for 28% of the differences between Black and White police killings (2020).

Individual Factors in Police Violence

Risk factors are not necessarily causal factors that are to be inferred to be true in every situation. This suggests that what may be true for some people may not have the same impact on others. However, experts contend that their presence often increases the likelihood that certain behavior will occur. Cuncic (2023) reports that there are several individual-level risk factors that influence PV. Some police studies reveal that problems may exist between police and the people they serve because police officers often come from different cultural backgrounds and have specific characteristics that include education, stereotypes, attitudes, prejudices, moods, and personalities that may increase opposing views toward the minority residents they encounter. Moreover, many police experts and scholars contend that police officers engage in brutality because of problems that originate from within such as the quality of their mental health fitness since research has established a link between PV and officers who suffer from depression, anxiety, and *PTSD* which can lead some officers to increased startle response, suspicion, and aggressive behavior. In its examination of PV, the *United Nations Human Rights* (2023) provides that police officers' mental health is affected by several factors such as work overload, racism, and racial discrimination they are presented with inside police departments. Moreover, officers who face other personal problems such as their economic woes and politics are often susceptible to using violence compared with other officers who struggle with the same issues. Another individual factor is racial profiling either in the form of religion, socioeconomic status, or others. For example, research supports the notion that some police officers are influenced by racism and implicit biases that are directed against young Black and Latino males, and members of the *LGBTQ+* community without defining their attitudes, beliefs, and actions as racist or homophobic. Consequently, they often perceive these groups as armed and dangerous more than Whites.

Relationship Factors in Police Violence

Police scholars argue that the institutional culture in American police organizations and the relationships that officers form with each other that begins with their training at the academy and later are reinforced in the field and department tends to socialize officers (e.g., recruits, new, and veterans) into believing that they can only trust and depend on other officers. Woods (2019) reports that some of the dominant training narrative tactics police receive at the academy often distort their perception of on-the-job dangers such as routine traffic stops that require a hypervigilance response by officers is instructive in explaining the mindset of officers who may already be stressed. Additionally, relationships with fellow police officers teach them that they must protect each other even if it means ignoring violence and crime committed by fellow police officers. It is the culture of policing that they are exposed to that teaches them that they are the *"thin blue line"* that protects society from crime, disorder, and lawlessness. This is the case even when what is being informally taught to officers is racist, discriminatory, and anti-*LGBTQ+*. Some experts contend that it is difficult to expect police officers to respect and protect human rights when it is not taught or reinforced in the culture (United Nations Human Rights, 2023). Their relationships reinforce that the demands of law enforcement may require a willingness to shield and hide the truth when fellow officers break the law. As such, they maintain a *"code of silence"* to protect fellow others when they cross the line that separates them from criminals. It is the culture itself that insulates corrupt police from being held accountable for violence since officers value and protect group loyalty and solidarity.

Community Factors in Police Violence

Studies show that some neighborhood risk factors that influence police use of violence include those areas that are characterized as socially disorganized and suffer economic disadvantages, high crime rates, a lack of group cohesion, and a lack of informal mechanisms of control that make residents conform their behavior to community standards. In these areas, police often overpolice residents by making routine stops, frisks, and arrests and engage in acts of violence and fatal shootings compared with high-income areas. Low-income neighborhoods are inhabited by vulnerable populations such as the chronically unemployed, those lacking educational attainment, and people without meaningful prospects for the future. Some experts report that these areas are rundown with abandoned apartments or low-income houses that are often used as fronts for drug sales, gangs, fencing stolen goods, or serving as places for sex work. Because these neighborhoods are socially disorganized, most residents stay to themselves and do not assist law enforcement efforts to solve crime or capture fugitives. Policing scholars suggest that law enforcement work is stressful, but it is exacerbated and could lead to violence when police are assigned to work in stressful work environments. In these areas, police officers perceive residents are hostile toward their work, unsympathetic, and appear to lack interest in crime solving. In a study that examined police use of fatal violence and neighborhood characteristics, Zare and colleagues (2022) contend that PV is influenced by factors that include race/ethnicity, neighborhood, structural inequality, and racism. They analyzed data that focused on the racial composition of communities and neighborhoods, and the nexus to police involved violence and fatal shootings that occurred between 2000 and 2020. The authors relied on 24 panel studies to conduct their study. They used seven cross-sectional studies, five time-series studies, seven studies that relied on official data, and eight studies that used *Mapping Police Violence* data. These studies provided data in the areas of a number of arrests, stops/stops and frisks, and incidents of violence and fatal shootings. The results were twofold. First, Blacks and Latinx citizens were disproportionately searched by police when stopped, arrested, and were victims of fatal police shootings. Second, the victims were residents of low-income neighborhoods with high rates of poverty and high levels of crime (Zare et al., 2022; Davis & Whyde, 2018).

Societal Factors in Police Violence

Racism is a major societal factor that influences PV (Cuncic, 2023). It is institutional and structural and has a profound effect on all aspects of one's life. Grimshaw (2020) contends that institutional racism is a tolerance of attitudes and working practices designed to racialize Black people, other people of color, and marginalized groups in disadvantaged positions. Within the context of criminal justice, its primary institutions (e.g., police, courts, and corrections) participate in adverse practices that are responsible for systemic forms of racism that are fueled by stereotypes, emotions, and assumptions about certain people that are reproduced in group practices (Phelan & Link, 2015). Even though similar rates of drug use among racial and ethnic groups have been evident in the literature (Bailey et al., 2022; *Human Rights Watch*, 2009), a stereotype that many police officers, prosecutors, and politicians have formulated is that drug users and dealers are disproportionately young people of color. The *War on Drugs* in general, but the battles waged against the *crack cocaine* epidemic fought in minority communities of color in the 1980s and early 1990s is instructive in this regard. Research reports that racism and differential enforcement owing to structural inequality were captured in disparate drug laws when the *Anti-Drug Abuse Act of 1986* mandated that the possession of five grams of crack cocaine commonly used by poor Blacks would follow a five-year prison sentence in federal prison, while people in possession of 500 grams of powder cocaine commonly used by wealthy Whites would receive the same sentence (*H.R. 5484-99th Congress*, 1986). Some scholars contend that whether they are aware, their attitudes, beliefs, experiences, and training either informed by racism or implicit biases, heighten their suspicion when young minorities are profiled, stopped, searched, and taken into police custody for formal processing (Rothestein, 2017). Other scholars argue that racism affects minoritized communities (Rothstein, 2017; Gee & Hicken, 2021). Bailey and colleagues (2022) argue that differential exposure to policing and the justice system is structural racism that harms the targeted community by exposing it to aggressive police, prosecutors, and more prisons (Raphling & Austin-Hillery, 2021).

Gruber (2021) reports that the literature on policing in America has well established that it has never been conducted in a fair and neutral manner, but rather it has always been characterized as being tainted by its racist legacy. Unfortunately, its legacy continues. In a recent study by DeAngelis (2024) that examined systemic racism in police killings, his investigation used data collected by *Mapping Police Violence Database* from 2013 to 2021 that included information on types of police killings (by on and off-duty police officers), race of the victim, whether the victim show signs of mental illness, or attempted to flee the moments before the killing, as well as the zip code, state, and neighborhood (e.g., urban, suburban, or rural) where the killing occurred. The results of the nationwide database revealed that systemic racism exists in police killings in the U.S. and Black victims were overrepresented among people killed by police compared to their White counterparts. The study found that Blacks were less likely than White victims to exhibit signs of mental illness or brandish a weapon at the scene of their killings. Some other distinctions were that Blacks were more likely to flee the scene while being killed by police. Similarly, Hispanics were less likely than Whites to exhibit signs of mental illness, but not any more likely to be armed with a weapon or flee the scene. Despite those killed by police, Whites posed a greater threat to police officers' safety compared with their Black and Hispanic counterparts. The study attributes the disparity in deaths to who police perceived as dangerous and warranted the use of lethal force. The study concludes that it is because of systemic pro-White and anti-Black racism that exists nationally (DeAngelis, 2024). This finding is echoed in a report from the *United Nations Human Rights* (2023) which finds that systematic racism is pervasive in American policing and its entire system of justice since these institutions share similar values and reproduce racist attitudes, and stereotypes as other institutions in the country. It noted that people in the U.S. of African descent are 3 times more likely to be killed by police compared to Whites and are 4.5 times more likely to be sentenced to a place of confinement. It reported that while there are more than 1,000 police killings yearly, only 1% of police officers are held criminally responsible. Critics contend that policing in America continues to struggle with a lack of diversity that is needed to prevent predominantly White police forces from developing an us versus communities of color mentality (Legewie & Fagan, 2016; Ba et al., 2021).

Police Violence Is a Criminal Justice Issue

PV is a criminal justice issue since police shooting and violence data estimate that 250,000 Americans experience physical injuries and another 1,000 are killed by police annually owing to gunshot wounds (Ludwig, 2023). Statistics show that the victims are disproportionately Black and Latinx and tend to be between the ages of 15 and 34 years old (Feldman et al., 2016; Ludwig, 2023). Of those who receive nonfatal injuries, an estimated 85,000 cases require hospital treatment (*Law Enforcement Epidemiology Project*, 2024). Furthermore, CDC data reveal that Blacks are more than twice as likely as their White and Latinx counterparts to be killed by police and five times more likely to sustain injuries that require hospitalization (DeGue et al., 2016; Ludwig, 2023). Considering this, Ludwig (2023) reports that CDC federal data on violent deaths committed by police officers suggest that thousands of cases where people die in police custody and in local jails are missing from these data. Despite this, some scholars argue that PV is a criminal justice issue for several other reasons. First, it violates citizens' constitutional rights, namely the *Fourth, Eighth,* and *Fourteenth Amendments.* The *Fourth Amendment* allows citizens to be free from unreasonable searches and seizures. The *Eighth Amendment* prohibits citizens from being subjected to excessive force and acts that can be defined as cruel and unusual punishment (del Carmen, 1991). The *Fourteenth Amendment* ensures that state officials must provide all citizens with due process and equal protection under the law. As such, when police fail to do so, they are not operating in a constitutionally correct manner, and should be held accountable and face charges of false arrest, unlawful detention, and where applicable, using excessive force that is likely to result in death when that amount of force is unreasonable to take a non-threatening person into custody.

Second, PV is a criminal justice issue because when it occurs, it erodes public trust and confidence in those who are sworn to serve and protect them from violence (Lyle & Esmail, 2016). This is particularly concerning since police are supposed to be trustworthy given that they are constitutionally mandated to uphold and enforce the laws in the U.S. (Gaines & Kappeler, 2008). In an investigation that used an uninterrupted time series design to replicate a study that focused on how communities react in the aftermath of police deadly shootings of Black men, Strom and Wire (2024) reported that after police are involved in fatal violence that raise issues of the legality of use of force in Black neighborhoods, there is also a corresponding decline in the number of 911 calls for service which suggests that fatal incidents of police shooting's impact residents' behavior when they no longer trust police and question whether they function with legitimate authority. Some criminal justice scholars report that PV has the effect of producing more violence and crime brought on by the fact that when community residents fail to report criminal activity owing to not trusting police, it alienates the community, undercuts cooperation, and allows offenders to continue wreaking havoc in their neighborhoods which leads residents to take matters into their own hands by engaging in retaliatory gun violence (Desmond et al., 2016; Desmond-Harris, 2015). Noray (2024) contends that in the aftermath of the police shooting death of *Michael Brown*, many states experienced the *"Ferguson Effect"* or an increase in retaliatory crimes against police brutality that included an increase in the murder rate. Other researchers have reported similar increases in national crime rates after police killings of unarmed Black men. The research suggests that when the officer is White and the victim is Black, there is a 2.1% increase in the total number of crimes in the month following the shooting death. They also argue that after these racially charged incidents, there is an appreciable large, short-term increase in arrest rates (Gold, 2015; Lopez, 2016). This has led some observers to argue that the criminal justice system routinely fails surviving family members of those who were either injured or killed by PV when grand juries decide not to indict police since many officers are not held criminally responsible for their wrongdoing (Breen, 2023). Third, PV harms the community since research reveals the physical and psychological impact found in neighborhoods where PV occur that affects surviving victims, their families, friends, and other residents. Community residents suffer elevated stress levels.

Police Violence Is a Public Health Issue

Both the CDC and WHO have declared assaultive violence a public health issue because of the short- and long-term health consequences associated with experiencing violence (Dahlberg & Mercy, 2009). In fact, the CDC and WHO report that after experiencing violence, some victims are treated for trauma and stress, physical injuries, and mental health issues (Alang et al., 2017). Sometimes, the experience can adversely affect their family members in ways that also require physical and mental health treatment (Fix, 2021; Krug et al., 2002). Recently, researchers have reported that *Black Lives Matter* and *SayHerName* protests are linked to PV that often results in death, physical injuries, acute racial stress, and other injuries primarily to young Black Americans. They also argue that the constant threat of PV poses a serious health risk to the Black community because of the stress associated with being a potential victim of PV and the level of force (e.g., excessive/deadly) shown on television of fatal Black shootings (Edwards et al., 2019; APHA, 2018). Health professionals contend that police encounters with Blacks are so violent that they affect the Black community's physical and mental well-being (Sandoiu, 2020).

Experts argue that while achieving health equality has always been the primary mission of public health, many groups in public health including epidemiologists were reluctant to list police use of excessive force as a major health risk and threat to people of color (APHA, 2018). Some scholars contend that despite the statistics showing a nexus between race and PV, the matter had been ignored by public health officials even when the evidence was clear that after encounters with police, minorities' physical and psychological health was negatively impacted. Critics reported that public health investigators produced little research criticizing the police for engaging in behavior that poses a threat to certain segments of the U.S. population (Copper et al., 2005). The public health system has been accused of taking even longer to address the nature and prevalence of PV perpetrated against Black women and gender-variant women (Fedina et al., 2018; APHA, 2018).

PV is a public health issue that affects the physical, mental, and sexual well-being of millions of people globally, especially marginalized populations in poor communities who receive inequitable exposure to police officers that negatively impact their ability to acquire basic rights such as housing, education, economic opportunities, and fair access to health services (*APHA*, 2018). The literature suggests that since PV affects the public, it requires public health approaches and interventions, rather than criminal justice responses for people who need hospitalization, medication, physical therapy, counseling, and treatment in the aftermath of violent police behavior. Studies report this type of violence adds a financial strain on people who can least afford the burden of having to defray the expensive costs of medical, legal bills, and funerals (Beyer & Kaine, 2021). Moreover, PV is a public health concern because it threatens the entire community's well-being and the sense of safety for those impacted by it. Some human rights advocates and watch groups contend that it has created collective insecurity that has rendered millions of people worldwide from trusting police actions owing to the belief that PV is state-sponsored (*Amnesty International*, 2024). Its violence not only impacts adults, but research shows that children and teens living in overly policed areas are also adversely affected. A research investigation revealed that children and teenagers exposed to violence and killings experience more absenteeism and decreased GPAs in the aftermath that lasts several semesters. Furthermore, some students are less likely to finish high school, and others are more likely to forgo attending college which diminishes their opportunity for success and reduces their economic worth as adults (Harding, 2009; Finkelhor et al., 2015). Research also evidence that after PV occurs, it leaves behind a host of victims including those who experienced the victimization firsthand and others who experienced it vicariously. Alang and colleagues (2017) reported that PV has a far-reaching effect that ripples across families, communities, and society by increasing parental stress, caregiver responsibilities, employment loss, and adding economic hardships to families. Reports from the CDC (n.d.) indicate that the overall costs of fatal and nonfatal injuries committed by law enforcement officers reported in 2010, including medical costs, hospitalization, and lost work was estimated at $1.8 billion.

International Comparative Statistics

Reports reveal that worldwide, police use aggressive tactics to disburse crowds of protesters who advocate peace and a recognition of their basic rights (Cheatham & Maizland, 2022). Human rights experts at the *United Nations* (UN) have declared it a global health problem and have called for an end to police brutality after examining rampant PV against peaceful protesters worldwide. UN experts have spoken out against police use of excessive force, police brutality, inhuman and degrading acts, torture, sexual violence, arbitrary detention, and enforced disappearance of peaceful protesters located in every region of the world. As was the case in France, where police have targeted Black and Arab people which led to rampant protests in 2018. Additionally, human rights experts and activists contend that state-sponsored violence has not only targeted protesters, but it has also singled out journalists covering protests and has been responsible for countless injuries, deaths, and devastation. As a result, UN officials warn that while PV is often motivated by racial, political, social, ethnic, religious, and other tensions that are unique to a particular regional or national situation, these actions perpetrated by police not only violate human rights and dignity, but they also violate the rule of international law. It contends that a common theme that follows PV and abuse is encouragement by divisive narratives and the support of political leaders and local authorities that insult the behavior with impunity (*United Nations Human Rights*, 2021). Similarly, officials at *Amnesty International* (2024) argue that it is difficult to get accurate data on police killings because many governments do not collect or publish these data, and what is known often comes from human rights watch groups. These data reveal that globally, police are quick to use force to respond to protests as evidenced by what occurred in *Hong Kong* from 2019 to 2020 when police deployed weapons and attacked peaceful protesters. In 2020, Nigerian police opened gunfire on a group of peaceful demonstrators and killed 12 people who were demanding police reform (Cheatham & Maizland, 2022). Another incident occurred between women protesters and the *Turkish* police in *Istanbul* in 2021 when police fired teargas into a crowd of women protesting femicide and domestic violence. Research also shows that in *Iran*, in 2019, protesters were confronted by armed police who shot and killed hundreds who were not posing a threat or risk to officers. It was revealed that at least 23 children were among the dead. In another case that occurred in the *Philippines*, witnesses recounted seeing local police shoot and kill people who were suspected of either using or selling drugs. Reports also indicate that Canadian police killed 254 people during encounters between 2013 and 2020 (Cheatham & Maizland, 2022).

In some of the most egregious cases, *Amnesty International* (2024) as well as the *Council on Foreign Relations* reported that in *Greece, Italy,* and *North Macedonia*, police have engaged in arbitrary detaining, torturing, and abusing refugees and migrants. There are also reported cases of death of Indigenous *Australians* while in police custody (Cheatham & Maizland, 2022). In *Brazil*, police officers kill people (e.g., young Black men) with impunity even when they do not pose a threat partly because such killings rarely get investigated or prosecuted. Experts estimate that in 2019, police killed 1,800 people or engaged in five killings each day in *Rio de Janeiro, Brazil*. Other examples include the following: in *Kenya*, police officers murdered 122 people; in *Iraq*, police killed 600 protesters between 2019 and 2020; and in *Jamaica*, an estimated 500 people were killed by police and another 300 were shot and seriously wounded by police. In *France* in 2015, evidence suggests that police engaged in thousands of discriminatory raids and house arrests that targeted Muslims solely based on their religious beliefs, and in the *Russian Republic of Chechnya* in 2017, police staged campaigns against *LGBTI* members resulting in many abductions, tortures, and deaths committed in secret places. Similarly, transgender sex workers in the *Dominican Republic* experienced various forms of abuse by police including beatings, humiliation, and rapes (*Amnesty International*, 2024). Moreover, existing data have allowed researchers to isolate reported cases of global police killings and create a list of the nations with the highest recorded incidents. The top ten countries and the number of police deaths as recently as 2024 are as follows: Philippines (6,069), Brazil (5,804), Venezuela (5,286), India (1,731), Syria (1,497), U.S. (1,096), El Salvador (1,087), Nigeria (841), Afghanistan (606), and Pakistan (495). Scholars and experts point out that of the top countries, the U.S. is the only one that is categorized as an advanced nation, while the others on the list are considered developing countries (*World Population Review*, 2024). This finding has prompted scholars to examine how the number of U.S. police killings compares with police killings in other wealthy democracies. A study conducted by Cheatham and Maizland (2022) has been instructive in this regard. According to their investigation that relied on data collected in 2019, they reported that when compared with other wealthy democracies, the U.S. is not only the leader in killings by police officers, but the behavior often goes unpunished. Their study provides the country, killings per 10 million people, and the total number of killings. They present the following outcomes: U.S. (33.5 and 1,099), Canada (9.8 and 36), Australia (8.5 and 21), the Netherlands (2.3 and 4), New Zealand (2.1 and 1), Germany (1.3 and 11), England and Wales (0.5 and 3), Japan (0.2 and 2), Iceland (0 and 0), and Norway (0 and 0).

Public Health and Social Work

Intersection of Public Health and Social Work

Police misconduct and violence have been linked with contributing to the dehumanization of racially and ethnically marginalized persons (Grills et al., 2016) and have been shown to have particularly detrimental effects on the health and social development of African-American teens and young men (Staggers-Hakim, 2016). As therapists, social workers can be trained to recognize and assess race-based trauma and to use trauma-informed best practices to assist clients in healing (Williams et al., 2022). One such best practice is the healing racial trauma protocol. There are many therapeutic techniques within the intervention that include the following:

- Assessing racial trauma and stress,
- Validating experiences and offering support,
- Providing psychoeducation on racism and its link to mental health,
- Assessing and strengthening coping skills,
- Teaching and encouraging self-care and self-compassion,
- Assisting in the development of external supports,
- Teaching mindfulness techniques,
- Providing psychoeducation about colorism to combat internalized racism,
- Cognitive restructuring and defusion from internalized racism,
- Ethnic and racial identity development/identity-affirming practices,
- Processing racist experiences,
- Recounting traumatic racism-related experiences,
- Skills building in confronting racism,
- Post-traumatic growth and meaning-making, and
- Social action and activism.

Social work advocates for strategies to achieve community reinvestment, pre-arrest diversion, and innovative approaches to 911 emergency responses (Wilson & Wilson, 2020). If "social workers can develop collaborative partnerships working with law enforcement agencies–in crisis response systems" (p. 3), they can participate in deflection and diversion programs. In this collaborative effort, social workers can:

- Respond to calls for service with a focus on mental illness, substance abuse, and homelessness,
- Refer individuals to treatment, housing, and other social services as appropriate through mobile crisis units,
- Counsel crime victims and refer them to social services agencies as needed,

- Assist with county-level reentry efforts, and
- Address law enforcement officers' trauma and mental health needs, and make referrals as needed.

This is the juncture at which social work and public health begin to intersect. Public health can assist in reducing the damage of policing through public health-informed alternative response programs. One approach is to develop public health-informed alternative response teams to respond to non-violent circumstances such as mental health and substance abuse crises and low-level offense calls. Experts contend that having interprofessional teams that include medics, trained community members, and social workers to perform crisis intervention may prove effective at de-escalating potentially explosive and violent situations. Public health and social work can also partner at the significant governmental and societal levels as discussed in the section below on *public health and social work approaches*.

Health Disparities and Health Equities

In this chapter's discussion on the nature and extent of police brutality, it was revealed that not only are Black, Indigenous, and People of Color disproportionately killed by police (Nix & Shjarback, 2021; Lett et al., 2020), but they are also excessively victimized by police brutality at a higher rate compared with Whites and Asian/Pacific Islanders. PV, physical and sexual, has also been found at higher rates among the LGBTQ community (Alang, 2020). Research finds that experiencing higher rates of brutality makes these populations more vulnerable to PV-related health inequities (Alang et al., 2023). These inequities include physical and mental health injuries, conditions, and diagnoses. Since inequity in police killings has been discussed, we will focus on other health issues.

Health inequities associated with police killings and other forms of PV include lower self-reported general health among Black and Hispanic adolescents compared with White youth (McFarland et al., 2019), increased risk of diabetes, high blood pressure, and obesity (Sewell, 2017), general poor health and asthma episodes (Sewell & Jefferson, 2016), and sleep disturbances (Testa et al., 2021). Moreover, mental health disorder inequities have been reported to include depression and anxiety symptoms (Alang et al., 2021; Bacak & Nowotny, 2020; Bowleg et al., 2022), general psychological distress (Del Toro et al., 2019; Dennison & Finkeldey, 2021), suicidal ideation and suicide attempts (DeVylder et al., 2017b), psychotic experiences (DeVylder et al., 2017a), and PTSD (Geller et al., 2014). The severity of depression was discovered to be stronger among Black and Latino persons (Alang et al., 2021), as was lowered self-efficacy, suicide ideation, and drug use (Dennison & Finkeldey, 2021). Additionally, allostatic load theory (McEwen, 2006) proffers that repeated and chronic stressors, such as police brutality, lead to the wearing of the body down over time and are associated with biological aging, increased risk of mortality, increased cognitive decline, and various other adverse health outcomes (Rodriquez et al., 2019). Since PV is more commonly committed in communities of color, there is evidence that suggests members of African-American and Black communities have a higher allostatic load compared with Whites ages 35–64 (Duru et al., 2012; Geronimus et al., 2006).

Negative Health Consequences of Police Violence

PV brings negative health consequences to people living in overly policed communities (Sewell & Jefferson, 2016; Davis & Whyde, 2018). Some documented health issues include physical and mental health problems that must be addressed and treated by non-criminal justice personnel since they are not properly trained and lack the necessary resources, and skillsets needed to assist victims of PV. Therefore, public health officials argue that what is needed are experts, professionals, counselors, and first responders who are trained in medicine and public health solutions since PV leads to short and long-term trauma that stems from personal injuries, psychological harm, and even death (Spolum et al., 2023). Moreover, while Nembhard and colleagues (2022) acknowledge that not every police encounter involves physical violence, they pointed out that police interventions with minorities often result in adverse health consequences such as depression, anxiety, PTSD, suicide, and increased rates of cardiovascular disease and premature mortality for its victims, their families, and bystanders. Several studies find that even in police stops viewed as unfair, discriminatory, or intrusive there is the potential of adversely impacting victims' mental health outcomes and can cause symptoms that include anxiety, depression, mood disorders, and PTSD (Geller et al., 2014). Other experts report that PV inflicted by racism causes more health problems such as panic attacks, hypervigilance, avoidance, psychotic experiences, substance abuse, self-harming, and difficulty focusing and functioning (Bryant-Davis & Ocampo, 2005). In other studies, Bor and colleagues (2018) and Deivanayagm and colleagues (2021) found that overpolicing in Black and Latinx neighborhoods does not mean effective or equitable policing, but rather it is linked to several health-related outcomes associated with daily aggression and systemic oppression that include fatal injuries, adverse physiological responses that increase morbidity, psychological stress, poor school performance, incomplete high school education, and the intersecting oppressive structures that are linked to disempowerment. Sewell and Jackson (2016) and Sewell (2017) report that in neighborhoods that experienced a high level of police stops and frisks followed by the use of force, all men in the neighborhood exhibited elevated levels of psychological distress, and an increased risk of diabetes and obesity.

Research by DeVylder and colleagues (2022) reveals that when police officers anywhere kill Blacks, it has a devastating effect on the Black community everywhere that is not as visible as when physical victimizations occur, yet it is more pervasive since it destabilizes the community's quality of mental health. This effect occurs even when residents have no direct contact with the police or are victims of violence (DeVylder et al., 2020). Both groups experience trauma and fear that this type of violence can happen again. A study by Smith and Rodriguez (2020) posits that in the aftermath of every police killing of a person of color, there is a reported increase in poor mental health of Blacks including chronic stress, depression, and lower life expectancy. Other studies find that PV in minority communities often leads to post-traumatic stress disorder and an increase in substance abuse, as well as suicidal ideation (Sewell, 2017).

Criminal Justice Approaches to Police Violence

There are several criminal justice approaches that can be used to prevent PV from occurring in the future. To that end, we suggest police departments nationwide adopt proactive methods to recruit better-qualified officers, provide police proper training to create greater police–community relations, and use body and dash cameras and create a mandatory federal database. Another approach is that victims of excessive force can file a *Section 1983 Litigation and Wrongful Death Lawsuit* when their civil or constitutional rights are violated.

Recruit Better-Qualified Police Officers

The duties and responsibilities of policing a diverse society have become more complex. As such, agencies should proactively recruit and properly train qualified candidates. Today, policing in the U.S. is different compared to decades ago. Police and criminal justice experts contend that because of increased diversity in nearly every locality in the country, changing cultural dynamics, changes in the use of technology, the threat of domestic as well as international terrorism, and other complicated matters, police officers are now required to do more than any other time in the history of policing (Gaines & Kappeler, 2008). Consequently, police work requires a rigorous recruitment and hiring process designed to attract more educated, diverse, and psychologically stable officers (Worrall, 2001). In fact, the *Center for Policing Equity* has recently initiated efforts to recruit new officers from different racial and ethnic backgrounds in policing given the diversity in society (Abrams, 2020).

Need to Provide Proper Training to Police

Because of the complexity of the problems police officers confront, extensive training is needed to build trust and reduce violence in the communities they serve. Owens and colleagues (2018) study discovered when police receive training in performing in a procedurally correct manner, it reduces the use of force by between 15% and 40%. As such, criminal justice experts argue police must receive ethical training in the academy by establishing clear standards for proper policing, making sure training is updated via continued education programs and in-service training, and being familiar with departmental policies governing aspects of policing, namely the use of force. Payne and colleagues (2016) posit this will allow avenues for police to be successful in servicing minority communities. Moreover, residents in Black and Latinx communities should not feel that police function with racist or implicit biases toward them. A failure to properly train officers could be used as evidence against police and their municipalities as a show of *deliberate indifference* to the plight of those they serve. Research reveals that implicit biases impact police behavior since it is based on cumulative perceptions that police construct of other people (Greenwald et al., 2015; Glaser & Knowles, 2008). The evidence finds that stereotypes of race and ethnicity influence the perception of threat. Police are socialized and trained to see young Black and Latinx men as more threatening and dangerous. Therefore, they are more likely to use excessive force without deliberation (Goff et al., 2008).

Experts contend that implicit biases are always present and exist outside people's conscious awareness and control. To some experts, this suggests that whether police officers are racists or homophobic is influenced by their experiences, exposures, upbringing, politics, and other individual, relational, cultural, and societal factors they acquire before, during, and after employment (Devine, 1989; Lee et al., 2022). To address implicit biases, as part of officers' training, experts recommend discussions and role-playing designed to help departments reduce high-discretion techniques and hold officers accountable for disparate treatment (Abrams, 2020). They also suggest that policymakers (e.g., police chiefs and others) work to diversify law enforcement agencies and offer intervention training programs such as intergroup contact, counter-stereotypic exemplars, stereotype negation training, and multifaceted interventions. While most police departments offer training in cultural competency, the addition of implicit bias training can help to reduce the effect of cultural biases and stereotypes that often influence policy decisions (Lee et al., 2022). Other important areas of training that are required to reduce violence and use of excessive force are crisis intervention team training or CIT, de-escalation training, and mental health training. This will teach police officers to quickly recognize people with mental health issues and de-escalate potentially dangerous encounters by diverting them to a social service agency for treatment (Parker, 2018).

Use Body and Dash Cameras

Police agencies nationwide should use body and dash cams to show transparency (Peak & Everett, 2017; Buchler, 2017). Experts contend that they can serve as a form of effective oversight that indicates to the public that police favor accountability. These devices could prove to be an effective and beneficial tool for policing for several reasons. First, they could provide training opportunities since they would reveal the encounters between police and citizens. When made accessible to the public, they will show what transpired if an officer is accused of engaging in unnecessary or excessive force. As a pedagogical tool, they can illustrate what is an appropriate action to take given the circumstances. Second, they can be used by prosecutors who go before grand juries seeking an indictment against an officer accused of using excessive force. Third, they could prove to be invaluable when an officer and his respective police department face civil litigation. Events captured by video can reveal whether an officer followed proper procedure during encounters with suspects. If an officer has been wrongfully accused of operating in a manner that exceeds his scope of authority, a body or dash camera can help to exonerate him and potentially save his police agency large sums of money in damage awards (Lee et al., 2022).

Mandatory Federal Database

A mandatory federal database of police shootings is needed. Currently, police departments report officer-involved shootings on a voluntary basis to the *Federal Bureau of Investigations* (FBI). Critics contend these reports are vague, lack details, and are categorized only as "justified" or "unjustified." Because they do not offer enough detail, the criminal justice system should create a federal database that resembles *42 U.S. Code §13031* which requires those in a professional capacity (including law enforcement personnel, see section B6) who engage in activities within federal jurisdictions to report the "facts that give reason to suspect that a child has suffered an incident of child abuse" or face federal criminal proceedings. A similar reporting system can be created that compiles accurate and timely data on officer-involved shootings. Advocates posit that such a database can be instrumental in monitoring officers with a history of shootings in one jurisdiction but later relocate to another jurisdiction since investigations sometimes reveal that officers have managed to leave their shooting histories behind when they become employed in another jurisdiction. The benefits of creating this database include facilitating justice, transparency, and restoring public confidence and trust in policing. Some experts believe that this database can be used to break the code of silence that is entrenched within the police culture (Lee et al., 2022).

Section 1983 Litigation and Wrongful Death Lawsuits

Because reports from *Mapping Police Violence* indicate that from 2013 to 2022, 98% of police killings failed to result in officers being held accountable for their criminal misconduct, some experts argue that victims or their surviving families should seek civil justice (*The Guardian*, 2024). A popular form of legal redress is found in *Title 42 of the United States Code, Section 1983: Civil Action for Deprivation of Civil Rights*. It allows citizens who had their civil and constitutional rights violated by government officials to bring a civil suit to recover monetary damages (del Carmen, 1991; Gaines & Kappeler, 2008). In a *Section 1983* claim, a victim (plaintiff) of excessive force, can bring a lawsuit in federal court against a police officer alleging that his constitutional rights were violated while the officer was acting under color of law. They require the victim to establish two basic elements: (1) the police officer (defendant) acted under the color of law, and (2) a violation of a constitutionally or federally protected right (del Carmen, 1991). In the case of excessive force, if a state or local law enforcement officer misuses his power or authority derived from his employment as a law enforcement officer, he has acted under color of law and can be held liable in a civil rights lawsuit. The plaintiff must show that a right granted by the U.S. Constitution or a federal law was violated. In cases where suspects are shot and killed and it is later determined that they were unarmed or retreating from police and did not pose a significant threat of death to the officer, nor posed danger to others, these matters are likely to be ruled as civil rights and constitutional rights violations.

 Section 1983 claims can also include municipal liability. In *City of Canton v. Harris* (1989, p. 1205), the Court ruled that inadequate police training may serve as the basis of liability under *Section 1983* if that failure amounts to "deliberate indifference" to the rights of persons with whom the police come into contact and those deficiencies in their training program are closely related to the victim's injuries. The Court stated that

> it may happen that in light of the duties assigned to specific officers or employees, the need for more or different training is so obvious, and the inadequacy so likely to result in violations of constitutional rights, and the policymakers of the city can reasonably be said to have been deliberately indifferent to the need.

Consequently, these lawsuits name the officer, his immediate supervisor, the police chief, the agency, and members of the city council as parties (del Carmen & Walker, 2004).

Wrongful Death Lawsuits

In a wrongful death lawsuit, surviving family members of the deceased can file a tort action alleging the death of their family member was caused by a police officer. These suits are brought for damage awards associated with pain, suffering, and the costs of the funeral and hospitalization. Experts contend that to prevail in a wrongful death lawsuit, the plaintiff must demonstrate that the death of a family member was unjustified (del Carmen, 1991).

Civil litigation is common in the U.S. and can be expensive. Thomas-DeVeaux and colleagues (2021) examined public records on police settlement spending in 31 of the 50 cities with the highest police-to-civilian ratios on data obtained by *FiveThirtyEight* and *The Marshall Project* and discovered in the past ten years, an estimated $3 billion have been paid out on lawsuits alleging police misconduct. Of the settlements that occurred during this period, records show that the largest amounts were paid out in New York City ($1,704,120,487), Chicago ($467,586,464), and Los Angeles ($329,925,620). The next two cities with the highest settlements for police misconduct include Washington, DC, and Philadelphia. Data collected on settlements for Washington, DC, is for a nine period at ($114,841,449), while data on Philadelphia police misconduct cases cover settlements for an 11-year period at ($116,881,088), respectively.

Public Health Approaches to Police Violence

Public health officials criticize criminal justice approaches to preventing crime and violence for several reasons, chief among them is that the system is reactive, rather than proactive, and its primary goal is to apprehend and punish offenders. Public health officials contend that the criminal justice system has historically failed society because of its limitation, namely it ignores the root causes of violence and crime. According to public health experts, criminal justice practitioners view the cause of crime and violence as a personal decision (owing to some moral failing) that offenders make prior to engaging in crime. As a result, they fail to consider that violence and crime stem from complex factors such as racism, discrimination, poverty, lack of access to jobs and social services, mental health challenges, and environmental factors. They argue that the failure to address the root causes perpetuates violence and produces more victims and offenders. Public health officials agree that a paradigm shift must occur whereby, crime and violence are viewed through different lenses. Even criminal justice historians and policymakers argue that increasing recidivism rates and more crime indicate that justice measures are flawed (Reddington & Bonham, 2019). Crime and violence must be seen as a public health issue that requires public health approaches, rather than continuing with failed reactive justice policies. When the public health approach is used, researchers bring a multidisciplinary approach to crime and violence that addresses the many facets that one discipline alone cannot provide. It also views them as a disease that adversely impacts certain segments of people in a community. Therefore, they advocate early proactive emphasis should be placed on prevention and stopping the spread of violence that can escalate from the individual to the neighborhood and later to the community in the same manner as a disease spreads throughout the population. Public health experts suggest that early prevention efforts that are evidence-based should be used as intervention strategies that facilitate collaboration with community stakeholders.

When it comes to addressing PV and preventing the devastation that it causes in the U.S., APHA (2018) posits that public health approaches should be adopted for two reasons: they are associated with reduced community trauma and improved community health and safety via preventative interventions, and they rely on evidence-based research that shows the determinants that increase the likelihood PV will occur including officers mental health, systemic racism, and racial discrimination that some officers experience within the context of the police academy. This combined with the masculine and militarized culture in police departments typically translates into them engaging in overpolicing that often manifests into violence that is disproportionately inflicted on disadvantaged populations including Blacks, Latinos, gender-variant women, and others who are members of the *LGBTQ+* community (see also *United Nations Human Rights*, 2023). Public health officials argue that efforts should be made to reduce and eliminate violence. Some key areas of focus should be on training police officers, providing police with mental health support, and working to improve police–community relations. Unlike other strategies designed to prevent violence, the public health approach recognizes that police brutality is a complex problem with historical roots that require experts to understand and consider determinant factors such as poverty, systemic inequalities, and mental health challenges. Because of the nature and enormity of the problem, those seeking to prevent PV should focus on prevention, collaboration, and evidence-based intervention by forming partnerships and collaborations with social service agencies, educational institutions, grassroots community organizations, and police departments to create and develop proactive rather than reactive responses to violence before it escalates (Gilmore, 2010). The inclusion of minority communities that are disproportionately the target of overpolicing is essential to any successful response given the need to build trust that can only emerge from community-engagement collaboration, especially in problem-solving efforts. Public health experts contend that this will facilitate effective communication, and cooperation, as well as result in safer neighborhoods. They also argue it addresses the reported high levels of fear, stress, and strain that contribute to the poor psychological health of many Blacks, Latinos, *LGBTQ+* members, and others who experience routine police intervention (Gilmore, 2010). This type of primary intervention addresses the need to improve police–community relations. Research finds that it helps reduce the number of excessive and deadly force cases in Black communities (Williams, 2018). Experts report that when police and residents participate together in community events such as youth mentoring programs and problem-solving events, it helps to establish mutual understanding and respect that creates positive relationships that encourage community residents to take a proactive approach by sharing their concerns with police (Gilmore, 2010).

According to DeVylder and colleagues (2018), research reveals that providing swift and adequate mental health support to officers who have experienced trauma can reduce the likelihood that they will use excessive force. Others find that community residents who receive mental health treatment will not suffer from stress, strain, and other injuries that diminish their quality of mental health and their lives (Williams, 2018). Furthermore, it encourages positive community engagement, experts believe that it can lead to improved morale, job satisfaction, and ultimately reduce high levels of police stress that improve their overall wellness (DeVylder et al., 2018). Another important reason to engage in a public health approach to reduce PV is that crime tends to saturate marginalized areas that experience systemic inequality including health disparities (Gilmore, 2010). The public health approach encourages police to partner and collaborate with public health and community organizations to provide officers with first-hand knowledge and experience with the inequalities that exist in society to dispel implicit biases, stereotypes, and preconceived notions about the minorities they encounter. This approach allows officers to objectively observe how some people are adversely impacted by social isolation, lack access to education, employment, housing, and limited access to health care (Gilmore, 2010). They also learn how poor segments of the population cope with systemic racism. It also reveals what is needed to improve the well-being of the community (APHA, 2018).

Public Health and Social Work Approaches

Public health and social work professionals are invested in creating safer and healthier communities. Both professions believe that one way to achieve health equity is to implement alternatives to traditional police response, sometimes referred to as *community response models*, though public health officials refer to them as *alternatives to police involvement* (Spolum et al., 2023). Nevertheless, public health and social work recommend three strategies for guiding alternative response models: (1) involving impacted communities directly in model design, (2) creating programs that work independently of the police, and (3) securing adequate funding for programs and social services. These community alternative efforts would also include those most affected by PV participating in community engagement and empowerment activities and employing community members to make significant program decisions, spearhead program implementation, and assist in designing key evaluation measures (Spolum et al., 2023). Some experts suggest that program designs should include pre-arrest and diversion solutions (Wilson & Wilson, 2020). More specifically, some advocates contend that this may also involve expanding already established programs such as "existing pre-arrest diversion programs, crisis intervention responses, and behavioral health interventions that are not law enforcement-centric" (p. 9). A successful example is the Law Enforcement Assisted Diversion (LEAD) implemented in King County of Seattle, Washington. The program yielded the following benefits:

- Reduced burden on the criminal justice system to solve public health and social challenges,
- Reduced crime,
- Reduced drug use,
- Better outcomes during crisis encounters,
- Lives saved, lives restored,
- Building police–community relations,
- Building (more) police–public relations,
- health/behavioral health relations,
- Correct movement of citizens into/away from the justice system,
- Cost savings,
- Kept families intact, and
- Addressed racial disparity.

Creating programs that exist separate from law enforcement and the criminal justice system necessitates the need for supportive public health and social services to help address the many different "concerns, needs, and power of local advocates and the responsiveness of government officials" (Spolum et al., 2023, p. S39). An example is the San Francisco Street Crisis Response Team (CRT). An alternative to police involvement, CRT requires funding, and one source of its funding comes from monies that were diverted from police-enforced programs (not only for program implementation), to employ community members who participated in the program's design, implementation, evaluation, and oversight. The program has met with success. Some other efforts to reduce police-inflicted harm include social work practice within police departments, offering crisis intervention training to police, diverting police response away from calls that involve homeless people, school discipline, neighbor conflicts, and other non-violent issues, and lobbying for systemic policing policy reform that includes training in the areas of crowd management and violence de-escalation (Wilson & Wilson, 2020).

Integrating Skills of Social Epidemiology to Address Disparities and Achieve Equity

Public health researchers and practitioners argue that most people are unaware of the impact that social determinants have on the epidemiology of disease as well as assaultive violence (Turabi et al., 2022). They contend that people from disadvantaged backgrounds living in various regions worldwide experience different health outcomes compared with those who have relative affluence and make up a nation's majority (Wallerstein et al., 2011; Turabi et al., 2022). McDonough and colleagues (1997) reported that people from lower socioeconomic positions experience virtually every disease and type of violence compared with others. When examining different diseases and violence, surveillance data reveal that they are distributed differently globally. This suggests that there are risk factors (e.g., structural inequality) within populations that increase the likelihood that disease and violence (e.g., health inequities) will occur. For epidemiologists, observing inequities provides a basis for intervention since these risk factors affect the population's health (Wallerstein et al., 2011). Because of this, researchers view the progression of health conditions as complex and health inequities present themselves via a lack of access and unmet needs that are saturated in poor underserved communities disproportionately inhabited by Blacks and Latinos (Turabi et al., 2022; Spolum et at., 2023). Epidemiologists advocate that health equity is essential to healthy living. They also contend that two concepts (health equity and health disparity) must be explored to fully understand the role that epidemiology plays in improving the overall health of a population. Epidemiologists argue that health equity occurs when everyone, regardless of region or country, is provided access to health despite the social detriments they face such as race, ethnicity, social class, and neighborhood. Alarmingly, health disparities cause different health outcomes among people with respect to region and nation. The literature is replete with findings that establish a disparity exists in PV and the overall health of Blacks, Latinx, Indigenous people, and transgenders in the U.S. compared with Whites (Spolum et al., 2023). It reveals the victims of PV are disproportionately poor, Black, of a certain age, and suffer negative health consequences after police encounters. Evidence shows that Black and Latinx young men experience more long-term physical and psychological trauma, acute stress, *PTSD*, poor mental health, and even death at the hands of police compared with others. In areas that are overly policed, researchers find higher rates of diseases (e.g., obesity, heart disease, hypertension, diabetes) that are distributed unequally in Black and Latinx neighborhoods compared with White communities (Turabi et al., 2022; Spolum et al., 2023).

Experts argue that public health and social service agencies, along with other partners will face challenges presented by social determinants found in areas that experience PV and advance health equity to improve the health outcomes for those that are impacted by the behavior. The same experts contend that this will require a collective effort that is data-driven and includes enlisting the help of researchers and others to empower communities that are most affected. Hence, communities nationwide must be educated and made aware of the disparities that exist regarding overpolicing and how it impacts their overall health. Community residents should be encouraged to seek counseling and treatment for mental health issues when needed least they risk suffering the long-term consequences of undiagnosed and untreated negative health conditions associated with chronic stress, heart diseases, and others. They must also mobilize and create grassroots programs designed for community activism that keep its issues at the forefront. To that end, community leaders must work with politicians, law enforcement, social workers, and public health officials to bring reforms to overpolicing and assisting community residents who are impacted by PV and the resources they need before and in the aftermath of state-sponsored violence. To improve health outcomes, some experts recommend that community engagement scholars form alliances with leaders to help identify informal structures and norms within minority communities that foster powerlessness. Wallerstein and colleagues (2011) argue that institutional racism in lower-class communities remains a by-product of historical systematic racism that must be addressed. When it is discovered, engagement scholars should help to eradicate any discriminatory practices in business or governmental agencies (e.g., overpolicing) that are involved with the community. Health experts also posit that it is important to point out that the areas where PV typically occurs have experienced historical inequities owing to systemic racism that has resulted in certain segments of the population being denied equal access to resources such as jobs, health care, educational attainment, and have served to perpetuate health disparities in the U.S. since unfairness impedes good health. By working together with public health and social service agencies, police organizations, and politicians, underserved communities will experience better health outcomes (Turabi et al., 2022).

How Can PV Be Prevented?

For critics of the justice system (who observe militarized PV used on citizens who exercise a constitutionally protected right to engage in peaceful protests), this action perpetuates racial disparities in the criminal justice system since it disproportionately targets marginalized groups. Critics contend that police reform is needed to prevent discriminatory practices that inevitably lead to disparate treatment and biased practices that often account for overpolicing in minority communities that often end in the use of fatal violence (Johnson & Johnson, 2023). Some police experts agree that while racial profiling is prohibited by law, police officers are allowed to engage in pretextual stops to enforce the law. However, when these stops occur, police are typically acting on racial stereotypes and biases for minor infractions under the pretext of a routine check, while their true purpose is to acquire consent to conduct a search in the hope that it will lead to probable cause to justify an arrest. This causes people of color to fear being stopped by police and has served to create distrust since they expect the worst to ensue from police encounters (Johnson & Johnson, 2023). Experts contend that to prevent inequitable practices and potential violence, police agencies must use evidence-based practices that are oriented toward public safety instead of engaging in low-level stops and arrests since they send the message that police are disproportionately targeting and monitoring Blacks and other minorities to arrest. These encounters can quickly escalate into physical violence and even death in some cases (Johnson & Johnson, 2023). To effect real change, the *Council on Criminal Justice's Task Force on Policing* contends that meaningful reforms can only occur when the *U.S. Department of Justice* creates a national clearinghouse of data collected on the number of people killed by police, implements departmental policies that mandate mandatory reporting when police officers engage in misconduct, teach police officers trauma-informed strategies that convey to how citizens view and respond to them, implement national training standards that encourage de-escalation of potentially violent situations, and implement a national decertification registry that lists and monitor law enforcement officers who were involved in shootings and received complaints in an effort to prevent them from transferring to another department in the aftermath of engaging in police misconduct. The *Task Force* also stated that police agencies must conduct thorough, independent, impartial, and transparent investigations of police use of excessive and lethal force cases (Johnson & Johnson, 2023; *Amnesty International*, 2005).

Public health experts argue that criminal justice responses to PV have failed and what is needed is public health-informed alternative response teams that can address situations such as mental health, substance abuse crises, non-violent situations, and even low-level offenses that may include trespass, indecent exposure, traffic incidents, and loitering complaints (Spolum et al., 2023). Health experts recognize that police contribute to violence so instead of overly relying on the justice system to address every situation that arises in a community, other groups such as social workers, medics, mental health workers, and community residents can be trained to provide crisis intervention or de-escalation services that can achieve a more favorable non-violent outcome compared with police intervention (Nembhard et al., 2022). A public health-informed alternative response strategy is primarily concerned with community safety, and it includes having people most affected by it as part of the conversation as well as involved in the decision-making process (Nembhard et al., 2022). As such, alternative responses target communities that have been directly impacted and harmed by PV. While these public health-informed alternative teams are designed to reduce police intervention, they are community-focused and inclusive of residents in their design, implementation, oversight, and evaluation (Spolum et al., 2023). Advocates contend that this includes a broad range of community engagement that places community residents center of the programs. In San Francisco, California, and Eugene, Oregon pilot programs entitled the *Street Crisis Response Team* and *Crisis Assistance Helping Out on the Streets* were created and launched by community-based organizations and residents who were victims of PV. Both programs have shown success in assisting victimized community residents with the resources needed in PV (Spolum et al., 2023).

Alang and colleagues (2017) contend that public health-informed alternative response programs must not resemble the justice system's approach of using punitive and harmful elements, but rather, they must focus on reducing their impact and offer supportive public health and social services. These programs should not include police officers in any capacity, not even as first responders, or co-respond with police (Spolum et al., 2023). Some experts advocate implementing community-based violence prevention programs that rely on interrupters to defuse potentially violent situations. These community-based responses would be composed of teams of residents who are trained to intervene in situations that often end in tragedy in the aftermath of law enforcement responses. Community teams can assist in calls regarding the homeless, mentally ill residents, and some domestic abuse situations (Smith & Rodriguez, 2020). Another suggestion is to reallocate funding at the local, state, and federal levels for programs and social services by diverting monies from police and the prison industrial complex to education, employment, and restorative justice programs (Smith & Rodriguez, 2020).

Policy Recommendations

Criminal justice and public health experts argue that to prevent PV, efforts should be made to address its root causes as well as hold police responsible for engaging in misconduct (Anderson et al., 2022; del Carmen, 1991). Because PV has historical roots stemming from systemic racism, efforts must be made to address the long-term impact that structural inequities have on health disparities and how certain groups' physical health, mental health, and quality of life continue to be adversely affected. Nevertheless, there are immediate strategies that can be implemented to reduce PV in the U.S. and help improve the quality of health for those who suffer PV. We recommend training in policing protests and community health and violence-reduction strategies.

National reports from watchdog groups show that police response to protests escalated volatile situations into violence and excessive use of force because officers lacked professional training in how to manage large protests. The reports stated police intervention during protests escalated tensions, rather than reduced them since they emphasized disorder control which escalates tense situations and leads to the use of force (Barker et al., 2021). Scholars report that nationally, police respond to protests as if they are riots as shown in the use of riot gear they wear when confronting civil protests. PV can be reduced when officers are trained to manage large crowds of protesters and form working relationships with community leaders who can put them in contact with members and protest organizers who can sensitize police departments to the concerns and needs of protesters as well as foster better police–community relations. Others suggest that police leaders should develop better ways to supervise crowd control and only use militarized responses as the last resort (Barker et al., 2021).

Public health experts argue health departments can play a critical role in reducing PV by partnering with communities to build mutual trust. Collaboratively, they can create solutions and interventions that address PV. Health departments must understand American policing and acknowledge and recognize that police often engage in violence in minority communities. Together with the community, health departments can address PV by conducting public health research that accurately frames racism, power imbalances, and structural inequities that influence PV. Experts contend that health departments must also have a clear understanding of social determinants of health. After building relationships with communities, health departments can use their authority, voice, and position to present the realities about how police use of force negatively affects the health of Black and Latinx community residents. Research reports that health departments are in the unique position to inquire and advocate for better data and reporting procedures on PV. As such, health departments can advocate for policies, practices, and budgets that could prioritize reducing the role of police and using their budgets to invest in social determinants of health (Barna, 2020). The *American Public Health Association* (APHA) presented a viable public health strategy to address PV. It recommends diverting funds from some areas of law enforcement by shifting monies into community-based programs designed to invest in social determinants of health such as employment initiatives and affordable housing. This strategy is designed to alleviate stressors that are placed on police officers such as having to serve the community as untrained social workers, counselors, and mental health professionals. APHA's strategy enlists the help of trained social workers, counselors, and mental health professionals by expanding the shareholders who will be responsible for keeping the community safe.

Summary

PV is a serious criminal justice as well as public health problem that has received national and international attention due in part to visual images shown on television and news reports of police violently responding to protesters in the aftermath of untimely deaths of young minority males. Literature shows that while anyone can be a victim of PV, those who are disproportionately affected are Black protesters, Black males, women of color, the *LGBTQ+* community, members of the media (e.g., reporters, camera crews), and medics. PV is a complex issue with equally complex root causes, but chief among them is its historical link to systemic racism given the institution of policing grew from slave patrols in early America. Experts argue that there are social determinants that increase the likelihood that PV will occur. They include factors such as the role that inequity plays in PV. Others include individual, relationship, community, and societal factors. Because PV is widespread, justice experts contend that it is a justice issue with serious ramifications. Some experts argue that PV increases the crime rate in certain communities. In fact, those communities that are overpoliced and experience violence at the hands of law enforcement officers report more physical and mental health problems and their residents experience a diminished quality of life compared to those that do not. International and comparative statistics report that PV is a global problem with similar risk factors, mainly income and health inequities. Experts report that social workers can assist both the victims and perpetrators of PV to help alleviate the problem. Negative health consequences of PV cannot be treated by police agencies, but rather, they require assistance from experts trained in medicine and health care to provide victims with the care needed in the aftermath of stress, obesity, and chronic heart disease that are linked to violent encounters with police. Because it is a justice and public health issue, solutions must come from both areas. Some suggest that the justice system provides inadequate training to recognize and manage protests without viewing them as an occasion to resort to militarized riot control and violence. They must also be trained not to engage in implicit race bias when encountering non-White citizens. However, those advocating public health approaches prefer strategies that are proactive and empower community residents, especially those directly impacted by PV to be stakeholders in proactive measures that are funded with monies that are shifted from police budgets. The idea is to allow communities to perform calls for low-level services that it can do better than police while ensuring community safety.

Discussion Questions

1 Why is police violence both a criminal justice and public health issue?
2 What are some determinant factors that can explain police violence?
3 List and explain three criminal justice responses to police violence.
4 How has systemic racism in the U.S. impacted police use of violence and lethal force?
5 Why should public health approaches be used to prevent police violence?
6 Why is a national clearinghouse on police misconduct needed in the U.S.?

References

Abrams, Z. (2020). What works to reduce police brutality. *American Psychological Association*, 51(7). www.apa.org/monitor/2020/10/cover-police-b rutality

Abramson, D., & Denenberg, A. (2024). What is the main cause of police brutality? File:///C:/Users/Owners/Downloads/What Is the Main Cause of Police Brutality_.htm

ACLED. (2020, September 3). Demonstrations and political violence in America: New data for summer 2020. https://acleddata.com/2020/09/03/demonstrations-political-violence-in-america-new-data-for-summer-2020/

Adler, F., Mueller, G.O.W., & Laufer, W.S. (1994). *Criminal justice*. McGraw-Hill, Inc.

Alang S. (2020). Police brutality and the institutional patterning of stressors. *American Journal of Public Health*, 110(11), 1597–1598. https://doi.org/10.2105/AJPH.2020.305937

Alang, S., Haile, R., Hardeman, R., & Judson, J. (2023). Mechanisms connecting police brutality, intersectionality, and women's health over the life course. *American Journal of Public Health*, 113(S1), 529–536. https://doi.org/10.2105/AJPH.2022.307064

Alang, S., McAlphine, D., McCreed, E., & Hardman, R. (2017). Police brutality and black health: Setting the agenda for public health scholars. *American Journal of Public Health*, 107, 622–665.

Alang, S., Pando, C., McClain, M., Batts, H., Letcher, A., Hager, J., Person, T., Shaw, A., Blake, K., & Matthews-Alvarado, K. (2021). Survey of the health of urban residents: A community-driven assessment of conditions salient to the health of historically excluded populations in the USA. *Journal of Racial and Ethnic Health Disparities*, 8(4), 953–972. https://doi.org/10.1007/s40615-020-00852-1

American Civil Liberties Union. (2024). New report finds harassment & mistreatment fuels mistrust among LGBTQ people toward police. www.aclu.org/press-releases/new-report-finds-harassment-mistreatment-fuels-mistrust-among-lgbtq-people-towards-police

American Psychiatric Association. (2018). APA Official Actions: Position statement on police brutality and black men and boys. www.psychiatry.org/getattachment/6494c34d-26ea-47f1-956e-c45a99464247/Position-Police-Brutality-and-Black-Males.pdf

American Public Health Association. (2018). Addressing law enforcement violence as a public health issue. https://nccdh.ca/resources/entry/addressing-law-enforcement-violence-as-a-public-health-issue

Amnesty International. (2005). *Stonewalled: Police abuse and misconduct against lesbian, gay, bisexual and transgender people in the U.S.* www.amnesty.org/en/documents/AMR51/122/2005/en/

Amnesty International. (2020). USA: Law enforcement violated Black Lives Matter protestors' human rights, document acts of police violence and excessive force. www.amnesty.org/en/latest/press-release/2020/08/usa-law-enforcement-violated-black-lives-matte-protestors-human-rights/

Amnesty International. (2024). Police violence. www.amnesty.org/en/what-we-do/police-bruality/

Anderson, J.F., Lee, T.P., Langsam, A.H., & Reinsmith-Jones, K. (2022). Police violence against black protesters: A public health issue. *International Journal of Social Science Studies*, 10(2), 26–34.

Ba, B.A., Knox, D., Mummolo, J., & Rivera, R. (2021). The role of officer race and gender in police-civilian interactions in Chicago. *Science*, 371(6530), 696–702.

Baćak, V., & Nowotny, K.M. (2020). Race and the association between police stops and depression among young adults: A research note. *Race and Justice*, 10(3), 363–375. https://doi.org/10.1177/2153368718799813

Bailey, J.A., Jacoby, S.F., Hall, E.C., Khatri, U., Whitehorn, G., & Kaufman, E.J. (2022). Compounding trauma: The intersections of racism, law enforcement, and injury. *Current Trauma Report*, 8, 105–112.

Bailey, Z.D., Feldman, J.M., & Bassett, M.T. (2021). How structural racism works-racist policies as a root cause of US racial health inequities. *The New England Journal of Medicine*, 384(8), 768–773.

Barker, K., Baker, M., & Watkins, A. (2021). In city after city, police mishandled Black Lives Matter protests. www.nytimes.com/2021/03/20/us/protests-policing-george-floyd.html

Barna, M. (2020). Ending police violence requires public health-based approach: APHA statement guiding work, 32 outreach. *The Nation's Health*, 50(6), 1–14.

Beirne, P., & Messerschmidt, J. (1991). *Criminology*. Harcourt Brace Jovanovich College Publishers.

Beyer, D., & Kaine, T. (2021). *CNBC – Police misconduct can be deadly: It also costs taxpayers millions every year*. Washington. https://beyer.House.gov

Biondi, L. (2000). Police brutality: Causes. www.fdle.state.fl.us/FCJEI/Programs/SLP/Documents/Full-Text/Biondi,-Louis-paper.aspx

Bittner, E. (1970). *The functions of the police inn modern society.* U.S. Government Printing Office.

Blain, K.N. (2020). A short history of black women and police violence. The Conversation. File:///C:/Users/Owners/DownloadsA short history of black women and police violence.html

Blauner, R. (1972). *Racial oppression in America.* Harper and Row.

Bor, J., Venkataramani, A.S., Williams, D.R, & Tsai, A.C. (2018). Police killings and their spillover effects on the mental health of black Americans: A population-based, quasi-experimental study. *Lancet*, 392, 302–310.

Bowleg, L., Boone, C.A., Holt, S.L., del Río-González, A.M., & Mbaba, M. (2022). Beyond "heartfelt condolences": A critical take on mainstream psychology's responses to anti-black police brutality. *The American Psychologist*, 77(3), 362–380. https://doi.org/10.1037/amp0000899

Braunstein, M.D. (2017). The five stages of LGBTQ discrimination and its effects of mass incarceration. *University of Miami Race & Social Justice Law Review*, 7, 217–248.

Breen, K. (2023). Settlements for police misconduct lawsuits cost taxpayers from coast to coast. www.cbsnews.com/news/police-misconduct-lawsuits-settlements-taxpayers/

Bryant-Davis, T., & Ocampo, C. (2005). The trauma of racism: Implications for counseling, research, and education. *The Counseling Psychologist*, 33, 574–578.

Buchanan, L., Bui, Q., & Patel, J.K. (2021). *Black Lives Matters may be the largest movement in U.S. history.* The New York Times. www.nytimes.com/interactive/2020/07/03/us/george-floyd-protests-crowd-size.html

Buehler, J.W. (2017). Racial/ethnic disparities in the use of lethal force by US police, 2010-2014. *American Journal of Public Health*, 107(2), 295–297.

Carmichael, J.T., & Kent, S.L. (2014). The persistent significance of race an economic inequality on the size of municipal police forces in the United States, 1980-2010. *Social Problems*, 61(2), 259–282.

CDC (n.d.). Cost of injury module help. WISQARS: Web-based Injury Statistics Query and Reporting System. www.cdc.gov/injury/wisqars/cost/index.html.

Champion, D.J. (2005). *The American dictionary of criminal justice* (3rd ed.). Roxbury Publishing Company.

Chaudhary, M.J., & Richardson, J. (2022). Violence against Black Lives Matter protestors: A review. *Current Trauma Reports*, 8, 96–104.

Cheatham, A., & Maizland, L. (2022). How police compare in different democracies. *Council on Foreign Relations*. www.cfr.org/backgrounder/how-police-compare-different-democracies

Chicago Citizen. (1997). *Police culture causes police brutality.* Greenhaven Press.

Cooper, H., Moore, L., Gruskin, S., & Krieger, N. (2005). Characterizing perceived police violence: Implications for public health. *American Journal of Public Health*, 94(7), 1109–1118.

Crenshaw, K.W., & Ritchie, A.J. (2014). Say her name: Resisting police brutality against black women (2014). *African American Policy Forum*. www.researchgate.net/publication/305346077_SayHerName

Cuncic, A. (2023). Understanding what police brutality is and why it occurs. *Race and Social Justice*. www.verywellmind.com/the-psychology-behind-police-bruality-5077410

Dahlberg, L., & Mercy, J. (2009). History of violence as a public health issue. *AMA Journal of Ethics*, 11(2), 167–172.

Davenport, C., Soule, S., & Armstrong, D. (2011). Protesting while black? The differential policing of American activism,1960 to 1990. *American Sociological Review*, 76(1), 152–178.

Davis, E., & Whyde, A. (2018). *Contacts between police and the public, 2015.* U.S. Department of Justice, Office of Justice Programs, Bureau of Justice Statistics.

DeAngelis, R.T. (2024). Systemic racism in police killings: New evidence from the mapping police violence database, 2013-2021. *Race and Justice*, 14(3), 413–422.

DeGue, S., Fowler, K.A., & Calkins, C. (2016). Deaths due to use of lethal force by law enforcement. *American Journal of Preventive Medicine*, 51(5 Suppl 3), S173–S187.

Deivanayagam, T.A., Lasoye, S., Smith, J., & Selvarajah, S. (2021). Policing is a threat to public health and human rights. *BMJ Global Health*, 6, e004582. https://doi.org/10.1136/bmjgh-2020-004582

del Carmen, R.V. (1991). *Civil liabilities in American policing: A text for law enforcement personnel.* Brady a Prentice Hall Division.

del Carmen, R.V., & Walker, J.T. (2004). *Briefs of leading cases in law enforcement* (5th ed.). Anderson Publishing.

Del Toro, J., Lloyd, T., Buchanan, K.S., Robins, S.J., Bencharit, L.Z., Smiedt, M.G., Reddy, K.S., Pouget, E.R., Kerrison, E.M., & Goff, P.A. (2019). The criminogenic and psychological effects of police stops on adolescent black and latino boys. *Proceedings of the National Academy of Sciences – PNAS*, 116(17), 8261–8268. https://doi.org/10.1073/pnas.1808976116

Dennison, C.R., & Finkeldey, J.G. (2021). Self-reported experiences and consequences of unfair treatment by police. *Criminology (Beverly Hills)*, 59(2), 254–290. https://doi.org/10.1111/1745-9125.12269

Desmond, M., Papachristos, A., & Kirk, D.S. (2016). Police violence and citizen crime reporting in the black community. *American Sociological Review*, 81(5), 857–876.

Desmond-Harris, J. (2015). Are black communities overpoliced or under policed? Both. *The Trace*. www.vox.com/2015/4/148411733/black-community-policing-crime

Devine, P.G. (1989). Stereotypes and prejudices: Their automatic and controlled components. *Journal of Personality and Social Psychology*, 56(1), 5–18.

DeVylder, J.E., Anglin, D.M., Bowleg, L., Fedina, L., & Link, B.G. (2022). Police violence and public health. *Annual Review of Clinical Psychology*, 9(18), 527–552.

DeVylder, J., Fedina, L., & Link, B. (2020). Impact of police violence on mental health: A theoretical framework. *American Journal of Public Health*, 110, 1704–1710.

DeVylder, J.E., Cogburn, C., Oh, H.Y., Anglin, D., Smith, M.E., Sharpe, T., Jun, H., Schiffman, J., Lukens, E., & Link, B. (2017a). Psychotic experiences in the context of police victimization: Data from the survey of police-public encounters. *Schizophrenia Bulletin*, 43(5), 993–1001. https://doi.org/10.1093/schbul/sbx038

DeVylder, J.E., Frey, J.J., Cogburn, C.D., Wilcox, H.C., Sharpe, T.L., Oh, H.Y., Nam, B., & Link, B.G. (2017b). Elevated prevalence of suicide attempts among victims of police violence in the USA. *Journal of Urban Health*, 94(5), 629–636. https://doi.org/10.1007/s11524-017-0160-3

DeVylder, J.E., Jun, H.J., Fedina, L., et al. (2018). Association of exposure to police violence with prevalence of mental health symptoms among urban residents in the United states. *JAMA Network Open*, 1(7), e184945. https://doi.org/10.1001/jamanetworkopen.2018.4945

Dreyer, B.P., Trent, M., Anderson, A.T., Askew, G.L., Boyd, R., & Coker, T.R., & Montoya-Williams, D. (2020). The death of George Floyd: Bending the arc of history towards justice for generations of children. *Pediatrics*, 146(1), 1–13.

Dunn, L. (2020). Who is most at risk for police violence? www.keranews.org

Duru, O.K., Harawa, N.T., Kermah, D., & Norris, K.C. (2012). Allostatic load burden and racial disparities in mortality. *Journal of the National Medical Association*, 104(1–2), 89–95.

Edwards, B. (2015). At least 5 black women have died in police custody in July, WTF? *The Roots*. www.theroot.com/at-least-5-black-women-have-died-in-police-custody-in-j-1790860695

Edwards, F., Lee, H., & Esposito, M. (2019). Risk of being killed by police use-of-force in the U.S. by age, race/ethnicity, and sex. *Proceedings of the National Academy of Sciences*, 116(34), 16793–16798.

Fedina, L., Backes, B.L., Hyun, J.J., Shah, R., Boyoung, N., Link, B.G., & DeVylder, J.E. (2018). Police violence among women in four U.S. cities. *Preventive Medicine*, 106, 150–156.

Feldman, J. (2020). Class and racial inequalities in police killings. *People's Policy Project*. file:///C:/Users/Downloads/Class and Racial Inequalities in Police Killings-People's Policy Project.html

Feldman, J., Chen, J.T., Waterman, P.D., & Krieger, N. (2016). Temporal trends and racial/ethnic inequalities for legal intervention injuries related to emergence departments: US men and women ages 15-34, 2001-2014. *Journal of Urban Health*, 93(5), 797–807.

Fileborn, B. (2019). Policing youth and queerness: The experiences and perceptions of young LGBTQ+ people from regional Victoria. *Current Issues in Criminal Justice*, 31(3), 433–451.

Finkelhor, D., Turner, H., Shattuck, A., Hamby, S., & Kracke, K. (2015). *Children's exposure to gun violence, crime, and abuse: An update.* U.S. Department of Justice, Office of Juvenile Justice and Delinquency Prevention. https://bit.ly/2tK7ah6

Fix, R.L. (2021). Mental and physical health consequences of police brutality toward Black community members in the United States. *Public Health in Practice*, 2, 100188.

Fyfe, J.J. (1991). Thinking about crime: Gains on the problem of police brutality. *The Public Prospective*, 8–9.

Gaines, L.K., & Kappeler, V.E. (2008). *Policing in America* (6th ed.). Anderson Publishing.

GBD 2019 Police Violence U.S. Subnational Collaborators. (2021). Fatal police violence by race and state in the USA, 1980-2019: A network meta-regression. *The Lancet*, 398(10307), 1239–1255. https://doi.org/10.1016/S0140-6736(21)01609-3

Gee, G.C., & Hicken, M.T. (2021). Commentary-structural racism: The rules and relations of inequity. *Ethnicity & Disease*, 31(Supplement 1), 293–300.

Geller, A., Fagan, J., Tyler, T., & Link, B.G. (2014). Aggressive policing and the mental health of young urban men. *American Journal of Public Health (1971)*, 104(12), 2321–2327. https://doi.org/10.2105/AJPH.2014.302046

Geronimus, A.T., Hicken, M., Keene, D., & Bound, J. (2006). "Weathering" and age patterns of allostatic load scores among Blacks and Whites in the United States. *American Journal of Public Health*, 96(5), 826–833. https://doi.org/10.2105/ajph.2004.060749

Gilmore, J. (2010). Policing protest: An authoritarian consensus. *Criminal Justice Matters*, 82(1), 21–23.

Glaser, J., & Knowles, E.D. (2008). Implicit motivation to control prejudice. *Journal of Experimental Social Psychology*, 44(1), 164–172.

Goff, P.A., Eberhardt, J.L., Williams, M.J., & Jackson, M.C. (2008). Not yet human: Implicit knowledge, historical dehumanization, and contemporary consequences. *Journal of Personality and Social Psychology*, 94(2), 292–306.

Goff, P.A., & Rau, H. (2020). Predicting bad policing: Theorizing burdensome and racially disparate policing through the lenses of social psychology and routine activities. *The Annals of the American Academy*, 687, 67–88.

Gold, A. (2015). Why has the murder rate in some US cities suddenly spiked? *BBC News*.

Gottbrath, L.W., & Strickland, P. (2020). Blinded, arrested: Police attack journalists covering U.S. protests. *Al Jazeera*. www.aljazeera.com/features/2020/6/16/blinded-arrested-police-attack-journalists-covering-us-protests

Greenwald, A.G., Banaji, M.R., & Nosek, B.A. (2015). Statistically small effects on the Implicit Association Test can have societally large effects. *Journal of Personality and Social Psychology*, 108(4), 553–561.

Grills, C.N., Aird, E.G., & Rowe, D. (2016). Breathe, baby, breathe: Clearing the way for the emotional emancipation of black people. *Cultural Studies, Critical Methodologies*, 16(3), 333–343. https://doi.org/10.1177/1532708616634839

Grimshaw, R. (2020). *Institutional racism in the police: how entrenched has it become?* Centre for Crime and Justice Studies. www.crimeandjustice.org.uk/resources/institutional-racism-police-how-entrenched-has-it-become

Gruber, A. (2021). Policing and "bluelining." *Houston Law Review*, 58(4), 867–936.

Harding, D.J. (2009). Collateral consequences of violence in disadvantaged neighborhoods. *Social Forces*, 88(2), 757–784.

Harris, L.K., & Cortes, Y.I. (2022). Police violence and black women's health. *The Journal for Nurse Practitioners*, 18(5), 589–590.

Hauss, B., & Nelson, T. (2020). *Police are attacking journalists at protests. We' re suing.* ACLU. https://aclu.org/news/free-speech/police-are-attacking-journalists-at-protests-were-suing

Hinton, E., & Cook, D. (2021). The mass criminalization of black Americans: A historical overview. *Annual Review of Criminology*, 4(1), 261–286.

H.R. 5484-99th Congress. (1986). Anti-Drug Abuse Act of 1986. www.congress.gov/bill/99th-congress/house-bill/5484

Human Rights Watch. (2009). Race, drugs, and law enforcement in the United States. www.hrw.org/news/2009/06/19/race-drugs-and-law-enforcement-united-states

International Association of Chiefs of Police. (2011). Addressing sexual offenses and misconduct by law enforcement officers: An executive guide. Alexandria, VA. www.theiacp.org/sites/default/files/all/a/AddressingSexualOffensesandMisconductbyLawEnforcementExecutiveGuide.pdf

Jackman, T., & Juvenal, J. (2015). Fairfax jail inmate in Taser death was shackled. *Wash Post.* www.washingtonpost.com/local/crime/fairfax-jail-inmate-who-died-was-fully-restrained-when-tasered-four-times/2015/04/11/ede0957c-decd-11e4-be40-566e265afe5_story.html

Jacob, D., & Britt, D. (1979). Inequality and police use of deadly force: An empirical assessment of a conflict hypothesis. *Social Problems,* 26(4), 403–412.

Jahn, J.L., & Schwartz, G.L. (2024). Who are the "police" in "police violence"? Fatal violence by U.S. law enforcement agencies across levels of government. *Injury Epidemiology,* 11, 13. https://doi.org/10.1186/s40621-024-00496-3

Johnson, T., & Johnson, N. (2023). If we want to reduce deaths at hands of police, we need to reduce traffic stops. *Time.* https://time.com/6252760/reducing-fatal-police-encounters-traffic-stops/

Kahn, K.B., Goff, P.A., Lee, J.K., & Motamed, D. (2021). Protecting witnesses: White phenotypic racial stereo typicality reduces police use of force. *Social Psychological and Personality Science,* 7(5), 403–411.

Kajeepeta, S., & Johnson, D.K.N. (2023). *Police and protests: The inequity of police responses to racial justice demonstrations.* Thurgood Marshall Institute.

Kappeler, V. (2014). A brief history or slavery and the origins of American policing. https://ekuonline.eku.edu

Kraska, P.B., & Kappeler, V.E. (1995). To serve and pursue: Exploring police sexual violence against women. *Justice Quarterly,* 85, 85–112.

Kratcoski, P., & Cebulak, W. (2000). Policing in democratic societies: An historical overview. In D. Das & O. Maremin (Eds.), *Challenges of policing democracies: A world perspective* (pp. 23–41). Gordon and Breach Publishers.

Krug, E.G., Dahlberg, L.L., Mercy, J.A., Zwi, A.B., & Lozano, R. (2002). *World report on violence and health.* World Health Organization.

Lambda Legal. (2014). Police: Protected and served? New York, NY. www.lambdalegal.org/protected-and-served

Law Enforcement Epidemiology Project. (2024). *Facts and Figures on Injuries caused by law enforcement.* School of Public Health, University of Illinois Chicago.

Lee, T.P., Anderson, J.F., Langsam, A.H., & Hatter, S. (2022). Disparate law enforcement practices against women of color and gender variant women: The More things change, the more they stay the same. *Journal of Law and Criminal Justice,* 10(1), 1–13.

Legewie, J., & Fagan, J. (2016). Group threat, police officer diversity, and the deadly use of police force. *Columbia Public Law Research Paper* No. 14-512, 75(4), 1–4. https://doi.org/10.1136/jech-2020-215097

Lett, E., Asabor, E.N., Cobin, T., & Boatiagght, D. (2020). Racial inequity in fatal U.S. police shootings, 2015-2020. *Journal of Epidemiology and Community* Health. . https://doi.org/10.1136/jech-2020-215097

Lopez, G. (2016, January 20). *Why violent crime increased in the first 6 months of 2015?* Vox. www.vox.com/2015/9/8/9273139/murder-rates-rising-sharply

Ludwig, M. (2023). *CDC report recognizes police-perpetrated killings as major cause of violent death.* Truthout. https://truthout.org/articles/cdc-report-recognizes-police-perpetrated-killing-as-majr-cause-of-violent-death/

Lyle, P., & Esmail, A.M. (2016). Sworn to protect: Police brutality-a dilemma for America's police. *Race, Gender & Class,* 23(3–4), 155–185.

Mallory, C., Hasenbush, A., & Sears, B. (2015). *Discrimination and harassment by law enforcement officers in the LGBT community.* The William Institute. www.escholarship.org/uc/item/5663q0w1

McDonough, P., Duncan, G., Williams, D., & House, J. (1997). Income dynamics and adult morality in the United States, 1972 through 1989. *American Journal of Public Health*, 87(9), 1476–1483.

McEwen, B.S. (2006). Protective and damaging effects of stress mediators: Central role of the brain. *Dialogues in Clinical Neuroscience*, 8(4), 367–381. https://doi.org/10.31887/DCNS.2006.8.4/bmcewen

McFarland, M.J., Geller, A., & McFarland, C. (2019). Police contact and health among urban adolescents: The role of perceived injustice. *Social Science & Medicine (1982)*, 238, 112487–112487. https://doi.org/10.1016/j.socscimed.2019.112487

Miller, T.R., Lawrence, B.A., Carlson, N.N., Hendrie, D., Randall, S., Rockettt, I.R., & Spicer, R.S. (2017). Perils in police action: A cautionary tale from US datasets. *Injury Prevention*, 23(1), 27–32.

Nadal, K.L., Skolnik, A., & Wong, Y. (2012). Interpersonal and systematic microaggressions towards transgender people: Implications for counseling. *Journal of LGBT Issues in Counseling*, 6(1), 55–82.

National Coalition of Anti-Violence Programs (NCAVP). (2012). Lesbian, gay, bisexual, transgender, queer and HIV-affected hate violence in 2012. http://avp.org/wpcotent/uploads/2017/04/ncavp_2012_hvreport_final.pdf

Nembhard, S., Perez, R., Jagannath, J., & Robin, L. (2022). *Understanding the harms of police violence can help build community safety*. Urban Institute. www.urban.org/urban-wire/understsanding-harms-police-violence-can-help-build-community-safety

Nix, J., & Shjarback, J. (2021). Factors associated with police shootings mortality: A focus on race and a plea for more comprehensive data. *PLoS One*. https://dio.org/10.1371/jounral.pone.0259024

Noray, K. (2024). Police brutality, law enforcement, and crime: Evidence from Chicago. *Journal of Urban Economics*, 141. https://doi.org/10.1016/j.jue.2023.103630

Owens, E., Weisburd, D., Amendola, K.L., & Alpert, G.P. (2018). Can you build a better cop? Experimental evidence on supervision, training, and policing in the community. *Criminology & Public Policy*, 17, 41–87.

Park, E. (1970). From constabulary to police society. *Catalyst*, 5, 76–97.

Parker, A. (2018). Interagency collaboration models for people with mental health in contact with the police: A systematic scoping review. *BMJ Open*, 8e, 019312.

Payne, B.K., Oliver, W.M., & Marion, N.E. (2016). *Introduction to criminal justice: A balanced approach*. Sage Publications.

Peak, K.J., & Everett, P.M. (2017). *Introduction to criminal justice: practices and process* (2nd ed.). Sage.

Phelan, J.C., & Link, B.G. (2015). Is racism a fundamental cause of inequalities in health? *Annual Review of Sociology*, 41(1), 311–330.

Platt, L.F., & Lenzen, A.L. (2013). Sexual orientation microaggressions and the experiences of sexual minorities. *Journal of Homosexuality*, 607(7), 1011–1034.

Quinn, K. (2015). *Woman accuses officer of going too far during stop*. ABC13.com. http://abc13.com/news/woman-accuses-officer-of-going-too-far-during-traffic-stop/905180/

Rahr, S. (2023). The myth propelling America's violent police culture. *The Atlantic*. www.theatlantic.com

Raphling, J., & Austin-Hillery, N. (2021). Poverty, pandemic, police violence: Ongoing crisis demand he US address pervasive racism. *Human Rights Watch*. www.hrw/world-report/2021/essay/poverty-pandemic-police-violence-in-us

Reddington, F.P., & Bonham, G. (2019). *Flawed criminal justice policies: At the intersection of the media, public fear and legislative responses* (2nd. ed.). Carolina Academic Press.

Ridgeway, G. (2015). Risk factors associated with police shootings: A matched case-control study. www.crim.sas.upenn.edu/sites/default/files/2015-10.0_Ridgeway_PoliceShooting%281%29%281%29.pdf

Ritchie, A.J. (2016). #Sayhername: Racial profiling and police violence against black women. *The Harbinger*, 41, 11–23.

Ritchie, A.J. (2017). *Invisible no more: Police violence against black women and women or color*. Beacon Press.

Rodriquez, E.J., Kim, E.N., Summer, A.E., Napoles, A.M., & Perez-Stable (2019). Allostatic load: Importance, markers, and score determination in minority and disparity populations. *Journal of Urban Health: Bulletin of the New York Academy of Medicine*, 96(Suppl 1), 3–11. https://doi.org/10.1007/s11524-019-00345-5

Rothstein, R. (2017). *The color of law: A forgotten history of how our government segregated America*. Liveright Publishing.

Sandoiu, A. (2020, June 22). Police violence: Physical and mental health impacts on Black Americans. www.medicalnewstoday.com/articles/police-violence-physical-andmental-health-impacts-on-black-americans

Schindler, M., & Kittredge, J. (2020). *A crisis within a crisis: Police killings of black emerging adults*. The Brookings Institute. www.brookins.edu/articles/a-crisis-within-a-crisis-police-killings-of-black-emerging-adults/; www.communitycommons.org/entites/6e8ae5d5-0fc6-4ed3-87c8-df9ee5967695

Schwartz, S.A. (2020). Police brutality and racism in America. *Explore*, 16, 280–282.

Serchen, J., Doherty, R., Atiq, O., & Hilden, D. (2020). Racism and health in the United States: A policy statement from the American College of Physicians. *Annals of Internal Medicine*, 173, 556–557.

Serpe, C.R., & Nadal, K.L. (2017). Perceptions of police: Experiences in the trans* community. *Journal of Gay & Lesbian Social Services: The Quarterly Journal of Community & Clinical Practice*, 29(3), 280–299. https://doi.org/10.1080/10538720.2017.1319777

Sewell, A.A. (2017). The illness associations of police violence: Differential relationships by ethnoracial composition. *Sociological Forum*, 32(S1), 975–997.

Sewell, A.A., & Jefferson, K.A. (2016). Collateral damage: The health effects of invasive police encounters in New York City. *Journal of Urban Health*, 93(1), 42–67.

Skolnick, J.H., & Fyfe, J.J. (1993). *Above the law: Police and the excessive use of force*. The Free Press.

Smith, M., & Rodriguez, R. (2020). Police brutality is not just a criminal justice issue, but a public health issue too. National Community Reinvestment Coalition. https://ncrc.org

Spolum, M.M., Lopez, W.D., Watkins, D.C., & Fleming, P.J. (2023). Police violence: Reducing the harms of policing through public health-informed alternative response programs. *American Journal of Public Health* (1971), 113(S1), S37–S42. https://doi.org/10.2105/AJPH.2022.307107

Staggers-Hakim, R. (2016). The nation's unprotected children and the ghost of mike brown, or the impact of national police killings on the health and social development of African American boys. *Journal of Human Behavior in the Social Environment*, 26(3–4), 390–399. https://doi.org/10.1080/10911359.2015.1132864

Statista. (2024). People shot to death by U.S. police 2017-2024, by race. File:///C:Users/Owner/Downloads/People shot to death by U.S. police, by race 2024_Statista.html

Stinson, P.M., Liederbach, J., Brewer, S.L., & Mathna, B.E. (2014). Police sexual misconduct: A national scale study of arrested officers. Lambda Legal, Protected and served? Survey of LGBT/HIV contact with police, courts, prisons, and security. www.lamdalegal.org/proteectedandserved

Stoddard, G., Fitzpatrick, D.J., & Ludwig, J. (2024). *Predicting police misconduct. Research Brief*, Becker Friedman Institute for Economics. The University of Chicago.

Strom, K.J., & Wire, S. (2024). *The impact of police violence on communities: Unpacking how fatal use of force influences residents calls to 911 and police activity. RTI Press Publication No. RR-0050-2401*. RTI Press. https://doi.org/10.3768/rtipress.2024.rr.0050.2401

Sullum, J. (2015). The war on drugs encourages roadside sexual assaults by cops. www.reason.com/2015/05/08/the-war-on-drugs-encourages-roadside-sex/

Testa, A., Jackson, D.B., & Semenza, D. (2021). Unfair police treatment and sleep problems among a national sample of adults. *Journal of Sleep Research*, 30(6), e13353. https://doi.org/10.1111/jsr.13353

The Guardian. (2017). *Young black men again faced highest rate of US police killings in 2017.* The Counted Project.

The Guardian. (2023). One in 20 U.S. homicides are committed by police-and the numbers aren't falling. www.theguardian.com>us-news

The Guardian. (2024). 2023 saw record killings by US police: Who is most affected? file:///C:/Suers/Owner/Downloads/2023 saw record killings by US police. Who is most affected_ _US policing_ The Guardian.html

The Lancet. (2021a). Fetal police violence in the USA: A public health issue. www.thelancet.com; https://doi.org/10.1016/S0140-6736(21)02145-0

The Lancet. (2021b). Fatal police violence by race and state in the USA, 1980-2019: A network meta-regression. 398(10307), 1239–1255.

Thomas-DeVeaux, A., Bronner, L., & Sharma, D. (2021). Cities spend millions on police misconduct every year. Here's why it's so difficult to hold departments accountable. https://fivethirtyeight.com/features/police-misconduct-costs-cities-millions-every-year-but-thats-where-the-accountability-ends/

Tucker, J.M., Brewster, M.P., Grugan, S.T., Miller, L.M., & Mapp-Matthews, S.M. (2019). Criminal justice students' attitudes toward LGBTQ individuals and LGBTQ police officers. *Journal of Criminal Justice Education*, 30(2), 165–192.

Turabi, A.E., Menon, A., Perez, L., & Tolub, G. (2022). Health equity: A framework for the epidemiology of care. *Life Sciences* www.mckinsey.com/industries/life-sceinces/our-insights/health-equity-a-framework-for-the-epidemolgy-of-care

United Nations Human Rights. (2021). UN experts call for an end to police brutality worldwide. www.ohchr.org/en/press-releases/2021/08/un-expertd-call-end-police-brutality-worldwide

United Nations Human Rights. (2023). Systemic racism pervades US police and justice systems, UN mechanism on racial justice in law enforcement says in new report urging reform. www.ohchr.org/en/press-release/2023/09/systemic-racism-pervades-us-police-and-justice-systems-un-mechanism-racial

Wallerstein, N.B., Irene, H., & Syme, L. (2011). Integration of social epidemiology and community-engaged interventions to improve health equity. *American Journal of Public Health*, 101(5), 822–830.

Williams, D.R. (2018). Stress and the mental health of populations of color: Advancing our understanding of race-related stressors. *Journal of Health and Social Behavior*, 59(4), 466–485.

Williams, M.T., Faber, S.C., Nepton, A., & Ching, T. (2022). Racial justice allyship requires civil courage: behavioral prescription for moral growth and change. *American Psychologist*. Advance online. https://doi.org/10.1037/amp0000940

Wilson, A., & Wilson, M. (2020). *Reimagining policing: Strategies for community reinvestment pre-arrest diversion; and innovative approaches to 911 emergency responses.* National Association of Social Workers (NASW). Washington, D.C.

Wolff, K.B., & Cokely, C.L. (2007). 'To protect and to serve?': An exploration of police conduct in relation to the gay, lesbian, bisexual, and transgender community. *Sexuality & Culture*, 11(2), 1–23.

Woods, J. (2019). Policing, danger narratives, and routine traffic stops. *Michigan Law Review*, 117(4), 635–712.

Woods, J.B., Galvan, F.H., Bazargan, M., Herman, J.L., & Chen, Y. (2013). Latina transgender women's interaction with law enforcement in Los Angeles County. *Policing: A Journal of Policy and Practice*, 7(4), 379–391.

World Population Review. (2024). Police killings by country 2024. https://worlpopulationreview.com/country-rankings/police-killings-by-country

Worrall, J.L. (2001). *Civil lawsuits, citizen complaints, and policing innovations.* LFB Scholarly Publishing.

Zare, H., Meyerson, N., Delgado, P., Spencer, M., Gaskin, D.J., & Thorpe, R.J. (2022). Association between neighborhood and racial composition of victims of fatal police shootings and police violence: An integrated review (2000-2020). *Social Sciences*, 11(4), 153. https://doi.org/10.3390./socsci11040153

Zennie, M., Greig, A. (2013). Pictured: The two women suing police after they were subjected to humiliating roadside cavity searches as they wore only their bikinis. *Daily Mail*. www.dailymail.co.uk/news/article-2356618/Pictured-The-women-suing-police-unconstitutional-roadside-cavity-search.html#ixzz42HIXOoak

Cases Cited

City of Canton v. Harris, 489 U.S. 378 (1989)

11

TEENAGE BULLYING AND PUBLIC HEALTH

Introduction

Phoebe Prince was 15 years old when she became another senseless tragedy in the long history of bully-suicide (bullycide) victims. Her problems began when she emigrated from her native country of Ireland about a year before her death and then had the unfortunate luck of catching the eye of a popular boy, whom she briefly dated. This apparently drew the ire and resentment of some of the other girls, who started bullying her relentlessly thereafter. Being an immigrant to the U.S., she no doubt stood out from her peers. She had also been bullied in Ireland, and her mother (a teacher) had taken the initiative to inform the school ahead of time, letting them know about this bullying history and that she was very vulnerable to its effects. She went so far as to ask them to keep an eye out for this, since Phoebe would likely internalize its effects rather than talk about it. Much was made of the cyberbullying Phoebe experienced, but Phoebe's mother says that cyberbullying was only a small fraction of what Phoebe went through, and most of that occurred after her death. What she did experience was relentless bullying at and on her way to and from school. There was some physical bullying, but most of it was emotional: Calling Phoebe names, spreading rumors about her, humiliating her, using peer exclusion, and writing swear words or racial slurs next to her name in the library. One of the bullies, shortly before her death, was overheard saying, "Why doesn't someone just convince her (Phoebe) to kill herself?" In one of her final text messages, Phoebe ominously wrote about the hurt she felt over the fact that her former boyfriend seemed to be overtly supporting what was taking place: "I think Shawn condoning this is one of the final nails in the coffin...it would be much easier if he or one of them would just hand me a noose." In addition to talking with school staff during enrollment, Phoebe's mother complained twice to school staffers, but to no avail. On a Thursday, Phoebe was hounded by bullies in the library, the cafeteria, and the hallways. Walking home from school that day, she had a can of Red Bull thrown at her from the window of a passing car. Unable to take any more, she went home and hung herself with the scarf she'd been given for Christmas. Phoebe's little sister was the one who found her body hanging in a stairwell.

DOI: 10.4324/9781003373001-11

This case study was retrieved from Keep Your Child Safe.org (The Phoebe Prince Bullying Case—Keep Your Child Safe.org), 2025.

Teenage Bullying Defined

According to the Centers for Disease Control and Prevention (CDC) (2024b), *bullying* is defined as:

> Any unwanted aggressive behavior(s) by another youth or group of youths who are not siblings or current dating partners that involves an observed or perceived power imbalance and is repeated multiple times or is highly likely to be repeated. Bullying may inflict harm or distress on the targeted youth including physical, psychological, social, or educational harm.

Bullying can include physical acts (e.g., hitting, kicking, and tripping); verbal assaults such as name-calling and teasing; social intimidation through gossip and exclusion; property damage; and cyberbullying (CDC, 2024b). Closely related to bullying, and sometimes used synonymously, is *harassment*, although harassment does not always connote repeated victimization (Volk et al., 2014).

Nature and Extent of Teenage Bullying

During 2021–2022, the weekly occurrence of bullying of youth at school was reported by more middle schools (28%) compared with 15% of high/secondary schools and 10% of elementary schools (Burr et al., 2024). Weekly cyberbullying at school or off campus was reported by 37% of middle schools and 25% of high/secondary schools, but only 6% of elementary schools. More traditional public schools (14.5%) than charter schools (12%) reported student bullying. Approximately 16.2% of public schools reported that bullying of minority students was 50% or higher. Overall, 15.6% of public schools reported cyberbullying, 1.6% sexual harassment, and 2.1% harassment because of sexual orientation or gender identity.

According to the United States Government Accountability Office (U.S. GAO) (2021), alcohol, drugs, weapons, and gangs are factors in school bullying. For academic year 2018–2019, 5.2 million students reported being bullied. Of these, 33% reported being a bully-victim by the presence or availability of drugs and alcohol, 54% by the presence of guns brought by others, 42% in a school that has gang presence, and 49% in the presence of those who could get loaded guns. These factors speak to an elevated risk of danger associated with teen bullying.

Characteristics of students bullied at school reveal greater details about victims. It was estimated that during 2018–2019, approximately 1.3 million students were bullied because of race, disability, religion, gender, sexual orientation, gender expression, and ethnicity or national origin (U.S. GAO, 2021). Available data (CDC, 2024a; Thomsen et al., 2024) show that students identifying as two or more races have been bullied at a higher rate (21%–30.1%) compared with students identifying as White (21.6%–23%), Hispanic or Latino (16.4%), Black (14%–17.0%), Asian (9.0%–11%), American Indian/Alaskan Native (AI/AN) (17%), and Native Hawaiian/Pacific Islander (6%). Middle schoolers were victimized more beginning in 6th grade through 8th (29.9%, 26.3%, and 25.1%, respectively). The percentage of LGBTQIA students reporting being bullied/harassed at school varied from 29% (2024a) to 83.1% (Kosciw et al., 2022). Being bullied for having a disability was reported by 9.7% of student victims in 2022 (Thomsen et al., 2024). However, higher percentages were reported previously: 20% for 2014–2015, 29% for 2016–2017, and 33% for 2018–2019 (U.S. GAO, 2021). A non-school-based study (Green et al., 2024) found that teens with a disability were at higher risk for all forms of bullying *and perpetration* compared with peers without disabilities.

For academic years 2014–2019, up to 47% of school youth reported being bullied *with hate speech* because of race, 26% due to ethnicity, 18% owing to sexual orientation, and 16% as a result of gender (U.S. GAO, 2021). According to the U.S. GAO (2021), schools reporting hate crimes have almost doubled from 3,166 (AY 2015–2016) to 5,732 (AY 2017–2018) and were overwhelmingly motivated by race.

Those students from households with annual incomes ranging from $49,999 and less appear to be targeted at a higher rate than students from higher-earning homes. Geographics are also a factor. For example, students living in rural and town areas are bullied more frequently than those in suburban or city areas. Physical space determines where youth are targeted (Thomsen et al., 2024). Most bullying occurs in classrooms, hallways and stairwells, cafeterias, outside on school grounds, or by text and online. Physical bullying was reported less (4.9%) than name-calling and teasing (11.9%).

The reports and prevalence of bullying vary widely. Lai and Kao (2018) found that immigrants and racial and ethnic minorities are likely to report bullying at lower levels than White and female youth. Reasons proffered include problems with the word "bullying," as many students may not define qualifying behaviors as such. Similarly, it was found that African American boys and girls and Asian American boys underreported victimization compared to White peers (Sawyer et al., 2008). Underreporting was thought to be associated with the wording of questions. Also considered is that some teens were unwilling to identify with the behavior of bullying due to cultural differences and social norms affecting their perception of bullying (Lewis et al., 2015), as well as possible cultural pressures to appear unaffected by behavior identified as bullying (Sawyer et al., 2008).

Cyberbullying

Nearly 46% of U.S. teens ages 13–17 reported experiencing at least one of six cyberbullying behaviors (Vogels, 2022), such as name-calling (32%), false rumors being spread about them (22%), receiving uninvited sexually explicit images (17%), stalking behavior defined as "Constantly being asked where they are, what they're doing, or who they're with by someone other than a parent" (15%), physical threats (10%), and unconsented sharing of sexually explicit photos of them (7%). Additionally, 28% of teens reported being bullied in more than one tactic. Youth from homes with annual income less than $30,000 report twice the bullying than those from households making $75,000 or more yearly. Moreover, across all methods of cyberbullying, girls between the ages of 15 and 17 are targeted more than younger girls and males, both younger and same-aged. White youth are reported as being victimized more by name-calling and having false rumors spread about them; Black teens are targeted more by receiving uninvited explicit images, physical threats, and having explicit photos of them shared without consent; and Hispanic teens are more often bullied by constantly being asked about their whereabouts and actions by a non-parent (Vogels, 2022). Bullied teens believe that they are targeted because of their physical appearance, gender, race, sexual orientation, and/or political views. Black youth particularly feel victimized because of ethnicity. In fact, cyberbullying has been identified as one of seven factors associated with the rise in suicide behaviors among Black middle schoolers (CDC, 2020).

Types of Teenage Bullying

Against Blacks

Black students faced a 203% higher risk of being bullied compared to White students and are 439% more likely to be bullied based on their race (Gage et al., 2021). African American, as well as Asian, youth who do not hold to cultural stereotypes or who are average academically have been found to be bully-victims (Wang et al., 2016). However, racial minority students were also discovered to be bullied at a greater rate when they participated in school extra-curriculars, as this behavior may have been interpreted by the racial majority as "acting 'White'" (Peguero et al., 2015, p. 344). The odds of being bullied also increased for Black students who had White friends (Peguero & Jiang, 2016). However, the likelihood of Black students being bullied decreased as the number of Black students in a school increased (Gage et al., 2021).

Against Asians

Among those in school who are victimized by bullying and harassment, Asian students, more so than other racially/ethnically diverse students, were found more likely (57%) to report experiencing racism in school (CDC, 2024a). In a study (Green et al., 2024) using survey responses from 639 teens between the ages of 13 and 17 years old, 43.5% of Asian youth reported bias-based harassment. However, data show that Asian students were less likely to be sexually assaulted or bullied/harassed than other racial/ethnic groups. The immigration experience is a factor: for first- and second-generation U.S. Asian students, common reasons for being bullied included language barriers, different appearance, and immigrant status (Qin et al., 2008). Others reported being bullied for not excelling academically (Wang et al., 2016), for being aggressive (Menzer et al., 2010), and for being involved in extracurricular activities (Peguero et al., 2015).

Against LGBTQIA

The percentage of LGBTQIA students who reported being bullied/harassed at school varied from 29% to 83.1% (Kosciw et al., 2022). The disparities in these percentages are likely due to the nature of the survey being used: one is a general survey about violence in schools, and the other (The Gay, Lesbian, and Straight Education Network [GLSEN] National School Climate Survey) is specific to hostile experiences of LGBTQ youth at school and, therefore, reports direct input from LGBTQ+ students. The latest GLSEN report is the result of participation by 22,298 students between the ages of 13 and 21 for the year 2021–2022 (Kosciw et al., 2022). According to the survey, 83.4%–97% of students *heard* negative words or phrases used about their gender identity or sexual orientation, and 76%

experienced direct verbal bullying and harassment. Approximately 31% of students were physically bullied/harassed based on sexual orientation, gender expression, or gender, and 53.7% were sexually bullied/harassed based on sexual orientation, gender expression, or gender. LGBTQ+ students were also bullied/harassed based on other characteristics: 34.4% because of perceived or visible disabilities, 29% as a result of religion (also see Green et al., 2024), and 23.3% due to race or ethnicity. Online hybrid and online-only learners also experienced bullying/harassment at considerable rates.

Bullying/Harassment prevalence also varied due to student personal demographics, such as sexual orientation, gender, and race/ethnicity (Kosciw et al., 2022). Green and colleagues (2024), in a study of 639 youth, found a higher rate of bullying reported by LGB teens due to sexual orientation and gender identity. Students identifying as pansexual (i.e., experiencing romantic, sexual, or emotional attraction disregarding gender identity) suffered the highest level of bullying/harassment and more discriminatory school policies (Kosciw et al., 2022). Transgender students were the targets of increased levels of bullying and harassment, particularly those who identified as transgender rather than male or female. While over 50% of LGBTQ+ students of color were bullied/harassed due to race or ethnicity, Native and Indigenous students experienced the greatest hostility and reported the lowest sense of belonging when compared to other students of color.

In addition to being bullied/harassed at school by other students, nearly 60% reported having experienced LGBTQ+ discriminatory policies and practices at school, such as not being allowed to use chosen pronouns or access gender-aligned bathrooms, being prevented from wearing clothing that matched their gender identity, receiving punishment for showing affection, being disallowed to talk about or do projects concerning LGBTQ+ issues, and not being able to form a Gay–Straight alliance student organization (Kosciw et al., 2022). Students (60.3%) reported that alerting school personnel to bullying and harassing behaviors resulted in no action being taken. At times, teachers were the perpetrators of bullying and harassment: 72% of students heard teachers and school staff make negative comments about gender expression.

Explaining the Roots of Teen Bullying

According to the United Nations Educational, Scientific and Cultural Organization (UNESCO) (2017), the roots of teen bullying lie in a community's gender norms and societal context, while also being linked to larger structural factors. "Discriminatory gender norms that shape the dominance of men and subservience of women and the perpetuation of these norms through violence are found in some form in almost every culture" (p. 16). This discrimination, within the context of gender inequality and high rates of violence against women, perpetuates and grows victimizations. With the female gender perceived as the weaker sex, domination of and showing violence toward others alleged or sensed as defenseless is a natural progression.

Social customs that support violence, notably patriarchal patterns against the vulnerable, have been discovered as perpetuating violence (Childress et al., 2024). Social norms that utilize violence for control are difficult for children to reject, as nonconforming can result in victimization at home and school (UNESCO, 2017). Violent behavior is often encouraged in schools through discriminatory practices, including discipline by teachers and staff, and through biased curricula and reading materials. By not reacting effectively to bullying and/or by not having protections and anti-policies in place (Olweus, 1993b), schools may willingly or unwillingly "reflect and reproduce environments that do not protect children and adolescents from violence and bullying" (UNESCO, 2017, p. 15).

The causes of bullying have been examined through many theoretical lenses, such as the social-ecological theory, family systems theory, group socialization theory, and social-cognitive theory. The *social-ecological theory* considers both the individual characteristics of bully and victim as well as bidirectional interactions between "family, school, peer, and community characteristics" (Thomas et al., 2018). For example, children may learn bullying behaviors from, and have them reinforced by, family (Olweus, 1993a), which is then supported by the peer group while disempowering the victim (Swearer & Espelage, 2011).

Family systems theory is similar to social-ecological theory: violent family patterns of behavior can be reinforced with positive feedback and become acceptable coping reactions (Minuchin, 1985). This teaches youth to act aggressively when protecting themselves. *Group socialization theory* helps to explain the power of peer groups as behavior reinforcers. While bullying may be perpetrated by a single aggressor, the act of bullying involves the bully, the victim, and peer witnesses who, through their responses to bullying, can either stop or reinforce the victimization (Salmivalli, 1999). Attached to group socialization are within-group and between-group processes. Within-group processes involve group similarity that develops through group selectivity based on common attitudes and behavior, as well as the similarity of those in the group. For example, perpetrators come together at first because of common characteristics but then become more alike because of the increasing time spent socializing (Kandel, 1978). Resultantly, their bullying becomes more frequent. The between-group process can increase bullying or biased behavior in group members because members seek to gain positive social acceptance—even by victimizing others (Tajfel & Turner, 1986).

According to Card and colleagues (2009), there are three cognitive elements to bullying or violent behavior: (1) knowing you can do the act, (2) believing that the violence will have a desirable outcome, and (3) the outcomes will be valuable to the aggressor. Morality, knowing that victimization is wrong, is a key component of this third element. While the bully perpetrator may recognize bullying as wrong when they are a victim, they may not recognize it as wrong when they are the perpetrator (Menesini et al., 2003). This construct is known as moral disengagement (Bandura, 2002). Many strategies are used to decrease the moral repercussions of bullying, such as rationalizing the behavior, blaming the victim, and minimizing or ignoring negative ramifications.

What Are the Risk Factors?

Role of Inequity in TB

Inequities in bullying have been documented for those students of gender and sexual minority status (Green et al., 2024; Kosciw et al., 2022; Thornton et al., 2024), students with disabilities (Gage et al., 2021; Thornton et al., 2024), students with lower academic achievement (Markkanen et al., 2021; Mundy et al., 2017), and students from lower-income families and disadvantaged neighborhoods (Elliott et al., 2019; Thornton et al., 2024). Campbell and colleagues (2019) found that lower-income children in the UK had a 20% greater chance of being bullied. Other disparities include age (i.e., younger) (Thornton et al., 2024), body appearance, student dwelling (urban or rural), and having caregiving responsibilities (D'Urso & Symonds, 2023; Hosozawa et al., 2021). These are not surprising findings, given that bullying has been defined as involving an imbalance of power (Olweus & Limber, 2018).

Internationally, Hosozawa and colleagues (2021) examined inequalities in bullying across 71 countries. They discovered that boys were victimized more than girls in all but two countries: Costa Rica and Moldova. However, Kennedy (2021) found that face-to-face bullying in the U.S. was declining among males and increasing among females. One reason for this anomaly could be the greater number of U.S. females graduating from high school and universities compared with males (Buchmann et al., 2008). Lower academic performance was also a factor for all countries with the exception of Korea and Japan. In fact, in Japan there was a reverse correlation for verbal victimization showing that higher academic achievers were bullied to a greater extent. Victimization based on socioeconomics was weak.

Individual Factors

Bias-based bullying and harassment refer to victimization that occurs because of personal characteristics that a person has no control over such as disability, race, gender identity, sexual orientation, ethnicity, and immigration status (Mulvey et al., 2018). In fact, "repeated and prolonged victimization from multiple perpetrators may make bias-based bullying a more psychologically harmful experience than non-bias-based bullying" (Xu et al., 2021, p. 19). Many victims of bias-based bullying report being bullied by more than one method and for more than one personal characteristic (Green et al., 2024). Bias-based bullying has also been identified with over three times the risk for suicide ideation and suicide attempts while also placing the victim at a higher risk for many mental health issues (Russell et al., 2012; Sinclair et al., 2012). Moreover, disability has been found to be significantly associated with bullying victimization. Students with disabilities have been found to be 282% more likely to be bullied than students without a disability. Students with a noticeable disability are more likely to be bullied in schools with a larger student body, secondary schools, and more male students (Gage et al., 2021). As noted previously, Black students are more likely than White students to be bullied (Cage et al., 2021). When compared to White students, Hispanic students are 119% more likely to be bullied, which is a lower probability than if they were Black. Hispanic students in schools with a larger minority student body are at a lesser risk of being bullied but at a greater risk when attending a predominately White school.

A child's behavioral functioning, such as whether they externalize or internalize problem behaviors, is also a predictor of becoming a bully or victim. Children who externalize behaviors can be more physically and verbally aggressive toward others, often leading to more peer rejection and a higher likelihood of becoming a bully or victim (Lebrun-Harris et al., 2019; Morgan et al., 2023; Oncioiu et al., 2020). Morgan and colleagues (2023) report that children who externalized problem behaviors during kindergarten to second grade would likely demonstrate bullying behaviors between third and fifth grades. This group of children is apt to be comprised primarily male youth (Maschi et al., 2008). Children who internalize behaviors, chiefly girls (Gallo et al., 2018), are more likely to be victims due to appearing anxious, shy, and fearful (Pouwels et al., 2019). Lower academic achievement and socioeconomic status may also be predictors of becoming a bully or victim

(Elliott et al., 2019; Mundy et al., 2017) due to academic frustration, lower social status that accompanies lower grades, and a child's ability/inability to regulate learning-related behaviors.

Relationship Factors

Sociodemographic factors such as family income and educational resources are theorized as being related to one's likelihood of being bullied, as these issues can be related to the parent–child relationship, such as quality of parenting, the amount of supervision provided by parents, and parental academic achievement (Oncioiu et al., 2020; Pouwels et al., 2019). Risks of becoming a bully have been associated with harsh parenting (Lee et al., 2021a; Saleh et al., 2021), unsupportive academic environments, deviant peers, and neighborhood chaos (Lee et al., 2021b). Some reasons for maladaptive parenting can include socioeconomic stress or abusive, neglectful, or distant caretaking tactics (Lereya et al., 2015). Comparatively, lenient parenting is found to be associated with victimization (Saleh et al., 2021). An extension of harsh parenting is parental physical violence (PPV). It can include maltreatment and severe violent punishment leading to death, injury, brain and nervous system impairment, negative coping and risky behaviors, and negative physical, emotional, and psychological health that impacts the victim, others, and communities (World Health Organization (WHO), 2022). PPV may also include implements of violence such as paddles, belts, and belt buckles that cause pain (United Nations Committee on the Rights of the Child, 2006). PPV is often in response to what a caregiver might refer to as misbehavior or disobedience. Children who experience PPV have a higher likelihood of demonstrating bullying behaviors (Fagan, 2020; Falla et al., 2022) toward peers (Lawrence, 2022; Li et al., 2021). This tendency is likely due to the development of hostility and aggression (Shackman & Pollak, 2014), leading to bullying others as a method of coping with feelings and retaliating against their circumstances (Jeong et al., 2021). Parental or caretaker violence or experiencing violence of any type in the home, especially for youth who have been poly-victimized, can lead to higher levels of impulsivity and lower levels of emotional regulation (Davis et al., 2018; Bosworth et al., 1999). Witnessing parental violence is also linked to becoming both a perpetrator and a victim (Lucas et al., 2016). Exposure to PPV can lead to the crossover of violence into other areas of a child's life.

Children experiencing PPV have been shown to exhibit violence and bullying in the classroom (Jang et al., 2024). If peers in the classroom accept bullying in the school environment, bullying is more likely to occur (Jang et al., 2024; Vel´asquez et al., 2021) and support for bully victimization is likely to decrease (Barhight et al., 2017). Male students, when exposed to PPV, are more susceptible than female students to display bullying (Falla et al., 2022; Lucas et al., 2016). Davis and colleagues (2020) found overlap in the roles of perpetrator and victim, meaning "it may be that youth who are typically labeled as only perpetrators may be experiencing victimization in other areas such as online, at home, or in the community" (p. 85).

Community Factors

Community violence is a significant factor in predicting the development of bullying. A high proportion of youth report more exposure to violence in the home than in the community (Davis et al., 2020; Finkelhor et al., 2015). However, elevated exposure to violence in the home combined with consistent high community violence has been associated with the development of bullying behavior (Davis et al., 2020; Low & Espelage, 2014), demonstrating the influence of community violence on classroom environment. Decreasing parental violence combined with heightened community violence during middle school has been associated with youth who became victims (Davis et al., 2020). Community violence has also been linked to lower school connectedness and poorer academic achievement (Borofsky et al., 2013). Relatedly, it is theorized that school environments are likely predictors of the development of both perpetrators and victims. Communities that have well-supported schools are viewed as likely to promote and teach prosocial behaviors and, therefore, decrease bullying (Hong et al., 2019). Well-resourced schools are also apt to have trained teachers and staff who intervene with acts of violence and prohibit victimization (Gage et al., 2014; Låftman et al., 2017). However, in underfunded schools, with possibly ineffective violence prevention policies and underqualified personnel, the opposite is likely true: student bullying behavior may be tolerated, even perpetrated by teachers and staff (Kosciw et al., 2022), and children are more likely to become victims (Azeredo et al., 2015; Grant et al., 2019). Such inadequately funded schools are more prone to having an atmosphere of fear (Bradshaw & Garbarino, 2004), engendering a low sense of school belonging, which can also lead students to become either engaged in or a victim of bullying (Nickerson et al., 2014). Poorly resourced schools typically have a higher percentage of students receiving free lunches, which is also a socioeconomic factor correlated with both being a bully and a victim (Morgan et al., 2023).

Criminal Justice Issue

Bullying is not a crime. However, when it involves physically injuring or attempting to injure someone, bullying becomes illegal and can result in assault, battery, or attempted assult. Criminal charges for bullying vary by state and depend on the severity of the act committed. Bullying has become a criminal justice issue in that the National Crime Victimization Survey (NCVS) reports findings on bullying in public and private schools in the U.S. from the School Crime Supplement (SCS). The NCVS is a household-based survey of nonfatal personal and property crimes conducted annually by the Bureau of Justice Statistics. The biennial SCS survey, sponsored by the National Center for Education Statistics (NCES), asks NCVS household members ages 12–18 who are enrolled in grades 6–12 to report on crime-related topics pertinent to their school experience, including bullying (Thomsen et al., 2024). A relatively new form of bullying has emerged. Cyberbullying involves bullying through electronic means by using a cell phone, computer, or electronic device to threaten and terrorize another online. Cyberbullying victimization online has become a focus of concern due to reported incidents of suicide linked to online bullying (El-Ghobashy, 2010; Schwartz, 2010). Nixon (2014) asserts that perpetrators of cyberbullying increase their use of illegal behaviors such as substance abuse, delinquent behavior, and aggression. Lee and colleagues (2020) assert that the literature is limited regarding individuals who are bullied at school. These researchers studied a sample of 2,670 middle and high school students in the U.S. and discovered that youth who were bullied or cyberbullied were more likely to engage in delinquent behavior. Depending on the nature of the act, all states have various criminal laws that might apply to bullying behaviors. For example, if someone physically injures another, an assault statute might apply depending on the state. All 50 states in the U.S. have anti-bullying laws that require schools to report, investigate, and document bullying within a specific time. The bullying law, in every state except Montana, requires schools to have a formal policy to assist with the identification of the behavior and discuss the formal/informal disciplinary response (Patchin & Hinduja, 2023). According to StopBullying.gov (n.d.), children and youth who bully others are more likely than those who do not to get into fights, vandalize property, steal, carry weapons, drop out of school, and use alcohol, cigarettes, and marijuana. StopBullying.gov cites the 2011 study of Lösel and Bender as well as the 2011 study of Ttofi and colleagues that suggests that those who bully others are also at a higher risk of becoming involved in antisocial and criminal behavior later in their lives.

Public Health Issue

According to Armitage (2021), bullying is a "major public health problem that increases the risk of poor health, social and educational outcomes in childhood and adolescence" (p. 1) with consequences following both bullies and victims well into adulthood, including depression, anxiety, suicide ideation, and suicidal behavior (Copeland et al., 2013). Moreover, bullying is recognized by the World Health Organization (WHO) as a form of youth violence or "violence that occurs among individuals ages 10–29 years who are unrelated and who may or may not know each other and generally takes place outside of the home" (Kieselbach & Butchart, 2015, p. 5). It is suggested that this form of youth violence be viewed as a pyramid with violent deaths represented at the top, injuries that bring children to the attention of medical providers and other care representing the middle, while the pyramidal base comprises bullying, which may never be reported. Bullying is also considered a global public health issue due to the ramifications, which are worse than physical violence because of the persistence of injury (Kieselbach & Butchart (2015).

Bullying victimization has been linked to health-related risky behaviors (e.g., smoking, alcohol, and drug use), poor mental health over the lifespan (e.g., depression, PTSD, anxiety disorders, and overall psychological dysfunction), and the likelihood of being involved in future violence (Kieselbach & Butchart, 2015). In addition, bullying has been shown to affect the lives of others associated with victims, including demonstrated depression, rule disobedience, physical aggression, threatening others, and drug and alcohol use (Mrug & Windle, 2010). Bullying comes at a high cost. In addition to educational underachievement (Borofsky et al., 2013), there is a high dollar cost to the schools where bullying occurs. One study (Baams et al., 2017) analyzed fiscal costs of bias-based bullying in California schools using high school and middle school survey data collected from 2011 to 2013. Costs ranged from approximately $49 million to $78 million annually: race or ethnicity ($77,985,020), religion ($54,573,624.82), gender ($54,598,635.30), sexual orientation ($62,795,337.10), and disability ($49,092,521.13). These financial losses were a direct result of students missing days at school because they felt unsafe.

A diminished quality of life for victims is also costly. A study in Germany (Jantzer et al., 2019) reported that the average annual healthcare cost to a non-bullied student ($3,242.83) was significantly lower compared with a student who was frequently bullied ($8,742.84). These costs covered direct care (e.g., psychotherapy, counseling, logo therapy, and occupational therapy) and indirect costs (e.g., transportation, parental time, contributions to insurance, private school lessons, and loss of parental participation in the workforce).

In Sweden, the 2022 cost of interventions from long-term public services for 140,000 child bully-victims was U.S. $4,235,915,000 (Gustafsson et al., 2022). In Australia, during 2016, $147 million ($92,168,788.01) was spent to treat bullying-related anxiety disorders and $322 million ($201,990,600) to treat bullying-related depressive disorders.

Another reason why bullying is a public health issue is the link between victim and perpetrator suicide. While there is a lack of direct causal evidence, there is a strong link. Espelage and Holt (2013) reported that middle school victims of bullying reported a three to five times higher rate of suicide ideation and attempts compared with non-victims. Similar results were found in a study of 6th, 9th, and 12th grade students (Borowsky et al., 2013): non-involved students reported a 1.2% suicide attempt rate compared with 5% by those who were sometimes verbally or socially bullied, 6.5% by those frequently verbally/socially bullied, and 11.1% for those who were both bully and victim of verbal/social bullying. Even students who observed bullying but who were not targeted victims were more likely than non-observers to report feelings of sensitivity, inferiority, and hopelessness (Rivers & Noret, 2013). Son and colleagues (2024) found an increased likelihood of suicide ideation among lower-income, less educated, migrant Korean mothers of victimized multicultural children, attesting to the spillover effects of victimization consequences. Across studies examining the bully-suicide nexus and across victims, perpetrators, and bully-victims, there was likely to have been a history of prior-year self-harm and emotional distress (Borowsky et al., 2013), as well as family dysfunction, poor caregiver monitoring and support, and living with one parent only as factors for victims (Cuesta et al., 2021). For victims and bully-victims, there was also a history of sexual abuse, mental health diagnoses, and having run away from home—which increased the likelihood of suicide ideation and attempts.

International Comparative Statistics

Research estimates that 246 million children experience bullying and other forms of school violence annually. UNESCO (2017) considers bullying to be synonymous with school violence yet reports on bullying separately because of the extensive occurrence of bullying. International bullying prevalence rates vary between less than 10% and over 65%, considering data from 18 countries. For example, Tajikistan reports a rate of 7% for all youth, but Samoa reports a high of 74%. UNESCO also found that school violence and bullying were reportedly three to five times greater for LGBT students, with 16%–85% of LGBT students experiencing school violence. Cyberbullying, as in the U.S., is a global concern, with a range of 5%–21% of children and teens being affected. Socioeconomically, lower-income youth in wealthy countries are more likely to be bully-victims. Like the U.S., school buildings and grounds are locations for most bullying behavior, although it does occur outside of the school. For example, in Korea, it was discovered that over 75% of bullying occurred inside educational facilities. Further emphasizing the seriousness of bullying on a global scale, Child Helpline International (CHI) (2024) reported that behavior identified as bullying was the top fourth reason (14% or 81,110 contacts) for adolescent requests for help, preceded only by physical violence (33%), psychological violence (17%), and sexual violence (15%). However, bullying was the most prevalent reason for calls in Europe (26%) and Asia-Pacific regions, while far less was reported in the Americas and the Caribbean. While girls reported sexual violence more often than boys, non-binary youth reported more psychological violence and bullying than girls or boys: 27% and 9.5%, respectively, in the

Americas and Caribbean, and up to 39% for bullying in Europe. In 2023, CHI received 6,368,322 child and youth contacts from over 130 countries, yet was able to assist only 2,302,244 due to several reasons that included insufficient staffing. Most contacts were from youth ages 13–15 years.

Public Health and Social Work

Intersection of Public Health and Social Work

Social workers intersect with victims of teen bullying in a variety of settings, such as schools, emergency rooms, community mental health centers, and private practices (Drucker, 2025). Social workers, as mental health experts, and especially in schools, can play a key role in both the prevention and intervention of bullying. They assist with teacher, student, and community education about bullying. They work on moderating student discussions about bullying and creating safe spaces for students to express feelings and fears. After students are identified (or self-identify) as either victim or perpetrator, social workers can provide evidence-based and trauma-informed support, counseling, or, if licensed, therapy to individuals or groups and make referrals for treatment to outside service providers. Social workers may also work with parents of bullied students, parents of perpetrators, or larger school-based groups of parents, teachers, and administrators to collectively and creatively address the behaviors for both intervention and prevention purposes.

Health Disparities and Health Equities

There are both childhood and adult detrimental health consequences found for both perpetrators and victims of bullying. Some research even suggests that health outcomes are worse for perpetrators due to prolonged involvement in violent behavior and criminal activity (Rose et al., 2015). In addition to the immediate negative health effects as consequences of bullying, including possible serious injury or death (CDC, 2024b), there are also demonstrated long-term effects strongly influencing adult health regardless of "social background and mediating factors of education, marriage, economic well-being, and social networks" (Momose & Ishida, 2024, p. 1). According to Momose and Ishida (2024), victims of bullying display disparities in poor psychological functioning and even restrictions in daily activities as adults, for men and women, due to resultant health conditions. These disparities in poor health have been discovered to persist into old age. Hu (2021) found that older persons previously victimized by bullying report more severe depression symptoms and life dissatisfaction than elders not victimized. Moreover, detrimental effects of bullying also impact adulthood educational attainment and diminished standard of living, leading to poorer health outcomes than adults not experiencing bullying victimization (Momose & Ishida, 2024). "Disadvantaged socio-economic status, especially lower economic well-being, acts as the key mediating factor" (p. 13). Similar findings were reported by Wolke and Lereya (2015), suggesting that victims of childhood bullying also exhibited lower-income earnings, increased job losses, and decreased money management skills. Victims were found less likely to find life partners and marry or to have supportive friends or social networks—both circumstances being associated with poorer health.

Negative Health Consequences of Teen Bullying

Teen bullying is associated with a host of negative health consequences such as alcohol, illicit drug, and tobacco use (Cardoso et al., 2018; Farrington & Baldry, 2010; Sanchez et al., 2024), physical injury and death (CDC, 2024b), self-harm, suicidal ideation, suicide attempts (Pan & Spittal, 2013; Cardoso et al., 2018), and sleep disturbance (CDC, 2024b). The additional stressor of trauma from race-based bullying may worsen poor health conditions (Jones et al., 2018). Moreover, negative mental health outcomes are common, especially for race-based harassment and bullying (de Oliveira et al., 2015). These mental health consequences include depression and anxiety (Cardoso et al., 2018; Lebrun-Harris et al., 2019; Pan & Spittal, 2013) and poorer psychological well-being (Kosciw et al., 2022). The physical and mental health negative outcomes are often compounded by social consequences such as social distress (CDC, 2024b), rejection (LeBrun-Harris et al., 2019), low self-esteem (Cardoso et al., 2018), strained relationships with family and friends (Thomsen et al., 2024), and a low sense of belonging (Kosciw et al., 2022). Likewise, perpetrators of bullying also experience negative health consequences. Research reveals that bullies have been found to engage in substance use and increased aggressive and violent behavior (Rose et al., 2015), to be at a higher risk of negative mental health and behavioral problems, and to continue criminal and violent behavior into adulthood (Farrington & Baldry, 2010). Perpetrators may also be more inclined to engage in child abuse and intimate partner violence (Renda et al., 2011).

Criminal Justice Approaches

Law enforcement officers often have good working relationships with school resource officers and the new Drug Abuse Resistance Education (DARE) programs that allow officers to assist in eliminating bullying in schools. Law enforcement agencies and officers take several approaches in addressing bullying. They include the following:

- Build positive relationships with students, teachers, parents, and others to help create a culture of tolerance and respect. Establishing rapport with students builds trust, and by building trust, law enforcement officers may prevent bullying.
- Engage in proactive activities to prevent bullying. By familiarizing themselves with best practices and common misdirections in bullying prevention and response, law enforcement personnel can actively engage in school and community initiatives designed to reduce bullying and improve peer relations. However, this approach cautions against avoiding zero-tolerance policies that are regarded as harsh and as imposing inflexible discipline strategies. Such policies have been found to harm student–adult relationships, weaken school climate, and contribute to poor student achievement. According to this approach, graduated sanctions should be used for rule violations that are appropriate for the developmental level of the child and the nature and severity of the bullying.
- Become experts on the state's bullying law(s). Most states currently have a law addressing bullying at school, and many of them address bullying online. Law enforcement officers who familiarize themselves with state bullying law(s) can share their knowledge with school officials, the community, and students so that they are aware of the differences between bullying, harassment, and discrimination.

- Provide supervision and be present and vigilant for warning signs. The mere presence of an adult is often enough to deter bullying, and it is important to be seen as a safe adult who can be relied on to stop bullying. Law enforcement personnel have skills in monitoring the behavior of large groups of individuals and being vigilant to signs of trouble; as such, they know what locations in the school or community are particular "hot spots" for bullying. Officers can increase supervision in these places but should be aware that bullying can migrate to new locations where adults are not present.
- Take part in efforts to investigate bullying and related behaviors so that when bullying or other problematic behaviors are reported or suspected within a school, community, or online setting, law enforcement personnel can work effectively with others to efficiently and thoroughly investigate the incident(s).
- Meet with involved students and parents, where appropriate. Depending on the situation, it may be helpful for law enforcement personnel to participate in meetings with youth who are involved with bullying, as well as with their parents.
- Take appropriate action if a crime is involved. If bullying behavior constitutes a crime, law enforcement officers should follow local laws and procedures to ensure public safety. Consider meeting with the local prosecuting attorney to explore the possibility of instituting a behavior intervention plan instead of filing formal charges against youth. Removal from the school setting should be a last resort option.

In addition to these approaches, the U. S. Department of Justice Office of Juvenile Justice Delinquency Prevention (OJJDP) (n.d.) established a national initiative in 2021 to prevent youth hate crimes and identity-based bullying. The goal is to build protective factors in youth, change the attitude and behavior of hate crime offenders, and help individuals working with youth to better understand the potential of advanced communications technologies to break cultural barriers and address bias. This approach increases awareness of bullying; identifies best practices and evidence-based strategies to build protective factors in youth and assist youth in resisting and disengaging from extremist hate groups; ensures that youth have a voice on the topic of hate crime; and the initiative partners with communities, middle and high schools, youth confined in the juvenile justice system, and those at risk for involvement (www.stopbullying.gov/communityguide).

Public Health Approaches

The widespread consequences of bullying, as well as its link to other unhealthy and potentially lethal behavior, such as suicide, demonstrate the necessity of applying public health approaches to problem intervention and prevention. The preferred public health intervention and prevention model is the primary, secondary, and tertiary-level action framework. Not only must prevention strategies target a specific concern, but these strategies must be synergistic to produce population-sized outcomes (Office of California Surgeon General, 2020. First, *primary* prevention approaches to bullying should include collaborative processes that address the root causes of bullying (Office of California Surgeon General, 2020). These measures are often referred to as *universal* (Rivara & Le Menestrel, 2016). If it is known that students likely to be bullied are from lower-income homes, disadvantaged communities, and communities where there is frequent violence, measures should be taken to address household financial security and community safety and cohesion. Many school-wide bullying prevention programs have been piloted and integrated into curricula to enhance school climate (Vreeman & Caroll, 2007). One such program type is *bystander* training, where students are taught the skills for intervening in bullying behavior and how to support victims (Forsberg et al., 2018). Programs that target other macro and meso determinants of bullying might focus on community access to alcohol by minors and illicit drug sales via public education campaigns. Since it is known that family violence influences bullying in schools (Jeong et al., 2021; Shackman & Pollak, 2014), primary intervention may include free parenting classes, after- or during-school mentoring programs, and community-based organized activities to connect youth with a network of caring adults. Next, *secondary* prevention involves early detection of bullying determinants and/or behavior and responsive actions to reduce the impact or level of harm (Office of California Surgeon General, 2020). This also includes the "use of surveillance of population-level indicators" (p. 150). For example, there may be referrals of at-risk families to public assistance or for parents to job training. If a child is acting out at school, there may be a referral for a home visit, to a support group, or to other tailored programs that utilize "intensive social-emotional skills training, coping skills, or de-escalation approaches" (Rivara & Le Menestrel, 2016, p. 184). For communities beginning to experience violence, neighbors and businesses may want to consider a community watch program or other law enforcement intervention. Third, *tertiary* interventions are for managing the harm caused by a problem (Public Health Scotland, 2024) across the lifespan (Office of California Surgeon General, 2020). Sometimes referred to as *indicated preventive intervention* (Rivara & Le Menestrel, 2016), these measures are tailored. For a child suffering detrimental effects of bullying, tertiary interventions may be private therapy, school-based therapy groups, or a change of schools. These same interventions can also be valuable for perpetrators since they too have been found to suffer from mental health conditions (Farrington & Baldry, 2010) and home or parental violence (Lee et al., 2021a). Such programs utilize "teachers, education support professionals, school resource officers, families, health care professionals, and community members" from across multiple ecological levels (Rivara & Le Menestrel, 2016, p. 184).

Public Health and Social Work Approaches

Public health and social work approaches combine forces to bridge primary, secondary, and tertiary bullying interventions for accessibility by individuals, groups, organizations, and communities. Public health officials play a myriad of roles in bullying prevention at the population level: they assess relevant bullying-related state laws and policies; collect, analyze, and disseminate data; provide training and technical assistance to public health and other professionals; facilitate collaborations between relevant organizations and professionals; and assist in developing, implementing, and evaluating interventions (Children's Safety Network, 2011). For example, public health can help integrate bullying prevention into Department of Health programs such as Maternal Child Health, provide guidance and resources to the medical community and health and human services providers, confer with Child Death Review teams to ensure that bullying is considered when reviewing deaths, and develop and conduct population-level education campaigns. Additionally, public health and social work can partner at the secondary level to provide assistance and training to law enforcement, parent groups, teachers, and families. For example, social workers educate schoolteachers, staff, and housekeepers about identifying the signs of bullying and provide best practice skills to manage bullying behavior. Public health officials and social workers together can partner with school leaders to review and/or establish bullying prevention and intervention policies. At the tertiary level, social workers and public health can work cooperatively in determining which bullying intervention measures are most effective for children and in developing professional support networks and training programs to maximize assistance for both perpetrators and victims (United States Department of Health and Human Services, n.d.).

Integrating Skills of Social Epidemiology to Address Disparities and Achieve Equity

Social epidemiology is a branch of public health that focuses on social conditions and structures (i.e., "economic systems and inequality, systemic racism, and residential segregation") as major factors of the development of poor physical and psychological health at the population level (Roux, 2022, p. 80). These structures also include "social class, gender, race and ethnicity, discrimination, social network, social capital, income distribution, and social policy" (Honjo, 2004, p. 194). According to social epidemiology, intervention in any of these areas should bring about positive change. More specifically, bullying is not exempt from the social epidemiology's reach. According to WHO (2015), several social processes are key factors in the development of youth violence behavior: youth access to alcohol, illicit drug markets, access to firearms, poverty, and inequality (p. 14). These and other factors are also determinants correlated with bullying, a form of youth violence. For example, studies have found that children from lower-income families (Mundy et al., 2017) and disadvantaged communities are more likely to be victims of bullying. According to social epidemiology, interventions such as income distribution equality and creating neighborhood cohesion should improve health and, therefore, decrease the rate of bullying. Children with disabilities have been found to be 282% more likely to be bullied (Gage et al., 2021). Creating cultures of equity and inclusion in schools—changing the learning environment—is believed to have a positive effect by lowering the rate of bullying victimization of students with disabilities. The established link between harsh parenting or PPV and the spillover effect of violence (i.e., bullying) in the classroom (Fagan, 2020; Falla et al., 2022) warrants epidemiological intervention. Public campaigns about the detriment to children from PPV, enhanced PPV surveillance methods, and increased avenues of detecting and reporting PPV are epidemiological interventions.

How Can Teen Bullying Be Prevented?

There are many bullying prevention programs, toolkits, and informational websites for bullying prevention. WHO (2015) reports that the most effective violence prevention programs have been school-based bullying prevention efforts and life and social skills development curricula. A 2014 systematic review (Evans et al., 2014) of bullying prevention trainings discovered that 11 of the 22 programs assessed led to decreased bullying perpetration, and 67% produced significantly less victimization. An additional review found that programs in general were successful with preventing perpetration by 20%–30% and victimization by 17%–20% (Farrington & Ttofi, 2009). More recently, Gaffney and colleagues (2021) conducted a review of 70 bullying prevention programs and 128 studies conducted globally. The results included 100 studies used in a meta-analysis of school-based programming effectiveness for reducing both bullying perpetration and victimization. It was discovered that school-based programs significantly reduced bullying perpetration by 19%–20%, meaning that student participants in prevention training were much less likely to engage in bullying behaviors. Bullying victimization was also found to be significantly reduced by 15%–16%, as prevention training participants were less likely to report being victimized. Cyberbullying prevention programs have been assessed separately from in-person programs. Gaffney and colleagues (2019), in a meta-analysis of anti-cyberbullying programs, discovered that cyberbullying prevention was successful in reducing perpetration by 9%–15% and victimization by 14%–15%.

School programs are by far the most popular and available for free through multiple websites. These include efforts such as restorative circles, peer mediation, programs that promote inclusion, social–emotional learning, and bullying/violence prevention (U.S. GAO, 2021). It was estimated that in 2017–2018, 51% of K-12 public schools offered mental health assessments, and 38% offered mental health treatment. The National School Climate Center offers programs that target children, parents, schools, and communities. The United States Department of Health and Social Services offers a robust bullying prevention program, stopbullying.gov/Espanol.StopBullying.gov promoting respect, reporting bullying, standing up for others who are bullied, and protecting oneself from cyberbullying. The CDC promotes the DASH (Division of Adolescent and School Health) program that focuses on safe environments. The School Social Work Association of America supports Olweus Bullying Prevention Program that teaches methods of intervening "on the spot" during a bullying situation. The GLSEN provides many resources for effective and age-appropriate prevention programs for improving school climate. As well, many support the use of restorative justice approaches.

Policy Recommendations

Bullying prevention policy recommendations can be implemented at the micro, meso, and macro levels of society. On a large scale, WHO (2015) has developed a policy brief describing victimization prevalence, the consequences of youth violence, and effective prevention programming. They also endorse national policy discussions that would lead to global/national educational resources, conferences, media campaigns, and better documentation of the long-term consequences of youth violence. When considering the establishment of a policy framework, WHO suggests considering the following: every national public health plan should include a section on youth violence prevention; each country's ministry or department of health should develop a national plan of action on violence prevention; there should also be a collaborative prevention plan developed by participating/relevant health, government, and business sectors; and all laws on youth violence should be reviewed. It is also proposed that collaborative networks, within and between countries, are necessary to effectively share information to help design policies.

All schools should have violence/bullying prevention and intervention policies. However, research reported by Kosciw and colleagues (2022) revealed that only 76.1% of students responding to the 2021 National School Climate Survey reported that their school had an anti-bullying policy, and only 12% reported their school had a comprehensive policy.

Additionally, only 8.2% of LGBTQ+ students reported attending a school with an official policy offering protection and support for transgender and nonbinary students. However, students attending schools with anti-bullying/anti-harassment policies reported much lower levels of negative verbiage targeting LGBTQ+ students, were more likely to report teacher/staff interventions of bullying behaviors, were more likely to report victimization, and reported less anti-LGBTQ+ victimization.

In response to reductions in bullying and harassing behaviors due to comprehensive school policy, it is recommended that educational environments adopt policies that educate and train supportive staff and that have curricular resources inclusive of LGBTQ+ students, students with disabilities, and students who may present as different due to income, home violence, or psychological challenges. Having staff present in hallways reduced bullying behavior (U.S. GAO, 2021). Policy recommendations that were suggested for LGBTQ+ students (Kosciw et al., 2022) are also pertinent for protecting all school children and youth. For example, policies should increase student access to appropriate and accurate information regarding diversity and support student groups and clubs that address specific student needs (e.g., Gay-Straight Alliances and Children of Alcoholics/Dysfunctional Families). For LGBTQ+ students, it is recommended that schools adopt and implement "comprehensive bullying/harassment policies that specifically enumerate sexual orientation, gender identity, and gender expression in individual schools and districts, with clear and effective systems for reporting and addressing incidents that [any] students experience" (p. xxiv). Kennedy (2021) also suggests that policymakers monitor bullying trends according to age for guiding implementation of programs and that more attention is given to the continuing rise in cyberbullying so that prevention measures will effectively address both face-to-face and online victimization.

Summary

Teen bullying is a public health issue that involves the perpetration of aggressive, unwanted behaviors (i.e., verbal attacks, physical assaults, property damage, and social intimidation), face to face or online (cyberbullying), against those who are considered vulnerable and lacking power. Bullying can cause physical, psychological, economical, and educational harm and serious injury or death. Bullying is a national and global problem. From 2021 to 2022, the weekly rates of youth bullying at school were reported by more middle schools (28%) compared to 15% of high/secondary schools and 10% of elementary schools (Burr et al., 2024). Weekly cyberbullying at school or off campus was reported by 37% of middle schools and 25% of high/secondary schools. From 2018 to 2019, 5.2 million students reported being bullied (U.S. GAO, 2021). In some cases, weapons, alcohol, and/or illicit drugs may have been involved. Students are bullied based on personal characteristics such as race (i.e., race-based bullying), ethnicity, disability, gender, gender expression, sexual orientation, and religion. Students are also bullied because of family income, the places they live (i.e., poorer neighborhoods), lower academic achievement, and body presentation. Most bullying occurs in school classrooms, hallways and stairwells, cafeterias, outside on school grounds, or by text and online (Thomsen et al., 2024). Those students with disabilities and others identifying as LGBTQ+ endure the most bullying victimization. Teen bullying is considered a form of youth violence with roots in global society's acceptance of violence against women and girls (UNESCO, 2017).

Social customs that support violence, notably patriarchal patterns against the vulnerable, have been discovered as perpetuating violence (Childress et al., 2024). School bullying is believed to be a spillover from PPV in the home (Fagan, 2020; Falla et al., 2022) and community (Davis et al., 2020). Children who are victims of parental violence can develop higher levels of impulsivity and lower levels of emotional regulation (Davis et al., 2018) and are believed to demonstrate bullying behavior as a way of mediating the effects of PPV and feelings of resentment (Jeong et al., 2021). Environments that are not well-resourced, lack comprehensive anti-bullying policies, and where teachers and staff are not trained to appropriately respond to bullying are likely to have an atmosphere of fear (Bradshaw & Garbarino, 2004) that leads to the development of both bully perpetrators and victims. Perpetrators and victims suffer detrimental health and psychological consequences such as mental health diagnoses and/or social rejection (Lebrun-Harris et al., 2019), poor psychological functioning (Kosciw et al., 2022), alcohol and drug use (Sanchez et al., 2024), low esteem, suicide ideation, suicidal behaviors (Cardoso et al., 2018), and strained relationships (Thomsen et al., 2024). Perpetrators are believed to endure even more harsh consequences due to increased aggressive and violent behavior (Rose et al., 2015), a higher risk of negative mental health and behavioral problems, and a continuation of criminal and violent behavior into adulthood (Farrington & Baldry, 2010). Victims of bullying report a continuation of negative health disparities even into older adulthood regardless of "social background and mediating factors of education, marriage, economic well-being, and social networks" (Momose & Ishida, 2024, p. 1). Hu (2021) found that older persons previously victimized by bullying reported more severe depression symptoms and life dissatisfaction compared with elders not victimized. Though bullying continues to be a worldwide problem, there are many programs that are accessible and effective at reducing school and cyberbullying. WHO (2015) reports that the most effective violence prevention programs have been school-based bullying prevention efforts and life and social skill development curricula. Gaffney and colleagues (2021) discovered that school-based programs significantly reduced bullying perpetration by 19%–20%, which suggests that student participants in prevention training were much less likely to engage in bullying behaviors. Bullying victimization was also significantly reduced by 15%–16%, as prevention training participants were less likely to report being victimized. Cyberbullying prevention has been successful in reducing perpetration by 9%–15% and victimization by 14%–15% (Gaffney et al., 2019).

It is recommended that all schools implement comprehensive violence prevention policies that include anti-bullying programs that are established at the national level of each country involving departments of ministries of health (WHO, 2015). Since programs have proven to be successful, it is surprising that only 76.1% of student respondents to the 2021 National School Climate Survey reported that their school had an anti-bullying policy, and only 12% reported their school had a comprehensive policy (Kosciw et al., 2022). The sheer number of bullying incidents that are reported each year demonstrates the importance of having a prevention policy that addresses this public health problem.

Discussion Questions

1 If you, or someone you know, has been the victim of bullying, what type of intervention do you now believe would have made the most difference at a younger age?

2 Are there neighborhood factors where you live now, or where you grew up, that you believe could lead to bullying? If so, what are some measures that you perceive might help to alleviate those conditions?

3 As a potential policymaker, who might you choose to invite to a discussion when writing school-based or community-based anti-bullying policy? What types of information do you foresee needing to develop an effective policy?

4 Are there anti-bullying/violence efforts at your university? If so, do you know about them well enough to be able to refer a friend who confides in you about victimization?

5 What actions make bullying a delinquent offense?

6 What social processes are key factors in the development of youth violent behavior?

References

Armitage, R. (2021). Bullying in children: Impact on child health. *BMJ Paediatrics Open*, 5(1), e000939. https://doi.org/10.1136/bmjpo-2020-000939

Azeredo, C.M., Rinaldi, A.E.M., de Moraes, C.L., Levy, R.B., & Menezes, P.R. (2015). School bullying: A systematic review of contextual-level risk factors in observational studies. *Aggression and Violent Behavior*, 22, 65–76. https://doi.org/10.1016/j.avb.2015.04.006 Baams, L., Talmage, C.A., & Russell, S.T. (2017). Economic costs of bias-based bullying. *School Psychology Quarterly*, 32(3), 422–433. https://doi.org/10.1037/spq0000211

Bandura, A. (2002). Selective moral disengagement in the exercise of moral agency. *Journal of Moral Education*, 31(2), 101–119. https://doi.org/10.1080/0305724022014322

Barhight, L.R., Hubbard, J.A., Grassetti, S.N., & Morrow, M.T. (2017). Relations between actual group norms, perceived peer behavior, and bystander children's intervention to bullying. *Journal of Clinical Child and Adolescent Psychology*, 46(3), 394–400. https://doi.org/10.1080/15374416.2015.1046180

Borofsky, L.A., Kellerman, I., Baucom, B., Oliver, P.H. & Margolin, G. (2013). Community violence exposure and adolescents' school engagement and academic achievement over time. *Psychology of Violence*, 3(4), 381–395. https://doi.org/10.1037/a0034121

Borowsky, I.W., Taliaferro, L.A., & McMorris, B.J. (2013). Suicidal thinking and behavior among youth involved in verbal and social bullying: Risk and protective factors. *Journal of Adolescent Health*, 53(1 Suppl), S4e12. https://doi.org/10.1016/j.jadohealth.2012.10.280

Bosworth, K., Espelage, D.L., & Simon, T.R. (1999). Factors associated with bullying behavior in middle school students. *The Journal of Early Adolescence*, 19(3), 341–362. https://doi.org/10.1177/0272431699019003003

Bradshaw, C.P., & Garbarino, J. (2004). Social cognition as a mediator of the influence of family and community violence on adolescent development: Implications for intervention. In J. Devine, J. Gilligan, K.A. Miczek, R. Shaikh, & D. Pfaff (Eds.), *Annals of the New York academy of sciences* (pp. 85–105, Vol. 1036, No. 1). Youth violence: Scientific approaches to prevention. New York Academy of Sciences. https://doi.org/10.1196/annals.1330.005

Buchmann, C., DiPrete, T. A., & McDaniel, A. (2008). Gender inequalities in education. *Annual Review of Sociology*, 34, 53–77. https://doi.org/10.1146/annurev.soc.34.040507.134551

Burr, R., Kemp, J., & Wang, K. (2024). *Crime, violence, discipline, and safety in U.S. public schools: Findings from the school survey on crime and safety: 2021–22* (NCES 2024-043). U.S. Department of Education. Washington, DC: National Center for Education Statistics. https://nces.ed.gov/pubsearch/pubsinfo.asp?pubid=2024043

Cage, E., Berridge, S., & Jones, L. (2021). Cyberbullying victimization among sexual minority youth: The role of family and school support. *Journal of Youth and Adolescence*, 50(12), 2415–2429. https://doi.org/10.1007/s10964-021-01490-2

Campbell, M., Straatmann, V.S., Lai, E.T.C., Potier, J., Pereira, S.M.P., Wickham, S.L., & Taylor-Robinson, D.C. (2019). Understanding social inequalities in children being bullied: UK millennium cohort study findings. *PLoS One*, 14(5), e0217162. https://doi.org/10.1371/journal. pone.0217162

Card, N.A., Isaacs, J., & Hodges, E. (2009). Aggression and victimization in children's peer groups: A relationship perspective. In A. Vangelisti (Ed.), *Feeling hurt in close relationships* (pp. 235–259). Cambridge University Press. http://dx.doi.org/10.1017/CBO9780511770548.013

Cardoso, J.B., Szlyk, H.S., Goldbach, J., Swank, P., & Zvolensky, M.J. (2018). General and ethnic-biased bullying among Latino students: Exploring risks of depression, suicidal ideation, and substance use. *Journal of Immigrant and Minority Health*, 20(4), 816–822. https://doi.org/ 10.1007/s10903-017-0593-5

Centers for Disease Control and Prevention (CDC). (2020). Youth risk behavior surveillance—United States, 2019. *Morbidity and Mortality Weekly Report: Supplement*, 69(1), 1–10. Youth Risk Behavior Surveillance — United States, 2019.

Centers for Disease Control and Prevention (CDC). (2024a). *Youth risk behavior survey data summary & trends report: 2013–2023*. U.S. Department of Health and Human Services. download (1).pdf.

Centers for Disease Control and Prevention (CDC). (2024b, October 28). *Bullying*. Bullying | Youth Violence Prevention | CDC.

Child Helpline International. (2024, November 20). *Voices of Children & Young People Around the World: Global Child Helpline Data from 2023*. Child Helpline International. https://childhelpli neinternational.org/global-child-helpline-data-from-2023/

Children's Safety Network. (2011, February). *Preventing bullying: The role of public health and safety professionals*. Child Safety Network National Resource Center. PreventingBullyingRolePublicHea lthSafetyProfessionals.pdf.

Childress, S., Shrestha, N., Kenensarieva, K., Urbaeva, J., & Schrag, R.V. (2024). The role of culture in the justification and perpetuation of domestic violence: The perspectives of service providers in Kyrgyzstan. *Violence against Women*, 30(5), 1198–1225. https://doi.org/10.1177/1077801223 1186814

Copeland, W.E., Wolke, D., Angold, A., & Costello, E.J. (2013). Adult psychiatric outcomes of bullying and being bullied by peers in childhood and adolescence. *JAMA Psychiatry (Chicago, IL)*, 70(4), 419–426. https://doi.org/10.1001/jamapsychiatry.2013.504

Cuesta, I., Montesó-Curto, P., Metzler Sawin, E., Jiménez-Herrera, M., Puig-Llobet, M., Seabra, P., & Toussaint, L. (2021). Risk factors for teen suicide and bullying: An international integrative review. *International Journal of Nursing Practice*, 27(3), e12930–n/a. https://doi.org/10.1111/ijn.12930

Davis, J.P., Dumas, T.M., Berey, B., Merrin, G.J., Tan, K. & Madden, D.R. (2018). Poly–victimization and trajectories of binge drinking from adolescence to young adulthood among serious juvenile offenders. *Drug & Alcohol Dependence*, 186, 29–35. https://doi.org/10.1016/j.drugalc dep.2018.01.006

Davis, J.P., Ingram, K.M., Merrin, G.J., & Espelage, D.L. (2020). Exposure to parental and community violence and the relationship to bullying perpetration and victimization among early adolescents: A parallel process growth mixture latent transition analysis. *Scandinavian Journal of Psychology*, 61(1), 77–89. https://doi.org/10.1111/sjop.12493

de Oliveira, W.A., Silva, M.A.I., de Mello, F.C.M., Porto, D.L., Yoshinaga, A.C.M., & Malta, D.C. (2015). The causes of bullying: Results from the national survey of school health (PeNSE). *Revista LatinoAmericana de Enfermagem*, 23(2), 275–282. https://doi.org/10.1590/0104-1169.0022.2552

Diez Roux, A.V. (2022). Social epidemiology: Past, present, and future. *Annual Review of Public Health*, 43(1), 79–98. https://doi.org/10.1146/annurev-publhealth-060220-042648

Drucker, E. (2025). Bullying and suicide: How social workers can help. *Social Work Today*. www.soci alworktoday.com/news/enews_0222_1.shtml

D'Urso, G., & Symonds, J. (2023). Risk factors for child and adolescent bullying and victimisation in Ireland: a systematic literature review. *Educational Review*, 75(7), 1464–1489. https://doi.org/ 10.1080/00131911.2021.1987391

El-Ghobashy, T. (2010, September 30). Suicide follows a secret webcast. *Wallstreet Journal, Eastern Edition*. A27. www.proquest.com/newspapers/suicide-follows-secret-webcast/docview/755708 867/se-2?accountid=10639

Elliott, S.N., Hwang, Y.S., & Wang, J. (2019). Teachers' ratings of social skills and problem behaviors as concurrent predictors of students' bullying behavior. *Journal of Applied Developmental Psychology*, 60, 119–126. https://doi.org/10.1016/j.appdev.2018.12.005

Espelage, D.L., & Holt, M.K. (2001). Bullying and victimization during early adolescence: Peer influences and psychosocial correlates. *Journal of Emotional Abuse*, 2(2–3), 123–142. https://doi.org/10.1300/J135v02n02_08

Evans, C.B., Fraser, M.W., & Cotter, K.L. (2014). The effectiveness of school-based bullying prevention programs: A systematic review. *Aggression and Violent Behavior*, 19(5), 532–544. https://doi.org/10.1016/j.avb.2014.07.004

Fagan, A.A. (2020). Child maltreatment and aggressive behaviors in early adolescence: Evidence of moderation by parent/child relationship quality. *Child Maltreatment*, 25(2), 182–191. https://doi.org/10.1177/1077559519874401

Falla, D., Ortega-Ruiz, R., Runions, K., & Romera, E.M. (2022). Why do victims become perpetrators of peer bullying? Moral disengagement in the cycle of violence. *Youth & Society*, 54(3), 397–418. https://doi.org/10.1177/0044118X20973702

Farrington, D., & Baldry, A. (2010). Individual risk factors for school bullying. *Journal of Aggression, Conflict and Peace Research*, 2(1), 4–16. https://doi.org/10.5042/jacpr.2010.0001

Farrington, D., & Ttofi, M. (2009). School-based programs to reduce bullying and victimization: A systematic review. *Campbell Systematic Reviews*, 5(1), i–148. https://doi.org/10.4073/csr.2009.6

Finkelhor, D., Turner, H.A., Shattuck, A. & Hamby, S.L. (2015). Prevalence of childhood exposure to violence, crime, and abuse. *JAMA Pediatrics*, 169(8), 746–754. https://doi.org/10.1001/jamapediatrics.2015.0676

Forsberg, C., Wood, L., Smith, J., Varjas, K., Meyers, J., Jungert, T., & Thornberg, R. (2018). Students' views of factors affecting their bystander behaviors in response to school bullying: A cross-collaborative conceptual qualitative analysis. *Research Papers in Education*, 33(1), 127–142. https://doi.org/10.1080/02671522.2016.1271001

Gaffney, H., Farrington, D.P., Espelage, D.L., & Ttofi, M.M. (2019). Are cyberbullying intervention and prevention programs effective? A systematic and meta-analytical review. *Aggression and Violent Behavior*, 45, 134–153. https://doi.org/10.1016/j.avb.2018.07.002

Gaffney, H., Ttofi, M.M., & Farrington, D.P. (2021). Effectiveness of school-based programs to reduce bullying perpetration and victimization: An updated systematic review and meta-analysis. *Campbell Systematic Review*, 17(2), e1143–n/a. https://doi.org/10.1002/cl2.1143

Gage, N.A., Katsiyannis, A., Rose, C., & Adams, S.E. (2021). Disproportionate bullying victimization and perpetration by disability status, race, and gender: A national analysis. *Advances in neurodevelopmental disorders*, 5(3), 256–268. https://doi.org/10.1007/s41252-021-00200-2

Gage, N.A., Prykanowski, D.A., & Larson, A. (2014). School climate and bullying victimization: A latent class growth model analysis. *School Psychology Quarterly*, 29(3), 256–271. https://doi.org/10.1037/spq0000064

Gallo, E.A.G., Munhoz, T.N., Loret de Mola, C., & Murray, J. (2018). Gender differences in the effects of childhood maltreatment on adult depression and anxiety: A systematic review and meta-analysis. *Child Abuse & Neglect*, 79, 107–114. https://doi.org/10.1016/j.chiabu.2018.01.003

Grant, N.J., Merrin, G.J., King, M.T., & Espelage, D.L. (2019). Examining within-person and between-person associations of family violence and peer deviance on bullying perpetration among middle school students. *Psychology of Violence*, 9(1), 18–27. https://doi.org/10.1037/vio0000210

Green, J.G., Ramirez, M., Merrin, G.J., & Holt, M.K. (2024). Bias-based harassment among US adolescents. *School Mental Health*, 16(2), 343–353. https://doi.org/10.1007/s12310-024-09648-8

Gustafsson, A., Loodberg, M., & Warg, F. (2022). Sexual harassment and bullying in the Nordic region: Research-based knowledge against sexual harassment and bullying among children and young people. *Friends*. NIKK-compressed.pdf.

Hong, J.S., Kim, D.H., & Hunter, S.C. (2019). Applying the social–ecological framework to explore bully–victim subgroups in South Korean schools. *Psychology of Violence*, 9(3), 267–277. https://doi.org/10.1037/vio0000132

Honjo, K. (2004). Social epidemiology: Definition, history, and research examples. *Environmental Health and Preventive Medicine*, 9(5), 193–199. https://doi.org/10.1007/BF02898100

Hosozawa, M., Bann, D., Fink, E., Elsden, E., Baba, S., Iso, H., & Patalay, P. (2021). Bullying victimisation in adolescence: Prevalence and inequalities by gender, socioeconomic status and academic performance across 71 countries. *eClinicalMedicine*, 41, 101142. https://doi.org/10.1016/j.eclinm.2021.101142

Hu, B. (2021). Is bullying victimization in childhood associated with mental health in old age. *The Journals of Gerontology. Series B, Psychological Sciences and Social Sciences*, 76(1), 161–172. https://doi.org/10.1093/geronb/gbz115

Jang, H., Son, H., Subramanian, S.V., & Kim, J. (2024). The spillover of violence: The gendered relationship between parental physical violence and peers' bullying victimization. *Children and Youth Services Review*, 166, 107978. https://doi.org/10.1016/j.childyouth.2024.107978

Jantzer, V., Schlander, M., Haffner, J., Parzer, P., Trick, S., Resch, F., & Kaess, M. (2019). The cost incurred by victims of bullying from a societal perspective: Estimates based on a German online survey of adolescents. *European Child & Adolescent Psychiatry*, 28(4), 585–594. https://doi.org/10.1007/s00787-018-1224-y

Jeong, J., Bhatia, A., Skeen, S., & Adhia, A. (2021). From ·fathers to peers: Association between paternal violence victimization and peer violence perpetration among youth in Malawi, Nigeria, and Zambia. *Social Science & Medicine*, 278(April), Article 113943. https://doi.org/10.1016/j.socscimed.2021.113943

Jones, L.M., Mitchell, K.J., Turner, H.A., & Ybarra, M.L. (2018). Characteristics of bias-based harassment incidents reported by a national sample of U.S. adolescents. *Journal of Adolescence (London, England)*, 65(1), 50–60. https://doi.org/10.1016/j.adolescence.2018.02.013

Kandel, D.B. (1978). Homophily, selection, and socialization in adolescent friendships. *American Journal of Sociology*, 84(2), 427–436. https://doi.org/10.1086/226792

Kennedy, R.S. (2021). Bullying trends in the united states: A meta-regression. *Trauma, Violence & Abuse*, 22(4), 914–927. https://doi.org/10.1177/1524838019888555

Kieselbach, B., & Butchart, A. (2015). *Preventing youth violence: An overview of the evidence*. World Health Organization. 9789241509251_eng.pdf.

Kosciw, J.G., Clark, C.M., & Menard, L. (2022). *The 2021 National School Climate Survey: The experiences of LGBTQ + youth in our nation's schools*. New York: GLSEN. NSCS-2021-Full-Report.pdf.

Låftman, S.B., Östberg, V., & Modin, B. (2017). School climate and exposure to bullying: A multilevel study. *School Effectiveness and School Improvement*, 28(1), 153–164. https://doi.org/10.1080/09243453.2016.1253591

Lai, T., & Kao, G. (2018). Hit, robbed, and put down (but not bullied): Underreporting of bullying by minority and male students. *Journal of Youth and Adolescence*, 47(3), 619–635. https://doi.org/10.1007/s10964-017-0748-7

Lawrence, T. (2022). Family violence, depressive symptoms, school bonding, and bullying perpetration: An intergenerational transmission of violence perspective. *Journal of School Violence*, 21(4), 517–529. https://doi.org/10.1080/15388220.2022.2114490

Lebrun-Harris, L.A., Sherman, L.J., Limber, S.P., Miller, B.D., & Edgerton, E.A. (2019). Bullying victimization and perpetration among U.S. children and adolescents: 2016 national survey of children's health. *Journal of Child and Family Studies*, 28(9), 2543–2557. https://doi.org/10.1007/s10826-018-1170-9

Lee, C., Patchin, J.W., Hinduja, S., & Dischinger, A. (2020). Bullying and delinquency: The impact of anger and frustration. *Violence and Victims*, 35(4), 503–523.

Lee, J.M., Kim, J., Hong, J.S., & Marsack-Topolewski, C.N. (2021a). From bully victimization to aggressive behavior: Applying the problem behavior theory, theory of stress and coping, and general strain theory to explore potential pathways. *Journal of Interpersonal Violence*, 36(21–22), 10314–10337. https://doi.org/10.1177/0886260519884679

Lee, J.M., Hong, J.S., Resko, S.M., Gonzalez-Prendes, A.A., & Voisin, D.R. (2021b). Ecological correlates of bullying and peer victimization among urban African American adolescents. *The*

Journal of Educational Research (Washington, DC), 114(4), 346–356. https://doi.org/10.1080/00220671.2021.1937914

Lereya, S.T., Copeland, W.E., Zammit, S., & Wolke, D. (2015). Bully/victims: A longitudinal, population-based cohort study of their mental health. *European Child and Adolescent Psychiatry*, 24(12), 1461–1471. https://doi.org/10.1007/s00787-015-0705-5

Lewis, C., Deardorff, J., Lahiff, M., Soleimanpour, S., Sakashita, K., & Brindis, C.D. (2015). High school students' experiences of bullying and victimization and the association with school health center use. *Journal of School Health*, 85(5), 318–326. https://doi.org/10.1111/josh.12256

Li, X., Huebner, E.S., & Tian, L. (2021). Vicious cycle of emotional maltreatment and bullying perpetration/victimization among early adolescents: Depressive symptoms as a mediator. *Social Science and Medicine*, 291(September), Article 114483. https://doi.org/10.1016/j.socscimed.2021.114483

Low, S., & Espelage, D. (2014). Conduits from community violence exposure to peer aggression and victimization: Contributions of parental monitoring, impulsivity, and deviancy. *Journal of Counseling Psychology*, 61(2), 221. https://doi.org/10.1037/a0035207

Lucas, S., Jernbro, C., Tindberg, Y., & Janson, S. (2016). Bully, bullied and abused. Associations between violence at home and bullying in childhood. *Scandinavian Journal of Public Health*, 44(1), 27–35. https://doi.org/10.1177/1403494815610238

Markkanen, I., Välimaa, R., & Kannas, L. (2021). Forms of bullying and associations between school perceptions and being bullied among Finnish secondary school students aged 13 and 15. *International Journal of Bullying Prevention*, 3(1), 24–33. https://doi.org/10.1007/s42380-019-00058-y

Maschi, T., Gibson, D., & MacMillan, T. (2008). family incarceration and bullying among urban African American adolescents: The mediating roles of exposure to delinquent peer norms, trauma, and externalizing behaviors. *Journal of Urban Social Work*, 2(1), 1–18.

Menesini, E., Sanchez, V., Fonzi, A., Ortega, R., Costabile, A., & Lo Feudo, G. (2003). Moral emotions and bullying: A cross-national comparison of differences between bullies, victims and outsiders. *Aggressive Behavior*, 29(6), 515–530. https://doi.org/10.1002/ab.10060

Menzer, M.M., Oh, W., McDonald, K.L., Rubin, K.H., & Dashiell-Aje, E. (2010). Behavioral correlates of peer exclusion and victimization of East Asian American and European American young adolescents. *Asian American Journal of Psychology*, 1(4), 290–302. https://doi.org/10.1037/a0022085

Minuchin, P. (1985.) Families and individual development: provocations from the field of family therapy. *Child Development*, 56(2), 289–302. https://doi.org/10.1111/j.1467-8624.1985.tb00106.x

Momose, Y., & Ishida, H. (2024). Bullying experiences in childhood and health outcomes in adulthood. *PLoS One*, 19(7), e0305005. https://doi.org/10.1371/journal.pone.0305005

Morgan, P.L., Farkas, G., Woods, A.D., Wang, Y., Hillemeier, M.M., & Oh, Y. (2023). Factors predictive of being bullies or victims of bullies in US elementary schools. *School Mental Health*, 15(2), 566–582. https://doi.org/10.1007/s12310-023-09571-4

Mrug, S., & Windle, M. (2010). Prospective effects of violence exposure across multiple contexts on early adolescents' internalizing and externalizing problems. *Journal of Child Psychology and Psychiatry*, 51(8), 953–961. https://doi.org/10.1111/j.1469-7610.2010.02222.x

Mulvey, K.L., Hoffman, A.J., Gönültaş, S., Hope, E.C., & Cooper, S.M. (2018). Understanding experiences with bullying and bias-based bullying: What matters and for whom? *Psychology of Violence*, 8(6), 702–711. https://doi.org/10.1037/vio0000206

Mundy, L.K., Canterford, L., Kosola, S., Degenhardt, L., Allen, N.B., & Patton, G.C. (2017). Peer victimization and academic performance in primary school children. *Academic Pediatrics*, 17, 830–836. https://doi.org/10.1016/j.acap.2017.06.012

Nickerson, A.B., Singleton, D., Schnurr, B., & Collen, M.H. (2014). Perceptions of school climate as a function of bullying involvement. *Journal of Applied School Psychology*, 30(2), 157–181. https://doi.org/10.1080/15377903.2014.888530

Nixon, C.L. (2014). Current perspectives: the impact of cyberbullying on adolescent health. *Adolescent Health, Medicine and Therapeutics*, *2014*(default), 143–158. https://doi.org/10.2147/AHMT.S36456

Office of California Surgeon General. (2020, December.). *Roadmap for resilience*: Primary, secondary, and tertiary prevention strategies in public health. https://osg.ca.gov/wp-content/uploads/sites/266/2020/12/Part-II-4.-Primary-Secondary-and-Tertiary-Prevention-Strategies-in-Public-Health.pdf

Olweus, D., & Limber, S.P. (2018). Some problems with cyberbullying research. *Current Opinion in Psychology*, 19, 139–143. https://doi.org/10.1016/j.copsyc.2017.04.012

Olweus, D. (1993a). *Bullying at school: What we know and what we can do*. Wiley-Blackwell.

Olweus, D. (1993b). Bullies on the playground: The role of victimization. In C.H. Hart (Ed.), *Children on playgrounds: Research perspectives and applications* (pp. 85–128). State University of New York Press.

Oncioiu, S.I., Orri, M., Boivin, M., Geofroy, M.C., Arseneault, L., Brendgen, M., Vitaro, F., Navarro, M.C., Galéra, C., Tremblay, R.E., & Côté, S.M. (2020). Early childhood factors associated with peer victimization trajectories from 6 to 17 years of age. *Pediatrics (Evanston)*, 145(5), 1. https://doi.org/10.1542/peds.2019-2654

Pan, S.W., & Spittal, P.M. (2013). Health effects of perceived racial and religious bullying among urban adolescents in China: A cross-sectional national study. *Global Public Health*, 8(6), 685–697. https://doi.org/10.1080/17441692.2013.799218

Patchin, J.W., & Hinduja, S. (2023). Bullying laws across America. *Cyberbullying Research Center.* https://cyberbullying.org/bullying-laws

Peguero, A.A., & Jiang, X. (2016). Backlash for breaking racial and ethnic breaking stereotypes: Adolescent school victimization across contexts. *Journal of Interpersonal Violence*, 31(6), 1047–1073. https://doi.org/10.1177/0886260514564063

Peguero, A.A., Popp, A.M., & Koo, D.J. (2015). Race, ethnicity, and school-based adolescent victimization. *Crime & Delinquency*, 61(3), 323–349. https://doi.org/10.1177/0011128713398021

Pouwels, J.L., Hanish, L.H., Smeekens, S., Cillessen, A.H., & van den Berg, Y.H. (2019). Predicting the development of victimization from early childhood internalizing and externalizing behavior. *Journal of Applied Developmental Psychology*, 62, 294–305. https://doi.org/10.1016/j.appdev.2019.02.012

Public Health Scotland. (2024). Public health approach to prevention: The three levels of prevention. https://publichealthscotland.scot/about-us/what-we-do-and-how-we-work/public-health-approach-to-prevention/the-three-levels-of-prevention/

Qin, D.B., Way, N., & Rana, M. (2008). The "model minority" and their discontent: Examining peer discrimination and harassment of Chinese American immigrant youth. *New Directions for Child and Adolescent Development*, 2008(121), 27–42. https://doi.org/10.1002/cd.221

Renda, J., Vassallo, S., & Edwards, B. (2011). Bullying in early adolescence and its association with anti- social behaviour, criminality and violence 6 and 10 years later. *Criminal Behaviour and Mental Health*, 21(2), 117–127. https://doi.org/10.1002/cbm.805

Rivara, F., & Le Menestrel, S. (Eds.). (2016). *Preventing Bullying Through Science, Policy, and Practice*. National Academies of Sciences, Engineering, and Medicine. National Academies Press (US). https://doi.org/10.17226/23482

Rivers, I., & Noret, N. (2013). Potential suicide ideation and its association with observing bullying at school. *Journal of Adolescent Health*, 53(1 Suppl), S32–S36. https://doi.org/10.1016/j.jadohealth.2012.10.279

Rose, C.A., Stormont, M., Wang, Z., Simpson, C.G., Preast, J.L., & Green, A.L. (2015). Bullying and students with disabilities: Examination of disability status and educational placement. *School Psychology Review*, 44(4), 425–444. https://doi.org/10.17105/spr-15-0080.1

Russell, S.T., Sinclair, K.O., Poteat, V.P., & Koenig, B.W. (2012). Adolescent health and harassment based on discriminatory bias. *American Journal of Public Health*, 102(3), 493–495. https://doi.org/10.2105/AJPH.2011.300430

Saleh, A., Hapsah, H., Krisnawati, W., & Erfina, E. (2021). Parenting style and bullying behavior in adolescents. *Enfermería Clínica*, 31(Supplement 5), S640–S643. https://doi.org/10.1016/j.enf cli.2021.07.009

Salmivalli, C. (1999). Participant role approach to school bullying: Implications for interventions. *Journal of Adolescence*, 22(4), 453–459. https://doi.org/10.1006/jado.1999.0239

Sánchez-Sánchez, A.M., Ruiz-Muñoz, D., & Sánchez-Sánchez, F.J. (2024). Research trends in the bias-based aggression among youth. *Children and Youth Services Review, 158*, 107444. https://doi.org/10.1016/j.childyouth.2024.107444

Sawyer, A.L., Bradshaw, C.P., & O'Brennan, L.M. (2008). Examining ethnic, gender, and developmental differences in the way children report being a victim of "bullying" on self-report measures. *Journal of Adolescent Health*, 43(2), 106–114. https://doi.org/10.1016/j.jadohea lth.2007.12.011

Schwartz, J. (2010, October 3). Bullying, suicide, punishment: Week in review desk *The New York Times*. www.proquest.com/newspapers/bullying-suicide-punishment/docview/756126880/se-2?accountid=10639

Shackman, J.E., & Pollak, S.D. (2014). Impact of physical maltreatment on the regulation of negative affect and aggression. *Development and Psychopathology*, 26(4), 1021–1033. https://doi.org/10.1017/S0954579414000546

Sinclair, K.O., Bauman, S., Poteat, V.P., Koenig, B., & Russell, S.T. (2012). Cyber and bias-based harassment: Associations with academic, substance use, and mental health problems. *Journal of Adolescent Health*, 50(5), 521–523. https://doi.org/10.1016/j.jadohealth.2011.09.009

Son, H., Ahn, E., & Kim, J. (2024). Children's bullying victimization and maternal suicidal ideation among multicultural families in south Korea: Heterogeneity by family socioeconomic status. *Social Science & Medicine (1982)*, 341, 116545–116545. https://doi.org/10.1016/j.socsci med.2023.116545

Stopbullying.gov. (n. d.). *Effects of bullying: Kids who bully others*. U.S. Department of Health and Human Services. Washington, D.C. Effects of Bullying | StopBullying.gov

Swearer, S.M., & Espelage, D.L. (2011). Expanding the social-ecological framework of bullying among youth: lessons learned from the past and directions for the future. In D.L. Espelage, & S.M. Swearer (Eds.), *Bullying in North American schools* (pp. 23–30). Routledge. https://doi.org/10.4324/9780203842898-7

Tajfel, H., & Turner, J.C. (1986). *An integrative theory of intergroup conflict. Psychology of intergroup relations*. Nelson-Hall.

Thomas, H.J., Connor, J.P., & Scott, J.G. (2018). Why do children and adolescents bully their peers? A critical review of key theoretical frameworks. *Social Psychiatry and Psychiatric Epidemiology*, 53(5), 437–451. https://doi.org/10.1007/s00127-017-1462-1

Thomsen, E., Henderson, M., Moore, A., Price, N., & McGarrah, M.W. (2024). *Student reports of bullying: Results from the 2022 school crime supplement to the National Crime Victimization Survey (NCES 2024-109rev)*. U.S. Department of Education. Washington, DC: National Center for Education Statistics. https://nces.ed.gov/pubsearch/pubsinfo.asp?pubid=2024109rev

Thornton, E., Panayiotou, M., & Humphrey, N. (2024). Prevalence, inequalities, and impact of bullying in adolescence: Insights from the #BeeWell study. *International Journal of Bullying Prevention*. https://doi.org/10.1007/s42380-024-00244-7

United Nations Committee on the Rights of the Child. (2006). *The right of the child to protection from corporal punishment and other cruel or degrading forms of punishment* (Arts. 19; 28, Para. 2; and 37, inter alia), 2 March 2007, CRC/C/GC/8. www.refworld.org/docid/460bc7772.html

United Nations Educational, Scientific and Cultural Organization (UNESCO). (2017). *School violence and bullying: Global status report*. GloPublished by the United Nations Educational, Scientific and Cultural Organization,7, place de Fontenoy, 75352 Paris 07 SP, France© UNESCO. School Violence and Bullying: Global Status Report (2017) | PDF | Bullying | Violence.

United States Department of Health and Human Services. (n.d.). *Understanding the roles of health and safety professionals in community-wide bullying prevention efforts*. Stopbullying.

gov. Understanding the Roles of Health and Safety Professionals in Community-Wide Bullying Prevention Efforts.

U.S. Department of Justice, Office of Juvenile Justice and Delinquency Prevention. (n.d.). *Preventing Youth Hate Crimes & Identity-Based Bullying Initiative.* Retrieved from https://ojjdp.ojp.gov/libr ary/publications/preventing-youth-hate-crimes-identity-based-bullying-initiative

United States Government Accountability Office (U.S. GAO). (2021, November). *K-12 education: Students' experiences with bullying, hate speech, hate crimes, and victimization in schools.* GAO@100. Highlights of GAO-22-104341, a report to the Chairman, Committee on Education and Labor, House of Representatives.

Velásquez, A.M., Saldarriaga, L.M., Castellanos, M., & Bukowski, W.M. (2021). The effect of classroom aggression-related peer group norms on students' short-term trajectories of aggression. *Aggressive Behavior, 47*(6), 672–684. https://doi.org/10.1002/ab.21988

Vogels, E. (2022). *Teens and cyberbullying 2022.* Pew Research Center. Teens and Cyberbullying 2022 | Pew Research Center.

Volk, A.A., Dane, A.V., & Marini, Z.A. (2014). What is bullying? A theoretical redefinition. *Developmental Review,* 34(4), 327–343. https://doi.org/10.1016/j.dr.2014.09.001

Vreeman, R.C., & Carroll, A.E. (2007). A systematic review of school-based interventions to prevent bullying. *Archives of Pediatrics & Adolescent Medicine*, 161, 78–88. https://doi.org/10.1001/archpedi.161.1.78. PMID: 17199071.

Wang, W., Brittain, H., McDougall, P., & Vaillancourt, T. (2016). Bullying and school transition: Context or development? *Child Abuse & Neglect, 51*, 237–248. https://doi.org/10.1016/j.chiabu.2015.10.004

Wolke, D., & Lereya, S.T. (2015). Long-term effects of bullying. *Archives of Disease in Childhood*, 100, 879–885. https://doi.org/10.1136/archdischild-2014-306667

World Health Organization (WHO). (2015). *Preventing youth violence: An overview of the evidence.* WHO: Management of Noncommunicable Diseases, Disability, Violence and Injury Prevention (NVI). 9789241509251_eng.pdf;jsessio

World Health Organization (WHO). (2022). *Violence against children: Types of violence against children.* Violence against Children.

Xu, S., Russell, S. T., & Kosciw, J. G. (2021). Exploring dimensions of bias-based bullying victimization, school fairness, and school belonging through mediation analysis. *Journal of School Psychology, 89*, 168–181. https://doi.org/10.1016/j.jsp.2021.09.006

12

WORKPLACE VIOLENCE AND PUBLIC HEALTH

Introduction

Karen and John are employees of an insurance company who have been secretly dating. John has just been demoted by his supervisor due to poor handling of an insurance claim. John and Karen decide to have lunch in the company's lounge to discuss why he was demoted. As they are having lunch, Karen leaves the table to congratulate Tim, a colleague who just received a promotion. When Karen returns to the table, John aggressively grabs her arm and questions her relationship with Tim. Overhearing this, Tim approaches the table and tries to assure John that nothing is going on between him and Karen. John disagrees and verbally threatens to kill Tim for taking the promotion that he assumed would have been his and for trying to take Karen from him. As Tim throws his hands up, leaving the table, John shoots Tim in the back and opens fire on everyone in the lounge, killing both Karen and Tim and seriously injuring 12 others. As John exits the lounge, he continues to shoot everyone in sight, including customers. John ends the shooting spree by shooting himself in the head. Cases of irate employees committing workplace violence (WPV) have become commonplace in local, state, federal, and global workplaces. WPV can cause psychological, physical, and financial loss to victims, their families, colleagues, witnesses, and the community. Therefore, it involves responses from employers, healthcare and social services professionals, and the community. Violence against employees can occur under any situation and can include robberies, assaults, threats/bullying, acts of sexual harassment, acts of frustration with customers/clients, acts perpetrated by disgruntled or former colleagues, as well as domestic and interpersonal violence incidents that spill over into the workplace.

Workplace Violence Defined

The U.S. Department of Labor Occupational Safety and Health Administration (2002) originally defined WPV as "violence or the threat of violence against workers." In 2015, the National Institute for OSHA broadened its original definition so that WPV now includes any act or threat of physical violence, harassment, intimidation, or other threatening

DOI: 10.4324/9781003373001-12

disruptive behavior that occurs at work (2015). This definition is used by the Centers for Disease Control, the Department of Labor, the Department of Justice, and many other agencies. Barling and colleagues (2009, p. 673) define WPV as a "distinct form of workplace aggression that comprises behaviors that are intended to cause physical harm." Cooper and colleagues (2011) define it as a long-term aggression carried out over time against someone who cannot defend themselves. Fute and colleagues (2015) and Arnetz and colleagues (2018) suggest that WPV is also referred to as occupational violence that manifests itself in the form of verbal abuse such as shouting or disrespecting others, or physical abuse/threat, which consists of hitting, beating, biting, throwing objects, strangling, pushing, kicking, or dragging. Occupational violence can also present itself in the form of sexual harassment, which can be displayed by attempting or forcing another to engage in sexual favors or threatening or blackmailing another to engage in sex by offering money, gifts, or special privileges.

WPV not only involves employees, but it can also involve clients, customers, and visitors to a workplace. The violence stemming from WPV can range from rape, murder, robbery, and assault against persons who are at work or on duty. The U.S. Bureau of Justice Statistics in collaboration with the Bureau of Labor Statistics and the National Institute of Occupational Safety and Health defines workplace homicide as "fatal violence against persons at work or on duty or fatal violence that was work-related." These organizations also define nonfatal WPV as violent acts, which include physical assaults and threats of assault, that are directed toward persons at work or on duty, or nonfatal violence that is work-related, such as an attack on a coworker away from work over a work-related issue (Harrell et al., 2022). This can include rape or sexual assault, robbery, aggravated assault, and simple assault. The various revisions in the definition of WPV may also signal how prevalent it has become.

Nature and Extent of Workplace Violence

In examining the extent of WPV in the U.S., Harrell and colleagues (2022) discovered that from 1992 to 2019, there were a total of 17,865 workers who were victims of workplace homicides in the U.S. In 2019, there were a total of 454 homicides in the U.S., which was a 58% decrease from a high of 1,080 in 1994. The researchers further found that the average annual rate of nonfatal WPV between 2015 and 2019 represented 8.0 million violent crimes per 1,000 workers aged 16 or older. Harrell and colleagues indicate that, according to the National Crime Victimization Survey (NCVS) data, approximately 1.3 million nonfatal acts of WPV occurred annually between 2015 and 2019. In addition, Harrell and colleagues assert that the National Electronic Injury Surveillance System – Occupational Supplement (NEISS-Work) data revealed there were approximately 529,000 injuries from WPV treated in hospital emergency rooms between 2015 and 2019. Between the years of 2015 and 2019, workers in corrections occupations had the highest average annual rate of nonfatal WPV of all the occupations examined (149.1 violent crimes per 1,000 workers aged 16 or older) between the years of 2015 and 2019.

In 2022, the U.S. Bureau of Labor Statistics Census of Fatal Occupational Injuries reported 5,486 work fatalities; of this number, homicides accounted for 61.7% of the fatalities, with 524 deaths. This was an 8.9% increase from 2021. Black fatalities accounted for 13.4% (734) of all fatalities in 2022 and represented 33.4% (175) of fatalities from homicides. Similarly, women accounted for 8.1% (445) of all workplace fatalities but accounted for 15.3% (80) of homicides in 2022. For protective service workers, there were 121 homicides and 17 suicides, which accounted for 41.2% of the fatalities (U.S. Bureau of Labor Statistics, 2022).

To determine the global prevalence of WPV and harassment, the International Labour Organization (2022), in collaboration with ILO-Lloyd's Register Foundation-Gallup Survey, conducted a joint analysis of worldwide data on individuals' experiences of violence and harassment at work. The survey data revealed that 22.8% or 743 million (i.e., more than one in five) employed people had experienced at least one form of violence and harassment in the workplace. The study's results displayed the global magnitude of WPV and harassment by examining physical, psychological, and sexual WPV and harassment. Of those who had experienced violence and harassment in the workplace, one-third or 31.8% revealed they had experienced more than one form, and 6.3% revealed they had experienced physical, psychological, and sexual violence and harassment in the workplace. This survey found that globally, men were more likely than women to report experiences of physical violence and harassment in the workplace. Approximately 8.5% or 277 million workers experienced physical violence and harassment during their work life.

For men and women, psychological violence and harassment were the most common forms of WPV experienced by both genders, with nearly 17.9% or 583 million workers, experiencing it throughout their work life. Among the forms of WPV and harassment, 6.3% or 205 million workers experienced sexual violence and harassment at work. Women were particularly more exposed to sexual violence and harassment than men, with women accounting for 8.2%, and men accounting for 5.0%. The survey displayed that violence and harassment are persistent and recurring. For example, most of the participants reported they had experienced WPV and harassment within the past five years of the study, and more than three in five victims stated it had occurred on multiple occasions. The results from these surveys indicate the global prevalence of WPV and the need to understand the categories of WPV.

Types of Workplace Violence

Many entities and researchers have proposed types of WPV. For example, in 2002, WHO developed categories of WPV that include physical violence and psychological violence, which includes verbal violence (World Health Organization [WHO], 2002). However, most organizations/agencies are based on the typologies of OSHA and the CDC (Wilkinson, 2001; Centers for Disease Control and Prevention [CDC], 2020), which suggests that researchers regard the four types of WPV to include the following:

- Criminal intent, which is the most common cause of homicide in the workplace, and the perpetrator does not have a legitimate relationship with the employee(s) or business and is usually committing a crime (i.e., robbery and shoplifting) in conjunction with the WPV.
- Customer/client/patient in which violence involves verbal threats to, or nonfatal assault on, an employee by a client, customer, patient, visitor, or inmate. This often occurs with incidents of violence in emergency rooms, psychiatric treatment settings, waiting rooms, and healthcare facilities. This is also referred to as "client-on-worker violence."

- Employee-on-employee is violence between coworkers and is referred to as lateral or horizontal violence. This includes bullying and can manifest into verbal and emotional abuse and result in homicide. This violence is more often a source of threat or assault at the workplace.
- Personal relationship or intimate partner is violence that spills over from an interpersonal dispute into the work environment but otherwise may not relate to work.

Although there are many types of WPV, for this chapter, we will explore the impact of domestic violence (DV), relationship or intimate partner violence (IPV)/love triangles, and disgruntled employee/coworker violence as an occupational hazard.

Domestic Violence

DV is defined as the actions or behaviors of an individual that dominate and control another. It can involve abusive, coercive, forceful, and threatening actions or words used by intimate partners, family members, or other members of a household against another (Work Safe BC, 2024). DV becomes WPV when the perpetrator attempts to harass, stalk, threaten, or injure a victim at work. It can affect employee productivity, lead to absenteeism, affect workplace morale, and place a workplace at risk. Limited research (Peek-Asa et al., 2013; Tiesman et al., 2014) has been conducted on the issue of DV in the workplace; most of the research regarding violence in the workplace tends to involve worker-on-worker violence and violence between workers and either clients, patients, or customers.

Showalter (2016) contends that violence by a partner not only impacts a female's chances of obtaining employment, but DV in the workplace appears to influence a females' wages as well as their ability to find another job. Likewise, Scott and colleagues (2017) imply that victims of DV in the workplace are impacted by low productivity and often have difficulty in finding jobs. Węziak-Białowolska and colleagues (2020) suggest that DV is a serious global issue that escalates outside the workplace, and little is known about its impact on one's work performance or WPV. Therefore, additional research needs to be conducted on the effect that DV may have on WPV (Adewumi & Danesi, 2017; Wathen et al., 2015; Lanctôt & Guay, 2014).

Relationship or Intimate Partner Violence (Love Triangle)

Gurm et al. (2020) suggests that relationship violence (RV) is a form of physical, emotional, spiritual, and financial abuse, negative social control, or coercion that is suffered by anyone who has a bond or relationship with the abuser. Livingston and colleagues (2021) and Gurm et al. (2020) note that RV also includes IPV, which can also occur in the workplace. The U.S. Department of Labor (2013) suggests that the most severe form of IPV results in homicide, with over one-third (38%) of all female murders in the U.S. workplace between 1982 and 2011 being committed by an intimate partner. The U.S. Bureau of Labor Statistics (2016) indicated that workplace homicides rose by 2% to 417 cases in 2015; approximately 43% of female decedents were fatally assaulted by a relative or domestic partner. A case in point occurred in 2017 in San Bernardino, California, when an elementary teacher, Karen Smith, was shot and killed by her husband at school; one student was murdered and another injured. In yet another case, Anthony McNaughton, the manager of a British Columbia Starbucks, was stabbed multiple times as he stepped between an employee and her ex-partner (Giesbrecht, 2022).

IPV affects all races, genders, and socioeconomic backgrounds and can be exhibited through physical, verbal, psychological, financial, emotional, economic, spiritual, and sexual abuse by a current or former partner (Brieding et al., 2015; Giesbrecht, 2022). Livingston further contends that IPV normally occurs privately but can be present in the workplace through acts of stalking. Traditionally, IPV had been uncommon in the workplace. IPV is growing in the number of individuals who report it, and workplaces are recognizing the impact it has on productivity due to its victims disclosing and seeking support from coworkers and supervisors (MacGregor et al., 2016).

Disgruntled Employee/Coworker

A disgruntled employee or coworker is an individual who is dissatisfied with some aspects of the organization, such as the company culture, being overworked, their duties, their pay, or they may feel overlooked by a superior. These workers pose threats or actual violence to the workplace. The threats can manifest in the form of creating a hostile working environment for other employees or instigating legal issues through complaints that negatively impact the organization. Spector and colleagues (2014) and Park and colleagues (2015) suggest that most disgruntled employees who commit WPV, aggression, violence, and hostility exist within the job environment. Wressell and colleagues (2018) suggest that the presence of discriminatory actions can cause employees to become unethical and commit acts out of rage.

Explaining the Roots of WPV

WPV is not a new phenomenon. There are historical connections between work organizations and violence. Early aspects of WPV were present in England, France, and the Caribbean when enslaved African men and women received physical violence, most often in the form of corporal punishment, and psychological abuse while working. Enslaved women were beaten and raped. This violence was conducted by the slave owner, overseer, or public authority. Violence was used to ensure slaves worked and followed their master's conditions of work (Vidal, 2020). At times, this violence was met with resistance from the slaves. For example, it is well documented that female slaves who prepared their owner's food often poisoned the owner and his family. Other acts of resistance resulted in breaking tools or slowing down the work rhythm (Evans, 2019). WPV occurred during the 19th century in Great Britain and involved the beating of child workers by their masters to control them. The masters assumed that beating the children would keep factory work steady and regular in intensity (Pollard, 1965). Violence and bullying were the primary forms of disciplining workers during this era.

In the 20th century, Taft and Ross (1969) regarded the American picket line as the bloodiest form of physical violence during the 1960s, with striking workers preventing plants from reopening. Attempts by the police and National Guard to stop the strikes resulted in over 700 deaths during labor disputes and over 160 occasions in which state and federal troops had to intervene. WPV also occurred among postal workers during the 20th century. Ames (2009) suggests that governmental policy changes contributed to the stress of postal workers and may have caused them to kill and injure others. One such policy change was former President Richard Nixon's signing of the Postal Reorganization Act of 1970, which banned postal employees from striking. During the early 1970s, National Guardsmen were commissioned to deliver mail because postal employees were striking due to low wages; Congressmen had given themselves raises but ignored postal workers (Rudio, 2021). Other incidents that led to postal strikes and WPV for postal workers were business deregulations and limiting the power of unions by former President Reagan. These and other economic policies, initiated by the Reagan administration, resulted in postal workers losing health and pension benefits, which caused further stress.

One of the first events that brought public attention to accounts of what Laden and Schwartz (2000) regard as the "New Workplace Violence" (e.g., previously, the focus of danger to work centered on the environmental hazards of unsafe working conditions) occurred in the U.S. in August of 1986 when a part-time letter carrier, Patrick H. Sherrill, facing possible dismissal after a troubled work history, shot 14 people in an Edmond, Oklahoma, post office, where he was employed. This was not the first WPV incident. Three years earlier, in 1983, postal employees were killed by present and former coworkers in separate shootings in Johnston, South Carolina; Anniston, Alabama; and Atlanta, Georgia (Johnson & Indvik, 1996). The violence in Edmond raised public awareness of acts of WPV.

In 1990, a man whose vehicle had been repossessed in Jacksonville, Florida, went to the dealership with a gun and killed nine victims, injuring six before killing himself. In 1999, Mark Barton, a day trader in Atlanta, Georgia, who had experienced financial hardships, not only killed his wife and two children but also shot 21 colleagues, killing nine. Again, the early 1990s were marked by incidents of WPV among postal employees. In 1991, Joseph Harris, a former postal employee, shot and killed two former coworkers at the post office in Richwood, New Jersey, and the previous night murdered his former supervisor and shot her fiancé at her home. Also, in 1991, Thomas McIlvane, a fired postal worker, killed four postal supervisors and left five wounded before killing himself (Campbell, 2020). Campbell notes that due to the 1991 attacks, a congressional investigation was launched and concluded with a report that job-related stress was a contributing factor in the shootings. Recommendations derived from the congressional report were to have better training of supervisors and better pre-employment screenings of employees. Despite these recommendations, additional postal shootings continued in 1993 in Michigan and California.

Reports of WPV incidents have been further heightened by the media, and as a result, the first half of the 21st century has been plagued with accounts of WPV. However, these accounts did not involve the postal service. For example, Campbell (2020) provides an account of 2018, when a female shot and wounded three employees at the headquarters of YouTube. The female had posted videos on a site and had allegedly held grievances regarding YouTube's policies. In February 2019, a man shot and killed five employees at a manufacturing business in Illinois after being informed that he was terminated. This historical analysis not only displays the seriousness of WPV but also furthers the need for it to be adequately addressed.

What Are the Risk Factors of Workplace Violence?

Gurm et al. (2020) suggests that individuals who are at a high risk of engaging in WPV display violent histories, have threatening/intimidating behavior, exhibit excessive stress, have a negative personality, exhibit mood changes, are socially isolated, are obsessed with their job, and demonstrate drug or alcohol abuse. A study conducted by the Canadian Centre for Occupational Health and Safety (CCOHS, 2020) suggests that work-related factors increase the risk of violence. These factors include the following:

- Working with customers or the public.
- Handling money, valuables, or prescription drugs (e.g., cashiers, pharmacists, veterinarians).
- Carrying out inspection or enforcement duties (e.g., government employees).
- Providing service, care, advice, or education (e.g., healthcare staff, teachers).
- Working with unstable persons (e.g., social services or criminal justice system employees).
- Working where alcohol is served (e.g., food and beverage staff).
- Having a mobile workplace (e.g., taxicab, salesperson, public transit).
- Working during periods of intense organizational change (e.g., strikes, downsizing).

In addition, CCOHS suggests that the risk of violence may be greater during the night or early morning hours; during certain seasons (e.g., tax return/refund time or holidays when the demand for a service is high); during the weekends in establishments that serve alcohol; or during performance evaluations on jobs. In the following section, we will examine additional risk factors for WPV, which include the role of inequity, individual factors, relationship factors, and community factors.

Role of Inequity in WPV

Discrimination and racism are globally systemic and are ever-present in the workplace. Sabri and colleagues (2015) examined racial/ethnic differences in risk factors related to WPV exposure and utilization of resources among nurses employed in four large healthcare institutions in a mid-Atlantic metropolitan healthcare workplace. Participants in the study were White, Black, and Asian nursing employees (N=2033). One of the risk factors reported for WPV was one's ethnic minority status. The study found that of the victims of WPV, Blacks and Asians were approximately 51% less likely than Whites to use formal resources to address WPV (OR=0.48–0.49; 15% within groups). When compared to Whites, a larger percentage of respondents with Black and Asian backgrounds either did not know about or were uncertain about the employers' WPV policies and procedures. This could result from employers' and supervisors' failure to inform Black and Asian workers of the policies and procedures, thus making them more vulnerable to issues of WPV, and perhaps, increasing their vulnerability of being a victim of hate crimes. Similarly, a survey conducted on WPV by the Institute of Finance and Management (IOFM) (2013) revealed that more than one-third of the organizations surveyed became aware of employee conflict in which cultural/racial differences were either the primary or contributing cause of WPV. This included 42% of the companies with more than 10,000 employees.

Practices and policies that produce inequalities on the job can result in an environment in which some employees are given privileges, which can develop into power dynamics that lead to workplace or RV on the job (Grum et al., 2020). For example, practices in organizations that promote a White male as police chief, when a Black female has proven she has more experience and is better qualified, or organizational practices that abided by Affirmative Action Policies that promote a Black female as police chief because her race and gender help the organization meet its quota of hiring additional females and minorities. While the Civil Rights Act in the U.S. petitioned the courts and the federal government to obtain relief from discriminatory practices and treatment, Mor Barak (2014) suggests that all nations do not have adequate laws or policies to address discrimination in the workplace. This is concerning because countries that grant such protection do not always abide by those protections. The mistreatment of workers from marinized groups whether in the U.S. or globally is a problem, especially when such groups are already subjected to civil, human, and labor rights violations.

Individual Factors

Individual factors such as working alone or in isolated areas, such as a store clerk or in a reception area, can place an employee at risk of WPV. In addition, one's gender and age may also pose individual risk factors, especially due to women who are victimized by sexual harassment more than men in the workplace. One's marital status is an individual risk factor because it can be an indication of domestic or interpersonal violence in the home, which can be brought into the workplace. Paul and Townsend (1998, p. 2) indicate that "personality conflicts with peers and supervisors, personal financial and health problems, alcohol and drug abuse, the inability to solve personal and family problems, as well as racial and ethnic prejudices are individual factors that can cause workplace violence." Peek-Asa and colleagues (2021) conducted a study that supports Paul and Townsend's notion that stress and financial problems are indicators of WPV. Their study used data collected between the years of 2013 and 2017 from the CDC and the National Violent Death Reporting System to examine characteristics and circumstances associated with work compared with non-work suicides. Work-related suicides included those regarded as such on the death certificates, or those in which the investigation acknowledged a work problem/crisis. The study indicated that of the 84,389 suicides, 12.1% were related to the decedent's work. The risk factors associated with work-related suicides were financial problems and home evictions. Peek-Asa and colleagues further suggest that job-related factors for suicide risk can be associated with service in the military, healthcare fields, mining, farming, and construction. Moreover, they indicate that work stress, job loss, and job-related financial stress have been identified as suicide risk factors.

Relationship Factors

DV in the workplace is considered a relationship risk factor. DV can cause difficult/strained relationships with coworkers and employers due to abusers contacting their partners' coworkers or employers (Wathen et al, 2015; McFerren, 2011). Wathen and colleagues (2015) contend that when the abuser, and the partner, are employed in the same workplace, the abuser can cause psychological and at times physical harm in the form of monitoring and harassing the victim due to the proximity to the victim. Capaldi and colleagues (2012) conducted an extensive, systematic search of findings of studies of risk factors for IPV, which include engaging in crime, deprivation including unemployment and low income, exposure to family or parental violence, and child abuse. These factors bring about psychosocial risk factors and socio-environmental risk conditions that include poverty, homelessness, isolation, feelings of powerlessness, and stressful environments. It is plausible that these risk factors may be present in the work environment.

Community Factors

Strubelle and colleagues (2020) suggest that many community factors can lead to the risk of WPV. Communities adjust to social changes in their makeup. These changes may be present in the form of race or multiculturalism in neighborhoods and workplaces. Individuals living and working in established communities have had to adapt to changes in the status quo; for many the change may not be easy, and WPV may erupt. For example, when Blacks reside, and work in communities that have historically been predominately White, racial riots may ensue. Working in hazardous communities and working under hazardous conditions in substandard communities can pose a risk of WPV. Strubelle and colleagues suggest that in depressed socioeconomic communities that are drug-infested, healthcare workers are placed at risk of WPV due to exposure to drug trafficking. It is plausible that in socioeconomically depressed areas, which are rampant with crime, family breakdown, unemployment, poor-performing schools, welfare dependency, and general decay in communities that constitute social blight and produce stress, WPV is present.

Criminal Justice Issue

WPV is a criminal justice issue. WPV includes threats, verbal abuse, physical abuse, and homicide. Once an act of WPV is committed, it involves the collective expertise and experience of various law enforcement agencies, including local and state police, federal law enforcement, security specialists, and criminal investigators. At times, in the case of such acts as sexual harassment, attempted murder, or homicide, it will also involve lawyers, the court system, and the correctional system.

The violence that stems from WPV ranges from rape, murder, robbery, and assault against a person(s) which all constitute violations of the criminal law, and thus, the commission of a criminal act. Any act or threat of violence is a crime. Therefore, violence that occurs in the workplace is also a crime. Cases of WPV were presented in the previous section on "Roots of WPV" and each of these cases constituted a crime. Most of the cases involved either first-degree murder or attempted murder, and in almost every jurisdiction in the U.S., first-degree murder involves an unlawful killing of a human being, and it must be committed intentionally, and with planning. The U.S. has no federal law to address WPV because the U.S. Department of Justice (DOJ) addresses WPV through a policy statement that is revised every five years through a federal workplace response to DV, sexual assault, and stalking. Excerpts of the purpose and scope of the response are below Figure 12.1 (U.S. Department of Justice, 2023).

While there is no federal law to specifically address WPV, the Bureau of Justice Statistics (2022) reports there were a total of 454 homicides in 2019. These statistics further revealed that for deaths by homicide in the workplace between 2015 and 2019, shootings accounted for 1,813 or 79%; stabbing, cutting, slashing, and piercing accounted for 199 or 9%; hitting,

---

DOJ POLICY STATEMENT

PURPOSE: This policy statement aims to (a) enhance workplace awareness and capacity to create a safe work environment for employees and contractors who are victims of domestic violence, sexual assault, and stalking, and their co-workers; (b) develop policies and procedures to assist victims and to support co-workers who may also be impacted by domestic violence, sexual assault, and stalking; and (c) provide guidance on taking corrective and disciplinary action to address the conduct of workers who commit domestic violence sexual assault, or stalking in the workplace.

SCOPE: This policy statement applies to all Department of Justice (DOJ) employees, including full-time, part-time, temporary, and probationary employees, as well as interns, detainees, fellows, and volunteers in federal workplaces, as defined below. The policy statement applies to contractors where they are explicitly included or when they are defined as victims.

FIGURE 12.1   U.S. Department of Justice Policy Statement.

kicking, and beating accounted for 149 or 7%. Of the 1.3 million workplace nonfatal violent crimes that occurred between 2015 and 2019, these crimes included 53,000 rapes or sexual assaults, 46,000 robberies, 186,000 aggravated assaults, and 979,000 simple assaults per year. Simple assaults accounted for 77% of nonfatal WPV; violent crimes accounted for 23%; aggravated assaults accounted for 15%; and robberies accounted for 4%, during this period.

When examining IPV in the workplace, Laharnar and colleagues (2015) contend that while there is no federal employment protection law for IPV victims in the U.S., several states have been working to provide protection. They further report that almost all states have workplace anti-discrimination laws for crime victims, but only four states have laws specifically for IPV victims. This limited number of states with laws addressing IPV victims is due to supervisors receiving limited training regarding methods to implement the law, and few employees having awareness that the law exists (Laharnar et al., 2015). Peterson and colleagues (2018) suggest that IPV becomes a criminal justice issue due to the impact it places on society for criminal justice-related costs of court and confinement for the perpetrator.

In the absence of federal legislation, many states have enacted laws with procedural rules allowing employers to seek injunctive relief from state courts, preventing future violent acts or threats at the workplace. These laws prohibit access to the workplace by potentially violent people, thus helping employers protect employees, customers, guests, and property. However, these laws only apply in instances where the employer or employee has been threatened, or received threats of violence at the workplace, or while performing a work duty (Reuters, 2024).

Some state laws require public employers to develop and implement programs to prevent WPV, and other states have enacted laws specifically for healthcare employers due to their unique risk. There are provisions in these laws that apply to most employers. States with some of these provisions are Arizona, North Carolina, Texas, New York, Louisiana, Kentucky, Illinois, and Colorado (Reuters, 2024). The state of Washington prohibits "any physical assault or verbal threat of physical assault against an employee of a health care setting on the property of the health care setting." The state of Washington's legislation addresses physical assault or verbal threats of assault with a weapon, including a firearm, or any object used as a weapon. The law originated in 2020 and covers hospitals, home health, including hospice and homecare agencies; evaluation and treatment facilities; behavioral health programs; and ambulatory surgical facilities (Brigham, 2023).

Public Health Issue

As has been seen, WPV can occur in all sectors of employment and involves injuries or death to not only the immediate victims but also to bystanders who are either in direct observance of the violence or the violence is communicated to them from another source. WPV and the injuries/deaths that it causes have become a rising global public health concern. Of particular concern is the growing prevalence of WPV in the healthcare field. For example, Jones and colleagues (2023) and the U.S. Bureau of Labor Statistics (2018) suggest that workers in the healthcare and social services fields were five times more likely to sustain injuries from WPV than other professions. The Bureau reported in 2018 that 73% of nonfatal WPV injuries involved healthcare workers and that this percentage may be higher due to the underreported incidence of WPV.

WHO (2022) suggests that the COVID-19 pandemic appears to be responsible for the rise in violence against healthcare workers, which has brought on physical and mental health risks and occupational stress. La Regina and colleagues (2021) add that the violence against healthcare workers spilled over into social media and created new forms of hate crime and harassment. Lu and colleagues (2020) contend that in a meta-analysis of 47 observational studies, the prevalence of WPV against healthcare professionals was 62.4%, with 61.2% representing verbal abuse, which had the highest majority, followed by 50.8% representing psychological violence, 39.5% representing threats, 13.7% representing physical violence, and 6.3% representing harassment. WHO (2022) suggests that when there is a crisis, emergency, or disaster that involves large groups who are overwhelmed with panic attacks, shock, uncertainties, and fear, violence in healthcare facilities worsens.

As a result of these growing statistics, the APHA (2018) addressed letters to the U.S. Senate and the House Education and Labor Committee in support of a Workplace Violence Prevention for Health Care and Social Services Workers Bill. This bill was proposed because there was no federally enforceable violence prevention act specifically covering healthcare and social services providers working in public facilities; these workers, in most cases, become on "the scene" victims of the WPV for which they have been called to assist. The bill was intended to require hospitals, residential treatment facilities, clinics at correctional and detention facilities, substance use disorder treatment centers, and other service facilities to develop and implement a violence prevention plan and protection for whistle-blowers. It would also protect nurses, social workers, psychiatric home health personnel, personal care aides, social service workers, and others who are placed at risk of assault when performing their duties. However, the bill was introduced and passed by Congress but never passed the Senate. Therefore, healthcare and social services workers have been left without the additional protection this bill could have provided.

The rising incidence of WPV in hospitals has also led The Joint Commission (TJC) (2021) to develop new accreditation requirements to guide hospitals in the event of a WPV crisis. These requirements focus on the development of effective hospital WPV Prevention Plans that include an annual workplace analysis that addresses WPV safety and security risks. TJC expects workplace analysis and best practices to drive improvements, including a review of policies, procedures, training, and education. The new standards of accreditation specifically require hospitals to include sections on leadership oversight, policies and procedures, reporting systems, data collection and analysis, post-incident strategies, training, and education to decrease WPV. According to Lim and colleagues (2022), if WPV is not addressed, particularly in the healthcare system, it will become a global phenomenon, undermining the peace and stability among the active communities while also posing a risk to the population's health and well-being.

International Comparative Statistics

International organizations have also defined WPV. The American Organization of Nurse Executives (AONE, 2022) suggests that the International Labour Organization defines WPV as, "Any action, incident or behavior that departs from reasonable conduct in which a person is assaulted, threatened, harmed, injured in the course of, or as a direct result of, his or her work." AONE also suggests that the WHO defines WPV as "The intentional use of physical force or power, threatened or actual, against oneself, another person, or against a group, or community that either results in or has the likelihood of resulting in injury, death, psychological harm, maldevelopment or deprivation."

Per the global prevalence of WPV and harassment, the International Labour Organization (2022) in collaboration with ILO-Lloyd's Register Foundation-Gallup Survey found that Americans had the highest incident rate of WPV with 34.3%, followed by the continent of Africa with 25.7%, Europe and Central Asia with 25.5%, Asia and the Pacific with 19.2%, and Arab States with 13.6%. According to the data, countries with high incomes had the highest prevalence of WPV and harassment. Moreover, globally, 61.2% of the victims revealed that they had experienced WPV and harassment more than three times during their work experience (International Labour Organization, 2022).

In Canada, DV is viewed as the most rapidly growing type of WPV. Employers and workers often do not recognize DV as a workplace hazard, and they view it as a personal issue, which makes it difficult for a victim to seek help (Public Services Health and Safety Association, 2019). In addition, findings of the first large-scale Canadian research survey on the prevalence and impact of DV in the workplace revealed that of a total of 8,429 participants, who completed a survey regarding its impact, more than half (53.5%, n=1515) reported that DV continued at or near work in the form of abusive phone calls, or text messages, and negatively affected their work performance (Wathen et al., 2015). Surveys from the countries of the Philippines, Australia, Mongolia, Taiwan, and Belgium revealed similar findings (Fos-Tuvera, 2015; McFerran, 2011; Olszowy et al., 2017a, 2017b; Saxton et al., 2017). Victims from these surveys reported either receiving threats from the abuser to come to the workplace, having car keys hidden, abusers actually coming to the workplace, and being stalked and harassed at or near work (Fos-Tuvera, 2015; McFerran, 2011; Olszowy et al., 2017a; Wathen et al., 2015; Galvez et al., 2011; Saxton et al., 2017).

Police data, collected from the province of Saskatchewan, Canada in 2017, indicate IPV's national rate is 313 victims per 100,000 populations (Burczycka, 2018). Included in the data were 4,949 (rate of 1,099) female victims and 1,250 (rate of 272) male victims. Further findings revealed that the rate in Saskatchewan is over double the national average, with 682 victims per 100,000 populations. In addition to Canadians experiencing IPV in the workplace, they also experience RV. The Canadian Centre for Occupational Health and Safety (CCOHS) (2020) conducted a systematic review that found that RV impacts 61.9% of employees, with many of the cases being connected with harassment, sexual harassment, and physical violence.

An analysis of the legislation on harassment and violence in the workplace in other countries revealed that, in Canada, all jurisdictions have legislation specific to harassment and violence in the workplace (2020). On January 1, 2021, the Treasury Board Secretariat of Canada released a new policy, *Directive on the Prevention and Resolution of Workplace Harassment and Violence,* to keep employees safe from violence and harassment. This policy ensures that harassment and violence are not tolerated or ignored in federally regulated workplaces. The directive requires all federal departments to better prevent and respond to harassment; to provide support for employees who have been affected by it; and to investigate, record, and report all complaints. Table 12.1 presents Canada's main sources of violence and harassment legislation according to jurisdiction, and a summary of the elements of the legislation (Canadian Centre for Occupational Health and Safety [CCOHS], 2022).

Public Health and Social Work

Intersection of Public Health and Social Work

The intersection of public health and social work on WPV is a matter of concern for worker safety. On April 19, 2021, the House of Representatives passed H.R. 1195 *Workplace Violence Prevention for Health Care and Social Service Workers Act* (Library of Congress, n.d.a). The act was later introduced on April 18, 2023, to the 118th Congress referred to as S.1176 *Committee on Health, Education, Labor, and Pensions*, but the measure failed to receive a vote (Library of Congress, n.d.b). The act intended to "direct the Secretary of Labor to issue an occupational safety and health standard that requires employers within the health care and social service industries to develop and implement a comprehensive workplace violence prevention plan, and for other purposes" (Library of Congress, n.d.c). The act contained three key provisions: (1) the establishment of WPV prevention plans, (2) the provision of employee training and education on WPV prevention, and (3) the recordkeeping of risk assessments and violence events (American Hospital Association, 2021). Currently, there are no federal laws to keep healthcare and social service workers safe. Despite the lack of federal action, some states have created laws that require employers to implement workplace safety standards, but most states have amended laws that protect first responders and have added healthcare providers and nurses (American Nurses Enterprise, 2021).

Health Disparities and Health Equities

While all workplaces are susceptible to violence, health care and social work overwhelmingly carry the burden of WPV vulnerability. Healthcare and social service workers experienced the highest levels of WPV in 2018. In fact, approximately 76% of all reported WPV injuries occurred among healthcare and social service workers since they are five times more likely

TABLE 12.1 Main Sources of Violence or Harassment Legislation in Canada

Jurisdiction	Legislation	Elements (general summary)
Canada	*Canada Labour Code, Part II* Workplace Harassment and Violence Prevention Regulations	• Workplace assessment • Workplace policy • Training • Response and resolution process, including investigation • Program review • Annual report
British Columbia	Occupational Health and Safety Regulation, B.C. Reg. 296/ 97, Part 4, Sections 4.22 to 4.31	• Risk assessment • Procedures and policies • Instruction of workers • Additional requirements for late-night retail workplaces
Alberta	Occupational Health and Safety Code, 2009 Part 27 Violence and Harassment	• Violence prevention plan, policy, and procedures • Harassment prevention plan, policy, and procedures • Response and investigation • Includes domestic violence • Program review • Training • Additional requirements for workplaces such as gas stations, other retail fueling outlets, and convenience stores
Saskatchewan	*Saskatchewan Employment Act,* S.S. 2013, c. S-15.1 Section 3-21, Duty re policy statement on violence and prevention plan Occupational Health and Safety Regulations, 1996, R.R.S., c. O-1, r. 1 Section 3-25, Harassment Section 3-26, Violence Section 3-27, Safety measures for retail premises	• Violence policy statement and violence prevention plan at prescribed workplaces • Harassment prevention policy (e.g., reporting, privacy, and procedures) • Implementation of policies • Additional requirements for late-night retail premises
Manitoba	Workplace Safety and Health Regulation, Man. Reg. 217/ 2006 Part 10 Harassment Part 11 Violence	• Harassment prevention policy • Workplace assessment for violence • Violence prevention policy • Investigation and implementation of control measures • Annual report

(*Continued*)

TABLE 12.1 (Continued)

Jurisdiction	Legislation	Elements (general summary)
Ontario	*Occupational Health and Safety Act*, R.S.O. 1990, c. O.1 Part III .0.1, Violence and Harassment	• Violence and harassment prevention policies • Violence prevention program • Assessment of risks of violence • Domestic violence • Duties regarding violence (e.g., provide workers with information and instruction, privacy) • Harassment prevention program • Duties regarding harassment (e.g., investigation, and annual review) • Information and instruction regarding harassment
Quebec	Act respecting labour standards, CQLR c. N-1.1 Chapter IV, Division V.2 Psychological Harassment Chapter V, Division II.1 Recourse Against Psychological Harassment	• Psychological harassment prevention and complaint processing policy • Filing a psychological harassment complaint with the Commission, and the Commission's inquiry
New Brunswick	General Regulation, N.B. Reg. 91-191 Part XXII.I Violence and Harassment	• Assess risk of violence • Code of practice for violence • Code of practice for harassment • Implementation • Privacy • Training • Review and update
Nova Scotia	Violence in the Workplace Regulations, N.S. Reg. 209/2007	• Violence risk assessment • Prevention plan • Prevention statement • Provide information to employees • Training and supervision for employees • Duty to report violence incidents • Documentation, investigation, and actions to prevent reoccurrence • Debriefing individuals involved
Prince Edward Island	*Occupational Health and Safety Act* General Regulations, EC180/87 Part 52 Violence Workplace Harassment Regulation, EC710/19	• Risk assessment • Informing workers • Confidentiality • Policies, programs, and work environment arrangements to eliminate or minimize risk of violence • Policy to prevent and investigate harassment • Investigation of incidents

TABLE 12.1 (Continued)

Jurisdiction	Legislation	Elements (general summary)
Newfoundland and Labrador	Occupational Health and Safety Regulations, 2012, N.L.R. 5/12 Part III, Sections 22 to 24.2	• Risk assessment • Procedures, programs, and work environment arrangements to eliminate or minimize the risk of violence • Family violence • Instruction to workers • Harassment prevention plan • Training (harassment prevention)
Yukon	Occupational Health and Safety Regulations (in force September 2021)	• Hazard assessment • Policy statements and procedures for preventing violence and harassment • Worker training • Incident investigation • Domestic violence
Northwest Territories	Occupational Health and Safety Regulations, R-039-2015 Section 34 Harassment Section 35 Violence	• Harassment prevention policy • Violence prevention policy • Identify and eliminate or reduce risks • Procedure for receiving and responding to harassment or violence complaints • Training for preventing and responding to potentially violent situations • Additional requirements for late-night premises
Nunavut	Occupational Health and Safety Regulations, R-003-2016 Section 34 Harassment Section 35 Violence	• Harassment prevention policy • Violence prevention policy • Identify and eliminate or reduce risks • Procedure for receiving and responding to harassment or violence complaints • Training for preventing and responding to potentially violent situations • Additional requirements for late-night premises

Notes:
According to Grum (2020), British Columbia has passed further legislation that covers relationship violence in the workplace, access to a copy of this legislation can be found by accessing the information below:
Canadian Human Rights Act., R.S.C., 1985, c. H-6.
British Columbia Human Rights Code [RSBC 1996] CHAPTER 210.
British Columbia Laws Bill 14 – The Workers Compensation Act, R.S.B.C. 1996, c. 492.
The Occupational Health and Safety Policies for BC (WorkSafe BC, n.d.).

to be assaulted at work compared with the rest of the labor force (U.S. Bureau of Labor Statistics, 2020a). Moreover, statistics reveal that healthcare workers accounted for 73% of all nonfatal WPV-related injuries in 2018: the number of reports for 2018 was 15, 230, an increase from 8,180 in 2011. During this timeframe, experts report that the industries where healthcare and social service workers were employed, for those experiencing the highest rates of injury, included psychiatric and substance abuse hospitals, healthcare and social assistance, hospitals, nursing and residential care facilities, and social assistance (U.S.

Bureau of Labor Statistics, 2020b). The workers employed by these industries tend to suffer the mental and physical health inequities from WPV. For example, disparate impact on healthcare workers is revealed in multiple studies and reported in several industry surveys, such as the 2022 *ACEP emergency department violence poll* with emergency physicians (Marketing General Incorporated, 2022). More specifically, of the 2,712 respondents who participated in the poll, 55% reported being assaulted and 79% reported witnessing an assault. Of those assaulted, 33% were injured. Because of that injury, 87% reported loss of productivity, 85% experienced emotional trauma and increased anxiety, 84% reported having less focus, 53% incurred physical harm, and 60% went on leave without being treated. In addition, 85% had been threatened with future harm. Of all healthcare providers, nurses reported being at a significantly higher risk of experiencing physical assault and verbal abuse compared with physicians (Cheung et al., 2018). In fact, nearly half of the nurses (53%) responding to the Minnesota Nurses Association (2022) survey reported they considered leaving the nursing profession owing to the fear of having violent encounters at work. Others, including social workers, have also expressed concerns for their personal safety. According to Whitiker and colleagues (2006), as early as 2004, an estimated 44% of 10,000 licensed clinical social workers reported having trepidations over safety concerns at work (Whitiker et al., 2006).

Research literature shows that healthcare workers who experience WPV were at a greater risk compared with other industry workers for developing higher levels of post-traumatic stress disorder (PTSD) symptoms including avoidance, intrusion, and hyperarousal (Chowdhury et al., 2023). Some health experts report that among health and social service providers, WPV take its largest toll by manifesting in the form of burnout and burnout symptomology. The literature is replete with studies that conclude nurses who experience WPV face a significantly higher risk of developing burnout syndrome that causes emotional exhaustion, depersonalization, and feelings of low professional accomplishment (Cao et al., 2022; Converso et al., 2021; Grinberg et al., 2022; Tsukamoto et al., 2022). In fact, one study revealed that 70% of 2,061 healthcare worker experienced moderate to high burnout due to WPV (Cao et al., 2022). Similarly, social worker burnout is also significant given that the nature of the work often places employees in potentially dangerous situations during encounters in child protective services, with persons experiencing mental health crises, and in healthcare settings, client homes, and in the community (National Association of Social Workers, 2022; Radey et al., 2024).

Negative Health Consequences of WPV

WPV causes mental disorders, which is supported by the evidence that exposure to very severe psychological trauma of a catastrophic nature may result in severe psychological disorders, such as PTSD (Utzon-Frank et al., 2014). Work-related violence is often prolonged or repeated, which may contribute to increased risk of mental disorders (Pihl-thingvad et al., 2019). Likewise, Bensiom (1994) asserted that stress produces WPV; accordingly, stress brings about a traumatic experience (e.g., a single major event or a smaller series of events), which creates a perception of an altered psychic state that has not been resolved, thus producing chronic anxiety. The traumatized individual blames the situation for his state of mind and begins to think only of himself without regard for others (e.g., the individual only seeks self-protection) and views violence as the only way out. This assessment is similar to Ames' (2009) earlier assessment of the postal shootings. (i.e., stress, anxiety, hypertension, stroke, and suicide).

Likewise, in the public health field, Sun and colleagues (2017) and Yang and colleagues (2018) suggest that there is a link between WPV and a reduced quality of life as well as stress, low self-esteem, and increased anxiety. Individuals and organizations suffer from WPV in many ways. These may include concerns for personal safety, coworker relationships, job insecurity, fear, lowered job performance, job satisfaction, commitment to the job, and the intent to leave the job which all bring about such health issues as psychological distress, emotional exhaustion, depression, increased anxiety, stress, physical well-being, interpersonal deviance, and organizational deviance (Piquero et al., 2013; Alexander, 2011). Similarly, Lanctôt and Guay (2014) identify the physical, emotional, and psychological illnesses, but also add PTSD as a health consequence of WPV.

Wathen and colleagues (2015) and McFerran (2011) suggest that victims who experience DV in the workplace may suffer physical and mental exhaustion from being restrained by their abuser. Futures Without Violence (2017) contends that, on average, two women in the U.S. are killed at work every month by an intimate partner. Health consequences of IPV that can spill over into the workplace include depression, substance abuse, chronic pain, gastrointestinal issues, physical injuries, and suicide (Sugg, 2015). It appears that the leading health consequence for victims of WPV is stress, which brings on anxiety, hypertension, stroke, and depression.

Criminal Justice Approaches

The DOJ views DV, sexual assault, and stalking as serious issues that affect individuals, families, and the community, and as such, the impact of the violence can be present in the workplace. The existing policy of the DOJ does not tolerate violence, threats, harassment, intimidation, or other disruptive behaviors that may be present in the workplace. Under the DOJ policy, services offered to victims of DV, sexual assault, and stalking that occur in the workplace are the following:

- *Responding to Employees and Enhancing Workplace Safety.* This offers and provides timely workplace support to employees to address WPV. This also covers an employee who is conducting work while traveling.
- *Protection and Restraining Orders.* This is offered to employees who are victims who disclose an existing protection or restraining order to department management to assist in the enforcement of the order in the workplace.
- *Non-Discrimination and Non-Retaliation.* The department's Equal Employment Opportunity policy may apply to circumstances of domestic or dating violence, sexual assault, or stalking in the workplace. As such, the Equal Employment Opportunity Policy describes the actions employees and managers should take. Actions for employees include such items as telling the harasser that the behavior is unwelcome and must cease immediately, reporting the behavior to the supervisor, seeking support from a colleague, keeping written documentation, discussing options with an Equal Employment Counselor, and filing a complaint. Actions for managers include setting an example by their own

conduct; making sure employees are not involved in harassment; communicating the policy on harassment to employees; making it clear that claims of harassment will be investigated immediately; and assuring employees that complaints will be treated seriously and fairly.
- *Victim Autonomy, Confidentiality, and Recordkeeping.* The Privacy Act of 1974 prohibits the DOJ from disclosing employee information without written consent from the employee. Therefore, DOJ staff must abide by the safe storage, retention, dissemination, and disposal of records.
- *Reporting by Employee Victims.* Any concern of DV, sexual assault, or stalking in the workplace should be brought to the attention of the employee's supervisor, their human resources officer, or someone identified by management to address such allegations.
- *Reporting by Contractor Victims.* Reports should be made to the contracting officer or the contracting officer's representative, who will work with their component's human resource office, security, and legal teams to address any issues by a contractor working in a DOJ workplace.

The policy also outlines the roles and responsibilities of the heads of components: resources, referrals, and points of contact for victims; safety planning; workplace flexibility for employees; workplace awareness and outreach; training; and monitoring and evaluating department responses. Included in the policy is a "Justice Management Division and Office on Violence Against Women" program, which is responsible for coordinating training and providing resources on DV, sexual assault, and stalking.

Although the federal policy exists with its services to the victims, local, state, and federal law enforcement agencies, along with emergency management personnel, are usually the first to respond to crises and engage in direct combat during instances of WPV. The role of law enforcement is to protect and serve by diffusing difficult situations. Most law enforcement officers use a diversion program known as the Crisis Intervention Team (CIT) model to interact with individuals with mental, emotional, or developmental challenges (Rogers et al., 2019). Officers are trained to notice the signs and symptoms of mental illnesses as well as types of mental health treatment needed; co-occurring disorders; legal issues the situation may involve; and the de-escalation techniques to use. Officers are also trained to determine if the perpetrator should be referred for additional services or transported to a mental health facility (Watson & Fulambarker, 2012).

Public Health Approaches

According to the CDC (2024), the public health approach to WPV is a multidisciplinary approach that provides the maximum benefit for the greatest number of individuals. It is a scientific method that is based on disciplines including the fields of medicine, epidemiology, sociology, psychology, criminology, education, and economics, which allow it to respond to a range of global public health issues. It also has input from such sectors as justice, social services, policy, and the private sector, which assist in addressing issues of violence. The public health approach is a four-step approach that consists of the following:

- Step 1: Define and Monitor the Problem
  The first step in preventing violence is understanding the "who," "what," "when," "where," and "how" associated with it. Obtaining the magnitude of the problem involves analysing data such as the number of violence-related behaviors, injuries, and

deaths. Data inform individuals of how frequently violence occurs, where it occurs, trends, and who the victims and perpetrators are. This data can be obtained from police reports, medical examiner files, vital records, hospital charts, registries, population-based surveys, and other sources.

- Step 2: Identify Risk and Protective Factors
What is important in this step is understanding what factors protect people or put them at risk for experiencing or perpetrating violence. Risk and protective factors help identify where prevention efforts need to be focused.
- Step 3: Develop and Test Prevention Strategies
Information revealed from the research literature and data from needs assessments, community surveys, key collaborator interviews, and focus groups is useful for designing prevention strategies. Using these data and findings is known as an evidence-based approach to program planning. Once prevention strategies are developed or existing strategies are identified, they are then evaluated to determine their effectiveness.
- Step 4: Assure Widespread Adoption
The strategies shown to be effective in step three are then implemented and adopted more broadly. Communities are encouraged to implement strategies based on the best available evidence and to continuously assess whether the strategy is a good fit with the community context and achieving its goal of preventing violence. Dissemination techniques to promote widespread adoption include training, networking, technical assistance, and evaluation.

This approach can be applied to WPV and other health issues that confront populations (CDC, 2024).

Public Health and Social Work Approaches

A viable approach that is recommended to prevent WPV is the four-step model used in public health to address all forms of violence that affect the health of the population. As such, it should be effective when targeting WPV. It recommends the following: (1) define and monitor the problem, (2) identify risk and protective factors, (3) develop and test prevention strategies, and (4) assure widespread adoption (CDC, 2024). In reaction to the increase in violence against healthcare workers, the *American Journal of Public Health* published several studies on violence and its effect on healthcare workers in 2022. There were several recommendations made, which include the following:

- Creating a national WPV reporting system for quantifying and describing the WPV (Ward et al., 2022),
- Training public health workers on responding to political conflict and improving support networks Ward et al., 2022; Yeager, 2022),
- Investing in the public health workforce, including funding, increased staffing, and better safety protections (Doucette et al., 2022; Ward et al., 2022),
- Establishing increased workplace communication after a WPV incident, including reporting the event to a designated official (Jeong & Kim, 2018).

The National Institute for Occupational Safety and Health (NIOSH) is part of the CDC. Both healthcare workers and social workers have benefited from NIOSH's Healthcare and Social Assistance Program created to "eliminate occupational diseases, injuries, and fatalities and optimize workers' health and well-being in healthcare and social assistance industries" (NIOSH, 2024). Among the aims of the program are identifying interventions that improve "work organization, safety culture, and well-being" to reduce "workplace stress, depression, anxiety, burnout, substance use disorders, and suicides," and reduce violence-related injuries. The social worker profession takes safety seriously and advocates that workers avoid making home visits alone, prevent visiting with clients in unpredictable circumstances and environments, acquire background information on clients they are meeting, be aware of potential violence warning signs when performing home visits, report incidences of violence when seeing or experiencing them, take a self-defense class, and be vigilant in not letting their guard down (Mustafa, n.d.).

The National Association of Social Workers (2013) has established standards for social worker safety in the workplace. The standards are guidelines for providing direction for developing agency policies and practices to improve worker safety. There are 11 standards:

Standard 1.   Organizational Culture of Safety and Security
Standard 2.   Prevention
Standard 3.   Office Safety
Standard 4.   Use of Safety Technology
Standard 5.   Use of Mobile Phones
Standard 6.   Risk Assessment for Field Visits
Standard 7.   Transporting Clients
Standard 8.   Comprehensive Reporting Practices
Standard 9.   Post-Incident Reporting and Response
Standard 10. Safety Training
Standard 11. Student Safety

While social workers acknowledge that client interaction is the cornerstone of practice, they also concede that some social work settings (e.g., child welfare, adult protective services, mental health, criminal justice, DV situations) present opportunities for violence. These guidelines are meant to support social workers in practice while not stereotyping any client population social workers serve.

Integrating Skills of Social Epidemiology to Address Disparities and Achieve Equity

Social epidemiology examines the patterns of social determinants of health and provides powerful systems approaches to population health. Individuals living and working in socioeconomically disadvantaged communities often suffer from environmental stressors, relationship issues, and gender and racial discrimination. At times, these stressors can lead to moments of aggression and rage, which in some cases spill over into the work environment, which is often filled with workplace injustices, particularly for socially disadvantaged individuals. Okechukwu and colleagues (2014) assert that workplace injustices are workplace-related discrimination, harassment, abuse, or bullying that occurs on the job or through interpersonal relationships. To address disparities and achieve equity, the Institute of Finance and Management (IOFM) suggests that to prevent racial and cultural differences from escalating into violence in the workplace, organizations can undertake the following actions (2013):

- Provide diversity training for supervisors, which includes threats based on race and ethnicity.
- Aggressively address complaints and threats of racial harassment.
- Appoint different WPV team members to represent different worker population groups and liaison with them.
- Track, analyse, and investigate all incidents/complaints of racial/ethnic harassment and bullying for any suggestions of discrimination. Diversity training should be provided for all employees.

To alleviate the disparities associated with WPV and promote safe and healthy environments, the Social-Ecological Model can be used (Smith et al., 2020). This model has four levels that influence violence and the intervention for promoting safe and healthy environments:

- *The Individual Level* examines such factors as an individual's biological and personal history, which may influence the risk of being a victim or perpetrator. Strategies of intervention at this level promote a person's attitudes, beliefs, and behaviors that prevent violence. Specific approaches to prevent violence may include conflict resolution and life skills training, social–emotional learning, and safe dating and healthy relationship skill programs (CDC, 2018).
- *The Relationship Level* examines interpersonal relationships that influence one's behavior and contribute to one being a victim or perpetrator of violence. Interventions at this level promote healthy, interpersonal relationships through using such strategies as conflict resolution, effective communication, and mentoring.
- *The Community Level* examines workplaces, schools, communities, and places where social relationships occur. Interventions include specific policies, resources, and environments that support healthy relationships. According to the CDC (2018), prevention strategies at this level focus on improving the physical and social environment by creating safe places where people live, learn, work, and play. This level also addresses other conditions that give rise to violence in communities (e.g., neighborhood poverty, residential segregation, instability, and high density of alcohol outlets).
- *The Societal Level* examines how societal and cultural norms, policies, and resources influence violence. The CDC (2018) suggests prevention strategies at this level should include efforts to promote societal norms that protect against violence as well as efforts to strengthen household financial security, education and employment opportunities, and other policies that affect the structural determinants of health.

The Department of Justice, through its Community Relations Service (CRS), is another program to address disparities and achieve equity. This program provides consultation, facilitation, mediation, and training services that improve communities' abilities to solve problems and build capacity to prevent and respond to disputes, conflicts, hate crimes, and incidents of violence. CRS is referred to as "America's Peacemaker," and services are provided confidentially and free of charge throughout localities in the U.S. The programs are designed to strengthen community and law enforcement partnerships. The goal of all CRS programs and services is to promote and restore peaceful relations among communities. These programs assist communities with learning about best practices for dispute resolution, obtaining available resources, and identifying and implementing solutions. CRS programs are tailored to a specific audience or setting (U.S. Department of Justice, 2025). All approaches in this section can be used by researchers, policymakers, health professionals, and community leaders to identify and address disparities that contribute to violence as a public health issue.

How Can WPV be Prevented?

CDC emphasizes input from the health, education, social services, justice, policy, and private sectors in addressing and preventing violence. Just as there are various categories of WPV, there are also various methods proposed to mitigate WPV. The IOFM (2013) questioned whether organizations having a policy on bullying and harassment in the workplace were enough to prevent WPV and suggest that organizations need to have more than just a policy to adequately address the issue. IOFM suggested the following recommendations for preventing bullying/harassment in the workplace:

- Educating employees as to unacceptable bullying/harassment behavior,
- Conducting tracking to identify trends and problem areas,
- Providing employees with a place to report the behavior other than the supervisor,
- Assessing how well management deals with employee discord,
- Regularly surveying employees or conducting focus groups to determine the prevalence of risk factors for bullying/harassment,
- In employee exit interviews, the supervisor should ask about workplace tensions and conflicts and investigate any incidents thoroughly and discipline employees according to organizational policy.

The CDC (2020), through the National Institute for Occupational Health (NIOSH), proposes dos and don'ts for employees to prevent WPV. These actions and non-actions include the following:

- Do attend all employer-provided training on how to recognize, avoid, and respond to potentially violent situations.
- Do report perceived threats or acts of violence to a manager or supervisor, following any existing policies that may be in place.
- Do remain aware of and support coworkers and customers if a threatening or violent situation occurs.
- Do not argue with a customer if they make threats or become violent. If needed, go to a safe area, ideally, a room that locks from the inside; use a second exit route; and have a phone or silent alarm.
- Do not attempt to force anyone who appears upset or violent.

To prevent WPV, American Nursing Association (2016) developed violence prevention guidelines based on industry's best practices. These guidelines provide recommendations for developing policies and procedures to eliminate or reduce WPV in a range of healthcare and social service settings. While there is no specific federal law that addresses WPV nor legislation requiring agencies to implement a plan, OSHA suggests that an effective approach for reducing WPV risk is for an organization to have a written prevention program. OSHA's Workplace Violence Prevention Plan states, "A comprehensive organizational violence prevention program should include a reporting and documentation system for acts of violence and a workplace violence prevention policy that includes specific strategies that can be instituted system-wide in the event of a violent incident, as well as post-event support and adequate training of personnel for pre- and post-event incident management" (U.S. Department of Labor Occupational Safety and Health Administration, 2022). Moreover, OSHA suggests that an effective WPV prevention program includes the following:

- *Management Commitment and Employee Participation.* Involved in this step is the complete support and visible involvement of all levels of management in promoting a WPV program. This includes the following:

  1 Allocating appropriate authority and resources to all responsible parties so that there is access to information, personnel, time, training, tools, or equipment.
  2 Assigning responsibility and authority to the various aspects of the WPV prevention program to ensure that all managers and supervisors understand their obligations.
  3 Maintaining a system of accountability for managers, supervisors, and workers.
  4 Supporting and implementing appropriate recommendations from the safety and health committees established by the agency.
  5 Establishing a comprehensive program of medical and psychological counseling and debriefing for workers who have experienced or witnessed assaults and other violent incidents, and ensuring that trauma-informed care is available.
  6 Establishing policies that ensure the reporting, recording, and monitoring of incidents and near misses and that no retaliation is made against anyone who does so in good faith. Workers can be involved by offering feedback as to the workplace policy prevention program; participating in the program's design, implementation, and evaluation; identifying activities that place workers at risk for WPV; and ensuring there is a way to report incidents.

- *Worksite Analysis and Hazard Identification.* This involves taking a step-by-step assessment of the workplace. This is conducted by the employer and employee to find existing or potential hazards that may lead to incidents of WPV. Those conducting the worksite analysis should inspect the workplace from time to time and evaluate the workers' tasks to identify hazardous conditions, operations, and situations that may lead to potential violence. To provide a different perspective and strengthen the program, advice may be solicited from health professionals, law enforcement, security specialists, and insurance safety auditors.
- *Hazard Prevention and Control.* After the worksite has been analysed, the employer should take steps to prevent or control the identified hazards. The employer should (1) identify and evaluate control options for workplace hazards; (2) select effective and feasible controls to eliminate or reduce hazards; (3) implement these controls in the workplace; (4) follow up to confirm that these controls are being used and maintained

properly; and (5) evaluate the effectiveness of controls and improve, expand, or update them as needed.

- *Safety and Health Training.* Primary elements of a workforce protection plan are training and education for all employees, including mid- and upper-level supervisors. Such programs help to ensure the employees that the organization is safe and that staff members are cognizant of potential hazards and how to protect themselves and their colleagues through established policies and procedures. This training includes de-escalation techniques. The purpose of training is to (1) help raise the overall safety and health knowledge across the workforce, (2) provide employees with the tools needed to identify workplace safety and security hazards, and (3) address potential problems before they arise and ultimately reduce the likelihood of workers being assaulted. There are various training topics, which may include the management of assaultive behavior, professional/police assault-response training, or personal safety training on how to prevent and avoid assaults. Training for supervisors and managers should involve recognizing high-risk situations and ensuring that workers are not placed in assignments that compromise their safety. Supervisors should train workers to report incidents and seek appropriate care after experiencing an incident. This training, according to OSHA, will reduce or eliminate WPV. A yearly evaluation of all training should be conducted and should involve supervisors and employee interviews, testing, observing, and reviewing reports of behavior of individuals involved in threatening situations.
- *Recordkeeping and program evaluation.* This is the final step in reducing or eliminating WPV and is done to determine the training's overall effectiveness and to identify any deficiencies so that changes can be made. It also involves the organization keeping proper records of injuries, assaults, patient histories, training, and incidents; these entities aid employers in determining the severity of the problem; identifying any developing trends or patterns in particular locations, jobs, or departments; evaluating methods of hazard control; and identifying training needs and developing solutions for an effective program.

According to OSHA (U.S. Department of Labor Occupational Health and Safety Administration, 2016), for those developing a WPV prevention program, it is always noteworthy to check applicable state requirements due to some states passing legislation and developing requirements for WPV. However, the guidelines and standards, especially the guidelines of OSHA, appear applicable to any organization that has incidents of WPV and either reduce or prevent such situations from occurring only if employees, management, employers, public health workers, and social service workers adhere to them. In addition, employers should ensure that, if an incident of WPV occurs, post-incident procedures and services are in place and immediately made available.

Policy Recommendations

WPV is a significant occupational issue for which the public, the media, regulatory and administrative agencies, legislative bodies, health care and social services, including law enforcement, continue to be confronted with. As was seen in the previous section, several methods have been proposed to prevent WPV, but there remains work to be done to reduce or eradicate it, especially for agencies that do not have violence-specific measures or reporting mechanisms in place, which can make it difficult to obtain comparable data on violence-related injuries. These agencies may be operating under violence prevention standards that are not research-based, thus leading to hazardous working conditions due to limited reliable resources for preventing and reducing WPV toward employers, employees, customers, clients, patients, and the public at large. In addition to OSHA's guidelines, what is needed is for employers to display leadership by providing a safe working environment with zero tolerance for violence and ensuring that those who commit WPV are held criminally accountable.

The recommended changes in legislation per the state and federal government are twofold. First, the "DOJ Policy Statement: Federal Workplace Responses to Domestic Violence, Sexual Assault, and Stalking" should be revised so that it's provisions have clear statements on all aspects of WPV in the federal government and not just address the issue of WPV through clauses on DV, sexual assault, and stalking. This policy should also address harassment, threats, bullying, IPV, violence among coworkers, and disgruntled worker violence. Second, the federal government should enact mandatory legislation in each state not only for the crime of WPV, but also for specific acts or types of WPV. The federal government should make it binding on states to ensure that all employees have the same access to protection and support; fines should also be imposed on employers who violate any part of this legislation (2013).

Employers should increase public awareness of all aspects of WPV. This can be done by formulating and implementing a WPV prevention plan (WVPP), which has a zero tolerance for WPV. This plan should be customized to fit the needs of the organization and should

1. Create/revise policies and procedures that support all employees as well as those who may be impacted by violent acts.
2. Require employees to participate in the formulation/revision of the plan; this ensures employee participation merely because they have assisted in either the plan's formulation/revision.
3. Ensure that the employer and top-level management promote awareness of WPV through the dissemination of information and the development of focus groups.
4. Require mandatory training sessions and workshops for employees at all levels of the organization. These training sessions should entail topics on recognizing signs and risk behaviors of violence; providing an effective response and sources of referral (such as information on a DV agency) for victims; diversity training; violence de-escalation tactics; active shooter training; and hostage situation training.
5. Provide information on instituting a workplace response plan along with the development of a response team to manage violent situations. This team would include healthcare and social services personnel who are on staff. If the organization cannot afford to hire a team, employees should be trained to provide temporary assistance until health care and social services arrive.
6. Require the employer to install doors that lock from the inside, closed-circuit cameras that are monitored by either law enforcement or security personnel, and panic buttons located in offices, breakrooms, restrooms, etc.
7. Assessing and evaluating incidents of violence stemming from employees, coworkers, patients, and visitors to determine the root cause of the violence and trend patterns.

8. Request a background check on all employees to determine if arrests or incidents involving violence have occurred.
9. Require all employees to evaluate and make additional recommendations yearly regarding the WVPP.

Agencies that follow these recommendations, as well as OSHA's guidelines, should see reductions in violence in the workplace. In addition to these recommendations, the APHA (2018) recommends that all agencies be involved and held accountable for preventing violence and the health effects it causes. Therefore, health sectors, schools, universities, nonprofit organizations, and the criminal justice system should share data on all forms of violence, identify protocols for screenings and referrals, develop and enhance programs and policies to prevent and reduce violence, and use available data to increase the efficiency and effectiveness of these efforts. Lim (2022) suggests WPV needs to be addressed more comprehensively, involving shared responsibilities from all levels. These include (1) government legislations; (2) the support of healthcare managers with clearly defined policies, reporting procedures, and training; (3) the healthcare workers' and social services agencies commitment to update their awareness and knowledge regarding WPV; and (4) the provision of technical support and assistance from professional organizations and the community.

Summary

Additional research on WPV needs to take place. While there seems to be a wealth of contemporary literature on WPV in the health sector, little can be found in other areas. A major challenge for employers has been controlling the impact of WPV and causing fear, stress, and uncertainty among employees. WPV continues to pose a serious problem that negatively affects the health of those directly involved, as well as those who may be coworkers, clients, or observe the aftermath through the media or other sources. On a global level, it may be helpful to advocate for a broader global conceptualization of WPV, which will promote greater awareness, understanding, and inclusiveness among employers, employees, public health officials, the criminal justice system, researchers, and policymakers. Moreover, it is the responsibility of governments, politicians, employers, and unions to create regulations that protect employees from WPV.

Discussion Questions

1. Discuss how the term "Going Postal" may have originated.
2. Discuss the definitions of workplace violence and how they differ. What definition, in your opinion, is more comprehensive for agencies?
3. Discuss the health consequences associated with workplace violence.
4. You were given a case scenario at the beginning of this chapter about John and workplace violence. Discuss and identify the type(s) of workplace violence presented in the scenario.
5. Discuss the prevalence of WPV in contemporary society.
6. Discuss the approaches you would use to prevent WPV.

References

Adewumi, O., & Danesi, R. (2017). Gender: A vulnerability factor or not? Exploring and investigating workplace bullying in Nigeria. *Journal of Economics, Business and Management*, 5(10), 324–330. https://doi.org/10.18178/joebm.2017.5.10.533

Alexander, P.C. (2011). Childhood maltreatment, intimate partner violence, work interference and women's employment. *Journal of Family Violence*, 26(4), 255–261. https://doi.org/10.1007/s10 896-011-9361-9

American Hospital Association. (2021). *House passes workplace violence prevention bill*. Legislation Update. www.aha.org/news/headline/2021-04-16-house-passes-workplace-violence-preventionb ill#:~:text=Apr%2016%2C%202021%20%2D%2002:,OSHA%20standards%20required%20 by%20H.R.

American Nurses Enterprise. (2021). *Workplace violence*. www.nursingworld.org/practice-policy/ advocacy/state/workplace-violence2/#:~:text=There%20is%20variation%20between%20sta tes,is%20limited%20to%20public%20employers

American Nursing Association. (2016). OSHA standards needed to prevent workplace violence.

American Organization of Nurse Executive. (2022). *Toolkit for mitigating violence in the workplace*. AONL-ENA_workplace_toolkit.pdf

American Public Health Association. (2018, November 13). "Violence is a public health issue: Public health is essential to understanding and treating violence in the U.S." Policy Number: 20185.

Ames, M. (2009, November 7). Going postal. *The Daily Beast*, www.thedailybeast.com/articles/2009/ 11/07/going-postal.html. Accessed February 27, 2017.

Arnetz, J., Hamblin, L.E., Sudan, S., & Arnetz, B. (2018). Organizational determinants of workplace violence against hospital workers. *Journal of Occupational and Environmental Medicine*, 60(8), Article 693.

Ball, J., & Pike, G. (2006). *At breaking point: A survey of the wellbeing and working lives of nurses in 2005*. Royal College of Nursing. [Google Scholar]

Barling, J., Dupré, K.E., & Kelloway, E.K. (2009). Predicting workplace aggression and violence. *Annual Review of Psychology*, 60(1), 671–692. https://doi.org/10.1146/annurev.psych.60.110 707.163629

Benismon, H. (1994, January). Violence in the workplace. *Training and Development*, 48, 27–32.

Breiding, M.J., Basile, K.C., Smith, S.G., Black, M.C., & Mahendra, R.R. (2015). *Intimate partner violence surveillance: Uniform definitions and recommended data elements, version 2.0*. National Center for Injury Prevention and Control, Centers for Disease Control and Prevention.

Bringham, G. (2023). Essentials for healthcare workplace violence prevention. *The Washington Nurse*, 53(2), 54–59. 6p. Spring/Summer 2023.

Burczycka, M. (2018). Family violence in Canada: A statistical profile. Section 2: Police-report intimate partner violence in Canada, 2018.

Campbell, J. (2020). *Workplace violence*. Salem Press Encyclopedia.

Canadian Centre for Occupational Health and Safety (CCOHS). (2020). Violence in the workplace. www.ccohs.ca/oshanswers/psychosocial/violence.html

Canadian Centre for Occupational Health and Safety (CCOHS). (2022). *Violence and harassment in the workplace*. www.ccohs.ca/oshanswers/psychosocial/violence/violence_legislation

Cao, Y., Gao, L., Fan, L., Jiao, M., Li, Y., & Ma, Y. (2022). The influence of emotional intelligence on job burnout of healthcare workers and mediating role of workplace violence: A cross-sectional study. *Frontiers in Public Health*, 10, 892421. https://doi.org/10.3389/fpubh.2022.892421

Capaldi, D., Knoble, N., Shortt, J., & Kim, H. (2012). A systematic review of risk factors for intimate partner violence. Partner Abuse The Partner Abuse State of Knowledge Project: Part 1 Vol 3 Issue 2, https://doi.org/10.1891/1946-6560.3.2.231

Caring for our Caregivers-Preventing Workplace Violence: A Road Map for Healthcare Facilities. Occupational Safety and Health Administration. (December 2015). https://oshce.uw.edu/sites/defa ult/files/documents/Caring%20for%20Caregivers%20Report.pdfAccessed November 9, 2018.

Centers for Disease Control and Prevention (CDC). (2018). *Violence prevention: The social-ecological model: A framework for prevention [Internet].* Centers for Disease Control and Prevention (US); Available from: www.cdc.gov/violenceprevention/publichealthissue/social-ecologicalmodel.html [Google Scholar]

Centers for Disease Control and Prevention (CDC). (2020). *Basic dos and don'ts for employees to prevent workplace violence.* National Institute for Occupational Safety and Health. https://stacks.cdc.gov/view/cdc/92425/cdc_92425_DS1.pdf

Centers for Disease Control and Prevention (CDC). (2024). *About the Public Health Approach to Violence Prevention.* www.cdc.gov/violence-prevention/about/about-the-public-health-approach-to-violence-prevention.html.

Cheung, T., Lee, P.H., & Yip, P.S.F. (2018). The association between workplace violence and physicians' and nurses' job satisfaction in Macau. *PLoS One, 13*(12), e0207577. https://doi.org/10.1371/journal.pone.0207577.

Chowdhury, S.R., Kabir, H., Das, D.C., Chowdhury, Hossain, A. (2023). Workplace violence against Bangladeshi registered nurses: A survey following a year of the COVID-19 pandemic. *International Nursing Review, 70*(2), 219–228. doi:10.1111/inr.12802.

Converso, D., Sottimano, I., & Balducci, C. (2021). Violence exposure and burnout in healthcare sector: Mediating role of work ability. *Medicina Del Lavoro, 112*(1), 58–67. https://doi.org/10.23749/mdl.v112i1.9906.

Cooper, J.R., Walker, J., Askew, R., Robinson, J.C., & McNair, M. (2011). Students' perceptions of bullying behaviours by nursing faculty. *Issues in Educational Research, 21*(1), 1–21.

Duan, X., Ni, X., Shi, L., Zhang, L., Ye, Y., Mu, H., Li, Z., Liu, X., Fan, L., & Wang, Y. (2019). The impact of workplace violence on job satisfaction, job burnout, and turnover intention: The mediating role of social support. *Health and Quality of Life Outcomes, 17*(1), 93–93. https://doi.org/10.1186/s12955-019-1164-3

Doucette, M.L., Surber, S.J., Bulzacchelli, M.T., Dal, B.C., Santo, C., & Crifasi, K. (2022). Nonfatal violence involving days away from work following California's 2017 workplace violence prevention in health care safety standard. *American Journal of Public Health, 112*(11), 1668–1675. https://doi.org/10.2105/AJPH.2022.307029

Evans, B. (2019). *Histories of violence. Slavery in America.* Los Angeles Review of Books. (lareviewofbooks.org)

Fos-Tuvera, A.L. (2015). Key findings of national survey on the impact of domestic violence on workers and in workplaces in the Philippines: Joint ITUC-AP/Philippine Aliates' report. Retrieved from http://dvatworknet.org/sites/dvatworknet.org/files/Philippine_Domestic_Violence_survey_key%20findings_September%202015.pdf

Fute, M., Mengesha, Z.B., Wakgari, N., Tessema, G.A. (2015). High prevalence of workplace violence among nurses working at public health facilities in Southern Ethiopia. *BMC Nursing, 14*(1), Article 9. https://doi.org/10.1186/s12912-015-0062-1

Futures Without Violence. (2017). Futures without violence unveils re-designed workplaces respond website. Futures without Violence. Retrieved from www.futureswithoutviolence.org/futures-without-violence-workplaces-respond-website/

Galvez, G., Mankowski, E.S., McGlade, M.S., Ruiz, M.E., & Glass, N. (2011). Work-related intimate partner violence among employed immigrants from Mexico. *Psychol Men Masculin, 12,* 230–246. [Google Scholar]

Giesbrecht, C.J. (2022). Toward an effective workplace response to intimate partner violence. *Journal of Interpersonal Violence, 37*(3–4), 1158–1178.

Grinberg, K., Revach, C., & Lipsman, G. (2022). Violence in hospitals and burnout among nursing staff. *International Emergency Nursing, 65,* 101230. https://doi.org/10.1016/j.ienj.2022.101230

Gurm, B., Salgado, G., Marchbank, J., & Early, S.D. (2020). *Making sense of a global pandemic: Relationship violence & working together towards a violence free society.* Kwantlen Polytechnic University. Ebook ISBN 978-1-989864-14-2 or Print ISBN 978-1-989864-13-5. https://kpu.pressbooks.pub/nevr/

Harrell, E., Langton, L., Petosa, J., Pegula, S., Zak, M., Derk, S., Hartley, D., & Reichard, A. (2022). *Indicators of workplace violence, 2019 (NCJ 250748; NIOSH 2022-124)*. Bureau of Justice Statistics, Office of Justice Programs, U.S. Department of Justice; Bureau of Labor Statistics, Office of Safety, Health, and Working Conditions, U.S. Department of Labor; and National Institute for Occupational Safety and Health, Centers for Disease Control and Prevention, U.S. Department of Health and Human.

Institute of Finance and Management (IOFM). (2013). *How will you stem the tide of workplace incivility (And Worse)?* Issue 13-05 p. 7. www.IOFM.Com/Security

International Labour Organization. (2022). *Experiences of violence and harassment at work: A global first survey*. ILO. https://doi.org/10.54394/IOAX8567 workplace violence/harassment at work/sexual harassment 13.04.5

Jeong, I., & Kim, J. (2018). The relationship between intention to leave the hospital and coping methods of emergency nurses after workplace violence. *Journal of Clinical Nursing*, 27(7–8), 1692–1701. https://doi.org/10.1111/jocn.14228.

Johnson, P.R. & Indvik, J. (1996). Stress and violence in the workplace. *Employee Counseling Today*, 8(1), 19–24.

Jones, C.B., Sousane, Z., Mossburg, S.E. (2023). Addressing workplace violence and creating a safer workplace. *Patient Safety Network*. https://psnet.ahrq.gov/perspective/addressing-workplace-violence-and-creating-safer-workplace#5

La Regina, M., Mancini, A., Falli, F., Fineschi, V., Ramacciati, N., Frati, P.,& Tartaglia, R. (2021). Aggression on social networks: What are the implications for healthcare providers? An exploratory research. *Healthcare (Basel)*, 9(7), 811. https://doi.org/10.3390/healthcare9070811.PMID:34203141;PMCID: PMC8304147

Laden, V.A., & Schwartz, G. (2000). Psychiatric disabilities, the Americans with Disabilities Act, and the new workplace violence account. *Berkeley Journal of Employment and Labor Law*, 21(1), 246.

Laharnar, N., Perrin, N., Hanson, G., Anger, W.K., & Glass, N. (2015). Workplace domestic violence leave laws: Implementation, use, implications. *International Journal of Workplace Health Management*, 8(2), 109–128. https://doi.org/10.1108/IJWHM-03-2014-0006

Lanctôt, N., & Guay, S. (2014). The aftermath of workplace violence among healthcare workers: A systematic literature review of the consequences. *Aggression and Violent Behavior*, 19(5), 492–501. https://doi.org/10.1016/j.avb.2014.07.010

Library of Congress. (n.d.a). H.R.1195 – Workplace *violence* prevention for Health Care and Social Service Workers Act. Congress.com. www.congress.gov/bill/117th-congress/house-bill/1195/text

Library of Congress. (n.d.b). S.1176 – Workplace *violence* prevention for Health Care and Social Service Workers Act. Congress.gov. www.congress.gov/bill/118th-congress/senate-bill/1176/all-actions.

Library of Congress. (n.d.c). S.1176 – Workplace *violence* prevention for Health Care and Social Service Workers Act. Congress.gov. www.congress.gov/bill/118th-congress/senate-bill/1176/text#:~:text=Introduced%20in%20Senate%20(04/18/2023)&text=To%20direct%20the%20Secretary%20of,plan%2C%20and%20for%20other%20purposes.&text=A%20BILL-,To%20direct%20the%20Secretary%20of%20Labor%2

Lim, M.C., Jeffree, M.S., Saupin, S.S., Giloi, N., & Lukman, K.A. (2022, May 13). Workplace violence in healthcare settings: The risk factors, implications and collaborative prevention measures. *Annals of Medicine and Surgery (London)*, 78, 103727. https://doi.org/10.1016/j.amsu.2022.103727. PMID:35734684;PMCID:PMC9206999

Livingston, B., Delavier, L., & Benaden, Y. (2021, February 24). Intimate partner violence is a workplace issue. *Harvard Business Review*. https://hbr.org/2021/02/intimate-partner-violence-9s-a-workplace-issue

Lu, L., Dong, M., bin Wang, S., Zhang, L., Ng, C.H., Ungvari, G.S., Li, J., & Xiang, Y.T. (2020). Prevalence of workplace violence against health-care professionals in China: A comprehensive meta-analysis of observational surveys. *Trauma Violence Abuse*, 21, 498–509. https://doi.org/10.1177/1524838018774429

MacGregor, J.C.D., Wathen, C.N., Olszowy, L.P., Saxton, M.D., & MacQuarrie, B.J. (2016). Gender differences in workplace disclosure and supports for domestic violence: Results of a Pan-Canadian Survey. *Violence and Victims*, 31(6), 1135–1154. https://doi.org/10.1891/0886-6708.VV-D-15-00078 [PubMed] [CrossRef] [Google Scholar]

MacQuarnie, B., MacPherson, M., Olszowy, L., Saxton, M. (2020*). Domestic violence and homicide in the workplace.* In P. Jaffe, K. Scott, A. Straatman (Eds.), *Preventing Domestic Homicides* (pp. 209-231). Academic Press.

Marketing General Incorporated. (2022). 2022 ACEP *emergency department violence poll results.* Marketing General Incorporated. www.emergencyphysicians.org/siteassets/emphysicians/all-pdfs/acep-emergency-department-violence-report-2022-abridged.pdf.

McFerran, L., & National Domestic Violence and the Workplace Survey. (2011). *Australia: Australian Domestic and Family Violence Clearinghouse, Australian Government; 201 (1) (PDF) The Impact of Domestic Violence in the Workplace: Results f*rom a Pan-Canadian Survey. Available from: www.researchgate.net/publication/279863879_The_Impact_of_Domestic_Violence_in_the_Workplace_Results_From_a_Pan-Canadian_Survey [accessed Apr 29 2024].

Minnesota Nurses Association. (2022). Keeping *n*urses at the *b*edside *a*ct. https://mnnurses.org/issues-advocacy/issues/top-legislative-issues/2023-legislative-session-recap/keeping-nurses-at-the-bedside-act/

Mor Barak, M.E. (2014). *Managing diversity; Toward a globally inclusive workplace* (3rd edition). Sage.

Mustafa, Y. (n.d.). 10 Safety tips for social workers: Importance of personal safety training for social workers. ROAR. www.roarforgood.com/blog/safety-tips-for-social-workers/

National Association of Social Workers. (2013). Guidelines for social worker safety in the workplace. www.socialworkers.org/Practice/NASW-Practice-Standards-Guidelines/Guidelines-for-Social-Worker-Safety-in-the-Workplace

National Association of Social Workers. (2022). *Protecting social workers and health professionals from workplace violence act (S. 4412/H.R. 8492). Issue Brief.* www.socialworkers.org/Advocacy/Policy-Issues/Social-Worker-Safety#:~:text=Addressing%20this%20growing%20epidemic%20of,mental%20health%20and%20health%20workforce

National Institute for Occupational Safety and Health. (2024). Healthcare and *s*ocial *a*ssistance *p*rogram. www.cdc.gov/niosh/research-programs/portfolio/hcsa.html.

Occupational Safety and Health Administration (OSHA). (2015). *Preventing workplace violence: A road map for healthcare facilities.* https://osha.washington.edu/sites/default/files/documents/Caring%20for%20Caregivers%20Report.pdf

Olszowy, L., Saxton, M.D., & MacQuarrie, B.J. (2017a). *National results survey on the impact of domestic violence on work, workers and workplaces in Taiwan: Joint CFL and ITUC-AP report.* Centre for Research & Education on Violence against Women and Children, London, ON. Retrieved from http://dvatworknet.org/sites/dvatworknet.org/files/dvatwork-taiwanese-surveyresults.pdf

Olszowy, L., Saxton, M.D., & MacQuarrie, B.J. (2017b). *National results survey on the impact of domestic violence on work, workers and workplaces in Mongolia: Joint CFL and ITUC-AP report.* Centre for Research & Education on Violence against Women and Children, London, ON. Retrieved from http://dvatworknet.org/sites/dvatworknet.org/files/dvatwork-taiwanese-surveyresults.pdf

Okechukwu, C.A., Souza, K., Davis, K.D., & de Castro, A.B. (2014). Discrimination, harassment, abuse, and bullying in the workplace: Contribution of workplace injustice to occupational health disparities. *American Journal of Industrial Medicine*, 57(5), 573-586. https://doi.org/10.1002/ajim.22221

Ontario Domestic Violence Death Review Committee (DVDRC). (2017). *Domestic Violence Death Review Committee 2016 annual report.* Office of the Chief Coroner.

Park, M., Cho, S.-H., & Hong, H.-J. (2015). Prevalence and perpetrators of workplace violence by nursing unit and the relationship between violence and the perceived work environment. *Journal of Nursing Scholarship*, 47(1), 87–95.

Paul, R., and Townsend, J. (1998). Violence in the workplace—A review with recommendations. *Employee Responsibilities and Rights Journal*, 11(1), 1–14.

Peek-Asa, C., Casteel, C., Rugala, E., Romanoa, S., & Ramirez, M. (2013). Workplace violence investigations and activation of the threat management team in a multinational corporation. *Journal of Occupational and Environmental Medicine*, 75(5), 870–876.

Peek-Asa, C., Zhang, L., Hamann, C., Davis, J., & Schwab-Reese, L. (2021, September 10). Characteristics and circumstances associated with work-related suicides from the National Violent Death Reporting System, 2013-2017. *International Journal of Environmental Research and Public Health*, 18(18), 9538. https://doi.org/10.3390/ijerph18189538. PMID: 34574474; PMCID: PMC8465410.

Peterson, C., Kearns, M.C., McIntosh, W.L., Estefan, L.F., Nicolaidis, C., McCollister, K.E., ... & Florence, C. (2018). Lifetime economic burden of intimate partner violence among U.S. adults. *American Journal of Preventive Medicine*, 55(4), 433–444. https://doi.org/10.1016/j.ame pre.2018.04.049 [PMC free article] [PubMed] [CrossRef] [Google Scholar]

Pihl-Thingvad, J., Andersen, L.L., Brandt, L.P., & Elklit, A. (2019, October). Are frequency and severity of workplace violence etiologic factors of posttraumatic stress disorder? A 1-year prospective study of 1,763 social educators. *Journal of Occupational Health Psychology*, 24(5), 543–555. https://doi.org/10.1037/ocp0000148

Pinkerton Consulting and Investigations. (2002). *Fortune*.

Piquero, N.L., Piquero, A.R., Craig, J.M., & Clipper, S.J. (2013). Assessing research on workplace violence, 2000–2012. *Aggression and Violent Behavior*, 18(3), 383–394. https://doi.org/10.1016/j.avb.2013.03.001

Pollard, S. (1965). *The genesis of modern management: A study of the Industrial Revolution in Great Britain*. Edward Arnold. Retrieved from http://dvatworknet.org/sites/dvatworknet.org/files/dvatwork-belgium-surveyresults-Sept18-2017.pdf

Public Services Health and Safety Association. (2019). *Addressing domestic violence in the workplace: A handbook for the workplace*. www.pshsa.ca

Radey, M., & Wilke, D. (2024). Client violence and emotional health among child protection services workers. *Occupational Health Science*. https://doi.org/10.1007/s41542-024-00212-z

Reuters, T. (2024). *Workplace violence prevention state laws: Overview*. Practical Law. https://anzlaw.thomsonreuters.com/w-041-9020?

Rogers, M.S., McNiel, D.E., & Binder, R.L. (2019, September). Effectiveness of police Crisis Intervention Training Programs. *Journal of the American Academy of Psychiatry and the Law Online*, JAAPL.003863-19; https://doi.org/10.29158/JAAPL.003863-19

Rubio, P.F. (2021). Unintended consequences: The U.S. Postal Service conundrum of service, business, labor, and politics. *Journal of Employment Responsible Rights*, 33, 125–141. https://doi.org/10.1007/s10672-021-09368-0

Sabri, B., St. Vil, N.M., Campbell, J.C., Fitzgerald, S., Kub, J., & Agnew, J. (2015, February). Racial and ethnic differences in factors related to workplace violence victimization. *Western Journal of Nursing Research*, 37(2), 180–196. https://doi.org/10.1177/0193945914527177. Epub 2014 Mar 20. PMID: 24658287; PMCID: PMC4169764.

Saxton, M.D., Olszowy, L., & MacQuarrie, B.J. (2017). *National Survey results on the impact of domestic violence on work, workers and workplaces in Belgium: Joint UWO and IEWM Report*. Centre for Research & Education on Violence Against Women and Children, London, ON.

Scott, K.L., Lim, D.M., Kelly, T., Holmes, M., MacQuarrie, B.J., Wathen, C.N., & MacGregor, J.C.D. (2017). *Domestic violence at the workplace: Investigating the impact of domestic violence perpetration on workers and workplaces*. University of Toronto. Retrieved from http://dvatworknet.org/sites/dvatworknet.org/files/PAR_Partner_report-Oct-23-2017dl.pdf

Showalter, K. (2016). Women's employment and domestic violence: A review of the literature. *Aggression and Violent Behavior*, 31, 37–47. https://doi.org/10.1016/j.avb.2016.06.017

Smith, C.R., Palazzo, S.J., Grubb, P.L., & Gillespie, G.L. (2020). Standing up against workplace bullying behavior: Recommendations from newly licensed nurses. *Journal of Nursing Education and Practice*. 10(7), 35. https://doi.org/10.5430/jnep.v10n7p35. PMID: 34136059; PMCID: PMC8205445

Spector, P.E., Zhou, Z.E., & Che, X.X. (2014). Nurse exposure to physical and nonphysical violence, bullying, and sexual harassment: A quantitative review. *International Journal of Nursing Studies*, 51(1), 72–84.

Strubelle, I., Pai, D., Tavares, J.P., de Trindade, L.L., Beck, C., & De Matos, V.Z. (2020).Workplace violence types in family health offenders, reactions, and problems experienced. *Revista Brasileira de Enfermagem*, 73(1), e2019005.

Sugg, N. (2015). Intimate partner violence: prevalence, health consequences, and intervention. *Medical Clinics of North America*, 99(3), 629–649. https://doi.org/10.1016/j.mcna.2015.01.012. Epub 2015 Mar 6. PMID: 25841604.

Sun, T., Gao, L., Li, F., Shi, Y., Xie, F., Wang, J., Wang, S., Zhang, S., Liu, W., Duan, X., Liu, X., Zhang, Z., Li, L., & Fan, L. (2017, December 7). Workplace violence, psychological stress, sleep quality and subjective health in Chinese doctors: A large cross-sectional study. *BMJ Open*. 2017;7(12), e017182. https://doi.org/10.1136/bmjopen-2017-017182. PMID: 29222134; PMCID: PMC5728267.

Swanberg, J.E., Logan, T., & Macke, C. (2005). Intimate partner violence, employment, and the workplace. *Trauma Violence Abuse*, 6, 286–312.

Taft, P., & Ross, P. (1969). Chapter 8: American labor violence: Its causes, character, and outcome. In *Violence in America: Historical and comparative perspectives* (pp. 281–395). Bantam Books.

The Joint Commission (TJC). (2021). *Workplace violence prevention standards.* www.jointcommiss ion.org/standards/r3-report/r3-report-issue-30-workplace-violence-prevention-standards

Tiesman, H.M., Hendricks, S., Konda, S., & Hartley, D. (2014). Physical assaults among education workers: Findings from a statewide study. *Journal of Occupational and Environmental Medicine*, 56(6), 621–627. https://doi.org/10.1097/JOM.0000000000000147

Tiesman, H.M., Hendricks, S., Wiegand, D.M., Lopes-Cardozo, B., Rao, C.Y., Horter, L., Rose, C.E., & Byrkit, R. (2022). Workplace violence and the mental health of public health workers during COVID-19. *American Journal of Preventive Medicine*, 64, 315–325.

Tsukamoto, S.A.S., Galdino, M.J.Q., Barreto, M.F.C., & Martins, J.T. (2022). Burnout syndrome and workplace violence among nursing staff: A cross-sectional study. *São Paulo Medical Journal*, 140(1), 101–107. https://doi.org/10.1590/1516-3180.2021.0068.R1.31052021

U.S. Bureau of Labor Statistics. (2016). Economic news release: Census of fatal occupational injuries.

United States Bureau of Labor Statistics. (2020). Injuries, illness, and fatalities. www.bls.gov/iif/fac tsheets/workplace-violence-healthcare-2018-chart1-data.htm

Utzon-Frank, N., Breinegaard, N., Bertelsen, M., Borritz, M., Eller, N.H., Nordentoft, M., Olesen, K., Rod, N.H., Rugulies, R., & Bonde, J.P. (2014). Occurrence of delayed-onset post-traumatic stress disorder: A systematic review and meta-analysis of prospective studies. *Scandinavian Journal of Work, Environment & Health*, 1, 40(3), 215–229. https://doi.org/10.5271/sjweh.3420

U.S. Department of Justice (2023). Chapter 2852.222-70 DOJ policy statement: Domestic violence, sexual assault, and stalking.

U.S. Department of Justice, Bureau of Justice Statistics. (2022, July). *Indicators of workplace violence, 2019.*

U.S. Department of Labor, Bureau of Labor Statistics (2013). *"Injuries, illnesses, and fatalities", Census of Fatal Occupational Injuries Charts, 1992-2011 (revised data).* Available at: www.bls. gov/iif/oshwc/cfoi/cfch0010.pdf

U.S. Department of Labor. (2024). *DOL.* www.dol.gov/agencies/oasam/centers-offices/human-resour ces-center/polices/workplace-violence-program

U.S. Department of Labor. Bureau of Labor Statistics. (2018). *Workplace violence in healthcare, 2018.* www.bls.gov/iif/factsheets/workplace-violence-healthcare-2018.htm

U.S. Department of Labor Occupational Health and Safety Administration. (2016). Prevention of workplace violence in healthcare and social assistance. 88147-88167.

U.S. Department of Labor Statistics. (2022). *Census of fatal occupational injuries for Year 2022.*

U.S. Department of Labor Occupational Safety and Health Administration. (2002a). *Workplace violence.* OSHA fact sheet.

U.S. Department of Labor Occupational Safety and Health Administration. (2022b). Guidelines for preventing workplace violence for healthcare and social service workers. 5–30.

Vidal, C. (2020). Violence, slavery and race in early English and French America. In: R. Anthony, S. Caroll, & C.D. Pennock (Eds.), *The Cambridge world history of violence* (pp. 36–54). Cambridge Press.

Violence Project. (2023, April 11). *Workplaces are the most common mass shooting sites, data shows.* National Institute of Justice. https.//abc11.com/Workplaces- are- the- most- common -mass-shooting- sites- data- shows/131138071/ ABC11 Raleigh-Durham

Ward, J.A., Stone, E.M., Mui, P., & Resnick, B. (2022). Pandemic-related workplace violence and its impact on public health officials, March 2020-January 2021. *American Journal of Public Health (1971)*, 112(5), 736–746. https://doi.org/10.2105/AJPH.2021.306649

Wathen, C.N., MacGregor, J.C., & MacQuarrie, B.J. (2015, July). The impact of domestic violence in the workplace: Results from a Pan-Canadian Survey. *Journal of Occupational and Environmental Medicine,*57(7), e65–e71. https://doi.org/10.1097/JOM.0000000000000499 PMID: 26147553; PMCID: PMC4676385.

Watson, A.C., & Fulambarker, A.J. (2012). The crisis intervention team model of police response to mental health crises: A primer for mental health practitioners. *Best Practices in Mental Health: An International Journal,* 8(2), 71–81.

Węziak-Białowolska, D., Białowolski, P., & McNeely, E. (2020). The impact of workplace harassment and domestic violence on work outcomes in the developing world. *World Development*, 126, 104732–110742. https://doi.org/10.1016/j.worlddev.2019.104732

Whitaker, T., Weismiller, T., & Clark, E. (2006). *Assuring the sufficiency of a frontline workforce: Executive summary.* National Association of Social Workers. www.socialworkers.org/LinkClick.aspx?fileticket=ESTCCZA4HAE%3d&portalid=0.

Wilkinson, C.W. (2001). Violence prevention at work: A business perspective. *American Journal of Preventive Medicine*, 20(2), 155–160. www.ajpmonline.org/article/S0749-3797(00)00292-0/pdf. Accessed November 9, 2018

World Health Organization (WHO). (2002). *World report on violence and health: Summary..*

World Health Organization (WHO). (2022). *Preventing violence against health workers.* WHO. Available at: www.who.int/activities/preventing-violence-against-health-workers

WorkSafeBC. (2024). *Domestic violence in the workplace.* www.worksafebc.com/en/health-safety/hazards-exposures/violence/domestic-violence

Wressell, J.A., Rasmussen, B., & Driscoll, A. (2018). Exploring the workplace violence risk profile for remote area nurses and the impact of organisational culture and risk management strategy. *Collegian*, 25(6), 601–606. https://doi.org/10.1016/j.colegn.2018.10.005

Yang, B.X., Stone, T.E., Petrini, M.A., & Morris, D.L. (2018). Incidence, type, related factors, and effect of workplace violence on mental health nurses: A cross-sectional survey. *Archives of Psychiatric Nursing*, 32(1), 31–38. https://doi.org/10.1016/j.apnu.2017.09.013.Return to ref 4 in article.

Yeager, V.A. (2022). The politicization of public health and the impact on health officials and the workforce: Charting a path forward. *American Journal of Public Health*, 112(5), 734–735. https://doi.org/10.2105/AJPH.2022.306744

13

FIREARM INJURIES AND PUBLIC HEALTH

Introduction

Six-year-old Nicole and her classmate Sidney are sitting at the kitchen table completing their homework when Nicole's 4-year-old brother Bryson enters the kitchen with his mother's gun. Bryson fires a shot, fatally hitting Sidney in the chest. When questioned as to where he found the gun, Bryson replied, "Under his mother's bed." Bryson's mother is charged with homicide. The usage of firearms is increasingly becoming a serious issue of concern in the U.S. Firearm use has ranged from firearm-related injuries from children having access to guns; the recent assassination attempt of President Donald Trump; mass shootings in schools, workplaces, and shopping malls; to drive-by shootings in neighborhoods which have resulted in either injury or death. Although firearm-related injury rates are difficult to measure due to challenges with collecting national injury data, studies by Kaufman and colleagues (2021) and Fowler and colleagues (2015) suggest that there are at least twice as many nonfatal firearm injuries as fatal firearm injuries.

Firearm Injuries Defined

Fowler and colleagues (2015) suggest that abstractor-coded data reveal that most nonfatal firearm injuries treated in emergency departments are the result of assaults, followed by unintentional injuries. The Centers for Disease Control and Prevention (CDC) (2024) suggests that "a firearm injury is a wound or penetrating injury from a weapon that uses a powder charge to fire a projectile. Weapons that use a powder charge include handguns, rifles, and shotguns." The CDC further argues that firearm injuries can be fatal or nonfatal and can include the following:

- Intentional/self-inflicted injuries such as suicide or nonfatal self-harm.
- Unintentional injuries, which can be fatal or nonfatal and occur while cleaning or playing with a firearm or other incidents of an accidental firing without evidence of intentional harm.

DOI: 10.4324/9781003373001-13

- Interpersonal violence, which occurs during a homicide or nonfatal assault injury.
- Legal intervention when an injury is inflicted by law enforcement agents acting in the line of duty.
- Undetermined intent, which occurs when there is not enough information to determine whether the injury was intentionally self-inflicted, unintentional, the result of legal intervention, or from an act of interpersonal violence.

Individuals own firearms for various reasons, which include protection, settling disputes, and engaging in violence. Others do not own them because they are viewed as the source of accidents. Injuries from firearms have a global effect on the health and safety of individuals and can impact any age, gender, race, or ethnicity. In 2022, the CDC reported that there were more than 48,000 firearm-related deaths in the U.S. according to mortality data. This was almost equivalent to 132 deaths daily from a firearm injury. Half of the firearm-related deaths were suicides, and more than four out of every ten were firearm homicides.

Nature and Extent of Firearm Injuries

Firearm injuries have resulted in mental and physical disabilities and death. In the U.S., firearm injuries are the leading cause of death among children and adolescents, surpassing motor vehicle crashes, cancer, drug overdose, and poisoning. Lee and colleagues (2022) argue that in 2020, firearms resulted in 10,197 deaths for individuals (youth) between 0 and 24 years of age. Similarly, Goldstick and colleagues (2022) suggest that more than 4,600 deaths of individuals under the age of 19 were due to gun violence in 2022. In comparing the rate of firearms deaths in the U.S. with other countries, Grinshteyn and Hemenway (2021) examined data for 2015 and discovered that 7,241 youth in the U.S. were killed by firearms compared with 685 youth in all other high-income countries combined. Cunningham and colleagues (2018) state that the U.S. has the highest rate of deaths by firearms in children and youth when compared with other high-income countries.

According to CDC (n.d.) data, nearly 500 people die each year from unintentional gun deaths. In 2019, 486 Americans died from unintentional firearm injuries. This is about 1.2% of total gun deaths. Unintentional shootings can be self-inflicted or inflicted by someone else. The Johns Hopkins Center for Gun Violence Solutions (2020) cites a 2002 study by Miller and Hemmingway, which found that children between the ages of 5 and 14 were more likely to die from unintentional gun injuries if they lived in states where guns are more prevalent. The Center further noted a 2016 study by Kalsen and colleagues, which found that a 2013 survey revealed that in New York, 10.3% of the adult population owns guns, while 48.9% of the adult population in Alabama owns guns; Alabama's unintentional firearm death rate is 48 times that of New York.

Bleyer and colleagues (2024) conducted polling that reveals that the majority of the public and the major political parties view mental health disorders as the cause of the high U.S. firearm death rate. Their study found that firearm deaths by suicide increased by 18% from the previous decade, and gun deaths by homicide increased by 39% since 2000. These researchers' study points to a different correlation; firearm deaths by suicide increased 18% over the past decade, and gun deaths by homicide increased 39% since 2000. They concluded that while the U.S. represents 4% of the world's population, 25% of the world's firearms are in U.S. households, as well as half of the world's non-military assault weapons. According to Bleyer and colleagues, this percentage is increasing.

Further examination about the nature and extent of firearm-related deaths between 2019 and 2020 show that the firearm homicide rate increased by approximately, 35% and the firearm suicide rate remained high with the largest increase in homicide rates being seen among Blacks (39%) and the largest increase in firearm suicides, (42%) occurring among American Indians and Alaskan natives. The year 2020 revealed that 79% of all homicides and 53% of all suicides involved a firearm (CDC, 2022). Data released by the CDC regarding firearm-related injuries for the year 2020 indicated that such injuries also constituted a major cause of death from unintentional injuries. The data show that there were 45, 222 firearm-related deaths in the U.S. in 2020, thus reaching a new peak (health. gov/news/202212/firearm-safety-and-public-health).

The CDC suggests that the COVID-19 pandemic brought about an increase in firearm homicide and suicide rates for some groups. In 2020, Black people had the highest rates of firearm homicide. The CDC argues that stressors during the Covid pandemic such as: changes to services and the disruption of education; mental and economic stressors such as difficulty covering expenses, job loss, and instability in housing; and social isolation may have led to the increase in firearm homicide rates for Black persons (CDC, 2022). This may have also impacted the rate for other persons of color.

The Surgeon General Advisory (Office of the U.S. Surgeon General, 2024) cited the results of a survey by Schumacher and colleagues, which examined the experiences of gun-related violence, injuries, and death among Americans. The study comprised 1,271 respondents and found that most of the adults or their family members (54%) had experienced a firearm-related incident. An examination of all respondents revealed that 21% had been personally threatened with a firearm, 19% had a family member who was killed by a firearm (including by suicide), 17% had witnessed a shooting, 4% had shot a firearm in self-defense, and 4% had been injured by a firearm. Moreover, almost six in ten adults stated that they worry "sometimes," "almost every day," or "every day," about a loved one becoming a victim of firearm violence.

Types of Firearm Injuries

Just as there are many types of firearm injuries, there are many circumstances and contexts in which those injuries occur. For example, those circumstances and categories can consist of firearm injuries as a result of a tool in the commission of a crime; random shootings; school shootings; mass shootings; homicides; and accidental deaths. These circumstances/ categories are explained below:

- *A Tool in the Commission of Crime*: Firearms can be used to commit a crime. For example, to assist in the commission of an armed robbery or kidnapping. Research indicates that most nonfatal firearm injuries treated in emergency departments are deemed to be a result of assaults, followed by unintentional injuries (Fowler et al., 2015).
- *Random Shootings*: Incidents where individuals are shot without there being a specific target or motive.
- *School Shootings*: Involves shootings in educational institutions, and students, staff, and faculty are shot. An example is the shooting at Apalachee High School in Georgia.

- *Mass Shootings*: The shooting of multiple victims at a public event. An example is a shooting at a concert that kills multiple people. Data published by Pierce (2024) revealed that the U.S. experienced more than 600 mass shooting incidents each year between 2020–2023, compared to an average of less than 400 annual mass shooting incidents between 2015 and 2018. As of September 4, 2024, there were 385 mass shootings in the U.S.
- *Homicides*: The intentional killing of one person by another with a firearm; for example, murder for hire.
- *Accidental Deaths*: The unintentional discharge of a firearm that results in fatalities, often due to negligence or mishandling. An example is someone cleaning a gun and unaware that it is loaded and accidentally killing someone in the path of the bullet.

Mass shootings, school shootings, and homicides appear to be on the rise daily in the U.S. The history, culture, and socioeconomic structure that exist in the U.S., with its roots in poverty and racism, often have led to violent acts, which have culminated with a firearm.

Explaining the Roots of Firearms

Firearms have been around for centuries in the U.S. as well as in other nations. One can conclude from the existence of the first colonial and state gun laws that guns existed in the U.S. as early as the year 1607. Firearms appear to have been ingrained in the U.S. culture. The ratification of the U.S. Constitution and the Bill of Rights granted U.S. citizens the right to bear arms. According to the Second Amendment, "A well-regulated Militia, being necessary to the security of a free State, the right of the people to keep and bear Arms, shall not be infringed." The wording of this Amendment was adopted from the constitution of the original 13 state constitutions, and to date is the centerpiece of much debate as to who has the right to bear arms; that is, was this right a collective or individual right?

Historians estimate that the origins of firearms, gunpowder, or black powder were discovered in China during 850 A.D. and were initially used for fireworks, but were soon used as weapons in initial form as cannons, grenades, and ultimately firearms (History.com Editors, 2023). By the 13th century, firearms had developed in Asia and spread to Europe, where they were developed into matchlocks, wheel locks, and flintlocks. Firearms arrived in the U.S. in the 15th century in the form of the German-made blunderbuss, an early version of the shotgun, and the matchlock musket (History.com Editors, 2023). Over the centuries, firearms have grown into an industry in the U.S. and have undergone several evolutions, which have included the Kentucky Rifle, the Colt.45 revolver, double-barrel shotguns, M1911 pistol, the Browning Automatic Rifle (BAR), the M2 .50 caliber machine gun, .22, AK-47 rifle, the AR-15, magazines, semi-automatic weapons, and various other types/brands (Weeks, 2013). Currently, there are illegal ghost guns, which are firearms assembled from parts that lack serial numbers, making them untraceable by law enforcement.

Americans' fascination with firearm violence or firearm-related violence can be traced to slavery, where they were used to control and ultimately kill runaway or disobedient slaves. Shufro (2021). It states that guns were also used after slavery to protect newly freed Black men and were later used to terrorize and kill Blacks if they attempted to vote. Firearms can further be traced to the American Revolution and men joining the local Militia, and to myths of the "Wild West" and firearm duels with "bad guys" being killed. After the

Civil War firearms became marketable due to small family-owned stores offering them for purchase and promoting the idea that owning a gun would help young boys become "sturdy" men (Shufro, 2021); it is ironic that the same notion is used by some gang members and young men in contemporary society to possess a gun. As a result, private firearm ownership flourished then just as it does today. In contemporary society, guns continue to be used as a weapon of racism by law enforcement officers to control persons of color.

In the political arena, the topic of firearms has been used to garner support from political parties to either abolish/alter firearm legislation or from groups to support firearm rights advocates, such as the National Rifle Association (NRA). The firearm fascination continues with firearm sales/marketing, racism, politics, concentrated poverty, gangs, income inequality, police brutality, permissive gun laws, fear, easy access to firearms, and other forces to blame. In addition, firearms are increasingly being used as weapons of fear or force in the commission of crimes; the infamous January 6th Insurrection is just one example.

What Are the Risk Factors?

Davis and colleagues cite a 2015 U.S. Department of Justice (DOJ) report, which found that U.S. firearm manufacturers increased annual production from 5.6 million firearms in 2009 to 10.9 million in 2013. They cite Steinbrook and Redberg, who found that exports of U.S. firearms in 2013 went from 195, 000 to 393,000. With the number of firearms in circulation, the risks of firearm violence in the U.S. pose significant problems; anyone can be at risk of a firearm injury. This section explores the various factors involved with the risk of firearms including: the role of inequity in firearms, individual factors, relationship factors, and community factors.

Role of Inequity in Firearms

According to the Educational Fund to Stop Gun Violence (EFSGV) (2020), policymakers must address the social and economic inequalities that cause gun violence. Reeves and Holmes (2015), as well as Soken-Huberty (2024), suggest that victims of firearms are more prone to have a lower socioeconomic status. Reeves and Holmes regard firearm violence as part of a vicious cycle of race and inequality that reflects social inequalities and assists in producing additional poverty and violence for most Black people. Reeves and Holmes contend that Whites comprise 77% of firearm-related deaths for suicides, and 82% of firearm-related deaths among Blacks are homicides. These researchers also suggest that among 20- to 29-year-old Blacks, racial disparity is the leading cause of firearm-related homicides, followed by Hispanics and then Whites. The CDC (2021) suggested that in 2021, among males, Black males had the highest age-adjusted rate of firearm-related homicide (52.9 deaths per 100,000 standard population), and Asian males had the lowest rate (1.5). Among females, Black females had the highest rate (7.5), and Asian females had the lowest rate (0.5). Males had higher rates than females across all racial and Hispanic origin groups.

Structural inequalities such as the discriminatory practice of redlining, impose residential segregation, which excludes certain racial populations from obtaining housing in wealthy neighborhoods, which are deemed by the government to be worthy of protecting from gun violence. Benns and colleagues (2020) suggest that underinvested communities historically experience higher rates of gun violence. Moreover, Branas and colleagues (2018) argue that impoverished/blighted neighborhoods with several dilapidated buildings and vacant lots are predictive of firearm violence. These items are primarily found in social-economically distressed communities.

Over the past two decades, the issue of racial inequality has reemerged as part of the national narrative. News media, as well as eyewitness accounts and video recordings of police shootings against Black females and males, have been credited with bringing heightened attention to racism and the need for criminal justice reform. Libresco (2015, p. 1) argues that within the scope of this phenomenon, one must realize that being arrested is almost twice as deadly for African-Americans compared to their White counterparts. African-American detainees also face a significantly higher rate of homicide-related arrests than Whites. These homicides are more likely to be committed by law enforcement officers than jail inmates. Libresco cites the DOJ, which reported that nearly 3,000 arrest-related homicides occurred between 2003 and 2009. Ninety-nine percent of these homicides were committed by law enforcement officers.

Villarreal and colleagues (2024) note data from the Everytown Research (2024), which suggests that 1,000 Americans are shot and killed by police each year. This database further notes that Black Americans are disproportionately impacted by police-involved shootings and killed at more than twice the rate of Whites. A report by Everytown Research (2024) found that Black people are victimized at disproportionate rates and those who reside in marginalized communities experience poor police-community relations, which furthers the tensions between the police and Black citizens (Morin et al., 2017).

Lee and colleagues (2022) cite the 2019 study of Edward and colleagues, which examined women's risk of being killed by police use of force. This study revealed that Black women and American Indian/Alaska native women face a higher risk of death compared to their White counterparts. Moreover, Latino and Asian/Pacific Islander women faced a lower risk of death compared to White women. The study also revealed that the age where risk of death peaked was between 20 and 35. More specifically, women between the ages of 25 and 29 faced the greatest risk; the median mortality risk was 0.12% per 100,000 for Blacks, 0.14% for American Indian/Alaskan native, and 0.02% for Asian/Pacific Islander; and 0.07% for Latinas and Whites, respectively. The mortality risk for women between the ages of 25 and 29 was 0.08% per 100,000. The researchers further note that for all deaths involving women between the ages of 20 and 24, police use of force accounted for 0.2% of Blacks; 0.2% of American Indian/Alaska native; 0.05% of Asian/Pacific Islander; 0.16% of Latina, and 0.11% of White women. In addition to racism, power differentials have emerged in patriarchal societies, in which Black, as well as sometimes White women, have become victims of inequalities and exploitation by male police officers who have been privileged by their gender status.

According to Villarreal and colleagues (2024), in 2022, Black youth between the ages of 1 and 17 had a gun death rate of approximately, six times higher than their White counterparts. Hispanic/Latino youth between the ages of 1 and 17 had similar gun death rates to their White counterpart in 2022; however, the death rate for Hispanic/Latino youth increased nearly twice as much as the rate for their White counterparts from 2013 to 2022. The gun homicide rate for Black teens in this age group was 18 times higher than the rate for their White counterparts. The gun homicide rate for Hispanic/Latino children and teens was over three times higher than that of their White counterparts. In 2022, more Black men between the ages of 15 and 24 died in gun homicides than from unintentional injuries, suicide, heart disease, COVID-19, cancer, non-firearm homicides, diabetes, congenital abnormalities, and chronic respiratory diseases, police shootings, cerebrovascular diseases, anemias, sepsis, influenza and pneumonia, and HIV combined (CDC, 2024).

Racial inequalities also exist for youth of color when it comes to gun violence. In examining the racial disparities in gun deaths, Villarrea and colleagues (2024) found that Black and Hispanic/Latino youth between the ages of 1 and 17 are disproportionately burdened by gun violence. These researchers found that in 2022, Black youth in this age bracket had a gun death rate that was approximately, six times higher than their White counterparts; while Hispanic/Latino youth between the ages of 1 and 17 had a similar gun death rate to their White counterparts in 2022. The Hispanic/Latino gun death rate increased almost twice as much as the rate for their White counterparts from 2013 to 2022. Other findings revealed that the gun homicide rate for Black teens in this age group was 18 times higher than the rate for their White counterparts, and the gun homicide rate for Hispanic/Latino children and teens was over three times higher than that of their White counterparts.

Panchal (2024) explains why youth and adolescents of color are more prone to experience injuries from firearms than their White counterparts by suggesting that the disparity between Black youth and their exposure to firearms has been exacerbated since the COVID-19 Pandemic. However, children of color are disproportionately exposed to firearms more often than their White counterparts due to living in poverty-stricken areas. In other words, due to the level of crime in impoverished neighborhoods, Black families own firearms for protection, and their children are disproportionately exposed to them. Johnson and colleagues (2004) and Kim (2018) suggest that children and adolescents have access to guns in their homes, which leads to injuries and violence from firearms.

Information regarding firearm violence in the Black community can have devastating impacts, even more so when the firearm violence involves a Black person being shot by law enforcement. While this violence directly causes harm to a small number of individuals, its impact is felt across the entire Black community due to past and present accounts of racial discrimination, segregation, and feelings of disinvestment inflicted upon the Black community by law enforcement. Therefore, law enforcement shootings are a constant, frightening reminder of what could happen to any person of color in daily interactions with law enforcement, reinforcing feelings of fear, stress, and loss. According to McLeod and colleagues (2020), Black people comprise 13% of the U.S. population and 23% of those who are fatally shot by law enforcement. Similarly, Johnson and colleagues (2019) state that highly segregated neighborhoods in which Black people reside, especially those with low resources, tend to experience fatal interactions with the police at a higher rate than those less segregated. As a result, Black people worry five times more often about police interactions compared to White people (Graham et al., 2020).

Individual Factors

Suicide is regarded as an individual risk factor for firearm injuries. Foley and colleagues (2006), later followed by Barrett and colleagues (2022), suggest that firearm access is an individual risk factor for firearm suicide. Rates of firearm-related suicides are higher among older adults (age 50–80) than those among younger adults; one-third of this population owns or keeps firearms (Carter et al., 2022). Older adults' risk of suicide can be compounded by issues of depression, illness, stressful life events, and loneliness (Carter et al., 2022; Betz et al., 2018).

Sullivan and colleagues (2015) suggest that suicide is the second leading cause of death among those aged 10–24. They also noted that firearms are the most common means of suicide in the U.S. In 2017, firearms were used in 41% of all suicides involving youth in the U.S. between the ages of 10 and 17 (CDC, 2019). Rivara (2015) contends that suicides by firearms are more lethal, with an approximately, 90% fatality rate, than many of the other most widely used suicide attempt methods (below 5% of fatality rate). Kann and colleagues (2018) suggest that in 2017, 4.8% of all high school students in the U.S. (7.7% male versus 1.9% female) reported carrying a gun at least one day during the past 12 months of that year for reasons other than hunting or sport.

In examining how youth gaining access to firearms shapes their development of suicide ideation, Kim (2018) conducted a study using a nationally representative sample of 9,973 U.S. adolescents from the National Longitudinal Study of Adolescent to Adult Health. This research involved a school-based, longitudinal study of the health-related behaviors of adolescents and their outcomes in young adulthood. Kim's findings revealed:

- Gaining access to guns at home increases suicidal thoughts for both male and female adolescents.
- Gaining access to household firearms may heighten abused males' risk for suicidal ideation and suicide attempts, especially as they enter the period of adolescence when they tend to act more impulsively and have more freedom in life choices.
- Males are more likely to view guns as a potential means of suicide than females and gaining access to household firearms may be more detrimental to suicidal ideation for male adolescents with suicidal motives (such as those with a history of childhood maltreatment) than their female counterparts.

Similarly, Byrne (2021) found that children who live in a home with a gun are at two times the risk of homicide and three times the risk of suicide. Byrne further found that increased gun sales, along with isolation during COVID-19, increased the risk of youth gun-related injuries. Depression is regarded as a major risk factor for suicide (CDC, 2022). A study by Hawton and van Heeringen (2009) indicated that 50% of the adolescents who died from suicide had a diagnosis of depression at the time of their death. Swanson and colleagues (2020) conducted research using data from the National Comorbidity Survey Replication Adolescent Supplement (NCSA), in which a cross-sectional study of 10,123 adolescents from the U.S. between the ages of 13 and 18 participated. The data was used to: (1) measure how adolescents who live in a home with a firearm differ from those who do not in ways related to their risk of suicide, and (2) incorporate these differences into an updated effect estimate of the risk of adolescent suicide attributable to living in a home with firearms. In addition to demographic questions, the respondents were assessed for lifetime psychiatric disorders, which included depression, anxiety, substance use, and eating disorders. Swanson and colleagues' findings revealed that approximately, one-third (30.7%) of the adolescents reported living in a home with one or more firearms. In addition, the distribution of demographic and mental health characteristics that were known to be risk factors for suicide was relatively similar among adolescents who lived in homes with firearms versus those who lived in homes without firearms. Relative to adolescents who did not report living in a home with a firearm, adolescents who reported living in a home with a firearm were somewhat more likely to meet the criteria for a substance use disorders. In fact, 2.3% versus 0.8% for alcohol dependence disorder and suicide plans or attempts (6.0%

versus 4.4%). Further findings indicated that an adolescent's suicide risk was increased if she lived in a home with versus without firearms, with the best estimate that the risk of dying by suicide is at least three times greater.

CDC (2022) reported that in more than half of the country's record 49,500 deaths by suicide in 2022, the data revealed that men, who traditionally die by suicide at a much higher rate than women, often do so using guns. However, a report by Garnett and Curtin (2024) for the CDC revealed that firearms were the leading means of suicide for women since 2020. Garnett and Curtin further revealed that for females, per Figure 13.1:

- The age-adjusted rate for firearm-related suicide increased for the years 2007 (1.4 deaths per 100,000 standard population) to 2016 (1.9), remained stable through 2020 (1.8), and then increased to 2.0 in 2022.

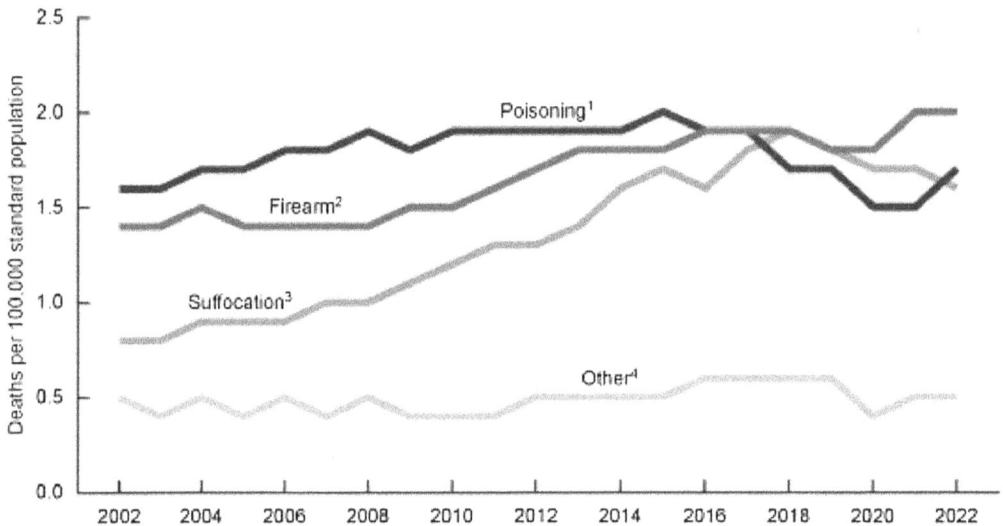

FIGURE 13.1 Age-Adjusted Female Suicide Rate, by Means of Suicide: United States, 2002–2022.

Notes:

[1]*Significant increasing trend from 2002 to 2016; no significant trend from 2016 to 2022 (p < 0.05) Rate was higher than for all other groups from 2002 to 2016 (p < 0.05).*

[2]*No statistically significant trend from 2002 to 2007; significant increasing trend from 2007 to 2016; no statistically significant trend from 2016 to 2020; significant increasing trend from 2020 to 2022 (p < 0.05) Rate was higher than for all other groups for 2021 and 2022 (p < 0.05).*

[3]*Significant increasing trend from 2000 through 2018; significant decreasing trend from 2018 to 2022 (p < 0.05).*

[4]*No statistically significant trend from 2002 to 2010; significant increasing trend from 2010 to 2017; significant. decreasing trend from 2017 to 2022 (p < 0.05).*

Notes: Suicide deaths are identified International Classification of Diseases, 10th Revision (ICD-10) underlying cause-of-death codes 103, X60–X84, and Y87.0. Means of suicide are identified using ICD-10 codes X72–X74 for firearm, X60–X69 for poisoning, and X70 for suffocation, "Other means" includes: cut/pierce; drowning; falls; fire or flame; other land transport; struck by or against; other specified, classifiable injury; other specified, not elsewhere classified injury; and unspecified injury, as classified by ICD-10. Age-adjusted death rates are calculated using the direct method and the 2000 U.S. standard population.

Source: CDC; "National Center for Health Statistics, National Vital Statistics System, Mortality Data File."

- Poisoning was the leading means of suicide between 2002 and 2015. The poisoning-related suicide rate was significantly lower than the firearm-related rate between 2020 and 2022 and was lower than the suffocation-related rate between 2018 and 2021.
- The rate of suffocation-related suicide (including hanging, asphyxiation, strangulation, and other means) for females increased from 0.8 in 2002 to 1.9 in 2018 but decreased to 1.6 in 2022.

Garnett and Curtin also reported that for males, firearms were the leading means of suicide across the period, with rates increasing between 2006 and 2022:

- Following a period of decline between 2002 (11.1 deaths per 100,000 standard population) and 2006 (10.3), the firearm-related suicide rate among males increased from 10.3 in 2006 to 13.5 in 2022 (Figure 13.2).
- The rate for suffocation-related suicide for males increased from 3.8 in 2002 to 6.7 in 2018 but decreased to 5.8 in 2022.

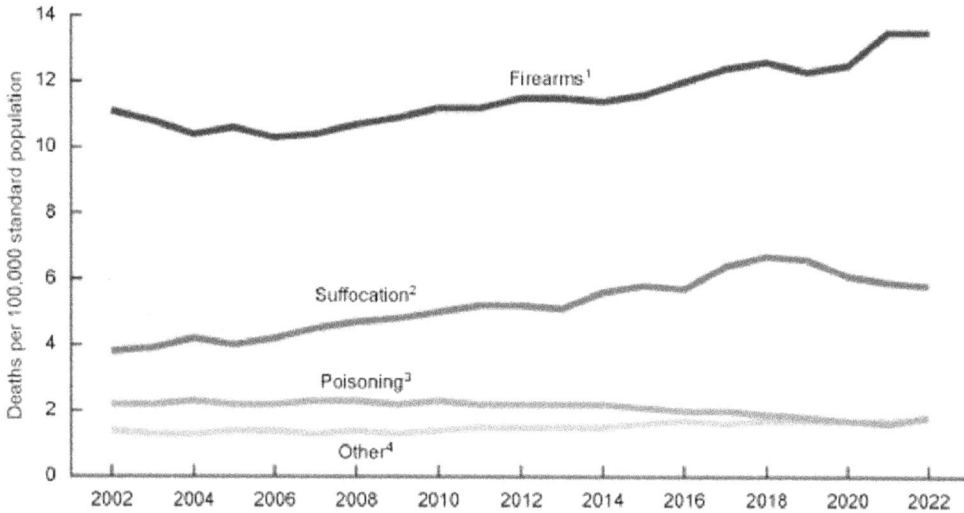

FIGURE 13.2   Age-Adjusted Male Suicide Rate, by Means of Suicide: United States, 2002–2022.

Notes:

[1]*Significant decreasing trend from 2002 to 2006; significant increasing trend from 2006 to 2022 (p < 0.05). Rate was higher than for all other groups for all years (p < 0.05). Of change; significant decreasing trend from 2018.*

[2]*Significant increasing trend from 2002 to 2018; with different rates to 2022 (p < 0.05).*

[3]*No statistically significant trend from 2002 to 2010; significant decreasing trend from 2010 to 2020, with different rates of change over time; no statistically significant trend from 2020 to 2022 (p < 0.05).* [4]*No significant trend from 2002 to 2009; significant increasing trend from 2009 to 2022 (p < 0.05).*

Notes: Suicide deaths are identified using International Classification of Diseases, 10th Revision (ICD-10) underlying cause-of-death codes U03, X60–X84, and Y87.0. Means of suicide are identified using ICD-10 codes X72–X74 for firearm, X60–X69 for poisoning, and X70 for suffocation. "Other means" includes: cut/pierce; drowning; falls; fire or flame; other land transport; struck by or against; other specified, classifiable injury; other specified, not elsewhere classified injury, and unspecified injury, as classified by ICD-10. Age-adjusted death rates are calculated using the direct method and the 2000 U.S. standard population.

Source: CDC; "National Center for Health Statistics, National Vital Statistics System, Mortality Data File."

- The rate of poisoning-related suicide for males was stable between 2002 (2.2) and 2010 (2.3), decreased through 2020 (1.7), and remained stable through 2022 (1.8).
- Firearms were the leading means of suicide for males across the period.

Although suicide deaths for children between the ages of 5 and 9 years are included in total numbers and age-adjusted rates, they are not shown as part of age-specific numbers or rates because of the small number of suicide deaths per year in this age group. This report also did not reveal if having access to a firearm was regarded as a risk. However, children who are placed at risk of having access to firearms have also unintentionally shot themselves or someone else. Cannon and colleagues (2023) examined data from the CDC (2021, 2023) between the years of 2015 and 2021, which revealed that 3,498 Americans died from unintentional gun injuries, including 713 children 17 years and younger. Miller and Azrael (2022) suggested that 4.6 million children live in households with at least one loaded and unlocked firearm. As a result, children have easy access to firearms, which leads to unintentional deaths or injuries. Cannon and colleagues extracted demographic and injury data of both the perpetrators and victims of unintentional shootings by children 17 and younger in the U.S. from January 1, 2015, through December 31, 2021, from the #NotAnAccident Index. A total of 2,448 unintentional shootings by children resulted in 926 deaths and 1,603 nonfatal gun injuries over seven years. Data revealed that 81% of the perpetrators and 76% of the victims were male. The mean age was 10.0 for shooters and 10.9 for victims. The majority of victims were under 18 years old (91%), and the shootings most often occurred in or around homes (71%) and with handguns (53%).

Figure 13.3 displays the age of the victims shot in unintentional shootings by children, by shooting type and age of shooter and victim, 2015–2021. According to the figure, children were as likely to shoot themselves as they were to shoot others (47%). Shooters between the ages of 0 and 5 years old, and adults 18 years and older were the next largest proportion of victims (30.4%). However, children between the ages of 6 and 13 were most likely to shoot children 0–5 (18.2%), and teenagers between the ages of 14 and 17 were most likely to shoot children between the ages of 6 and 13 (18.7%).

In addition to suicide, the availability of guns is a leading cause that encourages adolescents to engage in firearm-related crimes. Easy access to firearms tends to increase the level of violence, with some youth obtaining firearms through the black market, while others access these weapons through poor gun storage in their homes (Pear et al., 2023). The impulsive nature of youth and hostile confrontations may yield episodes of firearm violence. Unintentional accidents and suicides are individual risks, especially for children, that may be caused by having access to firearms, and if not prevented, may be on the rise.

Relationship Factors

Another population group that bears a significant burden of the risk of firearm violence is women. Domestic or intimate partner violence (IPV) involving firearms also puts women at heightened risk of death or life-altering injuries. A 2003 Office of Justice Factsheet argues that:

> compared to homes without guns, the presence of guns in the home is associated with a threefold increased homicide risk within the home. The risk connected to gun ownership

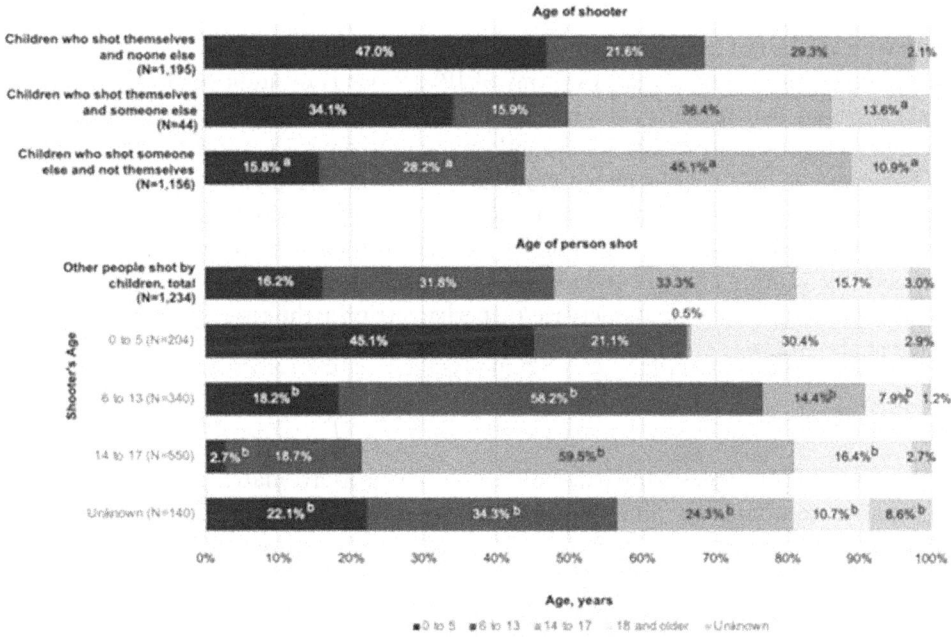

[a]P-value < 0.05 from chi-square test comparing this percentage to the percentage of children in this age category who shot themselves and no one else. [b]P-value < 0.05 from chi-square test comparing this percentage to the percentage of victims in this age category injured by 0 to 5 year-old shooters. *Source:* Everytown for Gun Safety Support Fund. #NotAnAccident Index, 2015–2021.

FIGURE 13.3   Age of Persons Shot in Unintentional Shootings by Children, by Shooting Type and Age of Shooter and Victim, 2015–2021.

Source: Everytown for Gun Safety Support Fund. #NotAnAccident Index, 2015–2021.

Notes: [a] p-value <0.05 from chi-square test comparing this percentage to the percentage of children in this age category who shot themselves and no one else. [b] p-value <0.05 from chi-square test comparing this percentage to the percentage of victims in this age category injured by 0 to 5-year-old shooters.

increases eightfold when the offender is an intimate partner or relative of the victim, and it is 20 times higher when previous domestic violence existed.

(Office of Justice Programs, 2003)

Zeoli and colleagues (2016) suggest that more than half of all female homicides involve a gun and that the use of firearms in IPV is widely recognized as a public health threat.

According to the CDC (2023), more than half of female homicide victims are killed by a current or former male intimate partner. The National Coalition of Domestic Violence argues that one in three women in the U.S. experiences physical violence, sexual violence, and/or stalking by a current or former intimate partner throughout their lifetimes. Tobin-Tyler (2023) noted the research of Smith and colleagues, which found that women who have been historically marginalized were at the greatest risk of IPV: 56.6% of multiracial women, 45.1% of Black women, and 47.5% of native women. Gollub and Gardner (2019) have shown that IPV is associated with an increased risk of homicide, with a firearm most commonly being the weapon of choice.

Traditionally, it has been men who kill or otherwise violate women as victims of IPV, especially with the use of a firearm, which has been used to threaten, coerce, and intimate women; however, some men are also victims of IPV. What is of additional risk to victims of IPV are the laws that regulate the use of guns. Tobin-Tyler argues that many of the gun laws have been inconsistent across states, and underenforced at the state and federal levels (2023). For example, the various interpretations of the Second Amendment along with the public-private dichotomy as to whether the right to own a gun should be a private matter without interference from the government. These inconsistencies place an added burden on marginalized IPV victims who are seeking refuge because the mere presence of a firearm in an abuse or non-abuse home may increase or perhaps trigger the risk of injury or murder (Campbell et al., 2022).

Community Factors

Soken-Huberty (2024) suggests firearm violence can disproportionately impact Blacks and boys in deprived communities. Similarly, Kravitz-Wirtz and colleagues (2022) suggest that community gun violence reflects inequalities in social, economic, and political systems that shape the daily living conditions of Black and Latinx youth who are disproportionately exposed to communities that experience high-risk factors associated with violence and low protective measures of safety. These researchers revealed that Black and Latinx youth were three to seven times more likely, depending on the exposure radius, to experience a previous-year gun homicide that was closer to their home than their White counterparts and, on average, experienced incidents more recently and closer to home. In examining differences in the probability of exposure of youth in all racial and ethnic groups, they found that in low versus high poverty households, the difference was approximately, 5–10 percentage points, while the difference between youth residing in low versus high disadvantage neighborhoods was approximately, 50 percentage points. Kravitz-Wirtz and colleagues conclude that Black and Latinx youth are disproportionately exposed to communities experiencing high-risk factors associated with violence and low protective factors associated with safety.

The EFSGV (2020) notes Hudley (Sonali et al., 2022), who contends that in addition to under-qualified instructors, poverty-stricken urban schools also face the problems of outdated curricula and dilapidated structures, which impact a child's development. The EFSGV regards this as a form of structural inequalities that are rooted in racism. To further this impact, Bergen-Cico and colleagues (2018) suggest that school systems in impoverished neighborhoods can also lead their students to exposure to community firearm violence. One's educational performance has been linked to firearm violence (Bergen-Cico et al., 2018). School systems in impoverished communities are usually underfunded by the government, and therefore, yield to poor educational performance, which can expose a child to firearm violence.

Barrett and colleagues (2022) and Spano and colleagues (2012) suggest that one's environment, which may influence the carrying of a firearm or having access to one in the event of perceived danger or due to peer influence, must be taken into consideration. This is especially true for those living in communities where firearms may be needed for gang involvement, drug use or dealing, violence, protection from violence, and other neighborhood disorders. However, the need to carry a firearm in a neighborhood ultimately places one at risk. Living in disadvantaged communities can increase the likelihood of getting involved with community firearm violence (Beardslee et al., 2021; Buggs et al., 2023).

Criminal Justice Issue

Butkus and colleagues (2018) assert firearm fatalities are any purposeful or accidental death that includes firearms as a vector. They are a common type of violent crime in the U.S., and every year, firearms claim the lives of 40,000 people. In 2020, with the COVID-19 pandemic and the racial tension following the murder of George Floyd, firearm background checks increased by over 30% to a peak of 39 million. A variety of strategies, methods, and laws have been implemented and enforced by law enforcement agencies over the years to combat firearm-related violence. Firearm-related violence has reached epidemic proportions in the U.S. and abroad. These epidemic portions have sparked questions and debates from citizens, organizations, and criminal justice practitioners to press legislatures and policymakers to create legislation and policies aimed at combating firearm violence.

Spitzer (2017) suggests gun laws and possession are as old as the U.S. and that by the end of the early 1900s, 43 states had laws restricting and, in some cases, prohibiting carrying firearms in public places. Some of these laws were:

Gun Ban Laws criminalized the sale or exchange of firearms, particularly pistols.

Brandishing Laws criminalized the threat to use a weapon or exhibit a deadly weapon rudely or angrily.

Gun Carry Restrictions were passed to prohibit individuals from wearing weapons because they introduced fear and fighting; however, travelers passing through areas were allowed to carry arms.

Restrictions on Dangerous or Unusual Weapons included weapons such as sawed-off shotguns, pistols, and anti-machine guns

Semi-Automatic Gun Restrictions were imposed on weapons such as machine guns, which fire singly or by separate trigger pressure, or fire by continuous trigger pressure.

Dueling Prohibitions prohibited public armed combat.

Felons, Foreigners, Others Considered Dangerous Laws prohibited guns from immigrants, children, felons, those who were inebriated, and non-state residents.

Firing Location Restrictions barred firing guns after dark, on Sundays, near roads, and in or near towns.

Hunting Restrictions barred hunting on private property and hunting deer. Most states require a hunting license to do so.

Gun Manufacture, Inspection, and Sale Restriction Laws required a state inspector to fire a firearm before it was sold to prove it could withstand the firing process. These laws also applied to gunpowder to keep loose gunpowder from igniting.

Militia Laws were enacted due to some states stipulating when, where, and under what circumstances firearms could be loaded/unloaded, and requiring men eligible for militia to obtain and maintain combat-worthy firearms along with gunpowder at their own expense.

Gun Access by Minors and Irresponsible Others Laws prohibited minors under the age of 12 and others deemed as irresponsible, including those of poor moral character, unsound mind, and convicts, from possessing a firearm.

Registration, Taxation Restrictions addressed gun sales, regulation, taxation, or dealer registration.

Race and Slavery Laws restricted slaves and freed Black men from firearm ownership.

Sensitive Areas restricted the discharge of firearms at communal gatherings, public places, entertainment events, cemeteries, near churches, bridges, homes, or state parks.

Sentencing Enhancement Laws occurred in some states that required the death penalty for those who committed a burglary or robbery with a gun, while other states increased sentencing time for using a gun during the commission of a crime.

Storage Regulations were placed on gunpowder and firearms stored in such places as barns, outhouses, shops, and warehouses; these items could be seized and sold at public auction.

Table 13.1 contains a partial list of colonial and state gun laws that have evolved since the Second Amendment to the Constitution throughout the U.S. until 1934:

On the national level, the National Firearms Act of 1934 was imposed and required the registration of sawed-off shotguns in the U.S. The Supreme Court Case of U.S. v. Miller, 307 U.S. 174, upheld this Act. Miller argued that the Supreme Court and most lower courts linked the right to bear arms to the maintenance of a "well-regulated militia", but did not convey in the Second Amendment a generalized right to citizens to own all types of firearms (Shrader, 1995).

By 1968, the Firearms Division of the Bureau of Alcohol, Tobacco, Firearms and Explosives (ATF) was given the responsibility of enforcing the Federal Gun Control Act. This Act regulated interstate and foreign commerce in firearms, including the importation of prohibited persons, and licensing provisions. The Gun Control Act was imposed after the assassinations of President John F. Kennedy, Attorney General Robert Kennedy, and Dr. Martin Luther King, Jr. This Act established new categories of firearm offenses and prohibited the sale of firearms and ammunition to felons and other prohibited people. The Act also imposed the first federal jurisdiction over "destructive devices," including bombs, mines, grenades, and other similar devices (ATF, 2022).

As of the 21st century, firearms remain an integral part of American society. Critics of America's firearm laws due to disappointment that many homicides, accidental shootings, mass shootings, and school shootings have not led to greater firearm legislation continue to spark debate/controversy among citizens, the National Rifle Association, and the Supreme Court over the vagueness of the Second Amendment to the U.S. Constitution. Throughout two rulings, the Supreme Court, in the case District of Columbia v. Heller (2008), ruled that the Second Amendment provides average citizens with a constitutional right to bear arms and that this right must be recognized at all levels of government. This rule prohibited felons and those with mental illnesses from purchasing or possessing firearms, and legal restrictions were placed on carrying firearms in schools and government buildings. Moreover, the ruling imposed conditions and qualifications on the commercial sale of arms and on the safe storage of firearms (Spitzer, 2017).

According to a Gallup survey, firearms can be found in 44% of the homes in the U.S. (Gallup, 2020). Individuals continue to use guns for recreation and protection, while others continue to use them to commit acts of violence. While the Second Amendment has protected the right to bear arms, many states have restrictions regarding the ease of possession, public carrying, and the right of self-defense.

TABLE 13.1 Numbers of Gun Laws in the States, and Numbers of State Gun Laws, by Categories, 1607–1934

Law type	1607–1790	1791–1867	1868–1899	1900–1934
Ban	0	0	7	0
Number of states	0	0	5	0
Brandishing	2	4	14	7
Number of states	2	3	13	7
Carry restriction	5	31	48	21
Number of states	4	19	28	18
Dangerous weapons	1	4	9	53
Number of states	1	4	8	35
Dueling	3	7	3	0
Number of states	2	7	3	0
Felons, foreigners, etc.	11	2	1	26
Number of states	5	2	1	19
Firing weapons	19	17	19	22
Number of states	9	14	17	20
Hunting	11	8	24	58
Number of states	8	5	21	43
Manufacturing, inspection	2	11	11	22
Number of states	2	10	9	17
Militias	23	15	2	0
Number of states	2	10	9	17
Minors etc.	0	2	15	21
Number of states	0	2	15	19
Registration, taxation	3	8	12	18
Number of states	2	6	11	15
Race/slavery[a]	5	18	0	0
Number of states	5	11	0	0
Sensitive areas etc.	11	23	30	35
Number of states	7	17	20	26
Sentencing enhancement	3	3	5	10
Number of states	3	3	5	10
Storage	2	7	2	0
Number of states	1	6	2	0

Source: Frassetto (2013). Though the table is labeled "State" gun laws, it also includes laws enacted when the states were colonies, and some local/municipal laws. The full category titles of gun laws from Frassetto's paper are: Bans on Handguns/Total Bans on Firearms; Brandishing; Carrying Weapons; Dangerous or Unusual Weapons; Dueling; Felons, Foreigners and Others Deemed Dangerous By the State; Firing Weapons; Hunting; Manufacturing, Inspection, and Sale of Gunpowder and Firearms; Militia Regulation; Possession by, Use of, and Sales to Minors and Others Deemed Irresponsible; Registration and Taxation; Race and Slavery Based Firearms Restrictions; Sensitive Areas and Sensitive Times; Sentence Enhancement for Use of Weapons; Storage.

Note

[a] *The small number of laws pertaining to slaves or race-based restrictions pertaining to guns is not meant to suggest that the legal regime in the pre–Civil War South was somehow not uniformly harsh but rather reflects the fact that express statutory restrictions were not necessary in all places, given the South's uniformly oppressive system of slavery.*

Peterson and Bushway (2021) note James's work in 2018, which suggests that the rate at which violent crimes are committed with guns saw a substantial decline over the past 30 years. They further note James as suggesting that the homicide rate, which usually involves firearms, dropped by 50% since 1980, with a large portion of that drop occurring between 1993 and 2014. Peterson and Bushway cite the 2013 work of Uggen and McElrath in which they suggest that part of this decline may have been due to the efforts of law enforcement. However, Leach-Kemon and Sirull (2022) suggest that the U.S. has the highest gun rate of any developed nation. The recent increases in the number of illegal firearms in circulation, mass shootings, individuals injured by a firearm, as well as deaths due to a firearm have always posed a major dilemma for those working in the criminal justice system; therefore, making firearm violence a criminal justice issue with public health ramifications due to the injuries and lives lost.

Firearm laws vary by state and jurisdiction. While the Second Amendment of the Constitution provides citizens with the right to bear arms, it has made it difficult for national gun control legislation to be passed. Therefore, many gun control laws are based on state legislation. The Gun Control Act still prevails as the legislation for the federal regulation of firearms. This Act is responsible for regulating the transfer of licensing, sale, possession, and use of firearms and ammunition, as well as establishing new categories of firearm-related offenses and restricting certain prohibited individuals, such as felons, fugitives, the mentally ill, and minors, from purchasing a firearm (Korhonen, 2024).

A law aimed at further controlling the possession of firearms is the Brady Bill. Before the enactment of this Law, individuals who were minors, drug users, convicted of a felony, or committed to a mental institution could not own a gun, but there was no national system in place to verify if a prospective gun owner fell into these categories. The Brady Bill was modified to include those dishonorably discharged from the military or convicted of certain misdemeanors or domestic violence crimes from purchasing a firearm. The Bill requires all federally licensed gun dealers to conduct background checks on customers through either the Federal Bureau of Investigation (FBI) or a local or state agency. To streamline the process of conducting those checks, the National Instant Criminal Background Check System, or NICS was instituted to quicken the process (Brownlee, 2023). However, in front of there are gun shops that slip through the cracks and allow individuals who are restricted by this Act to purchase a gun.

In a critique of the laws that are in place Santaella-Tenorio and colleagues (2016) suggest that criminal and civil laws are needed to address firearm ownership, but they fail to address the issue of firearm violence. Criminal laws seek punishment and deterrence of violent crimes, but fail to address the underlying social and behavioral factors that cause the violence. The researchers further state that criminal laws are inadequate in preventing suicide by firearm, and civil laws that regulate background checks and licensing are insufficient in addressing issues at the community level and fail to address unlicensed firearms already in circulation (2016). While none of the legislation appears to have been 100% effective in preventing anyone from acquiring illegal firearms or using firearms for violent means, the use of firearms for the commission of a crime(s) is well documented in the criminological literature due to its use in homicides, suicides, murder-suicides, and accidental deaths (Siegel & Worrall, 2018), thus making firearm violence a criminal justice issue.

Public Health Issue

Firearm violence is not only a crime, but it is also the cause of morbidity, mortality, and racial health disparities in the U.S. Criminal justice practitioners, social workers, epidemiologists, and other experts argue that gun violence is a public health issue that has reached epidemic proportions in the U.S. (Novella, 2018; Hemenway & Richardson, 2011; Moore et al., 1994). Gun violence is present in various forms, including suicide, homicide, and unintentional deaths, as well as nonfatal gunshot injuries, threats, and exposure to gun violence in communities and society. According to the CDC, every year, more than 23,000 Americans die by firearm suicide. Each year, 14,000 Americans die by firearm homicide (CDC, n.d.). More than half of female intimate partner homicides are committed with a gun. Approximately, 1,000 Americans are shot and killed by police every year (Zeoli et al., 2016).

Firearm-related violence has become an infectious disease; it has spread like a cancer that is growing on U.S. soil. To help combat this epidemic, the Biden-Harris Administration announced more executive actions to reduce gun violence. On June 25, 2022, Former President Biden signed the Bipartisan Safer Communities Act (BSCA) (The White House Briefing Room, 2024). This law was enacted in the aftermath of the mass school shooting in Uvalde, Texas, and the mass shooting at a grocery store in Buffalo, New York. The purpose of the Act is to make various changes to federal firearms laws, which include the expansion of background check requirements, broadening the scope of existing restrictions, and establishing new criminal offenses for firearms.

The issue with firearm violence is so dire that Former President Biden established the first White House Office of Gun Violence Prevention to be overseen by Former Vice President Harris. This initiative was formed to assist in the implementation of legislation that would provide leadership and reduction of the injuries caused by shootings (The Lancet, 2023). In 2024, the U.S. Surgeon General issued an advisory notice declaring firearm violence an urgent public health crisis; this was the first time a notice on firearm violence had come from the U.S. Surgeon General's Office. The goal of the notice was to reduce gun violence by 30% by the year 2030, which equates to 14,400 lives saved by the year 2022 (Office of the U.S. Surgeon General, 2024). Moreover, the Biden-Harris administration announced an executive order that aimed to treat gun violence as a public health crisis. This order would have directed federal agencies to improve school-based active shooter drills and combat the emerging threats of machinegun conversion devices and unserialized, 3D-printed firearms (The White House Briefing Room, 2024).

International Comparative Statistics

Data compiled by Small Arms Survey (2018) suggest that it is difficult to account for the number of firearms privately owned globally and asserts that the most reliable method for capturing the number of firearms globally owned is through official registration. However, not all individuals register firearms. As a result, the survey revealed that approximately, 100 million civilian firearms were reported as registered, accounting for about 12% of the global total. At the end of 2017, this data indicated there were approximately, 857 million civilian-held firearms in 230 states and autonomous territories. Tables 13.2 and 13.3 display national ownership rates, which vary significantly from a high of about 120.5 firearms for every 100 people in the U.S. to less than 1 firearm for every 100 residents in countries such as Indonesia, Japan, Malawi, and several Pacific Island states.

TABLE 13.2 Estimated Total Civilian-Held Legal and Illicit Firearms in the 25 Top Ranked Countries and Territories, 2017

United States	393,300,000	Turkey	13,200,000	Saudi Arabia	5,500,000
India	71,100,000	France	12,700,000	South Africa	5,400,000
China	49,7000,000	Canada	12,7000,000	Columbia	5,00,000
Pakistan	43,900,000	Thailand	10,300,000	Ukraine	4,400,000
Russian Federation	17,6000,000	Italy	8,600,000	Afghanistan	4,300,000
Brazil	17,500,000	Iraq	7,600,000	Egypt	3,900,000
Mexico	16,8000,000	Nigeria	6,200,000	Philippines	3,800,000
Germany	15,800,000	Venezuela	5,900,000	Yemen	14,900,000
Iran	5,900,000				

Source: Small Arms Survey (2018).

TABLE 13.3 Estimated Rate of Civilian Firearms Holdings in the 25 Top-Ranked Countries and Territories, 2017 (firearms per 100 residents)

United States	120.5	Iceland	31.7	Sweden	23.1
Yemen	52.8	Bosnia and Herzegovina	31.2	Pakistan	22.3
Montenegro	39.1	Austria	30.0	Portugal	21.3
Serbia	39.1	Macedonia[a]	29.8	France	19.6
Canada	34.7	Norway	28.8	Germany	19.6
Uruguay	34.7	Malta	28.3	Iraq	19.6
Cyprus	34.0	Switzerland	27.6	Luxembourg	18.9
Finland	32.4	New Zealand	26.3	Lebanon	31.9
Kosovo[b]	23.8				

Source: Small Arms Survey (2018).

Notes: This table excludes countries and territories with a population of under 150,000.
[a] Macedonia = the former Yugoslav Republic of Macedonia.
[b] The designation of Kosovo is without prejudice to positions on status and is in line with UN Security Council Resolution 1244 and the International Court of Justice Opinion on the Kosovo Declaration of Independence.

The rates of firearm violence in the U.S. are high when compared with other countries. This holds for high-income countries. Both the CDC and World Health Organization (WHO) in 2015 revealed that the firearm-related death rate was 11.4 times higher in the U.S. compared to 28 other high-income nations (Grinshteyn & Hemenway, 2019). These sources further found that the difference between the U.S. and peer nations was greater when examining firearm-related mortality among children and adolescents. Grinshteyn and Hemenway (2019) argue that of the 29 nations studied in 2015, more than nine in ten children (between the ages of 0 and 14) who died from firearm-related injuries lived in the U.S. (97% of children between the ages of 0 and 4, and 92% of children between the ages of 5 and 14). McGough and colleagues (2023), revealed data from the Institute for Health Metrics and Evaluation (IHME) which displayed that, in 2019, the rate of firearm mortality among children and adolescents (between the ages of 1 and 19) in the U.S. (36.4 per 1 million) was more than 5 times the rate of firearm mortality among the same age group in Canada (6.2 per 1 million), this was approximately, 18 times the rate of firearm mortality in Sweden (2.0 per 1 million), and more than 22 times the rate of firearm mortality in Australia (1.6 per 1 million).

Bleyer and colleagues (2024) suggest that more individuals are dying in the U.S. from bullets than from cancer. These researchers further examined mental health disorders and firearm data from between the years 2000 and 2019 from the IHME Global Health Burden and compared the U.S. to 40 countries with similar sociodemographic Index (SDI). The finding revealed that while the prevalence of mental health disorders in the U.S. is similar in all major categories to its 40 comparable SDI countries, death by firearms is 20 times greater. Findings further revealed that the difference between the U.S. and all other high SDI countries cannot be explained by differences in mental disorder prevalence; however, a significant proportion of the U.S. population attributes its firearm mortality and injury epidemic to inadequate care of its mentally disabled population (Bleyer et al., 2024).

Public Health and Social Work

Intersection of Public Health and Social Work

Both public health and social work are well-known for their efforts in gun violence and firearm injury prevention. Social workers have been referred to as "violence interrupters" (Bosco-Ruggiero, 2023) due to their work at the micro level that includes schools and other community venues where they interact with persons and populations that are typically viewed as being more at risk of getting involved with gun violence and sustaining firearm injuries. Social workers are trained to assist communities with violence prevention capacity building and to be community organizers. They discuss violence prevention, dispute resolution, and aspects of gun safety. Whether working with individuals, groups, or neighborhoods, social workers often teach safe gun storage practices and advocate for temporary transfers of gun ownership or storage during stressful periods (Abrams, 2022). Additionally, they often report the presence of firearms to law enforcement agencies when discovered in the homes of clients they deem to be a danger to themselves and others (Bosco-Ruggiero, 2023). They also work as advocates with violence-interrupter groups such as *Violence Interrupters* in Chicago.

As therapists, licensed clinical social workers can choose from a variety of research-based best-practice therapy techniques to use when working with clients who are impacted by gun violence (Kaplan, 2024). Some therapeutic techniques include the following:

- Trauma-Focused Cognitive Behavioral Therapy: an evidence-based counseling technique designed to help gun violence survivors understand the connections between their thoughts, feelings, and behaviors related to the incident.
- Eye Movement Desensitization and Reprocessing: an National Association of Social Workers (NASW)-endorsed counseling technique used for the treatment of trauma that involves having the gun violence survivor recall painful memories of the incident while undergoing a form of bilateral sensory stimulation such as eye movements.
- Narrative Exposure Therapy: a therapeutic technique that social workers can use to teach survivors how to integrate and process the traumatic events surrounding their experience of the gun violence incident into the larger context of their own life story.

- Group Therapy: a therapeutic technique that social workers can use to create a supportive environment where gun violence survivors can feel safe to share the traumatic effects of the incident with others going through the same experience.
- Play Therapy and Art Therapy: these are two age-appropriate therapeutic techniques that social workers can use with young children affected by gun violence to help them communicate their feelings connected to this type of traumatic experience more effectively than other, more traditional forms of verbal interaction between the clinician and the survivor.

Health Disparities and Health Inequities

Research shows that Black males and Black females disproportionately suffer from firearm violence (Reeves & Homles, 2015; CDC, 2021). We also discuss the disproportionality of firearm violence experienced by minority groups and argue that it extends to a host of injuries (e.g., fatal and nonfatal) in the section on *Negative Health Consequences of Firearm Injuries*. However, it is important to note that the reach of firearm injuries is far wider than the immediate victims and those nearby. In fact, Semenza and Kravitz-Wirtz (2024) suggest a three-tiered exposure (TTE) framework to better understand the full impact of gun violence and related injuries. The TTE framework demonstrates how "direct, indirect, and community exposure converge in local communities can shape population health outcomes" (p. 2). Figure 13.4 displays Semenza and Kravitz-Wirtz's (2024) "Three-Tiered

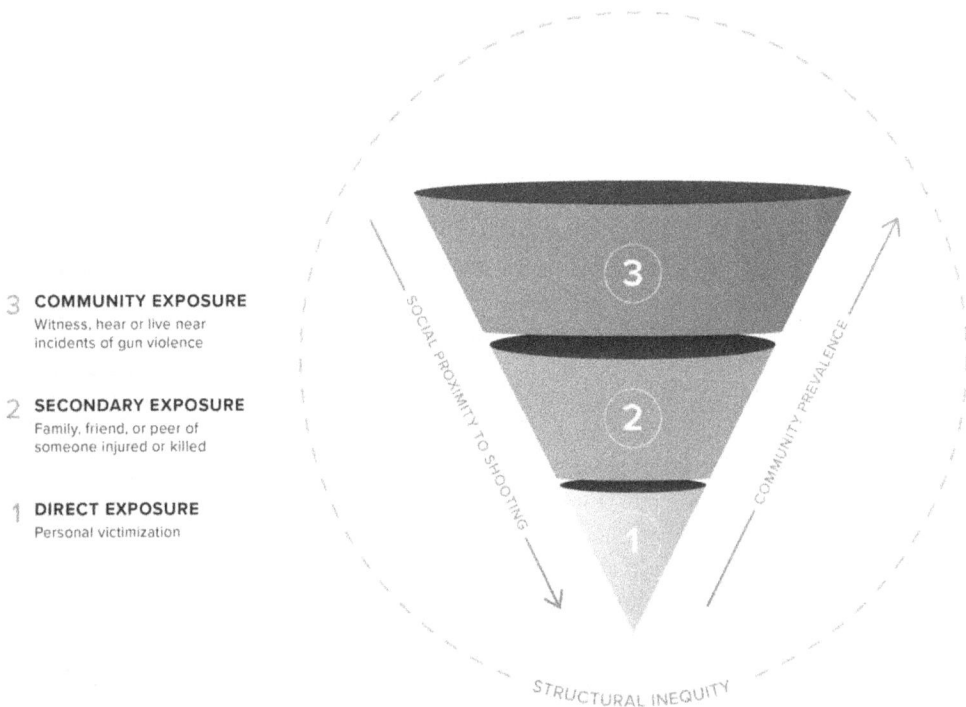

3 **COMMUNITY EXPOSURE**
Witness, hear or live near
incidents of gun violence

2 **SECONDARY EXPOSURE**
Family, friend, or peer of
someone injured or killed

1 **DIRECT EXPOSURE**
Personal victimization

SOCIAL PROXIMITY TO SHOOTING

COMMUNITY PREVALENCE

STRUCTURAL INEQUITY

FIGURE 13.4 Three-Tiered Exposure Framework.

Source: NIH; "Three-Tiered Exposure Framework."

Exposure Framework" which reveals the downward left arrow showing that "social proximity or personal involvement" is greater when moving from "community exposure (i.e., witnessing, hearing or living near an incident of gun violence) to direct victimization" (p. 2). Several studies support the notion that as the social and relational proximity to gun violence increases, so too, does the likelihood of a traumatic stress reaction from those who are aware of the presence of firearm violence (May & Wisco, 2016; Price et al., 2013). Moreover, the upward right arrow demonstrates how "the prevalence of a particular form of exposure within a given neighborhood increases when moving upwards from direct exposure to community-level exposure" (p. 2). The inverted pyramid depicts that the most typical form of exposure to firearm violence and injury is indirect from community exposure. Thus, the TTE framework symbolizes the broad impact of gun violence exposure and the consequential trauma exposure that damages the collective well-being of entire communities (Opara et al., 2020).

Firearm injuries not only affect people who are directly impacted, but rather, they also have a tremendous negative impact on others in the community at large because of how they affect collective behavior, mental health disorders, substance use and abuse patterns, and the likelihood that others will start arming themselves for self-protection (Song et al., 2023). Firearms experts report that the mere sound of a firearm going off or gunshots can cause traumatic reactions from those with direct or indirect experiences and exposures to firearm violence. For example, given the recent pervasiveness of gun violence in many schools in America, most school shooting research has focused only on shootings that occur on school campuses or property, while ignoring gun violence that occurs on the periphery of school campuses. Nevertheless, students are exposed to firearm violence when they hear gunshots daily often along the paths they walk to school. This is concerning given that research finds that traumatic aspects of firearm violence are related to impaired academic ability, mental health issues, and behavioral issues such as:

- Post-traumatic stress disorder (PTSD), depression, anger, and disassociation (Barboza, 2018),
- Poor psychological functioning and psychosocial adjustment including inability to regulate anger (Sharkey et al., 2014),
- Concentration problems (Mayer & Leone, 2007),
- Compromised student–teacher relationships (Bowen & Bowen, 1999),
- Weapon carrying (Beardslee et al., 2018),
- Involvement in drug use or distribution (Sheley et al., 1992), and
- Lower cognitive assessments and standardized test scores (Sharkey et al., 2014).

When spatial studies were conducted to determine the impact of gun-related homicides on selected communities in the last 12 months, the findings revealed that shooting deaths that occurred near the homes of youth were linked to high levels of anxiety and depression (Aubel et al., 2021; Leibbrand et al., 2020) particularly those homicides that occurred near the homes of low-income Black male youth (Rouhezamin et al., 2013). Beyond the direct impact of firearm violence, experts contend that those people who experience secondary trauma from firearm violence who may have been relatives or simply knew the victims of firearm fatalities, can also suffer extensive trauma and persistent feelings of betrayal, alienation, and loneliness (Magee et al., 2023). An interesting finding from firearm violence research is that Black survivors of homicide attempts, in particular, are at a higher risk of experiencing poor psychological health (Shrpe & Iwamoto, 2022). In fact, in the aftermath of their victimization, research reveals that the effects of trauma can cause them to engage in behaviors such as substance use and abuse, diet and exercise, and physical conditions such as chronic illness (Semenza et al., 2024).

Negative Health Consequences of Firearm Injuries

According to Abba-Aji et al. (2024), available estimates suggest that in 2016, there were approximately, 251,000 firearm-related fatalities outside of war zones worldwide, an increase from an estimate of 209,000 in 1990. In the U.S. alone, there were over 48,830 gun-related fatalities and 175,459 nonfatal injuries in 2021 (National Center for Injury Prevention and Control, 2023). Weaver and colleagues (2004) suggest that the risk of death in firearm-involved violent encounters is approximately, five times greater than the risk of other weapons, such as knives.

Survivors of firearm injuries may experience many mental and physical consequences. These consequences can range from memory problems, emotions, PTSD, physical disabilities from brain injury, and paralysis from spinal cord injuries (DiScala & Sege, 2004; Greenspan & Kellermann, 2002; Vella et al., 2020; Lowe & Galea, 2017). Kagawa and colleagues (2018) suggest that individuals injured by guns are at a significantly higher risk of PTSD, anxiety, depression, and substance use, compared to those injured through other violent means (Kagawa et al., 2018).

Song and colleagues (2023) examined data from commercial health insurance claims from 2007 to 2021, which suggests that children and adolescents, between the ages of 0 and 19, who survived a firearm injury experienced long-term negative health consequences. The researchers studied 2,052 child and adolescent survivors of gun injuries compared to 9,983 matched controls who did not incur firearm injuries, along with 6,209 family members of survivors compared to 29,877 matched controls, and 265 family members of decedents compared to 1,263 matched controls. They further revealed that in the year following a firearm injury, compared to matched controls who did not experience a firearm injury, the survivors experienced a 117% increase in pain disorders (e.g., musculoskeletal pain, headache, and other pain syndromes), a 68% increase in psychiatric disorders (trauma- and stress-related disorders such as major depressive disorders, and other psychiatric disorders), and a 144% increase in substance use disorders (i.e., alcohol or drug use disorders).

In examining mental health issues associated with firearm violence at different life stages, Shonkoff and colleagues (2012) argue that at the perinatal and infancy stages, exposure to accidental firearm discharges or domestic violence incidents involving a gun can lead to early trauma and developmental disruptions. Likewise, Panchal (2024) suggests that exposure to gun violence is linked to PTSD and anxiety, in addition to other mental health concerns among youth. According to Finkelhor and colleagues (2015), exposure to firearm violence during childhood and adolescence may also bring about experiences of long-term emotional well-being due to this period being marked by increased risk for violence and victimization in schools, neighborhoods, and homes. They further state that adults exposed to gun violence may experience heightened risks of PTSD, depression, and substance abuse. Abba-Aji and colleagues (2024) argue that the understanding of the mental health effects of gun violence remains limited. Perhaps this is because firearm violence may impact individuals in different ways.

Regarding police shootings of Black people, these shootings have broad impacts on entire communities, leading to trauma and worsening mental health. One study found that a police officer's killing of an unarmed Black person led to a significant increase in the number of poor mental health days for Black people living in proximity to the shooting in the following three months. The mental health burden of police shootings in Black communities is estimated to be nearly as large as the mental health burden associated with diabetes in these communities (Bor et al., 2018). Systemic racism in policing only reflects the need for a broader discourse on the structural and institutional racism that appears to be a constant in society.

Criminal Justice Approaches

Before the 21st century, various interventions and policies were developed by the criminal justice system to reduce and prevent firearm-related crimes and the violence imposed by them. Some of these policies were: (1) gun courts, (2) enhanced sentences for criminal use of firearms, and (3) problem-oriented policing. According to the National Academies of Sciences, Engineering, and Medicine (NASEM) (2005), while these interventions have had political support from both sides, they are the primary focus of the federal government's efforts toward reducing firearm-related violence. The research evidence, however, is mixed. In some cases, evidence revealed that the programs may be effective, and other evidence revealed that the programs might have negligible effects, while other evidence was lacking.

Peterson and Bushway (2021) identified several approaches used by the criminal justice system to reduce crime. These approaches are standard law enforcement approaches, proactive law enforcement approaches, and community-based approaches. Standard law enforcement approaches involve law enforcement officers performing random patrols, responding to 911 calls, investigating reported crimes with the hope of making an arrest, enforcing firearm possession laws, and prosecuting gun crimes. Peterson and Bushway contend that while the standard law enforcement approaches are good at deterrence and incapacitation, the extent to which such elements as the consistent enforcement of gun laws, improvements in the investigation of violent crime and clearance rates, or an increase in the role of federal enforcement activities need further research as it relates to violent crimes that are committed with guns.

According to Peterson and Bushway, evaluations of proactive law enforcement strategies fail to distinguish criminal violence from criminal violence involving a gun. Due to this limited information, the researchers had to rely on a report published in 2018 by NASEM on proactive policing. The report reveals that proactive law enforcement consists of the following approaches:

- **Place-Based:** Focuses on places where the most violent crimes are committed with guns occur. This assumes that violent crimes occur in small geographic areas such as neighborhoods and small portions of cities. However, this approach tends to ignore gun violence or other violence that could be happening in other areas because it covers crimes known as crime hot spots.

- **Problem-Solving:** Addresses the underlying cause(s) of violent crimes committed with guns. This concept uses third parties working along with the police to deter elements in communities that may be the underlying causes of gun violence. For example, having a landlord replace outside lights so that the neighborhood is brighter and more inviting, or having a security officer present on the premises so that individuals feel safer. Peterson and Bushway suggest that to improve intelligence gathering, conducting homicide and shooting reviews in which probation officers, medical examiners, social service workers, and district attorneys work along with law enforcement to assist in better understanding the factors present in homicide and shooting incidents, such as whether there was gang member involvement, or location features, such as gang territory or nuisance locations (e.g., hourly motels, problematic bars). These researchers note the 2019 work of Braga and colleagues (2019), who suggest that although guidance exists for conducting these reviews, more rigorous research is needed to demonstrate their value.
- **Person-Focused:** Focuses on individuals at high risk of being perpetrators or victims of violent crimes committed with guns. One such program is the Civil Gang Injunction (CGI), which prohibits gang members from engaging in a variety of legal and illegal behaviors, including associating with other gang members in public. CGIs allow for civil penalties against individuals engaged in prohibited behavior, which often includes possessing any firearms, ammunition, or illegal weapons, or being around others with such weapons.
- **Community-Based:** Uses community resources (and social connections) to counter violent crimes committed with guns and narratives supportive of such crimes.

Many criminal justice agencies do not run Community-Based Approaches, but often involves law enforcement in strategizing with such individuals as former gang members, criminals, and clergy, in developing a means to reduce violence in communities. Additionally, other approaches used by the criminal justice system involve slowing the illegal supply of guns, reducing the carrying of firearms in public areas, and stopping the possession of firearms by juveniles. Law enforcement officers play a pivotal role in these efforts. At the local and state level, law enforcement officers are responsible for responding to and investigating crimes involving firearms, they also enforce laws regarding the transfer and handling of firearms. At the federal level, law enforcement officers are responsible for handling licensing, inspections, and commerce; tracing crime guns; prosecuting crimes committed with guns; investigating trafficking, terrorism, and mass violence; running the National Integrated Ballistic Information Network (NIBIN); and running the National Instant Criminal Background Check System (NIC) (Peterson and Bushway, 2021). Two agencies at the federal level, the FBI and the Bureau of ATF, enforce regulations and perform investigations relevant to guns and gun crimes. The FBI oversees the NICS, which helps to ensure that those legally excluded from purchasing a firearm are detected during a background investigation. More than 25 million background checks in 2018 were conducted through the NICS. The ATF regulates federal firearms licensees (FFLs) by processing licenses, conducting inspections, and tracking national firearm commerce (Peterson and Bushway, 2021). Local and state law enforcement agencies also conduct background checks and issue concealed-carry permits.

Zeoli and colleagues (2022), suggest that the criminal justice system takes a logical approach to reducing firearm access by restricting population-specific laws which grant access to firearms to individuals who are regarded as high-risk (i.e., individuals who are mentally challenged, who have criminal convictions, or individuals who have a previous arrest for domestic violence). Only the court system is authorized to prohibit an individual from purchasing or possessing a firearm. The increase in the number of firearm injuries and violence, as well as the need for criminal justice policymakers to enact legislation that ensures background checks for purchasing firearms and issues concealed-carry permits, demonstrates that firearm violence is a criminal justice issue.

Approaches to reduce firearm-related violence were announced in a DOJ press release in a meeting convened by Former Attorney General Merrick Garland in which justice agencies discussed efforts to reduce violent crime and to combat the gun violence that often accompanies it. As a result of this meeting, a summary of those approaches was provided (Office of Public Affairs. U.S. Department of Justice [DOJ], 2023):

1 U.S. Attorneys are cracking down on illegal firearm trafficking pipelines to hold those with unlawful "ghost guns" accountable and investigate illegal gun dealing.
2 Under the BSCA background checks are being expanded to juvenile criminal and mental health records and local law enforcement contacts for prospective purchasers under the age of 21. Since the law's enactment, the FBI has conducted more than 100,000 enhanced background checks for purchasers under the age of 21. Those checks have kept nearly 1,000 firearms out of the hands of dangerous and prohibited people, including over 200 attempted transactions that were denied solely because of the changes made by BSCA. The FBI continues to engage in extensive education and outreach efforts to improve the state and local partnerships necessary for the success of these enhanced background checks, including hosting webinars attended by over 500 law enforcement agencies.
3 BSCA has expanded restrictions on firearm purchases by those convicted of misdemeanor crimes of domestic violence to include those convicted of assault in a "dating relationship." In August 2022, the FBI implemented the new "dating relationship" definition into its background-check system, and in October, the Department trained federal prosecutors and law enforcement agents on the expanded restriction. The Department also engaged in efforts to educate local and state law enforcement, prosecutors, and court personnel on the need to document "dating relationship" factors in police reports and court records.
4 BSCA created new criminal offenses for unlawful trafficking in firearms and for straw-purchasing (i.e., occurs when someone buys something on behalf of another person who is unable or unwilling to make the purchase themselves) a firearm on behalf of a prohibited person, and it expanded the definition of "engaging in the business" of dealing in firearms. In the months since BSCA's enactment, the Department held multiple training courses for federal prosecutors and law enforcement agents on these new provisions. U.S. Attorneys' Offices around the country charged more than 100 defendants with the new BSCA offenses of firearms trafficking and straw purchasing, and prosecutions for engaging in the business of dealing in firearms without a license have increased 52% over their FY2021 level.
5 BSCA authorized a total of $1.4 billion in funding for new and existing violence-prevention and intervention programs between 2022 and 2026. The Department awarded more than $231 million in Byrne State Crisis Intervention Program grants that will fund

state crisis intervention programs such as drug, mental health, and veterans' treatment programs, and extreme risk protection orders that were designed to keep guns out of the hands of those who pose a threat to themselves or others. This grant also funds State programs such as:

- Education, training, and public-awareness campaigns on extreme risk protection order ("red flag") laws;
- School resource officer training programs related to gun violence and youth mental health; and,
- Drug, mental health, and veterans' treatment courts and behavioral health responses such as crisis mobile response teams and stabilization facilities.

The DOJ also allocated $40 million in supplemental STOP School Violence grants; $20 million in supplemental Community Oriented Policing Services (COPS) School Violence Prevention Program grants; and $100 million in supplemental Community Violence Intervention (CVI) Grants (these funds were allocated to allow for the development and expansion of infrastructure needed to strengthen neighborhood and community safety). In 2022, the Department became more stringent on ghost guns and recovered 25,785 ghost guns in domestic seizures, and 2,453 through international operations. In 2023, it recovered more than 10,000 privately made firearms domestically and 1,000 internationally. In 2022, the National Tracing Center operated by the ATF conducted 622,735 traces for firearms associated with crimes, representing a 10% increase over 2021 and a 48% increase over 2017. As of June 2023, the National Tracing Center had conducted 299,319 traces. During this period, 10,000 law enforcement agencies were granted access to eTrace, the online system that allows participating agencies to submit firearm traces to ATF. Since June 2022, the ATF's NIBIN has generated approximately, 200,000 leads for law enforcement partners across the country.

According to the press release, the Department adopted an enhanced enforcement policy for federally licensed firearms dealers who willfully violate the law; for example, by refusing to run required background checks or selling guns with full awareness that they will end up in the hands of prohibited persons. The ATF published information on over 90 FFL revocations in 2023. In addition to the summation of the press release, the U.S. Attorneys initiated weekly, data-driven coordination with local law enforcement to identify shooters and other drivers of violent crime for federal prosecution. Surges in federal firearms prosecutions increased focus on prosecution for possession or use of machinegun conversion devices, which convert semi-automatic firearms into fully automatic machine guns.

According to Fatal Force Database (2020), Black Americans are disproportionately impacted by police-involved shootings and are killed at more than twice the rate as White Americans. Morin and colleagues (2017) suggest that 79% of Black civilians perceive police killings of Black Americans as signs of a broader problem rather than, isolated incidents. Due to the shootings of Michael Brown, Eric Garner, and Walter Scott, the public's confidence in the police has eroded. Ironically, none of the criminal justice approaches, initiatives, and laws address the many law enforcement officers who are charged with enforcing firearm laws, but are also guilty of committing the laws they are sworn to enforce, especially when it comes to the arrest of persons of color.

Public Health Approaches

According to the EFSGV (2020), a comprehensive public health approach is needed to address the gun violence epidemic. A population-level approach that is aimed at addressing access to firearms, as well as the factors that contribute to violence and protection from gun violence is needed as the public health approach to end firearm violence. Such approaches will bring together institutions and multidisciplinary experts to: (1) define and monitor the problem, (2) identify risk and protective factors, (3) develop and test prevention strategies, and (4) ensure widespread adoption of effective strategies. According to the American Public Health Association (APHA) (n.d.), gun violence is a major public health problem and a leading cause of premature death in the U.S. APHA suggests that it will take a public health approach to prevent death, disability, and injury from gun violence. They argue that this approach must involve data collection and surveillance, research to understand which policies and programs are effective in decreasing gun violence, initiatives to implement those measures that are shown to work, and continued surveillance and evaluation. APHA further states that this approach must be comprehensive and aimed at keeping families and communities safe.

The CDC (n.d.) and the WHO (n.d.) outline approaches to prevent violence that are based on four steps, which can be applied to firearm violence. A synopsis of these approaches appears below:

- *Step 1—Define and monitor the problem*
  This involves defining firearm violence through systematic data collection. To understand the scope of gun violence, researchers and policymakers need reliable data due to the varying types of firearms, which call for different prevention strategies. The public health approach requires collecting and distributing reliable firearm data to combat gun violence. Therefore, researchers need reliable and timely data regarding the number of firearm fatalities and nonfatal injuries that occur in the U.S. each year, and this data should include demographics of the victim and shooter (if applicable), the location and time of the shooting, and the type of gun violence that occurred. Databases should classify based on clear and standardized definitions the types of gun violence (suicides, IPV, mass shootings, interpersonal violence, police shootings, and unintentional injuries). This data should be free of charge, widely available, and easily accessible to the public.
- *Step 2—Identify risk and protective factors*
  Research is conducted in this step to find out why firearm violence occurs and who is affected by it. This step focuses on preventing and addressing population-level risk factors that lead to gun violence and the protective factors that reduce gun violence. An example is provided of a specific risk factor at the individual level that increases the likelihood of engaging in firearm violence. Having access to a firearm at the individual level increases the likelihood of engaging in firearm violence, which increases the likelihood of a dangerous situation becoming fatal. Therefore, policies and programs should be developed that mitigate risk factors and promote protective factors at the individual and community levels.
- *Step 3—Develop and test prevention strategies*
  This step involves designing, implementing, and evaluating interventions to determine what works. Interventions that address risk factors for firearm violence should be

addressed by policymakers and practitioners and should be tested often to ensure they are effective and equitable; rigorous evaluations should also be conducted on a routine basis. An example is given by the Foundation for Effective Gun Violence Prevention Policy, which is a universal background check law that ensures that each person who desires to purchase or transfer a firearm undergoes a background check before purchase. Universal background checks should be supplemented by a firearm purchaser licensing system, which regulates and tracks the flow of firearms, to ensure that firearms do not make it into the hands of prohibited individuals. Policymakers can build upon this and create interventions that target behavioral risk factors for firearm violence, and they can advocate for policies that address community risk factors that lead to violence (e.g., investing in community-based violence prevention programs). In addition to these gun violence prevention policies, several evidence-based strategies can reduce gun violence within communities. For example, community-based violence intervention programs work to de-escalate conflicts, interrupt cycles of retaliatory violence, and support those at elevated risk for violence.

- *Step 4— Ensure widespread adoption of effective strategies*
This involves scaling up effective and promising interventions and evaluating their impact and cost-effectiveness. CDC and WHO suggest that while it is essential to pass strong laws, it is equally important to enforce and implement these laws and to scale up evidence-based programs. Strong firearm violence prevention policies are only effective if they are properly implemented and enforced equitably. A key focus of the public health approach is ensuring that these strategies are not only effective, but that they also promote equity. CDC and WHO state that groups that have been historically disenfranchised should be involved in the implementation process to ensure that public health strategies do not have unintended consequences. For example, gun violence prevention policies should be consistently evaluated to ensure that they do not stigmatize individuals living with mental illness or perpetuate the discriminatory and racist practices embedded in the criminal justice system. The public health approach includes a focus on allocating funds for the implementation and evaluation of these firearm violence prevention strategies at the local, state, and federal levels. Funds should be allocated to train the proper stakeholders to ensure that new policies and programs are adopted and achieve measurable and equitable outcomes.

Below is a flow-chart of the CDC and WHO's Public Health Approach (Figure 13.5):
CDC and WHO suggest that following the steps outlined in the public health approach will reduce firearm violence and save lives. According to the U.S. Surgeon General's Advisory on Firearm Violence (2024):

during an emergency, such as that of firearm violence in the U.S., a public health approach requires combining the best available scientific evidence with scientific judgment and expertise to take life-saving action quickly. This involves simultaneously implementing promising prevention strategies and policies, continuing to gather more evidence, and iterating to improve interventions. This entire approach is continuous and iterative.

Public Health Approach

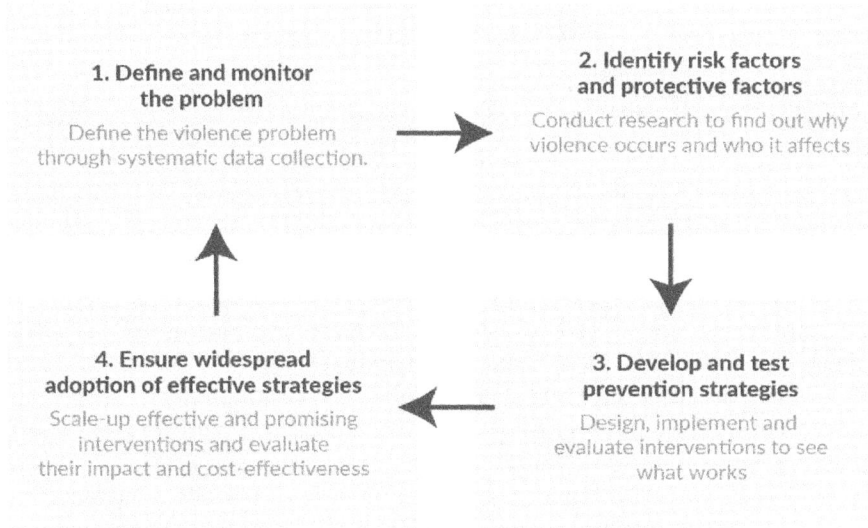

1. Define and monitor the problem

Define the violence problem through systematic data collection.

2. Identify risk factors and protective factors

Conduct research to find out why violence occurs and who it affects

4. Ensure widespread adoption of effective strategies

Scale-up effective and promising interventions and evaluate their impact and cost-effectiveness

3. Develop and test prevention strategies

Design, implement and evaluate interventions to see what works

FIGURE 13.5   CDC and Who Public Health Approach.

Source: CDC and WHO; "Pubic Health Approach."

Public Health and Social Work Approaches

Both social work and public health have similar approaches to addressing gun violence and firearm injuries. Public health and social workers act alongside public health community workers with designated populations as needed, in addition to the general population with an emphasis on preventing community violence, youth violence, and/or family violence related to firearm injury (Barbero et al., 2022). When helping communities with gun violence and firearm injury prevention, social workers often assist community health workers by providing cultural mediation, research and evaluation, health education, outreach, care coordination, individual and community advocacy, and individual and community capacity building.

The public health strategy of applying a four-step approach to address firearm violence and injuries, including a discussion on policy recommendations, is presented in this chapter's section on *Public Health Approaches*. That withstanding, social work also takes a strong stand on needed gun law reform. For example, federal background check law does not pertain to unlicensed gun sellers. Another federal law concern is the 2004 expiration of the federal ban on assault weapons which is a notable setback in reducing firearm injuries given that most mass shooters obtain their firearms and ammunition legally (Bosco-Ruggiero, 2023). To address this, the *NASW* and the Brady Campaign support the transparency of records on crime (Lanyi et al., 2019). Even though public health and social work rely on accurate and updated data to effectively guide firearm injury prevention efforts, the *Bureau of Alcohol, Tobacco, and Firearms* has been prevented from releasing data about crime guns and *bad apple dealers* by the 2005 *Protection of Lawful Commerce in Arms Act*. Because of this, some argue that what is needed is a collaborative endeavor to discover methods for circumventing the Act and obtaining crucial information. Another way that social workers can be effective at the community level and can act on policy matters is to empower victims of firearm violence at the grass-roots level to organize and advocate for stricter gun laws.

Integrating Skills of Social Epidemiology to Address Disparities and Achieve Equity

Firearm violence is a preventable public health epidemic that affects communities, particularly communities of color in the U.S. In socially deprived communities, exposure to firearm violence and the stress, fear, and depression that result from firearm violence extends from the individual who was directly injured/killed to the entire community. This is due to the close social proximity to individuals and communities that are disproportionally affected by violence almost daily. Personal victimization and indirect exposure to violence are well-documented in the criminal justice and social science literature as having detrimental impacts on adults' and adolescents' health and well-being and disproportionately affect low-income, urban-dwelling adults and youth of color (Bancalari et al., 2022). Similarly, the CDC (2022b) suggests that health disparities are common among socially disadvantaged populations who are exposed to firearm violence. These socially disadvantaged populations continue to suffer from the lack of generational investment in their communities to promote their safety and well-being.

Jay and Allen (2023) cite studies of Krieger and colleagues (2017) and Jay and colleagues (2022), both of which analyzed firearm violence as a function of racialized economic segregation. Each study used an indicator referred to as the index of concentration at the extremes (ICE) for race-poverty. ICE is a neighborhood-level measure of exposure to structural racism that captures race and class, the most interrelated dimensions of social stratification. Black-headed households were found at the low end of the measure with values closer to –1. Additional findings at this level were deprived neighborhoods, with Black-headed households that have incomes below the poverty line outnumbering White-headed households with incomes over $100,000/year. Privileged neighborhoods with values near 1 were found at the other end, where those proportions were reversed. According to Jay and Allen, the studies by Krieger and colleagues and Jay and colleagues found that racialized economic segregation was a strong predictor of firearm assaults. The Krieger and colleagues study revealed that living in a neighborhood in the most-deprived ICE quintile was associated with a 3.96 times greater risk of a firearm assault injury, compared to living in the most-privileged ICE quintile. The Jay and colleagues study found that neighborhoods in the most-deprived ICE quintile experienced an average of 36.1 shootings over six years, while neighborhoods in the most-privileged quintile experienced 2.9.

To better understand how social determinants of health (SDOH) such as residential racial segregation, income inequality, and community resilience impact firearm fatalities, Shour and colleagues (2023) conducted research in which they investigated the relationship between residential racial segregation and the likelihood of firearm fatalities in Wisconsin. The researchers collected and analyzed SDOH data on 72 counties in Wisconsin from the Agency for Health Care Research and Quality (the database is a project supported by the Patient-Centered Outcomes Research [PCOR] Trust Fund and generates linkable SDOH-focused data for use in PCOR research, it informs ways of addressing emergent health challenges, and contributes to improved health outcomes) for 2019. The number of firearm fatalities per county was used as the dependent variable and as a continuous variable. Residential racial segregation was used as the independent variable and was defined as the degree to which non-White and White residents lived across the counties, ranging from 0 (complete integration) to 100 (complete segregation); higher values indicated greater residential segregation (categorized as low, moderate, and high). The covariates were income inequality, ranging from zero (perfect equality) to one (perfect inequality), categorized as low, moderate, and high, community resilience risk factors (low, moderate, and high risks), and rural-urban classifications. The study's findings revealed that residential racial segregation and income inequality in Wisconsin were mostly low, compared to moderate and high. Community resilience was predominantly moderate risk and high risk when compared to low risk, and rural areas outnumbered urban areas. The adjusted model results indicated that the risk of firearm fatalities is 1.3 times higher in places with high residential racial segregation than in areas with low residential racial segregation after controlling for income inequality, community resilience, and rural-urban classifications. In the adjusted model, other SDOH variables were also significantly associated with an elevated risk of firearm fatalities. When compared to places with low-income inequality, the risk of firearm fatalities was 1.2 times higher in areas with high-income inequality. When compared to low-risk community resilience areas, the risk of firearm fatalities was 0.6 times greater in moderate-risk areas and 0.5 times higher in high-risk areas. Shour and colleagues further suggest that this implies that when community resilience is low, the risk of firearm fatalities increases. They measured community resilience by estimating the number of individuals who live with multiple risk factors. These individuals were categorized as having 0 risk factors (low risk), 1–2 risk factors (moderate risk), and 3 or more risk factors (high risk). The risk factors include income-to-poverty ratio, single or zero caregiver households, crowding, communication barriers, households without full-time year-round employment, disability, no health insurance, age 65 or older, no vehicle access, and no broadband internet access. Wisconsin's areas with high residential racial segregation also had high rates of firearm fatalities, which indicated that residential racial segregation influences firearm fatalities. The findings of Shour and colleagues' study were similar to Houghton and colleagues' (2021) study, which involved a cross-sectional analysis of 51 metropolitan areas in the U.S. between 2013 and 2017 and found that structural racism was associated with firearm homicide.

The studies reviewed in this section lend support to the argument of the Giffords Law Center to Prevent Gun Violence (2022) that multi-level approaches are needed to save lives, reflecting how no single cause or factor of firearm violence exists in isolation (Giffords Law Center to Prevent Gun Violence, 2022). Firearm violence disproportionately impacts communities of color and is associated with measures of structural racism. Therefore, public health interventions targeting gun violence must address these systemic inequities. What may be needed is a CVI program. According to the U.S. DOJ's Office of Justice Programs (2024), CVI is an approach that uses evidence-informed strategies to reduce violence through tailored community-centered initiatives. These multidisciplinary strategies engage individuals and groups to prevent and disrupt cycles of violence and retaliation and establish relationships between individuals and community assets to deliver services that save lives, address trauma, provide opportunity, and improve the physical, social, and economic conditions that drive violence.

The CVI focuses on reducing homicides and shootings by establishing relationships with people at the core of gun violence in their communities. These are individuals who are chronically alienated by, disconnected from, and distrustful of traditional structures of support, safety, and health (Boag-Munroe & Evangelou, 2012). CVI programs intend to change/instill positive life trajectories, facilitate healing, and promote abstinence from violence. Investments can be made at the community level that involves individuals who are skilled in the intervention and in supporting individuals to make positive changes. These are neighborhood change agents or life coaches who have credibility or standing in the communities where they work and can reach out to those at the center of gun violence in their communities, building relationships, and working to support healing and addressing conflict through nonviolent means, including de-escalation and mediation. In most cases, these individuals can relate to community members because they have been victims of shootings, survivors of loved ones who have been killed by a firearm, or they have been incarcerated or have a family member who has been incarcerated for violence involving a firearm (Dholukia, & Gilbert, 2021). Life coaches may also assist community members in finding affordable housing or in pursuing education or employment opportunities. Moreover, research has found that improvements in blighted areas in communities such as renovating dilapidated buildings and homes, and replacing dim street lights with brighter lights have led to a reduction in firearm violence (Branas et al., 2018; Hohl et al., 2019; Gobaud et al., 2022).

Counties with the highest levels of poverty in 2022 experienced firearm homicide rates 4.5 times as high, and firearm suicide rates 1.3 times as high, as counties with the lowest poverty levels (Simon et al., 2022). Firearm violence and injuries do not exist in isolation; many factors cause them, especially in marginalized communities of color. Policies are needed that address community investment. This investment must be provided in the form of programs designed to bring about positive social change for individuals living and working in marginalized communities.

How Can Firearm Injuries Be Prevented?

It is plausible, given the statistics, that the more access an individual, especially children, has to a firearm, the more firearm injuries, homicides, unintentional shootings, and deaths. Therefore, preventive measures must be in place to block access to firearms. Some of these measures include Lethal Means Restrictive Counseling, Anticipatory Guidance and Firearm-Retirement Counseling, Safe Storage and Personalized Smart Gun Technology, and Legislation.

Lethal Means Restrictive Counseling

According to the CDC, firearms are the most commonly used method of committing death by suicide, regardless of sex. The presence of a firearm in the home has been associated with a higher risk of being a victim of homicide and suicide among all household members, and an unlocked firearm in the home is associated with a higher risk of suicide and unintentional firearm injury among children and adolescents (Arglemyer et al., 2014; Grossman et al., 2005). Individuals at risk of having access to loaded firearms require removing firearms from the home or securing them with the unloaded firearm locked away separately from the ammunition; thus, preventing or reducing the lethality of an attempt, this is referred to as lethal means restriction (Dodginton, 2021). Lethal Means Restriction Counseling (LMRC) is a vital part of safety planning. It is a process to first assess whether patients are at risk for suicide, and then to work with them to restrict access to lethal means, to a firearm. The means chosen for a suicide attempt during a crisis are also strongly associated with their immediate availability, suggesting that reducing access to lethal means may delay an attempt long enough for patients to seek help or for the crisis to pass (Barber & Miller, 2014).

The National Suicide Prevention Resource Center, according to Hunter and colleagues (2021), considers LMRC as a program with evidence of effectiveness. To be successful, individuals and their families must be counseled regarding suicide risk and methods of effective LMRC before the onset of a suicidal crisis or subsequent attempts. Counseling should focus on enhancing locked-storage measures and planning for how to address risks if they emerge. LMRC should be provided once suicide risk is identified and should be reinforced at all subsequent healthcare visits. However, Hunter and colleagues (2021) recommend that LMRC should be modified based on the age, gender, and race of an individual.

Anticipatory Guidance and Firearm-Retirement Counseling

In addition to older individuals having the highest rate of suicide, possibly due to such issues as depression and loneliness, their cognitive abilities can decline and bring on dementia, which can bring on confusion and aggressive behavior with family and caregivers (Pinholt et al., 2014). Also, as individuals age, they may have arthritis, which may impede their ability to use firearm-locking devices. Therefore, it is recommended by clinicians that at-risk patients receive counseling to enhance their locked-storage practices and address their risk of suicide (Carter et al., 2018). As individuals age or cognition worsens clinical counseling interventions may progress from counseling regarding storage to supervised access to more intensive measures, such as reducing weapon lethality (e.g., removing the firearm's firing pin), transferring ownership, or removal of firearms from the household (Carter et al., 2022; Betz et al., 2018). The Alzheimer's Association (2024) recommends removing firearms from the home of someone living with dementia to prevent unintentional shootings, recognizing that storing or locking up a firearm may not be enough.

Safe Storage and Personalized Smart Gun Technology

According to the American Academy of Pediatrics policy statement, storing a firearm outside the home is the safest form of storage (2023). Schell and colleagues (2022) suggest that over one-third of households, representing 22.6 million children, own and store firearms in the home. Lee and colleagues (2022) present several safe options that can be used for storing firearms either inside or outside of one's home to prevent firearm injury or death.

Four key elements for safer firearm storage in the home are:

1 Store the firearm unloaded.
2 Store the firearm locked.
3 Store the ammunition separated from the firearm.
4 Store the ammunition locked separately from the firearm.

Each element of safe storage decreases the likelihood of youth inappropriately accessing firearms and decreases the risk of injury and death (Lee et al., 2022).

In addition, another means of preventing firearm injuries and death is technology using personalized "smart guns," which provide gun owners with the ability to secure their handguns by keeping unauthorized users from firing a firearm because these firearms are designed to recognize authorized users, either using proximity devices, such as paired radio frequency identification (RFID) watches or rings, or via built-in biometrics recognizing fingerprints or palmprints (Lee et al., 2022).

Legislation

Child Access Prevention (CAP) laws or Safe Storage Laws allow prosecutors to bring charges against adults who intentionally or carelessly allow children to have unsupervised access to firearms. CAP laws aim to reduce unintentional firearm injuries and deaths, suicides, and violent crime among youth chiefly by reducing children's access to stored guns (Gun Policy in America, 2024). Webster and colleagues (2004), Azad and colleagues (2020), and Gius (2020) found that CAP laws showed a 10% decrease in suicides among youth. These laws make it a civil or criminal offense for the firearm owner if a child is provided with access or could potentially access an improperly stored firearm.

The John Hopkins Center for Gun Violence (2020) suggests that Extreme Risk Laws are state laws that provide law enforcement and, depending on the jurisdiction, family members, health professionals, and school administrators, among others, a formal legal process to temporarily reduce an individual's access to firearms if they pose a danger to themselves or others. As of June 2021, these laws have been enacted in 19 states and the District of Columbia. Extreme Risk Laws often involve a civil court order, prompted by a petition by a family member or law enforcement officer and issued by a judge upon consideration of the evidence. The order temporarily prohibits a person from possessing or purchasing firearms and provides a process for the removal of firearms already in the person's possession. In some states, extreme risk laws also prohibit the possession of ammunition. These orders have been associated with decreased population-level firearm suicide rates and individual-level suicide risk (Betz et al., 2023).

Evidence was cited by the Johns Hopkins Center from peer-reviewed studies by Swanson and colleagues in Connecticut, Indiana, and California, which found that these laws have helped prevent firearm deaths. For example, an analysis of Connecticut's extreme risk law found that the passage of the law between 1999 and 2013 accomplished the following:

- A total of 762 firearm removal cases were issued, and police found firearms in 99% of cases, removing an average of seven guns per subject.
- Suicidality or self-injury was a less concerning issue in ≥61% of cases where such material was available.
- For every 10–20 firearm removals issued, one life was saved.

Parents, family members, clinicians, and policymakers must stay abreast of the best practices being used to prevent firearm injuries and deaths. However, no one method alone can prevent these injuries or death. Therefore, efforts to prevent firearm injuries and death must be guided by evidence-based research to prevent firearms from being introduced into families and communities.

Policy Recommendations

The International Network for Epidemiology in Policy (INEP) (Davis, 2018) developed a Policy Brief that seeks to ensure that those responsible for formulating firearm injury policy have access to information to inform policy decisions that are guided by evidence from epidemiological and social sciences research. As such, INEP makes the following recommendations:

- National and local governments should collect and make epidemiological and other scientific data relating to firearm-related morbidity and mortality publicly available for research;
- WHO and other global public health and human rights organizations should continue to encourage all member countries to collect and disseminate epidemiological and other scientific data about firearm-related deaths, injuries, disabilities, and associated costs, and to repeal any restrictions on collecting such data;
- National and local governments, private organizations, and nonprofit organizations should prioritize research funding specifically aimed at assessing the scale and scope of firearm violence and promote the development and evaluation of firearm violence prevention interventions through improved understanding of upstream determinants derivable from epidemiological and other scientific disciplines.
- Epidemiologists should engage in multidisciplinary firearm violence prevention research and, in designing and evaluating primary, secondary, and tertiary prevention and mitigation strategies, apply evidence-based injury prevention approaches to address and evaluate the multilevel factors of the hosts, agents, and vehicles, and their related physical, social, and environmental factors; and
- Public health educators should harness the epidemiological and other scientific evidence regarding the harms of firearm violence and incorporate this issue in the curriculum; they also should address how students of epidemiology can work with public health professionals and engage with relevant stakeholders (i.e., policymakers, public health practitioners, and the public).

The U.S. Surgeon General's Advisory Report on Firearm Violence (2024) argues that a public health approach to firearm violence prevention can curb the alarming trends of firearm-related injury and death in America and the resulting health impacts. Therefore, the following recommendations, some of which mirror the INEP recommendations, are made by the U.S. Surgeon General:

- Critical need to increase research funding. This involves:
  1 Improving data sources and data collection to inform prevention activities. Here, without proper data, the extent and severity of firearm violence outcomes as well as evaluations of prevention efforts and interventions will be limited. Prioritizing coordination across organizations that have access to firearm injury data (health systems, states, localities, public health agencies, nonprofits, law enforcement, etc.) will allow for a more complete analysis of firearm violence.
  2 Expanding research to examine short-term and long-term outcomes of firearm violence and evaluate specific prevention strategies. There are multiple research gaps regarding

firearm-related violence and injury prevention; therefore, research should also evaluate the health outcomes of individuals directly and indirectly exposed to firearm violence, including survivors, their families, and communities. Additionally, research should be expanded to evaluate the effectiveness of firearm violence prevention strategies in new settings or within subpopulations, and to support follow-up evaluations of the long-term outcomes associated with such strategies.

3 Conducting implementation science research to improve the effectiveness of prevention strategies. There are existing firearm violence prevention strategies that have evidence of effectiveness. However, expanding support and investment for implementation science research is necessary to improve the uptake of evidence-based strategies, policies, and practices in communities. Implementation science research can support the adoption, implementation, and sustainment of evidence-based prevention strategies and also help ensure that such strategies do not have any unintended impact.

- Community risk reduction and education prevention strategies, which involve entities such as:

4 Implementing CVI. These are approaches that are evidence-informed, multidisciplinary strategies that disrupt cycles of violence and connect individuals at risk of violence involvement with services that address trauma and improve physical, social, and economic circumstances (Office of Justice Programs, 2024). Under this approach, individuals are connected with health care, housing, employment, and other resources (Center for Gun Violence Solutions, n.d.).

5 Incorporating organizational violence prevention and emergency preparedness elements into safety programs. This approach involves establishing behavioral threat assessment and management (BTAM) teams, as well as emergency action plans to address the threat from firearm violence. With this approach, communities can facilitate the development of trauma-informed preparedness and response plans for schools and the implementation of student programs before, during, and after school to ensure safety.

6 Encouraging health systems to facilitate education on safe and secure storage. Here, healthcare systems can petition healthcare workers to talk with patients regarding safe gun storage and gun transfers during routine visits to protect family members who are children and those with dementia.

- Firearm risk reduction strategies which include:

7 Requiring safe and secure firearm storage, including CAP laws. Firearms should be stored, unloaded, and locked in a secure place that is only accessible to authorized users; ammunition should be stored separately from the firearm(s).

8 Implementing universal background checks and expanding purchaser licensing laws. Anyone who engages in the business of selling firearms should have a license and conduct universal background checks.

9 Banning assault weapons and large-capacity magazines for civilian use. Such weapons include automatic weapons and some semiautomatic weapons that may include military-style features that make the firearm more lethal, such as detachable large-capacity magazines.

10 Treating firearms like other consumer products, including requiring safety testing or safety features. There are no federal safety standards and regulations for firearms manufactured in the U.S.; therefore, all firearms may not undergo safety testing or include safety warning labels.

11 Creating safer conditions in public places related to firearm use and carry. This includes developing policies that govern who can carry a loaded firearm in public spaces, concealed or opened, and through rules around using deadly force with a firearm in public situations where the individual(s) could have safely retreated without firing a weapon.

- Mental health action and support, such as:

12 Increasing access to affordable, high-quality mental health care and substance use treatment. Health workers and community-based organizations can address the mental health consequences associated with firearm violence by providing trauma-informed care for individuals who experience firearm violence. Health systems and health workers can connect individuals at risk of suicide to timely mental health resources and care. Policymakers can provide support to sustain mental health access and crisis support services.

13 Building on investments to enhance safety measures and evidence-based violence prevention efforts in learning settings. This approach involves expanding school-based mental health to build a positive school climate along with the capacity and resources needed to connect students to mental health services.

In addition to the INEP and the Johns Hopkins Center for Gun Violence, we recommend the following:

- Institutions of higher learning provide a multidisciplinary program that educates and trains a diverse group of faculty and students with opportunities to teach and take new firearm-related courses that revolve around epidemiology, disparities, interventions, and policy analysis. Also, foster scholarly multidisciplinary collaboration across disciplines that engage in innovative projects focused on research, scholarship, and creative practice, and prepare teams for external funding opportunities to support future firearm injury prevention research. This program will work toward improving epidemiological data and strengthening social science-informed policy analysis. It will identify design applications and develop new safety technologies.

- Developing and strengthening community-based and hospital-based programs that provide early education and intervention about firearm-related injuries. This includes providing clinicians and other healthcare workers with information on the most effective ways to counsel patients and families on proper firearm safety, emphasizing evidence-based methods that are shown to reduce intentional and unintentional injuries (NASEM, 2019; Bulger, 2019). This is especially important for those individuals who may be impacted by such social determinants as residential racial segregation, income inequality, IPV, and exposure to violence. In addition, free public workshops on firearm safety and storage, as well as firearm violence, should be held at recreational centers, schools, and places of worship. These workshops should be accompanied by pamphlets on firearm-related injuries and prevention; the pamphlets can be disseminated to local shopping centers and physicians' offices.

- Addressing investments for structural determinants increases the risk of firearm-related injury and violence that are concentrated in poverty-stricken communities. These investments would increase funding to improve blighted areas which have dilapidated houses and structures, poor street lighting, and a lack of security personnel. Investment would also be made to provide access to education, employment, economic growth, and health care;
- Extending Extreme Risk Protection Laws so that they are universal, and all states are covered. This will temporarily restrict access to guns from individuals determined to be at elevated risk of harming themselves or others; and
- Implementing clear and unbiased laws for law enforcement officers who intentionally misuse a firearm to shoot and/or kill a person of color.

Summary

Addressing the issue of firearm injuries is complex, and it is the responsibility of the entire global society. Socioeconomic factors such as poverty, lack of educational opportunities, low levels of mental health accessibility, and residing in blighted communities, among other inequalities, play a large role in firearm-related injuries. The rise in firearm injuries has led to violence, mortality, and racial unrest. It has led the Surgeon General of the U.S. to issue a warning and regard firearm-related violence as a pandemic. The DOJ should continue to expand the availability and effectiveness of federal investigative resources to help local, state, and Tribal partners solve crimes and bring perpetrators of firearm-related violence to justice. Although further research, funding, evidence-based policies, and education are needed to better understand and prevent firearm injuries, it will take a societal effort to create safer and healthier communities.

Discussion Questions

1 What are the types of firearm injuries?
2 What are the community risk factors associated with firearm injuries?
3 Discuss the policies used by the Criminal Justice System to reduce firearm-related violence.
4 Discuss the impact that firearm-related injuries have had on the international community.
5 Discuss the impact of CVI Programs.
6 How can institutions of higher education assist in preventing firearm-related injuries?

References

Abba-Aji, M., Koya, S.F., Abdalla, S.M., Ettman, C.K., Cohen, G.H., & Galea, S. (2024). The mental health consequences of interpersonal gun violence: A systematic review, *SSM – Mental Health*, 5, 100302, https://doi.org/10.1016/j.ssmmh.2024.100302; www.sciencedirect.com/science/article/pii/S2666560324000070

Abrams, Z. (2022). Talking to patients about firearm safety: Providers can help reduce injuries and deaths by talking with patients about safe storage and temporary transfers during high-risk periods. *CE Corner. Monitor on Psychology*, 53(3), 34. CE Corner. www.apa.org/monitor/2022/04/ce-firearm-safety

Alzheimer's Association. (2024). Firearm safety and dementia. www.alzheimersdisease.net/resources/firearm-gun-safetyl.

American Academy of Pediatrics. (2023). Gun safety and injury. www.aap.org/en/patient-care/gun-safety-and-injury-prevention/. Accessed July 12, 2022.

American Public Health Association (APHA). (n.d.). Gun violence is a public health crisis. www.apha.org/topics-and-issues/gun-violence

Anglemyer, A., Horvath, T., & Rutherford, G. (2014). The accessibility of firearms and risk for suicide and homicide victimization among household members. *Annals of Internal Medicine*, 160(2), 101–110. https://doi.org/10.7326/M13-1301-73

Armenta, A., & Rosales, R. (2019). Beyond the fear of deportation: Understanding unauthorized immigrants' ambivalence toward the police. *American Behavioral Scientists*, 63(9), 1350–1369. https://doi.org/10.1177/0002764219835278

ATF. (2022, October 21). Gun Control Act of 1968. Gun Control Act | Bureau of alcohol, tobacco, firearms and explosives (atf.gov).

Aubel, A.J., Pallin, R., Wintemute, G.J., Kravitz-Wirtz, N. (2021). Exposure to violence, firearm involvement, and socioemotional consequences among California adults. *Journal of Interpersonal Violence*, 36(23–24), 11822–11838. www.pubmed.ncbi.nlm.nih.gov/33380237/

Azad, H.A., Monuteaux, M.C., Rees, C.A., Siegel, M., Mannix, R., Lee, L.K., Sheehan, K.M., & Fleegler, E.W. (2020, May 1). Child access prevention firearm laws and firearm fatalities among children aged 0 to 14 years, 1991–2016. *JAMA Pediatrics*, 74(5), 463–469.

Bancalari, P., Sommer, M., & Rajan, S. (2022). Youth exposure to endemic community gun violence: A systematic review. *Adolescence Research Review*, 7, 383–417.

Barbero, C., Hafeedh Bin Abdullah, A., Wiggins, N., Garrettson, M., Jones, D.S., Guinn, A., Girod, C., Bradford, J., & Wennerstrom, A. (2022). Community health worker activities in public health programs to prevent violence: Coding roles and scope. *American Journal of Public Health* (1971), 112(8), 1191–1201. https://doi.org/10.2105/AJPH.2022.306865

Barber, C., Cook, P.J., & Parker, S. (2022, December). The emerging infrastructure of U.S. firearms injury data. *Journal of Preventive Medicine*, 165(Pt A), 107129. https://doi.org/10.1016/j.ypmed.2022.107129. Epub 2022 Jul 5. PMID: 35803350.

Barber, C.W., & Miller, M.J. (2014). Reducing a suicidal person's access to lethal means of suicide: A research agenda. *American Journal of Preventive Medicine*, 47(Suppl 2), S264–S272.

Barboza, G.A. (2018). Secondary spatial analysis of gun violence near Boston schools: A public health approach. *Journal of Urban Health*, 95(3), 344–360. https://doi.org/10.1007/s11524-018-0244-8

Barrett, J.T., Lee, L.K., Monuteaux, M., Hoffmann, J.A., & Fleegler, E.W. (2022). Association of county-level poverty and inequities with firearm-related mortality in U.S. youth. *JAMA Pediatric*, 176(2), e214822.

Beardslee, J., Docherty, M., Mulvey, E., & Pardini, D. (2021). The direct and indirect associations between childhood socioeconomic disadvantage and adolescent gun violence. *Journal of Clinical Child & Adolescent Psychology*, 50(3), 326–336.

Beardslee, J., Kan, E., Simmons, C., Pardini, D., Peniche, M., Frick, P.J., Steinberg, L., & Cauffman, E.A. (2021). Within-individual examination of the predictors of gun carrying during adolescence and young adulthood among young men. *Journal of Youth Adolescence*, 50(10), 1952–1969. https://doi.org/10.1007/s10964-021-01464-6. Epub 2021 Jul 16. PMID: 34272654; PMCID: PMC8417009.

Beardslee, J., Mulvey, E., Schubert, C., Allison, P., Infante, A., & Pardini, D. (2018). Gun- and non-Gun – Related violence exposure and risk for subsequent gun carrying among male Juvenile Offenders. *Journal of the American Academy of Child and Adolescent Psychiatry*, 57(4), 274–279. https://doi.org/10.1016/j.jaac.2018.01.012

Benns, M., Ruther, M., Nash, N., Bozeman, M., Harbrecht, B., & Miller, K. (2020). The impact of historical racism on modern gun violence: Redlining in the city of Louisville, KY. *Injury*, 51(10), 2192–2198.

Bent-Goodley, T., St. Vil, C., Cuevas, C.A., & Abbey, A. (2022). Police, violence, and social justice: A call for research and introduction to the special issue. *Psychology of Violence*, 12(4), 195–200. https://doi.org/10.1037/vio0000438

Bergen-Cico, D., Lane, S.D., Keefe, R.H., Larsen, D.A., Panasci, A., Salaam, N., Jennings-Bey, T., & Rubinstein, R.A. (2018). Community gun violence as a social determinant of elementary school achievement. *Social Work Public Health*, 33(7–8), 439–448.

Betz, M.E., Bowen, D.M., Rowhani-Rahbar, A., McCourt, A.D., & Rivara, F.P. (2023). State reporting requirements for involuntary holds, court-ordered guardianship, and the US National Firearm Background Check System. *JAMA Health Forum*, 4(11), e233945–e233945.

Betz, M.E., McCourt, A.D., Vernick, J.S., Ranney, M.L., Maust, D.T., & Wintemute, G.J. (2018). Firearms and dementia: Clinical considerations. *Annals of Internal Medicine*, 169, 47–49.

Bleyer, A., Siegel, S.E., Estrada, J., & Thomas, C.R. Jr. (2024). Fallacy of attributing the U.S. firearm mortality epidemic to mental health. *PLOS One*, 19(8), e0290138. https://doi.org/10.1371/journal.pone.0290138

Boag-Munroe, G., & Evangelou, M. (2012). From hard to reach to how to reach: A systematic review of the literature on hard-to-reach families. *Research Papers in Education*, 27(2), 209–239.

Bor, J., Venkataramani, A.S., Williams, D.R., & Tsai, A.C. (2018). Police killings and their spillover effects on the mental health of black Americans: A population-based, quasi-experimental study. *Lancet*, 392(10144), 302–310. https://doi.org/10.1016/S0140-6736(18)31130-9

Bosco-Ruggiero, S. (2023). *Social work and gun violence resources*. A 2023 guide for social work and gun violence prevention. www.mastersinsocialworkonline.org/resources/gun-violence-prevention/ Masters of social work online. A 2023 guide for social work and gun violence prevention. https://mastersinsocialworkonline.org/resources/gun-violence-prevention/

Bowen, N.K., & Bowen, G.L. (1999). Effects of crime and violence in neighborhoods and schools on the school behavior and performance of adolescents. *Journal of Adolescent Research*, 14(3), 319–342. https://doi.org/10.1177/0743558499143003

Braga, A.A., Zimmerman, G., Barao, L., Farrell, C., Brunson, R.K., & Papachristos, A.V. (2019). Street gangs, gun violence, and focused deterrence: Comparing place-based and Group-based evaluation methods to estimate direct and spillover deterrent effects. *Journal of Research in Crime and Delinquency*, 56(4), 524–562. https://doi.org/10.1177/0022427818821716

Branas, C.C., & Morrison, C.N. (2022). Place-based interventions and the epidemiology of violence prevention. *Current Epidemiology Reports*, 9(4), 316–325.

Branas, C.C., South, E., Kondo, M.C., Hohl, B.C., Bourgois, P., Wiebe, D.J., & MacDonald, J.M. (2018). Citywide cluster randomized trial to restore blighted vacant land and its effects on violence, crime, and fear. *Proceedings of the National Academy of Sciences*, 115(12), 2946–2951.

Brownlee, C. (2023). How 30 years of federal background checks changed gun buying by the numbers. *Trace*. www.thetrace.org/2023/11/background-checks-gun-purchasing-brady/

Buggs, S.A.L., Kravitz-Wirtz, N.D., & Lund, J.J. (2023). Social and structural determinants of community firearm violence and community trauma. *The ANNALS of the American Academy of Political and Social Science*, 704(1), 224–241. https://doi.org/10.1177/00027162231173324

Bulger, E.M., Kuhls, D.A., Campbell, B.T., Bonne, S., Cunningham, R.M., Betz, M., Dicker, R., Ranney, M.L., Barsotti, C., Hargarten, S., Sakran, J.V., Rivara, F.P., James, T., Lamis, D., Timmerman, G., Rogers, S.O., Choucair, B., & Stewart, R.M. (2019). Proceedings from the medical summit on firearm injury prevention: A public health approach to reduce death and disability in the US. *Journal of the American College of Surgeons*, 229(4), 415–430. https://journals.lww.com/journalacs/fulltext/2023/06000/proceedings_from_the_second_medical_summit_on.34.aspx

Butkus, R., Doherty, R., & Bornstein, S.S. (2018). Reducing firearm injuries and deaths in the United States: A position paper from the American college of physicians. *Annals Internal Medicine*, 169(10), 704–707.

Byrne, A., Hagen, M.G., & Thompson, L. (2021). Gun safety for children. *JAMA Pediatric*, 175(3), 332.

Campbell, K.A., Ford-Gilboe, M., Stanley, M., & MacKinnon, K. (2022, May 18). Intimate partner violence and women living with episodic disabilities: A scoping review protocol. *Systematic Reviews*, 11(1), 97.

Cannon, A.D., Reese, K., Tetens, P., & Fingar, K. (2023, October 23). Preventable tragedies: Findings from the #NotAnAccident index of unintentional shootings by children. *Injury Epidemiology*, 10(Suppl 1), 52. https://doi.org/10.1186/s40621-023-00464-3

Carter, P.M., Losman, E., Roche, J.S., Malani, P.N., Kullgren, J.T., Solway, E., Kirch, M., Singer, D., Walton, M.A., Zeoli, A.M., & Cunningham, R.M. (2022). Firearm ownership, attitudes, and safe storage practices among a nationally representative sample of older U.S. adults aged 50 to 80. *Preventive Medicine*. https://doi.org/10.1016/j.ypmed.2022.106955. Epub 2022 Jan 21. PMID: 35065980.

Centers for Disease Control. (n.d.). Wonder. About provisional mortality statistics, 2018 through last month. Accessed September 7, 2022. https://wonder.cdc.gov/mcd-icd10-provisional.html

Centers for Disease Control and Prevention (CDC). (n.d.a). Wonder – Wide-ranging online data for epidemiologic research. Provisional mortality statistics. https://wonder.cdc.gov/mcd.html

Centers for Disease Control and Prevention (CDC). (2024). About firearm injury and death. Firearm injury and death prevention. www.cdc.gov/firearm-violence/about/

Centers for Disease Control and Prevention (CDC). (n.d.c). National center for health statistics. Underlying cause of death 1999–2019. Average based on years 2015–2019.

Centers for Disease Control and Prevention (CDC). (n.d.d). The national center for injury prevention and control, division of violence prevention. The Public Health Approach to Violence Prevention.

Centers for Disease Control and Prevention (CDC). (2019). Web-based injury statistics query and reporting system (WISQARS) [online]. www.cdc.gov/injury/wisqars

Center for Disease Control and Prevention (CDC). (2021). National Center for Health Statistics, National Vital Statistics System, mortality data, 2021. www.cdc.gov/nchs/nvss/deaths.htm

Center for Disease Control and Prevention (CDC). (2022a). Firearm deaths grow, disparities widen: Comprehensive strategies can prevent violence and help reduce racial ethnic disparities.

Centers for Disease Control and Prevention (CDC). (2022b). National violent death reporting system (NVDRS) coding manual revised [Online] 2021 National Center for Injury Prevention and Control. www.cdc.gov/nvdrs/about/nvdrs-data-acess.html

Centers for Disease Control and Prevention. (2023). Unintentional firearm injury deaths among children and adolescents aged 0-17 years-National Violent Death Reporting System, United States, 2003-2021. www.cdc.gov/mmwr/volumes/72/wr/pdfs/mm7250a1-h.pdf

Centers for Disease Control and Prevention (CDC). (2024). Fast facts: Firearm injury and death. www.cdc.gov/firearm-violence/data-research/facts-stats/

Center for Gun Violence Solutions. (n.d.). Community violence intervention. Johns Hopkins Bloomberg School of Public Health. Retrieved March 15, 2024. https://publichealth.jhu.edu/center-for-gun-violence-solutions/solutions/community-violence-intervention

Cunningham, R.M., Walton, M.A., & Carter, P.M. (2018). The major causes of death in children and adolescents in the United States. *New England Journal of Medicine*, 379(25), 2468–2475.

Davis, A.B., Gaudino, J.A., Soskolne, C.L., Al-Delaimy, W.K. (2018, August). The role of epidemiology in firearm violence prevention: A policy brief, *International Journal of Epidemiology*, 47(4), 1015–1019. https://doi.org/10.1093/ije/dyy059

Dholukia, N., & Gilbert, D. (2021). Community violence intervention programs, explained. *Vera Institute of Justice*, 1–4. https://vera-institute.files.svdcdn.com/production/inline-downloads/community-violence-intervention-programs-explained-report.pdf

DiScala, C., & Sege, R. (2004). Outcomes in children and young adults who are hospitalized for firearms-related injuries. *Pediatrics*, 113(5), 1306–1312.

Dodington, J. (2021). Safety devices for firearms. In L.K. Lee & E.W. Fleegler (Eds.), *Pediatric firearm injuries and fatalities: The clinician's guide to policies and approaches to firearm harm prevention* (pp. 179–192). Springer Nature.

Educational Fund to Stop Gun Violence (EFSGV). (2020). The public health approach to gun violence prevention. efsgv.org/PublicHealthApproachToGVP

Everytown Research and Policy. (2024). Gun violence in America. www.everytownresearch.org/rep ort/gun-violence-in-america/

Fatal Force Database (2020). Everytown research analysis of 2019 to 2023 Mapping police violence data.. www.everytownresearch.org/report/gun-violence-in-america/

Finkelhor, D., Turner, H.A., Shattuck, A., & Hamby, S.L. (2015). Prevalence of childhood exposure to violence, crime, and abuse: Results from the national survey of children's exposure to violence. *JAMA Pediatrics*, 169(8), 746–754.

Foley, D.L., Goldston, D.B., Costello, E.J., & Angold, A. (2006). Proximal psychiatric risk factors for suicidality in youth: The Great Smoky Mountains Study. *Archives of General Psychiatry*, 63(9), 1017–1024.

Fowler, K.A., Dahlberg, L.L., Haileyesus, T., & Annest, J.L. (2015). Firearm injuries in the United States. *Preventive Medicine*, 79, 5–14. https://doi.org/10.1016/j.ypmed.2015.06.002

Frassetto, M. (2013). Firearms and weapons legislation up to the early twentieth century. (unpublished manuscript), NOTE* – The contents of this document have been incorporated into the Duke Center for Firearms Law, Repository of Historical Gun Laws, available at https://firearmslaw.duke.edu/repository/search-the-repository/

Gallup Survey. (2020, November 13). What percentage of Americans own guns. https://news.gallup.com/poll/264932/percentage-americans-own-guns.aspx

Garnett, M.F., & Curtin, S.C. (2024). Suicide mortality in the United States, 2002–2022. NCHS Data Brief, no. 509. Hyattsville, MD: National Center for Health Statistics. https://dx.doi.org/10.15620/cdc/160504

Giffords Law Center to Prevent Gun Violence (2022). Passing gun safety laws isn't enough—These laws must be effectively and equitably implemented in order to save lives. https://files.giffords.org/wp-content/uploads/2022/10/22.10.18-GLC-Factsheet-Implementation.pdf

Gius, M. (2020). Examining the impact of child access prevention laws on youth firearm suicides using the synthetic control method. *International Review of Law and Economics*, 63, 1–9.

Gobaud, A.N., Jacobowitz, A.L., Mehranbod, C.A., & Sprague, N.L. (2022). Place-Based interventions and the epidemiology of violence prevention. *Current Epidemiology Reports*, 9(246142). https://doi.org/10.1007/s40471-022-00301-z

Goldstick, J.E., Cunningham, R.M., & Carter, P.M. (2022). Current causes of death in children and adolescents in the United States. *New England Journal of Medicine*, 386(20), 1955–1956. https://doi.org/10.1056/NEJMc2201761

Gollub, E.L., & Gardner, M. (2019). Firearm legislation and firearm use in female intimate partner homicide using National Violent Death Reporting System data. *Preventive Medicine*, 118, 216–219. https://doi.org/10.1016/j.ypmed.2018.11.007

Graham, A., Haner, M., Sloan, M.M., Cullen, F.T., Kulig, T.C., & Jonson, C. (2020). Race and worrying about police brutality: The hidden injuries of minority status in America. *Victims & Offenders*, 5(5), 549–573. https://doi.org/10.1080/15564886.2020.1767252

Greenspan, A.I., & Kellerman, A.L. (2002). Physical and psychological outcomes eight months after serious gunshot injury. *Journal of Trauma*, 53(4), 709–716.

Grinshteyn, E., & Hemenway, D. (2019). Violent death rates in the US compared to those of the other high-income countries, 2015. *Preventive Medicine*, 123, 20–26.

Grinshteyn, E., & Hemenway, D. (2021). Firearm violence in the pediatric population: An international perspective. In L.K. Lee & E.W. Fleegler (Eds.), *Pediatric firearm injuries and fatalities: The clinician's guide to policies and approaches to firearm harm prevention* (pp. 75–85). Springer Nature.

Grossman, D.C., Mueller, B.A., & Riedy, C. (2005). Gun storage practices and risk of youth suicide and unintentional firearm injuries. *JAMA*, 293(6), 707–714. www.pubmed.ncbi.nlm.nih.gov/15701912/

Hawton, K., & van Heeringen, K. (2009). Suicide. *The Lancet*, 373, 1372–1381. https://doi.org/10.1016/s0140-6736(09)60372-x

Hemenway, D., & Richardson, E.G. (2011). Homicide, suicide and unintentional firearm fatality: Comparing the United States with other high-income countries. *Journal of Trauma*, 70(1), 238–243. https://doi.org/10.1097/TA.0b013e3181dbaddf

History.com Editors. (2023, March 27). *Firearms.* A&E Television Networks. www.history.com/top ics/inventions/firearms

Hohl, B.C., Kondo, M.C., Kajeepeta, S., MacDonald, J.M., Theall, K.P., Zimmerman, M.A., Branas, C.C. (2019). Creating safe and healthy neighborhoods with place-based violence interventions. *Health Affairs*, 38(10), 1687–1694.

Houghton, A., Jackson-Weaver, O., Toraih, E., Burley, N., Byrne, T., McGrew, P., Duchesne, J., Tatum, D., & Taghavi, S. (2021). Firearm homicide mortality is influenced by structural racism in US metropolitan areas. *Journal Trauma Acute Care Surgery*, 91(1), 64–71. https://doi.org/10.1097/TA.0000000000003167

Human Rights Careers. (2024). 15 root causes of gun violence. *Human Rights Careers*. www.humanri ghtscareers.com/issues/root-causes-of-gun-violencewww.

Hunter, A.A., DiVietro, S., Boyer, M., Burnham, K., Chenard, D., & Rogers, S.C. (2021, September 13). The practice of lethal means restriction counseling in US emergency departments to reduce suicide risk: A systematic review of the literature. *Injury Epidemiology*, 8(Suppl 1), 54. https://doi.org/10.1186/s40621-021-00347-5

Jay, J., & Allen, K. (2023). Curbing the epidemic of community firearm violence after the *Bruen* decision. *Journal of Law and Medical Ethics*, 51(1), 77–82. https://doi.org/10.1017/jme.2023.42

Jay, J., Kondo, M.C., Lyons, V.H., Gause, E., & South, E.C. (2022). Neighborhood segregation, tree cover and firearm violence in 6 U.S. cities, 2015–2020. *Preventive Medicine*, 165. https://doi.org/10.1016/j.ypmed.2022.107256

John Hopkins Center for Gun Violence Solutions. (2020). Examining the gun suicide epidemic: Gun violence in the U.S. https://publichealth.jhu.edu/center-for-gun-violence-solutions

Johnson, O. Jr., St. Vil, C., Gilbert, K.L., Goodman, M., & Johnson, C.A. (2019). How neighborhoods matter in fatal interactions between police and men of color. *Social Science & Medicine*, 220, 226–235. https://doi.org/10.1016/j.socscimed.2018.11.024

Johnson, R.M., Coyne-Beasley, T., & Runyan, C.W. (2004). Firearm ownership and storage practices, U.S. households, 1992–2002: A systematic review. *American Journal of Preventive Medicine*, 27(2), 173–182. https://doi.org/10.1016/j.amepre.2004.04.015

Kagawa, R.M.C., Cerdá, M., Rudolph, K.E., Pear, V.A., Keyes, K.M., & Wintemute, G.J. (2018). Firearm involvement in violent victimization and mental health: An observational study. *Annuals of Internal Medicine*, 169(8), 584–585.

Kann, L., McManus, T., Harris, W.A., Shanklin, S.L., Flint, K.H., Queen, B., Lowry, R., Chyen, D., Whittle, L., Thornton, J., Lim, C., Bradford, D., Yamakawa, Y., Leon, M., Brener, N., & Ethier, K.A. (2018, June 15). Youth risk behavior surveillance – United States, 2017. *Morbidity and Mortality Weekly Report. Surveillance Summaries*, 67(8), 1–114. https://doi.org/10.15585/mmwr.ss6708a1. PMID: 29902162; PMCID: PMC6002027.

Kaplan, M. (2024). Working with gun violence survivors: The social worker's role in crisis intervention and prevention. In H. Belchior Rocha (Ed.), *Social work-perceptions for a new era*. IntechOpen. https://doi.org/10.5772/intechopen.111168

Kaufman, E.J., Wiebe, D.J., Xiong, R.A., Morrison, C.N., Seamon, M.J., & Delgado, M.K. (2021). Epidemiologic trends in fatal and nonfatal firearm injuries in the US, 2009-2017. *JAMA Internal Medicine*, 181(2), 237–244. https://doi.org/10.1001/jamainternmed.2020.669

Kim, J. (2018). Beyond the trigger: The mental health consequences of in-home firearm access among children of gun owners. *Social Science and Medicine*, 203, 51–59. https://doi.org/10.1016/j.socscimed.2017.11.044

Kivisto, A.J., & Phalen, P.L. (2018). Effects of risk-based firearm seizure laws in Connecticut and Indiana on suicide rates, 1981–2015. *Psychiatric Services*, 69, 855–862.

Korhonen, V. (2024). Gun laws in the United States-statistics and facts. *Statista, Crime and Law Enforcement*. www.statista.kkjtcon/topics/12578/gun-laws-in-the-united-states/#topicOverview

Kravitz-Wirtz, N., Bruns, A., Aubel, A.J., Zhang, X., & Buggs, S.A. (2022). Inequities in community exposure to deadly gun violence by race/ethnicity, poverty, and neighborhood disadvantage among youth in large US cities. *Journal of Urban Health*, 99(4), 610–625. https://doi.org/10.1007/s11 524-022-00656-0

Krieger, N., Feldman, J.M., Waterman, P.D., Chen, J.T., Coull, B.A., & Hemenway, D. (2017). Local residential segregation matters: Stronger association of census tract compared to conventional city-level measures with fatal and non-fatal assaults (Total and Firearm Related), using the index of concentration at the extremes (ICE) for racial, economic, and racialized economic segregation, Massachusetts (US), 1995–2010. *Journal of Urban Health*, 94(2), 244–258. https://doi.org/ 10.1007/s11524-016-0116-z

Lanyi, B., Gonzales, R., & Wilson, M. (2019). Tools for social workers to prevent gun violence – Social justice brief. Tools for social workers to prevent gun violence: Safe storage of guns in the home, extreme risk protection orders, and other methods of gun violence prevention. National Association of Social Workers. Washington, DC. www.socialworkers.org/LinkClick.aspx?filetic ket=YvR20CC6ORU%3d&portalid=0

Leach-Kemon, K., & Sirull, R. 2022. *On gun violence, the United States is an outlier*. Institute for Health Metrics and Evaluation. Available from www.healthdata.org/acting-data/gun-violence-uni ted-states-outlier. Accessed March 4, 2023.

Lee, L.K., Fleegler, E.W., Goyal, M.K., Doh, K.F., Laraque-Arena, D., & Hoffman, B.D. (2022). Firearm-related injuries and deaths in children and youth. *Pediatrics*, 150(6). https://doi.org/ 10.1542/peds.2022-060071

Lee, T.P., Anderson, J.F., Langsam, A.H., & Hatter, S. (2022). Disparate law enforcement practices against women of color and gender variant women: The more things change, the more they stay the same. *Journal of Law and Criminal Justice*, 10(1), 63–72.

Leibbrand, C., Hill, H., Rowhani-Rahbar, A., & Rivara, F. (2020). Invisible wounds: community exposure to gun homicides and adolescents' mental health and behavioral outcomes. *SSM – Population Health*, 12, 100689. https://doi.org/10.1016/j.ssmph.2020.100689

Libresco, L. (2015). Being arrested is nearly twice as deadly for African Americans as whites. *538ABCNews*. https://fivethirtyeight.com/features/being-arrested-is-nearly-twice-as-deadly-for-african-americans-as-whites/

Lowe, S.R., & Galea, S. (2017). The mental health consequences of mass shootings. *Trauma, Violence, and Abuse*, 18(1), 62–82.

Magee, L.A., Semenza, D., Gharbi, S., & Wiehe, S.E. (2023). Addressing mental health needs of secondary homicide survivors through a social determinants of health framework. *Homicide Studies*, 27(4), 435–453. https://doi.org/10.1177/10887679231163099

May, C.L., & Wisco, B.E. (2016). Defining trauma: How level of exposure and proximity affect risk for posttraumatic stress disorder. *Psychological Trauma*, 8(2), 233–240. https://doi.org/10.1037/ tra0000077

Mayer, M.J., & Leone, P.E. (2007). School violence and disruption revisited: Equity and safety in the school house. *Focus on Exceptional Children*, 40(1), 1. https://doi.org/10.17161/foec.v40i1.6863

McGough, M., Amin, K., Panchal, N., & Cox, C. (2023). Child and teen firearm mortality in the U.S. and peer countries. *KFF*. www.kff.org/mental-health/issue-brief/child-and-teen-firearm-mortal ity-in-the-u-s-and-peer-countries/ – endnote

McLeod, M.N., Heller, D., Manze, M.G., & Echeverria, S.E. (2020). Police interactions and the mental health of Black Americans: A systematic review. *Journal of Racial and Ethnic Health Disparities*, 7(1), 10–27. https://doi.org/10.1007/s40615-019-00629-1

Miller, M., & Azrael, D. (2022). Firearm storage in US households with children: Findings from the 2021 National Firearm Survey. *JAMA Network Open*, 5(2), e2148823. https://doi.org/10.1001/ jamanetworkopen.2021.48823

Moore, M.H., Prothrow-Stith, D., Guyer, B., & Spivak, H. (1994). Violence and intentional injuries: Criminal justice and public health perspectives on an urgent national problem. In A.J.

Reiss, Jr. & J.A. Roth (Eds.), *Understanding and Preventing Violence, Volume 4: Consequences and Control* (pp. 167–216). National Academy Press.

Morin, R., Parker, K., Stepler, R., & Mercer, A. (2017). Behind the badge: Amid protests and calls for reform, how police view their jobs, key issues and recent fatal encounters between blacks and police. *Pew Research Center*. https://assets.pewresearch.org/wp-content/uploads/sites/3/2017/01/06171402/police-report_find_web.pdf

National Academies of Sciences, Engineering, and Medicine (NASEM). (2005). *Firearms and violence: A critical review*. The National Academies Press. https://doi.org/10.17226/10881

National Academies of Sciences, Engineering, and Medicine. (2019). Taking action against clinician burnout: A systems approach to professional well-being. *The National Academies Press*. doi:10.17226/25521.

National Center for Injury Prevention and Control, Centers for Disease Control and Prevention. (2023). WISQARS Fatal and Nonfatal Injury Reports. https://wisqars.cdc.gov/reports/

National Coalition Against Domestic Violence. (2020). "Domestic violence," 2020, *available at* https://assets.speakcdn.com/assets/2497/domestic_violence-2020080709350855.pdf?1596811079991

Novella, S. (2018). Gun violence as a public health issue: Gun violence is a serious public health issue in America but is not getting the research it deserves. Retrieved from http://sciencebasedmedicine.org/gun-violence-as-a-public-health-issue

Office of Justice Programs. (2003). Fact sheet: Domestic violence. Archived. The President's Family Justice Center Initiative.

Office of Justice Programs. (2024). Community Violence Intervention: A collaborative approach to addressing community violence. U.S. Department of Justice. www.ojp.gov/topics/community-violence-intervention

Office of Public Affairs. U.S. Department of Justice (DOJ). (2023, June 14). Fact Sheet: Update on Justice Department's ongoing efforts to tackle gun violence.

Office of the U.S. Surgeon General. (2024). The U.S. Surgeon General's advisory on firearm violence: A public health crisis in America.

Opara, I., Lardier, D.T., Metzger, I., Herrera, A., Franklin, L., Garcia-Reid, P., & Reid, R.J. (2020). "Bullets have no names": A qualitative exploration of community trauma among black and Latinx youth. *Journal of Child and Family Studies*, 29(8), 2117–2129. https://doi.org/10.1007/s10826-020-01764-8

Panchal, N. (2024). The impact of gun violence on children and adolescents. *KFF* www.kfforg/mental-health/issue-brief/the-impact-of-gun-violence-on-children-and-adolescents

Pear, V.A., Wintemute, G.J., Jewell, N.P., Cerda', M., & Ahern, J. (2023). Community-level risk factors for firearm assault and homicide: The role of local firearm dealers and alcohol outlets. *Epidemiology*, 34(6), 789–806. https://journals.llw.com/epidem/fulltext/2023/11000/community_level_risk_factors_for_firearm_assault.6aspx

Peterson, S., & Bushway, S. (2021). Law enforcement approaches for reducing gun violence. In R. Ramchand & J. Saunders (Eds.), *Contemporary Issues in Gun Policy: Essays from the RAND Gun Policy in America Project* (pp. 77–96). RAND Corporation, RR-A243-2.. www.rand.org/pubs/research_reports/RRA243-2.html

Pierce, O. (2024). A decade of American gun violence: Here's how we analyzed 10 years of GVA Data. *The Trace*. www/thetrace.org/2024/03/gun-violence-archive-data-shootings

Pinholt, E.M., Mitchell, J.D., Butler, J.H., & Kumar, H. (2014). Is there a gun in the home? Assessing the risks of gun ownership in older adults. *Journal of American Geriatric Society*, 62, 1142–1146.

Poulson, M., Neufeld, M.Y., Dechert, T., Allee, L., & Kenzik, K.M. (2021). Historic redlining, structural racism, and firearm violence: A structural equation modeling approach. *Lancet Regional Health Americas*, 100052. https://doi.org/10.1016/j.lana.2021.100052. Epub 2021 Aug 20. PMID: 34888540; PMCID: PMC8654098.

Price, M., Higa-McMillan, C., Kim, S., & Frueh, B.C. (2013). Trauma experience in children and adolescents: An assessment of the effects of trauma type and role of interpersonal proximity. *Journal of Anxiety Disorders*, 27(7), 652–660. https://doi.org/10.1016/j.janxdis.2013.07.009

Reeves, R.V., & Holmes, S.E. (2015). *Guns and race: The different worlds of black and white Americans*. Brookings Institute. www.brookings.edu/articles/guns-and-race-the-different-worlds-of-black-and-white-Americans

Rivara, F.P. (2015). Youth suicide and access to guns. *JAMA Pediatrics*, 169(5), 429–430. https://doi.org/10.1001/jamapsychiatry.2014.1760.430

Rivara, F.P., Hink, A.B., Kuhls, D.A., Banks, S., Agoubi, L.L., Kirkendoll, S., Winchester, A., Hoeft, C., Patel, B., & Nathens, A. (2023). Firearm injuries treated at trauma centers in the United States. *Journal of Trauma and Acute Care Surgery*, 96(6), 955–964. https://doi.org/10.1097/ta.0000000000004172

Rosenberg, M. (2021). Considerations for developing an agenda for gun violence prevention research. *Annual review of Public Health*, 42(1), 23–41. www.annualreviews.org/content/journals/10.1146/annurev-publhealth-012420-105117

Rouhezamin, M., Paydar, S., Hasirbaf, M., Bolandparvaz, S., & Abbasi, H.R. (2013). The spatiotemporal pattern of trauma in victims of violence visited in emergency room of Rajaee hospital. *Bulletin of Emergency & Trauma*, 1(4), 141–146. https://doaj.org/article/be1033053bd04a08850eacb1ced34b04

Runyan, C.W. (2003). Introduction: Back to the future—Revisiting Haddon's conceptualization of injury epidemiology and prevention. *Epidemiological Review*, 25, 60–64.

Santaella-Tenorio, J., Cerdá, M., Villaveces, A., & Galea, S. (2016). What do we know about the association between firearm legislation and firearm-related injuries? *Epidemiological Review*, 38, 140–157.

Schell, T., Peterson, S., Vegetabile, B., Scherling, A., Smart, R., & Morral, A. (2022). State-level estimates of household firearm ownership. www.rand.org/pubs/tools/TL354.html

Schleimer, J.P., Buggs, S., McCort, C.D., Pear, V.A.; DeBiasi, A., Tomsich, E., Shev, A., Laquer, J.S., & Wintemate, G.J. (2022) Neighborhood racial and economic segregation and disparities in violence during the COVID-19 Pandemic. *American Journal of Public Health*, 112, 144–153. https://doi.org/10.2105/AJPH.2021.306540

Schnippel, K., Burd-Sharps, S., Miller, T., Lawrence, B., & Swedler, D.L. (2021). Nonfatal firearm injuries by intent in the United States: 2016–2018. Hospital discharge records from the healthcare cost and utilization project. *Western Journal of Emergency Medicine: Integrating Emergency Care with Population Health*, 22(3), 462–470.

Schrader, D. (1995). The assault weapons ban: Review of federal laws controlling possession of certain firearms. Congressional Research Report #95–108, December 1.

Semenza, D.C., Baker, N.S., & Vil, C.S. (2024). Firearm violence exposure and functional disability among black men and women in the United States. *Journal of Urban Health*, 101(3), 522–534. https://doi.org/10.1007/s11524-024-00866-8

Semenza, D.C., & Kravitz-Wirtz, N. (2024). Gun violence exposure and population health inequality: A conceptual framework. *Injury Prevention*, 1–8. https://doi.org/10.1136/ip-2023-045197

Sharkey, P., Schwartz, A.E., Ellen, I.G., & Lacoe, J. (2014). High stakes in the classroom, high stakes on the street: The effects of community violence on Student's standardized test performance. *Sociological Science*, 1(14), 199–220. https://doi.org/10.15195/v1.a14

Sharpe, T.L., & Iwamoto, D.K. (2022). Psychosocial aspects of coping that predict post-traumatic stress disorder for African American survivors of homicide victims. *Preventive Medicine*, 165(Pt A), 107277. https://doi.org/10.1016/j.ypmed.2022.107277

Sheley, J., Mcgee, Z., & Wright, J. (1992). Gun-related violence in and around inner-city schools. *American Journal of Diseases of Children (1960)*, 146(6), 677–682. https://doi.org/10.1001/archpedi.1992.02160180035012

Shonkoff, J.P., Garner, A.S., & Committee on psychosocial aspects of child and family health, committee on early childhood, adoption, and dependent care, & section on developmental and behavioral pediatrics. (2012). The lifelong effects of early childhood adversity and toxic stress. *Pediatrics*, 129(1), e232–e246. https://doi.org/10.1542/peds.2011-2663

Shour, A.R., Anguzu, R., Zhou, Y., Muehlbauer, A., Joseph, A., Oladebo, T., Puthoff, D., & Onitilo, A. (2023). Your neighborhood matters; an ecological social determinant study of the relationship between residential racial segregation and the risk of firearm fatalities. Open Access. *Injury Epidemiology*, 10(14). https://doi.org/10.1186/s40621-023-00425-w

Shufro, C. (2021). A brief history of guns in the U.S: How to explain Americans' astonishing personal arsenal? Start with politics, fear, and marketing. *John Hopkins Bloomberg Public Health Magazine*, Fall/Winter Issue. www.https://magazine.publichealth.Jhu.edu/2021/brief-history-guns-us

Simon, T.R., Kegler, S. R., Zwald, M.L. (2021). Notes from the field: Increases in firearm homicide and suicide rates-United States, 2020-2021. *Centers for Disease Control and Prevention, Morbidity and Mortality Weekly Report*, 71, 1286-1287. http://dx.doi.org/10/15585/mmwr.mm7140a4

Siegel, L.K., & Worrall, J.L. (2018). *Introduction to criminal justice* (16th ed.). Cengage.

Small Arms Survey. (2018). Estimating global civilian-held firearms numbers. Briefing Paper. Department of Foreign Affairs and Trade of Australia, pp. 1–12.

Smith, S.G., Zhang, X., Basile, K.C., Merrick, M.T., Wang, J., Kresnow, M., Chen, J. (2018). The National Intimate Partner and Sexual Violence Survey (NISVS): 2015 data brief – Updated release. Atlanta, GA: National Center for Injury Prevention and Control, Centers for Disease Control and Prevention.

Soken-Huberty. (2024). 15 Root causes of gun violence. Human Rights Careers. https://humanrightscareers.com/issues/root-causes-of-gun-violence/#:~:text=15%20Root%20Causes%20of%20Gun%20Violence%201%20%231.,%238.%20Weak%20gun%20control%20laws%20...%20More%20items

Song, Z., Zubizarreta, J.R., Giuriato, M., Koh, K.A., & Sacks, C.A. (2023). Firearm injuries in children and adolescents: Health and economic consequences among survivors and family members. *Health Affairs*, 42(11). https://doi.org/10.1377/hlthaff.2023.00587

Sonali, R., Reeping, P.M., Ladhani, Z., Vasudevan, L.M., Branas, C.C. (2022). Gun violence in K-12 schools in the United States: Moving towards a preventive (versus reactive) framework. *Preventive Medicine*, 165, Part A, https://doi.org/10.1016/j.ypmed.2022.107280

South, E.C., Hemenway, D., & Webster, D.W. (2022). Gun violence research is surging to inform solutions to a devastating public health crisis. *Preventive medicine*, 165, 107325. www.ncbi.nlm.nih.gov/pmc/articles/PMC9642971/

Spano, R., Pridemore, W.A., & Bolland, J. (2012, January). Specifying the role of exposure to violence and violent behavior on initiation of gun carrying: a longitudinal test of three models of youth gun carrying. *Journal of Interpersonal Violence*, 27(1), 158–76. https://doi.org/10.1177/0886260511416471

Spitzer, R.J. (2017). Gun Law History in the United States and Second Amendment Rights, 80. *Law and Contemporary Problems*, 55–83. http://scholarship.law.duke.edu/lcp/vol80/iss2/3

Sullivan, E.M., Annest, J.L., Simon, T., Luo, F., & Dahlberg, L.L. (2015). Suicide trends among persons aged 10-24 years—United States, 1994–2012. *Centers for Disease Control and Prevention: Morbidity and Mortality Weekly Report*, 64, 201–232.

Swanson, S.A., Eyllon, M., Sheu, Y.H., & Miller, M. (2020). Firearm access and adolescent suicide risk: Toward a clearer understanding of effect size. *Injury Prevention*, 27(3), 264–270.

The Lancet. (2023). Understanding global gun violence, and how to control it. *The Lancet*, 402, 1393. www.thelancet.com

The White House Briefing Room. (2024, September 26). FACT SHEET: President Biden and Vice President Harris announce additional actions to reduce gun violence and save lives.

Tobin-Tyler, E. (2023). Intimate partner violence, firearm injuries and homicides: A health justice approach to two intersecting public health crises. *Journal of Law Medical Ethics*, 51(1), 64–76. https://doi.org/10.1017/jme.2023.41

Vella, M.A., Warshauer, A., Tortorello, G., Fernandez-Moure, J., Giacolone, J., Sims, C., Schwab, C.W., & Reilly, P.M. (2020). Long-term functional, psychological, emotional, and social outcomes in survivors in firearm injuries. *JAMA Surgery*, 155(1), 51–59.

Villarrea, S., Kim, R., Wagner, E., Somayaji, N., Davis, A., & Crifasi, C.K. (2024). *Gun violence in the U.S. 2022: Examining the burden among children and teens* (pp. 1–20). John Hopkins University Center for Gun Violence Solutions.

Weaver, G., Wittekind, J., Huff-Corzine, L., Corzine, J., Petee, T., & Jarvis, J. (2004). Violent encounters: A criminal event analysis of lethal and nonlethal outcomes. *Journal of Contemporary Criminal Justice*, 20, 348–368.

Webster, D.W., Vernick, J.S., Zeoli, A.M., & Manganello, J.A. (2004). Association between youth-focused firearm laws and youth suicides. *JAMA*, 292(5), 594–601.

Weeks, L. (2013, April 6). *The first guns in America*. National Public Radio.

World Health Organization (WHO). (n.d.) *Violence prevention alliance*. The Public Health Approach. www.who.int./groups/violence-prevention-alliance/approach

Zeoli, A.M., Malinski, R., & Turchan, B. (2016). Risks and targeted interventions: Firearms in intimate partner violence. *Epidemiologic Reviews*, 38(1), 125–139. https://doi.org/10.1093/epirev/mxv007

Zeoli, A.M., Mccourt, A.D., & Paruk, J.K. (2022). Effectiveness of firearm restriction, background checks, and licensing laws in reducing gun violence. *The ANNALS of the American Academy of Political and Social Science*, 704(1), 118–136. https://doi.org/10.1177/00027162231165149

Court Cases

District of Columbia v. Heller, 554 U.S. 570 (2008).
Id. at 628–30, 635–36.

14

OPIOID ADDICTION AND PUBLIC HEALTH

Introduction

A 36-year-old man with opioid-use disorder was seen in the emergency room (ER) because of an opioid overdose. Approximately, four years before this evaluation, he had undergone an unspecified hand surgery. Immediately after the procedure, hydromorphone was administered. After being discharged to his home, he initially sought more prescription opioids and then switched to intravenous heroin because he found it to be less expensive and easier to obtain. During the next three years, he injected 1–2 grams of heroin each day. One year before this ER visit, after losing his job, he attempted to quit using heroin. He began to take methadone, which helped to reduce withdrawal symptoms and cravings, but he stopped taking it after ten days because he was concerned that weaning off methadone after a period of maintenance treatment would be associated with unacceptable adverse effects. He then resumed heroin use. Six months before this ER visit, he again stopped using heroin and was admitted to an inpatient, medically supervised detoxification program for the management of withdrawal symptoms. After two weeks, he was discharged home. He was later arrested, convicted, and jailed after a drug charge. Approximately, two months before his ER visit, he was released from jail and was admitted to a structured residential rehabilitation program, in which he participated in work therapy, attended regular Narcotics Anonymous meetings, and underwent random, intermittent urine toxicology screenings. He continued in the program and abstained from opioid use until three days before admission to the ER, when he resumed intravenous heroin use. He obtained the drug, which he believed to be mixed with fentanyl, from a single dealer and began to inject 0.5 grams at a time. Before the ER admission, he injected 0.5 grams at 10 a.m., followed by another 0.5 grams at approximately 1:30 p.m. He remembered subsequently walking around a park and calling a friend to arrange a meeting. At approximately, 3:00 p.m., emergency medical services personnel were dispatched to the park, where he was found lying on the ground in a puddle of slush, and unresponsive. His friend was present and reported that when he had found his friend, he had administered intranasal naloxone and then called for emergency medical assistance. First responders from the Fire Department had administered a second dose of

DOI: 10.4324/9781003373001-14

intranasal naloxone before emergency medical services personnel arrived. On examination, he appeared cyanotic, and he had a Glasgow Coma Scale score of 3 (on a scale ranging from 3 to 15, with lower scores indicating lower levels of consciousness). He was ventilated and revived. In the ER, he reported that the overdose was unintentional, that he had never had an overdose before, that this incident was a "wake-up call," and that he wanted help with managing his opioid addiction (OA). He had been feeling sad after the recent deaths of his mother and grandmother, and he thought that his relapse in opioid use might have been related to these stressors. He had no history of other medical conditions, took no medications, and had no known allergies. He was a high-school graduate and had worked as an electrician before he became unemployed. He was single and had no children. He had smoked a half-pack of cigarettes daily for the past four years and had smoked marijuana when he was younger. He did not drink alcohol or use illicit drugs other than heroin. There was no family history of depression, bipolar disorder, schizophrenia, dementia, or suicide (Raja et al., 2017).

Opioid Addiction Defined

Opioids are commonly used as pain relievers by reducing the perception of acute pain often associated with vehicle or occupational injuries, surgery, cancer treatment, palliative care, and end-of-life care (American Psychiatric Association [APA], 2022). There are three main types of opioids: (1) natural opiates such as morphine and codeine, (2) semi-synthetic opioids such oxycodone, hydrocodone, hydromorphone, oxymorphone, and heroin, and (3) synthetic opioids such as methadone, tramadol, fentanyl, buprenorphine, pethidine, and carfentanil (Memorial Sloan Kettering Cancer Center Library, 2025; U.S. Department of Health & Social Services, 2022). Natural opiates are derived from the poppy plant while semi-synthetic and synthetic opioids are lab-created and are intended to be stronger than natural opiates (APA, 2025). Along with the reduction in pain, opioids may also cause drowsiness, confusion, euphoria, nausea, constipation, and even death because of high doses.

An *opioid use disorder* (OUD) (i.e. abuse or addiction) can occur easily when using opioids because of the feeling of euphoria that is typically induced. Its continued use can cause tolerance to the drug, or rather, more is needed to get the relief or euphoric high that is sought, typically leading to increased use (Mayo Clinic, 2024b). Since opioid prescribers should prevent patient harm, they are reluctant to continue prescriptions. This often leads the patient to seek opioid procurement illegally or to switch to a more available and cheaper opioid such as heroin. When an opioid user is willing to face negative physical, psychological, and legal consequences to obtain opiates, they may be diagnosed with an opiate use disorder.

DSM-5-TR

The DSM-5 replaced the diagnoses of substance *abuse* and substance *addiction* with *substance use disorder(SUD)*, measuring the severity of the disorder on a scale from 2 to 3 symptoms (mild), 4–5 symptoms (moderate), and 6 or more symptoms (severe) out of a total of 11 symptoms (Robonson & Adinoff, 2016). An opiate use disorder is diagnosed according to the DSM 5-TR (APA, 2025) as: a problematic pattern of opioid use leading to problems or distress, with at least two of the following occurring within a 12-month period:

1 Taking larger amounts or taking drugs over a longer period than intended.
2 Persistent desire or unsuccessful efforts to cut down or control opioid use.
3 Spending a great deal of time obtaining or using the opioid or recovering from its effects.
4 Craving, or a strong desire or urge to use opioids.
5 Problems fulfilling obligations at work, school, or home.
6 Continued opioid use despite having recurring social or interpersonal problems.
7 Giving up or reducing activities because of opioid use.
8 Using opioids in physically hazardous situations such as driving while under the influence of opiates.
9 Continued opioid use despite ongoing physical or psychological problem likely to have been caused or worsened by opioids.
10 Tolerance (i.e., need for increased amounts or diminished effect with continued use of the same amount)
11 Experiencing withdrawal (opioid withdrawal syndrome) or taking opioids (or a closely related substance) to relieve or avoid withdrawal symptoms.

ICD

The international classification of diseases (ICD) is used globally as a way of coding primarily for billing, data collection, reporting, and analysis (World Health Organization [WHO], 2025). Unlike the DSM5-TR, the ICD does use differentiating classifications of opioid disorders including opioid dependence, opioid withdrawal, opioid-induced delirium, opioid-induced psychotic disorder, and certain specified opioid-induced mental or behavioral disorders (Find-A-Code, 2025). Opioid SUDs are unique compared to some others because of the brief period it takes to develop a severe level of use disorder as well as the acuteness of the withdrawal when stopping usage (APA, 2025).

Nature and Extent of Opioid Addiction

Approximately, 27.2 million persons aged 12 and older self-reported, via the 2023 National Survey on Drug Use and Health (NSDUH), that they were diagnosed with at least one drug use disorder (Richesson et al., 2024). Of those, 5.7 million who reported having an OUD, an estimated 316,000 were aged 12–17, 396,000 were between ages 18 and 25, and 5 million were 26 and older. This number does not include OUDs explicitly due to the use of illicitly manufactured fentanyl or prescription pain reliever use disorder (discussed in more detail in a section below). The survey did not reveal significant differences for OUD among racial groups. For survey participants aged 12 and older, 587,000 reported having a heroin use disorder (HUD) within the past year: 570,000 were aged 26 and older, and 17,000 were between ages 18 and 25. The survey results could not calculate the HUD estimate for youth between ages 12 and 17.

Adolescent opioid use is a major concern, although levels of youth drug use decreased largely after the COVID-19 pandemic (Miech et al., 2024). This was established through survey data from 24,257 8th, 10th, and 12th-grade students from 272 private and public schools. For heroin use, the percentage of young users has been consistently low with a yearly prevalence rate that is never greater than 2%. Non-prescription Oxycontin use, however, has increased for 12th graders even though use has remained low at 1.1%. Non-prescription use of Vicodin increased among 10th graders, but remain less than 1% for all grades. A 2024 survey data identified respondents by race/ethnicity and gender: 14% were Black/African-American, 35% Hispanic, 37% White, 4% Asian, 1% American Indians/Alaskan Native (AI/AN), 1% Middle Eastern, 47% male, 49% female, and 1% other. Despite the low self-reported use of opioids, overdose deaths among teens have increased since 2010 (Friedman et al., 2022). Moreover, reported use and misuse of opioids for youth between ages 12 and 18 appears to be problematic according to data collected by the annual National Surveys on Drug Use and Health (see in sections below on prescription opioid misuse).

Types of Opioid Addictions

While there may be subtle differences in how specific opiates and opioids impact the brain, such as naturally occurring opiates versus lab-made opioids, they lead to pain reduction and a *euphoria* interpreted as pleasurable. It is the euphoria that leads people to misuse prescription opioids, or to use illicit opioids, which can lead to an OUD—possibly overdose, and death (National Institutes of Health [NIH], 2018). Naturally occurring opiates (opiates produced by our bodies) work by activating opioid receptors in the brain that healthily modulate behavior. However, man-made opiates "distort" behavior that leads to "pathology," or rather, diagnosable disordered use (Stoeber et al., 2018, p. 963). These opioid receptors are found not only in the brain, but also throughout the body, including in the respiratory system, the autonomic nervous system (gastrointestinal tract), on cardiac tissue, and even on immune cells (Dhaliwal & Gupta, 2023). When used for extended periods of time, tolerance develops, and current dosages become ineffective. Naturally occurring opiates that work to relieve pain may become rendered useless when taking prescription opioids. Therefore, when tolerance to opioid medications or illicit opioids occurs, it is a natural progression for user to seek a higher dose, creating a dependence or reliance on the drug and eventually to a moderate or severe OUD. In addition to OUD, there is also prescription OUD (POUD), or rather, prescription opioid disorder.

Prescription Medications

Prescription opioids can be manufactured directly from the opium poppy plant (opiates), and others are lab-made using the same chemical structure (National Institute on Drug Abuse [NIDA], 2021). They are most often prescribed to treat pain and sometimes coughing and diarrhea. Some common opioid prescription drugs include hydrocodone (Vicodin), oxycodone (OxyContin, Percocet), oxymorphone (Opana), morphine (Kadian, Avinza), codeine, fentanyl, and a class of synthetic opioids called benzimidazole-opioids, or rather, nitazines. Nitazines were developed as an alternative to morphine, but were never released because of overdose potential (Drug Enforcement Administration [DEA], 2024a). Some nitazines are even more potent than fentanyl (DEA, 2024b). However, nitazines are sold illicitly and often mixed with other drugs including fentanyl.

Prescription opioid use can lead to prescription opioid (legal and illegal) misuse, which is described as using the medication in a manner other than what it is prescribe for. For example, if a patient is prescribed an opioid for pain, but uses it only for euphoric reasons.

This is misuse. Some other ways to misuse a drug include taking larger doses than prescribed, taking it in a different form than prescribed (pill crushing, inhaling, injecting), and taking someone else's medication (National Library of Medicine, 2025). The continued use or misuse of opioids can lead to tolerance, which, as previously stated, can lead to a moderate to severe OUD (NIDA, 2021). However, this is not always the case.

An analysis of data collected by the 2021 NSDUH demonstrated that only 38% of 4.8 million U.S. adults with a diagnosed POUD reported prescription opioid misuse (Han et al., 2024). Data from the 2023 NSDUH showed that among 8.6 million persons aged 12 and older who misused pain relievers in the past year, 3.6 million misused hydrocodone (opioid) products, 2.6 million misused oxycodone (opioid) products, and 2.0 million misused codeine products (Richesson et al., 2024). Most of those who misused opioids were aged 26 and older (7.5 million) compared with those aged 18–25 (846,000 people) or youth aged 12–17 (574,000 people). There were no significant differences in race found. Moreover, nonmedical prescription opioid use has been linked to the development of non-injection heroin use by youth, but not to heroin injection use (Goldman-Hasbun et al., 2019). The 2023 NSDUH data also revealed the source of misused prescription pain relievers. It appeared that 47% of misused pain relievers are either prescribed by or were stolen from a healthcare provider, 39.1% were bought or stolen from friends and relatives, 8% were purchased from a drug dealer or stranger, and 5.8% were procured by another method (Richesson et al., 2024). Registered prescribers of opioid pain relievers reported "fraudulent use of their registration numbers and identities on prescriptions submitted via e-script in locations across the country" (DEA, 2024a, p. 43). The United States Drug Enforcement Agency (DEA) encourages people to remove unused and unneeded drugs from their homes to prevent them from being stolen and sold on the street or taken inappropriately by other residents. This is important when considering prevention strategies, and school/community safety and resilience.

Opioid misuse, including heroin, is slightly higher than prescription pain reliever and is misused by 8.9 million, which include those misusing opioid pain relievers. Of opioid misusers, there were 342,000 with heroin use only, and 336,000 misused prescription pain relievers and used heroin (Richesson et al., 2024). Prescription opioid use has been linked to the start of heroin use, which is believed to be a predisposition to polydrug use (Muhuri et al., 2013). Research has also found that persons who often use opioid prescription drugs and those diagnosed with OUD, have a higher likelihood of transitioning to heroin (Jones et al., 2015). Prescription fentanyl misuse was discovered to be less, but also more deadly. Fentanyl is 50–100 times more potent than morphine, and therefore, brings much higher overdose risks. In 2023, among those aged 12 and older, 828,000 misused fentanyl in the last 12 months (668,000 people aged 26 and older, 110,000 aged 18–25, and 50,000 youth aged 12–17) (Richesson et al., 2024).

Link between Opioid Use, Violence, and Crime

Opioid use, particularly the use of heroin, nitazines, controlled prescription drugs, and fentanyl, is seated at the center of extensively networked crime cartels. Synthetic opioid drugs "have transformed not only the drug landscape in the United States, with deadly consequences... [but] have also transformed the criminal landscape in the United States, as the drug cartels... reap huge profits" (DEA, 2024b, p. 1). Fentanyl, alone, is the largest drug threat in the U.S., with an estimated 38,000 deaths that occurred in the first half of 2023 largely because of violent gangs. For example, the Mexican Sinaloa Cartel and the Jalisco Cartel are the most notorious drug manufacturers, controlling smuggling corridors into the U.S. and maintaining "large network 'hubs' in U.S. cities, along the Southwest Border, and other key locations across the United States" (p. 1). They are drug manufacturers and traffickers, arms traffickers, migrant smugglers, sex traffickers, and are involved in many other crimes. Fentanyl and other synthetic opioids are easily produced in laboratories anywhere the cartels have reached, especially in U.S. communities where they employ "wholesale-level" traffickers and street dealers to get their drugs on the market via social media and other messaging apps (p. 1). These cartels operate extensively worldwide. Reports reveal they have taken control over the U.S. drug market, producing and delivering illicit opioids, such as illegal fentanyl, "by the tons" (DEA, 2024b, p. 2). This has allowed them to establish a presence in every state employing "precursor chemicals production facilities, . . . international shippers, cross-border transporters, corrupt officials, tunnel builders, shell companies, [and] money launderers" (DEA, 2024b, p. 2). The Sinaloa Cartel has trafficked "multi-ton quality drug loads—mainly cocaine and heroin—to the U.S." (p. 10) through networks of corrupt law enforcement, military, and police in exchange for millions of dollars in bribes. Furthermore, the greatest presence of the cartels is seen in California, Arizona, Texas, Florida, and Illinois followed closely by New Mexico, Oregon, Georgia, North Carolina, and Maine (DEA, 2024b). Much of the illicit fentanyl sold in the U.S. is in pill form to mimic legal fentanyl and is obtained on the street by unsuspecting buyers. While not operating on the same scale as the Sinaloa cartel with fentanyl production, the Jalisco cartel controls extensive networks of fentanyl smuggling hubs in major cities such as Atlanta, Georgia. In addition to lab-made drugs, the Sinaloa Cartel continues to be a major trafficker of heroin in the U.S. with its connections to opium poppy growers to produce heroin.

Both the Sinaloa and Jalisco cartels are responsible for most of the heroin trafficked in the U.S. with Southwest Border entry points, most often in California (DEA, 2024b). Between 2019 and 2023, U.S. heroin seizures fell by 70%, while fentanyl seizures increased by 451%. Fentanyl is easier to produce compared to the growing process needed for heroin. Experts report that fentanyl looks like heroin in its powdered form, and therefore, the two can be combined without detection unless by forensic analysis. Heroin ranked fifth in drug-related deaths for 2023, however, 82% of all heroin-related deaths involved fentanyl during the first half of 2023 (Tanz et al., 2024).

The DEA's 2023 *Operation Last Mile* consisted of 1,436 investigations that resulted in 3,337 arrests (DEA, 2024b). Intelligence gathered during Operation Last Mile confirmed that the cartels used violent street gangs, local criminal groups, and others to flood U.S. communities with drugs and untimely deaths. Nearly, 44 million fentanyl pills, more than 6,500 pounds of fentanyl powder, and over 8,000 firearms were confiscated (Drug Enforcement Agency [DEA], 2023). Street gangs rely on weapons to enforce payment for drugs, to protect their drugs, to gain "streetcred," and to commit robberies, assaults, murders, and carjackings (DEA, 2024b). Despite this, some experts argue it can be difficult to pinpoint a precise measure of how drug abuse impacts crime rates. A novel way of exploring the substance abuse-crime nexus was demonstrated by Bondurant and colleagues (2018) in their study on the effects of substance abuse treatment (SAT) facilities on local county crime. They discovered that having SAT in a county, decreased the annual rates of homicide, aggravated assault, robbery, motor theft, and burglary. They also demonstrated that the decrease in these offenses reduced the county's costs associated with crime by approximately, $2.9 million. On an individual level, opiate users were found to have significantly greater rates of lifetime prior sanctioned offending than nonusers (Pearce et al., 2017). It was also revealed that existing levels of serious offending were made worse upon initiation of opioid use for males and non-serious offending for females.

Illegal/Street Drugs

While morphine is derived naturally from poppies, heroin is a semi-synthetic opioid drug that is derived from morphine and is most often found as a street drug (Tracy, 2025). It can be injected, smoked, ingested, snorted, or inserted in suppository form. Heroin is known by various street names such as Big H, China white, hell dust, horse, smack, and skunk (Peterson, 2025). Opium is also a synthetic opioid derived from the poppy plant and is highly addictive (DEA, n.d.). It is better known as Ah-pen-yen, Aunti, Aunti Emma, Big O, Black pill, Chandoo, Chandu, Chinese Molasses, Chinese Tobacco, Dopium, Dover's Powder, and Dream Gun among other street names. Opium is most often smoked, injected, or taken in pill form.

Illegal fake prescription pills containing fentanyl are another factor in opioid deaths. In 2021, the DEA warned of international and domestic drug networks that produced and sold fake prescription pills in the U.S. that contain methamphetamine and fentanyl (DEA, 2021). With prescription medication costs soaring, illegal prescription drugs, purchased on the street, seem a viable alternative to people who lack insurance to cover the pharmacy cost. DEA-seized pills containing fentanyl increased by 430% between 2019 and 2021. In fact, one of every two pills contained at least 2 milligrams of fentanyl—enough to be deadly. Most of the counterfeit pills were made to look like common prescription opioids: Oxycontin, Percocet, Vicodin, and Xanax.

The transition from the nonmedical use of prescription drugs to heroin has been extensively studied with most studies demonstrating a link between the two. Heroin is cheaper than pharmacy-purchased prescription drugs, so some people make the switch. In 2011, it was reported that approximately, 80% of heroin users first misused prescription opioids (Carlson et al., 2015; Muhuri et al., 2013). Moreover, heroin has been the first drug regularly used by one-third of patients in treatment for OUD (Cicero et al., 2017).

Explaining the Roots of OA

The roots of OA and the opioid crisis are complex and range from obvious causes, such as over-prescribing to hidden community-level factors. Notwithstanding, the roots of the opioid problem witnessed today took hold in the U.S. during three distinct phases. The *first phase* began in the 1980s with the proliferation of the opiate propoxyphene prescribed for pain, making it the second most-prescribed drug in the U.S. (Schnoll, 1982). Under-treated pain, attributed to musculoskeletal disorders of aging, obesity, injury and cancer survivorship, and complexities of surgery (Institute of Medicine, 2011), brought opportunities to pharma companies as insurance plans reduced coverage for cognitive behavioral therapies once relied on to treat pain. Pharmaceutical innovations for opioid medication dispensing included "extended-release formulations, transdermal patches, nasal sprays, and oral dissolving strips as well as pain-modulating implants" (Dasgupta et al., 2018, p. 182). Pharmaceutical companies minimized the addiction risks of OxyContin (Griffin & Miller, 2011), leading to the promotion of "off-label" drugs such as *Actiq*, or rather, fentanyl citrate, which was created to be used only for breakthrough cancer pain (United States [U.S.] Department of Justice [DOJ], 2008). As a result, overdose deaths caused by prescription opioids began to increase around 1999, spiking in 2011 (Paulozzi et al., 2011), and have since decreased, currently responsible for an estimated 12.7% of overdose deaths (CDC, 2024a). Moreover, the second phase began with heroin overdose deaths tripling between 2010 and 2015 (CDC, 2014). Some experts theorized that deaths had increased due to a large population of prescription opioid users developing dependency and tolerance who later turned to the cheaper alternative of heroin (Mars et al., 2014). By 2024, only 5.5% of overdose deaths were attributed to heroin (CDC, 2024a). The third phase started in 2013 with the use of illegally made fentanyl which quickly accounted for approximately, 70% of the opioid overdose deaths in 2024. As mentioned earlier, the spread of fentanyl has been attributed to drug cartels and the establishment of extensive distribution networks throughout the U.S. (DEA, 2024b, p. 1).

Opioid medication dispensing rates declined from a rate of 46.8 prescriptions per 100 persons in 2019 to 37.5 per 100 persons in 2023 (CDC, 2024c). While opioid over-prescribing has played a significant part in the OA and overdose death surge, overdose deaths continue despite the decrease in opioid prescribing. "Social distress" is likely an underlying factor (Dasgupta et al., 2018, p. 183). In addition to socioeconomic inequality, there are other factors such as race, mental illness, behavioral risk, and access to care (Dwyer-Lindgren et al., 2016). These issues, and others, are examined more closely in the next section about risk factors.

What Are the Risk Factors?

Role of Inequity in OA

Racial Inequity

In 2021, an extensive review of the root causes of health inequities of drug overdoses and the related social detriments of health was conducted by the Division of Overdose Prevention (DOP), National Center for Injury Prevention and Control (NCIPC) at the Centers for Disease Control and Prevention (CDC), and the National Association of County and City Health Officials (NACCHO). Four primary categories of inequity were established: *social inequities* such as class, race, immigration status, gender, and self-identification within the LGBTQIA+ community; *institutional inequities*: "law and regulation, organizations, and media [narratives]"; *living conditions*: physical, work, social, and service environments; and *individual-level factors*: history of overdose, polysubstance use, co-morbidities, and mortality (p. 4).

As highlighted by the CDC (2022), the number of U.S. drug overdose deaths increased from 48,261 in 2020 to 68,239 in 2023. Of these deaths, approximately, 77% were from all opioids, and 75% were attributed specifically to illegal fentanyl. Very little of the total deaths were attributed to heroin. Furthermore, nearly 35%–47.5% of the overdoses were linked to opioids alone (no stimulants), and around 45%–46.5% were linked to both opioid and other stimulant use. Overwhelmingly, overdose victims were male (44%–49.5%) and either AI/AN (39.5% in 2020–70% in 2023), or Black (41.6% in 2020–63.7% in 2023). In 2020, overdoses were greater for ages between 35 and 44, followed closely by both 25–34-year-olds, and 45–54-year-olds, with other age ranges lagging. However, by 2023, drug use was less delineated by age, increasing in every age category for males except for ages less than 15 and between 15 and 24. For females, drug use across the age ranges remained steady, and even decreased, except for a reported an increase of use for those 65 and older (4.0 in 2020 to 6.3 in 2023). As these statistics show, race is the largest inequity by far.

The rise in opioid deaths among African-Americans (an increase of 198% between 2013 and 2018) began rivaling White opioid users (77%) during the same period (2020–2023) (Furr-Holden et al., 2021). The media portrayed "deaths of despair" as a White, middle-aged, low-income phenomenon in places such as the Appalachians, partly associated with an increase in physical pain and opioid poisoning (Case & Deaton, 2015). However, in 2015, deaths of despair trended sharply upward for Blacks, and by 2022, the number had almost tripled to 103.81 deaths per 100,000 compared with Whites at 102.63 per 100,000 (Friedman & Hanson, 2024). At the same time, the rate for AI/AN rose to 241.70 deaths per 100,000. In 2023, misuse of opioids was at 5.9% for AI/NA, 5.3% for bi-racial and multi-racial individuals, 3.3% for Whites, 3.9% for Blacks, 3.3% for Hispanics, and 1.8% for Asians, respectively (Substance Abuse and Mental Health Services Administration [SAMHSA], 2024a).

Economic Inequality

In 2008, the Mental Health Parity and Addiction Act was passed. It prohibited insurance companies from denying coverage for mental health and SAT. However, barrier such as economic disparities to receive services continued. For example, research revealed that AI/AN communities were under-resourced for treating OUD, leading to underfunding Indian Health services and a lack of buprenorphine prescribers (Venner et al., 2018). Policies that examine and address economic inequality are necessary to address social investment. It is worth noting that most AI/NA people live in geographical areas that pose other barriers to needed services and resources for fighting opioid overdose. Often these economically disadvantaged communities are experiencing generational trauma.

Individual Factors

Personal Economics

People who were economically disadvantaged typically reside in poor neighborhoods due to limited finances to afford housing in other, less impoverished areas. According to data from a Mortality Disparities in American Community (MDAC) Study, those hardest hit by the opioid epidemic, in addition to living in resource-scarce communities, were those who were never married, unemployed, or otherwise, not in the labor force, to have only a high school education or general educational development (GED) diploma to rent, rather than own, and live in non-rural areas (Altekruse et al., 2020). For those with income, an estimated 24.6% were at less than 100% above the poverty level, 33% were within the 100%–299% poverty level range, 20.3% within the 300%–499% range, and 15.9% within the 500%–999%.

Nearly, 80% of decedents were White, 8.2% Black, and 7.3% Hispanic. Persons with disabilities were at a higher risk for opioid overdose compared with non-disabled persons.

Justice System-Involved

Being involved in the justice system either institutionalized or on probation, is a high-risk factor for opioid overdose (Brinkley-Rubinstein et al., 2018a) due to the lack of OUD treatment in prison (Iheanacho & Jordan, 2020), the conditions of confinement exacerbate use (Austin et al., 2023), and heightened the risk of overdose (at a 3-8-fold increase) during the first two weeks of release for individuals who have not used while in prison (Human Impact Partners & WISDOM, 2012). Research also suggests that ineffective community re-entry programs that do little to assist parolees find jobs, housing, and other resources lead to impoverished conditions that are likely triggers for previous opioid use pre incarceration (Brinkley-Rubinstein et al., 2018b).

LGBTQ+ Identity

As opioid misuse, use, and overdose decreased among the U.S. general population between 2015 and 2018, disparities continued for persons identified as GLBTQ (Morgan et al., 2020) and especially for those identifying as bisexual, for both youth (Pitzer et al., 2020; Wilson et al., 2020) and adults (Anderson-Carpenter et al., 2020; Capistrant & Nakash, 2019). In fact, opioid use differences were significant between bisexual and heterosexual women (Anderson-Carpenter et al., 2020; Schuler et al., 2019) revealing a higher likelihood of past month or past 12-month prescription opioid misuse (Duncan et al., 2019). Moreover, bisexual women demonstrated a higher likelihood of lifetime injection heroin use and past 12-month OUD compared with heterosexual women (Schuler et al., 2019). Despite these findings, other studies report higher disparities for gay men compared with heterosexual men for past 12-month prescription opioid misuse (Morgan et al., 2020; Schuler et al., 2019). Among 10,736 LGBTQ+ youth responding to an online survey in 2022, illicit drug use was found to be less than in the general population (Freeman et al., 2025). Approximately, 2.2% of youth disclosed misusing opioid prescription drugs.

Other Personal Factors

While not considered root causes of the surge in opioid use and overdoses, individual-level factors, play a significant role in who is at risk for misuse, abuse, addiction, and death. These factors include family history of drug use, male gender, comorbid mental health conditions, isolation from family, homelessness, and peer pressure (Frankenfeld & Leslie, 2019; Saloner et al., 2018), as well as having a history of physical or sexual abuse, heavy tobacco use, and thrill-seeking behavior (Mayo Clinic, 2024b). While being a male (gender identified at birth) is a risk factor for OUD and opioid overdose, research shows that females (gender at birth) were more likely to have chronic pain and be prescribed opioid pain relievers, not only for a longer duration, but also, in higher doses than males (Campbell et al., 2020; Tanz et al., 2022). It was also discovered that persons experiencing nonfatal overdoses, were likely to be young females who had taken non-prescription opioids (Chatterjee et al., 2019). In addition, certain factors put users at a high risk of overdose such as having a history of substance abuse, including illicit and prescription drugs, elevated opioid use, methadone use, coprescribing of benzodiazepines and antidepressants, polysubstance abuse, higher pain intensity, heart or pulmonary complications, and age (middle age ranges) (Dasgupta et al., 2016; Zedler et al., 2018). For persons with a past-year OUD, the rates of co-occurring mental illness are high with approximately, 64% having *any* mental illness (AMI) in the past 12 months and nearly, 27% having a serious mental illness within the past 12 months (Jones & McCance-Katz, 2019). This also raises the possibility of at least a portion of opioid overdoses being suicide attempts. In fact, between 2006 and 2011, 53.3% of overdoses seen in emergency departments were deemed unintentional, leaving another 46.5 to be viewed as either intentional suicides, or undetermined (Tadros et al., 2015).

Another individual-level factor in opioid abuse that is being studied is *genetics*. Although still in the beginning stages, genetic links have been found in connection to substance use in general, and in only a few instances with specific substances, including alcohol, tobacco, cannabis, and opioids (Hatoum et al., 2023). While SUDs are heritable, their genetic expression is influenced by other genes and environmental factors. In addition to a genetic pattern being linked to general addiction risk, it can also predict a higher risk of psychiatric disorders, suicide, chronic pain, and other physical conditions. With further genetic data gathering, especially from ancestral groups, it is believed that more accurate, personal, and effective prevention and interventions can be accomplished through personal genomic medicine.

Relationship Factors

Both direct relationship factors such as intimate partner violence (IPV), and indirect relationship trauma, as with adverse childhood experiences (ACES), have been linked to opioid misuse, along with perceived stress, pain intensity, and depressive symptoms (Williams et al., 2020). Accumulated exposure to intimate partner trauma (IPT) and early experience of IPT, especially in the form of IPV, was positively correlated with opioid prescription and opioid misuse. Among the women involved with IPV being subjected to childhood abuse increased their odds of misusing opioids because of their history of physical symptoms that caused them to seek pain relief treatment. IPV is also a factor reported in opioid use among AI/AN and Native Hawaiian (NHPI) college students (Qeadan et al., 2021). Responses given in the 2015–2019 American College Health Association National College Health Assessment II survey demonstrated that additional factors such as family problems, and difficult social relationships played a part in decisions on opioid misuse. Relationship variables were also discovered to be significant in the misuse of opioids among older adults. More specifically, isolation associated with divorce or never being married increased the odds of combined opioid and benzodiazepine misuse by three times that of older persons who were married or widowed (Day & Rosenthal, 2019). Moreover, not attending religious services was also a factor in opioid misuse for this demographic, possibly implying a spiritual isolation component to misuse.

Community Factors

Community Overdose Response Inequity

One finding from the National Association of County and City Health Officials (NACCHO) (2021) study was institutional overdose response inequity. In other words, effective overdose strategies and resources were not reaching communities of color as they were White communities. According to Weerasinghe and colleagues (2020) harmful policies, such as the War on Drugs, led to damaged and ineffectual community infrastructure, preventing the establishment of adequate drug treatment options. In turn, insufficient resources created long-term negative economic and health effects for community residents. This discrepancy is attributed to historical racism and especially the biased thinking that Black people have a higher pain tolerance, and therefore, do not have a legitimate medical need for prescription pain medication (Villarosa, 2019). As well, some individuals may be unable to adequately gauge their pain using a numeric scale and, therefore, under-report what they are experiencing (Curtin & Goldstein, 2010). Despite monies appropriated from the U.S. Senate and House to combat the opioid crisis in 2017, the resources are not required to be culturally and linguistically appropriate for communities of color (Weerasinghe et al., 2020).

An inequity in access to legal effective pharmacological pain relief is a global problem: there exists a "40-fold difference in the availability of opioids per capita for pain management and palliative care between high-income and low- and middle-income countries," which means that approximately, 86% of persons worldwide do not have sufficient access to legal prescription opioids for pain relief (United Nations Office on Drugs and Crime [UNODC], 2023b, p. 18). The lack of sufficient legal prescription pain management is what leads to self-medication with illegal prescription pills and street drugs. To elucidate this point, despite a low decrease of 38 overdose deaths in New York City in 2018, the poorest boroughs of New York City (Bronx, East Harlem, Crotana-Tremont, and Hunts Point Mott-Haven) experienced the highest rate of overdose deaths per 100,000 residents (34.1%, 49.2%, 49.1%, and 56.1%, respectively), effecting Latino New Yorkers the greatest (New York City Department of Health and Mental Hygiene, 2019).

Supporting the finding that poor neighborhoods have the least resources and the most overdose deaths is an additional discovery demonstrating that U.S. counties investing the most money per capita to address social determinants of health, have the least overdose deaths (Lindenfeld et al., 2025). This investment includes cleaning up deteriorating neighborhoods, a factor in higher overdose death rates. These investments include street cleaning, fixing or demolishing vacant, dilapidated buildings, and improving home utilities. It was also revealed that decreasing overdose deaths were related to increasing investments in health care, public safety, social services, and in education. Research also finds that even when there are medical facilities available, there may not be a provider who is registered to prescribe opioids for pain and/or OA medications. Apprising the opioid overdose death epidemic as a structural failure, rather than, a moral failure shifts the responsibility of decreasing these deaths back to community systems, "considering the factors that influence these outcomes, such as economic opportunity, social cohesion, racial disadvantage, and life satisfaction" (NACCHO, 2021, p. 44). To treat persons of color effectively, practitioners must have *structural competence* to recognize and consider the structural barriers that patients experience not only for receiving treatment, but also, for maintaining a non-drug using life. Showing compassion and understanding to those who are opioid addicted, rather than, a criminalization and institutional racism approach is particularly important for communities of color that already have a deep distrust of the medical system.

To help ameliorate some of the barriers, the final rule from the DEA and (SAMHSA) within the Department of Health and Human Services allows providers to use telehealth to prescribe six months' of OUD treatment, buprenorphine, through telehealth (Hellman & Raman, 2025). Afterward, to continue prescribing buprenorphine, providers can see the patient in person or continue using telehealth for conducting a more thorough evaluation. This allowance is to improve OUD treatment to outlying, rural areas. The *Community Opioid Overdose Reversal Medications (OORMs) Planning Toolkit* (SAMHSA, 2025) is designed to help communities expand access to opioid overdose remedies such as naloxone to reduce overdose fatalities, guiding community leaders, public health professionals, and others to create effective overdose prevention and response strategies. Furthermore, an additional factor driving ineffective community opioid crisis response is neighborhood economic hardship (Adler & Newman, 2002). An example of this is the city of Chicago. Rushovich and colleagues (2020) found that rates for opioid overdose deaths in high economic-hardship neighborhoods were estimated at 36.9 per 100,000 compared with 20.5 per 100,000 in medium-hardship neighborhoods and 12.3 per 100,000 in low economic-hardship neighborhoods. Affluence and poverty were also linked to the type of drugs that decedents used at the time of death. Consequently, more affluent areas saw increases in deaths associated with oxycodone and benzodiazepines, whereas low-income deaths were typically due to an overdose of methadone and cocaine (Visconti et al., 2015), as well as fentanyl, especially in economically distressed mining and service-sector communities (Monnat, 2019).

Criminal Justice Issue

According to Caulkins and colleagues (2021), the opioid epidemic is dominating the criminal justice system. Before the 1980s and 1990s, the criminal justice system was plagued with the illegal use of heroin which was believed to cause crime, particularly property crime. During this period, the illegal drug of choice for most individuals was cocaine and concern about crime and drug connection shifted to violence which led to the criminal justice system responding with punitive measures such as mandatory sentences and cracking down on street drug markets.

The criminal justice system through the Department of Justice (DOJ) controls the opioid supply through law enforcement; regulation of manufacturers, distributors, and dispensers; and grants to state and local agencies. According to the Congressional Research Services Report (2019), the U.S.' efforts to target opioid trafficking have centered on law enforcement initiatives such as:

- The Organized Crime Drug Enforcement Task Force (OCDETF) program which targets major drug trafficking and money laundering organizations with the intent to disrupt and dismantle them. Federal agencies that participate in this program include the DEA; Federal Bureau of Investigation (FBI); Bureau of Alcohol, Tobacco, Firearms, and Explosives (ATF); U.S. Marshals; Internal Revenue Service (IRS); U.S. Immigration and Customs Enforcement (ICE); U.S. Coast Guard; Offices of the U.S. Attorneys; and the DOJ's Criminal Division. These federal agencies also collaborate with state and local law enforcement on task forces.
- The FBI investigates opioid trafficking as part of its efforts to counter transnational organized crime and gangs, cybercriminals, fraudsters, and other malicious actors. The FBI participates in investigations that range from targeting drug distribution networks bringing opioids across the Southwest border to prioritizing illicit opioid distributors leveraging the Dark Web to sell their drugs.

- The Offices of the U.S. Attorneys are responsible for prosecuting federal criminal and civil cases, which include cases against prescribers, pharmaceutical companies, and pharmacies involved in unlawful manufacturing, distributing, and dispensing opioids as well as illicit opioid traffickers. Other enforcement agencies such as the ATF and U.S. Marshals may also be involved in seizing illicit opioids while carrying out their official duties.

The U.S. Department of Homeland Security (DHS) also plays a role in controlling illicit opioid use (Congressional Research Services Report, 2019). The control of opioids comes from the following agencies:

- U.S. Customs and Border Protection (CBP) works to counter the trafficking of illicit opioids (among other drugs), along the U.S. borders as well as via mail carriers. To help detect and interdict these substances, CBP employs tools such as nonintrusive inspection equipment (including x-ray and imaging systems), canines, and laboratory testing of suspicious substances. The agency also uses information and screening systems to help detect illicit drugs, targeting precursor chemicals, equipment, and the drugs themselves.
- U.S. Postal Inspection Service (USPIS) is the law enforcement branch of the U.S. Postal Service. It shares responsibility for international mail security with other federal agencies, and because of the opioid epidemic, it has dedicated more resources to investigating prohibited substances in the mail.

The DEA also conducts law enforcement activities such as investigating illicit opioid trafficking and regulating the flow of controlled substances in the U.S. The Controlled Substances Act (CSA) requires the DEA to establish and maintain a closed system of distribution established by Congress. This requires the regulation of anyone who handles controlled substances, including exporters, importers, manufacturers, distributors, health care professionals, pharmacists, and researchers to register with the DEA. Registrants must keep records of all transactions involving controlled substances, maintain detailed inventories of the substances in their possession, and periodically file reports with the DEA, as well as ensure that controlled substances are securely stored and safeguarded. The DEA uses its criminal, civil, and administrative authorities to maintain a closed system of distribution and prevent the diversion of drugs, such as prescription opioids, from legitimate purposes (U.S. DOJ, 2023).

In addition to the criminal justice agencies that are charged with controlling opioid drugs, one's criminal justice involvement plays a role in OA, becoming a criminal justice issue. An examination of a report from the SAMHSA (2017) using the 2016 NSDUH revealed that one in four individuals with an OUD had contact with the criminal justice system during the prior year. Further findings revealed that these individuals had significantly higher rates of OUD compared with those without criminal justice involvement (i.e., 8.5% versus 0.8%). Winkelman and colleagues (2018) found that the severity of opioid use revealed a strong association with increased criminal justice involvement after controlling for socio-demographic, mental, and physical health issues, and abuse of other substances.

For inmates who are released into the community and have previously used opioids, untreated OUDs are linked to returning to criminal activity, reincarceration, as well as spreading HIV and hepatitis B and C infections (Zaller et al., 2013). Likewise, Keen and colleagues (2020) suggest that after release from incarceration, individuals with OUD are at high risk of opioid relapse and overdose, and recidivism once released into the community. Binswanger and others (2007), suggest that the risk of death of former inmates within the first two weeks of release is more than 12 times that of other individuals, with the leading cause of death being a fatal overdose. Similarly, death risk from opioid overdose is high in the period immediately following prison release with one study showing a 40-fold increase in risk of opioid overdose fatality among parolees in the two weeks following prison release (Ranapurwala et al., 2018).

WHO (2009) suggests that individuals who are incarcerated should receive adequate health care and that opioid withdrawal, agonist maintenance, and naltrexone treatment should be available in prison settings, but prisoners should not be forced to accept treatment. Although studies (Moore et al., 2019; Gordon et al., 2014) have shown the benefits of having medication-assisted treatment (MAT) in criminal justice treatment programs, many states do not offer access to or utilize medications to treat OUD among arrestees or inmates. The National Institutes of Health (2020) contends that one of the challenges facing inmates and former inmates who are addicted or have prior addictions to opioids is the need for comprehensive follow-up support in the form of medication, counseling, wraparound services, and overdose education. However, further research that examines the association between criminal justice involvement and public health to reduce opioid-related morbidity and mortality rates needs to be conducted (Winkelman et al., 2018).

Paradigm Shift

Lessons Learned from the Crack Cocaine Epidemic of the 1980s and 1990s

The *War on Drugs* began in 1971 when President Richard M. Nixon declared drug use as "public enemy number one" (Richard Nixon Foundation, 2016). It was later intensified by President Ronald Reagan in 1981 who facilitated a boom in the nation's jail and prison populations. This would be carried to another level with the George Bush Senior and William Clinton Administrations accounting for today's prison industrial complex. Nevertheless, beginning in the 1980s and throughout the 1990s, the "get tough" approach emerged as a viable strategy to curb crime. However, it was largely fueled by the media's portrayals of communities "under siege by violent gangs that used extreme violence to control turf needed to sell drugs, namely crack cocaine, and engage in other criminal activities" (Anderson et al., 2017, p. 34). The Violent Crime Control and Law Enforcement Act dramatically increased the number of incarcerated individuals by requiring mandatory imprisonment for anyone convicted of a third violent felony (Krisberg et al., 2015). In most cases, the felonies were non-violent drug-related convictions as states were allowed to decide which crimes would be considered under the law (Donzinger, 1996). Drug officials contend that this coincided with the *first phase* of the opioid epidemic, credited to the proliferation of prescribing the opiate propoxyphene for pain (Schnoll, 1982). The U.S. prescription opioid overdose death toll rose from 3,444 in 1999 to 17,029 in 2017 and overdose deaths involving any opioid, including heroin and fentanyl rose from less than 10,000 to 47,600 during the same period (CDC, 2024b). By 2022, overdoses by any opioid had nearly doubled to 81.806. The war on drugs did not work.

In the early 2000s, ER visits for opioid misuse increased by more than 98% since 2004 (FDA, n.d.). The beginning of public education about the dangers of prescription drug use began in 2001, and label warnings about the dangers of Oxycontin were established. From the first FDA approval in 2014 to the present day, medication-assisted OUD treatment is the standard (Rollston et al., 2021)—when available. The federal government began taking more progressive actions beginning with the Drug Addiction Treatment Act of 2000, followed by the Comprehensive Addiction and Recovery Act of 2016, and the recently renewed SUD Prevention that Promotes Opioid Recovery and Treatment (SUPPORT) for Patients and Communities Act of 2018. While the legal system continues to incarcerate persons with OUDs, who many times go without treatment, the 1976 U.S. Supreme Court case, *Estelle v. Gamble*, established that withholding medically necessary care from prisoners is cruel and unusual punishment, a violation of the Eighth Amendment, and further, violated the Americans with Disabilities Act. While still having a long journey ahead, a shift has begun from seeing drug addiction as a moral shortcoming to viewing it as a disease. This perspective is gaining ground with recent genetic findings, as discussed earlier.

During the *crack cocaine* epidemic that was fought in minority communities, legislation and laws were created that criminalized crack cocaine use as well as its users. Unfortunately, it devastated and destabilized the black community by removing males (e.g., fathers, brothers, sons, and the community's future) and giving them long prison sentences for being dealers or crack addicts. The correctional system is still negatively impacted by the influx of inmates that were brought into the system during the 1980s and 1990s. It created issues such as violence, overcrowding, geriatric populations, and others. Critical scholars argue that the war on drugs was in fact, a war against the poor since its causalities in and out of the prison systems were targeted from the start of the war. However, with the advent of the opioid crisis that has emerged of late, most abusers of this drug are disproportionately White. Consequently, there has been a paradigm shift in how the criminal justice system views and responds to drug addiction. For example, their behavior is not criminalized or demonized, but instead, it is defined and viewed as a public health issue that deserves treatment and not punishment. As a result, they receive humane approaches to alleviating and treating their addiction instead of being victims of mass incarceration.

Public Health Issue

In 2017, the opioid crisis was declared a public health emergency under Section 319 of the Public Health Service Act, and that declaration was renewed most recently in June 2024 (Federal Communications Commission [FCC], n.d.). The scope of this crisis deems it a public health issue. A few sobering facts attest to the enormity of the opioid problem in America. For example, an estimated 650,000 persons have died from opioid-involved overdoses since the 1980s. Presently, over 220 people die each day by opioid overdose, and yearly, opioid overdose deaths remain more than six times greater than in 1999 (CDC, 2024c). The impact of the crisis was exacerbated by COVID 19 which led to increased alcohol and substance misuse and poorer mental health (FCC). Moreover, opioid overdoses increased from 47,885 in 2017 to 80,926 in 2021. While the social burden of these deaths and the tremors they send throughout communities is tremendous, nonfatal overdoses burden governments, health systems, communities, and families (FCC, n.d.) as captured by ER visits owing to opioid misuse and overdose. For example, in 2023, there were approximately, 881,556 ER opioid-related visits, a nearly 4% decrease from 2022 (SAMHSA, 2024b). Visits were highest for those aged 26–44 years, males (336,000 per 100,000), Black (425 per 100,000), and non-Hispanic or Latino individuals (272,000 per 100,000). White and Native Hawaiian/Pacific Islander (NH/PI) individuals shared comparable rates at 206 per 100,000 and 210 per 100,000 respectively. The most common opioid-related ER visit was for a prescription opioid (47.7%, an increase of 16.5% since 2022), fentanyl (31.5%, a 46% increase since 2022), and heroin (27%, a 40.8% decrease since 2022). The decreased heroin visits are likely due to the increased use of fentanyl and fentanyl analogs, or rather, chemical structural alterations of fentanyl. Opioids were also involved in polysubstance use ER visits. In 2023, heroin was involved in 47.5% of polysubstance visits, fentanyl in 60.7%, and prescription opioids in 45.3% of polysubstance ER visits.

The opioid crisis has been expensive. Experts report that not counting the costs to emergency departments nationally in terms of staff, time, medication-assisted overdose treatments, and bedspace, particularly related to caring for the uninsured, has been the cost to government programs such as Medicaid and Medicare for treating a crisis, rather than, being spent on active treatment or recovery programs. In 2016, the cost of the opioid crisis to the U.S. gross domestic product (GDP) was estimated at $504 billion or nearly 2% of GDP (Florence et al., 2016). In 2020, the cost of the epidemic to the U.S. was estimated at $1.5 trillion, using the CDC's original estimate that accounted for "costs of health care, public safety, lost productivity, lower quality of life, and lives lost due to opioids" (Joint Economic Committee Democrats, 2020, p. 2). In terms of public safety, the opioid crisis cost the criminal justice system an estimated $8 billion in 2017, of which nearly, $270 million was related to crime laboratory costs (Ropero-Miller & Speaker, 2019).

International Comparative Statistics

Globally, opioid use remained relatively stable from 2019 to 2021 and held steady with an estimated 60 million users, or an annual user prevalence rate of approximately, 1.2 (UNODC, 2023b). Those regions that reported high past-year use include North America (2021 annual prevalence of 3.3), Near and Middle East/South-West Asia (3.19 annual prevalence), and Oceania (2.39 annual prevalence). While Asia has more numbers of opiate users, North America has more opioid users. From data provided by 61 countries, opiates appeared more than any other drug in post-mortem toxicological testing. Overall, deaths attributed to drug use increased by 17.5% from 2010 to 2019. Furthermore, from 1990 through 2020, it was revealed that opioid use directly accounted for the most years of healthy living losses. Gender differences were significant between opiate users and nonmedical users of prescription opioids. In fact, 75% male and 15% female versus 53% male and 47% female, respectively (UNODC, 2023a). Moreover, globally, OUDs have had the greatest impact on the U.S. in terms of years of lost life per 100,000 for ages 0–19 (111.5 years), followed by Canada (39.28 years), and Guatemala (22.32 years) (Pan American Health Organization, 2021). The country least impacted is Jamaica (1.03). For ages 20–24, the U.S. is again most burdened (1,046.32 lost years), as well as for ages 25–29 (1398.96), 30–34 (1,1445.99), 35–39 (1,527.23), and so on. Canada is the second most affected country, but far less so than the U.S. Countries comprising 20% of the highest opioid mortality rates for 2019 included the U.S., Canada, Bolivia, Guyana, Peru, Guatemala, and Honduras. The U.S., Canada, Bolivia, Peru, Uruguay, Brazil, and Guyana had the highest rates of disability-adjusted life years in 2019.

Public Health and Social Work

Intersection of Public Health and Social Work

Where public health uses approaches to address problems that can be applied at a population level, social approaches to intervene with OA occur primarily at an individual, family, and community level. The United States Department of Labor Statistics (2023) estimates that 123,200 social workers are employed in the mental health and substance abuse field, and work in outpatient clinics, individual and family services, health practitioner offices, local government agencies, and care facilities. Additionally, 365,900 social workers are employed in child, family, and school social work, which often involves working with those experiencing substance use or have families who are substance-involved. After receiving specialized training, social workers perform psychosocial and substance use assessments, develop treatment plans, and participate in prevention, harm reduction, recovery efforts, counseling, and case management services (Royall, 2024). Social work identifies key determinants of health that can interfere with SUD treatment and works with individuals to address issues such as co-occurring mental health diagnoses, financial and employment concerns, legal problems, housing, and complex health conditions (Vanderplasschen et al., 2007). The treatment methods and evidence-based interventions often used by social workers are brief intervention strategies, cognitive behavioral therapy, motivational interviewing, individual and group counseling, dialectical behavioral therapy, family treatment approach, and others (National Association of Addiction Treatment Providers, 2023).

Health Disparities and Health Equities

Racial bias in health care is likely responsible for disparities in how users are assessed, who receives treatment, and how they are treated (Siddiqui & Urman, 2022). Research shows that in care systems, people of color are more likely to be under or inadequately treated for pain (Mossey, 2011). Stereotyping is more likely to occur in stressful and busy environments and when there is insufficient information for a physician to use for making an informed decision. While Whites have traditionally been shown to most likely die from opioid use, Native American overdose deaths were at a rate of 33.1 for fentanyl compared to 24.6 for Whites (Spencer et al., 2023). However, due to myths about pain, and discrimination toward people of color, minority communities do not receive the care they need to both prevent and intervene with OUD. For example, the criminalization of drug use, an opportunity used by the media to portray minority community members as addicts and criminals, fueled the healthcare system's discriminatory practices (Netherland & Hansen, 2016). Moreover, a healthcare area where discrimination has been particularly noticed is in the prevention and management of OUD in the surgical setting. In a study of postpartum pain, Black women reported high levels of pain, yet they received significantly lower levels of pain management medication in the hospital, as well as were less likely to be prescribed prescription opioids for pain at discharge (Badreldin et al., 2019). Similar results were found by Johnson and colleagues (2019) in a postpartum study where Black and Hispanic women reported significantly higher levels of pain compared with White women. However, the White patients received more pain evaluations and received higher levels of both Oxycodone and over-the-counter pain relievers than did the women of color.

Correctional Facilities and Inmate Access to Treatment

While access to treatment as a disparity was discussed earlier in this chapter, the plight of the inmate with an OUD is worth revisiting. While almost two-thirds of jail and prison populations are diagnosed with a SUD (Bronson & Stroop, 2020), less than half of these facilities offer medication-assisted OUD treatment. A recent county-level study demonstrated that 21% of overdose descendants had been in jail shortly before their deaths. This reinforces findings from the CDC (2022) that in 2021, 67.2% of the overdose deaths had at least one opportunity for intervention such as the decedent was currently in treatment for a SUD (7.1%), the drug overdose was witnessed (8.2%), the decedent had shown signs of a mental illness (29.4%), there had been a potential bystander at the overdose (44.0%), the decedent has experienced a prior overdose (13.8%), *and the decedent was recently released from institutional care (9.1%)*. "The criminal justice system is a crucial point of intervention in the overdose crisis" (NIDA, 2024). Jails and prisons with medical staff or at least some hybrid form of care, were more likely to prescribe OUD treatment medication in the form of buprenorphine (69.9%), naltrexone (54.5%), and methadone (46.6%) (Flanagan et al., 2024).

Age as a Factor in Receiving Substance Use Treatment

In 2023, 19.1% or 54.2 million people in the U.S. needed SAT, most were ages 18–25 (28.7%), followed by 12 or older (19.1%), 12–17 (11.2%), and 26 or older (18.6%) (SAMHSA, 2024b). The need for substance use treatment was highest among AI/NA persons (30.6%), followed by multi-racial persons (26.2%), non-Hispanic Whites (19.9%), Blacks (19.7%), Hispanic (17.5%), and Asians (10.5%). Of those who needed treatment, persons aged 18–25—the largest group —were less likely to receive treatment. Of those classified as needing treatment in 2023, only 14.6% received it, leaving the other 85.4% without services (e.g., inpatient, outpatient, telehealth, or in jail/prison). Persons with severe SUD were more likely to receive any treatment compared to those with mild to moderate disorders. Having a dual-diagnosis of a mental health disorder and SUD brings a higher likelihood of receiving treatment for one or the other disorder. In 2023, among the 856,000 youth 12–17 years old with a co-occurring major depressive episode (MDE) and SUD in the past 12 months, 71.1% received treatment. Of the 20.4 million adults aged 18 and older in 2023, with AMI and a SUD, 62.4% received treatment.

AIDS and Blood-Borne Disease Risk

Approximately, 13.2 million persons globally were known to inject drugs in 2023, an increase of 18% from 2020. North America has the highest rate of PWID, or rather, persons who inject drugs (United Nations [UN], 2023a). Injecting drugs places the user at a higher risk of developing Hepatitis C and a 35 times higher risk for contracting AIDS. According to the UN, liver disease associated with Hepatitis accounts for over 50% of deaths attributed to drug use. Moreover, injection use increases the risk for blood-borne diseases such as endocarditis (United States Department of Health and Human Services [USDHHS], Office of the Surgeon General, 2018) and bacterial and antibiotic-resistant infections such as methicillin-resistant *Staphylococcus aureus* or MRSA (Jackson et al., 2018). While more men than women inject drugs, females who inject are at an elevated risk for abuse from law enforcement, IPV, and rape.

Negative Health Consequences of Opioid Addiction

In addition to death by overdose, opioid use carries additional physical and psychological consequences, such as suicide. As mentioned earlier, not all opioid overdose deaths can be classified as accidental since some users may be contemplating suicide due to life circumstances (Tadros et al., 2015). Research has long established the link between suicide and opioid use. For example, people using opioids are 14 times more likely to commit suicide than non-users (Harris & Barraclough, 1997; Wilcox et al., 2004) with rates of suicide among those with an OUD ranging from 17% to 48% (Dark et al., 2015; Kazour et al., 2016). More recently, the association between OUD and suicide was found in a 2023 study with OUD treatment patients (Lent et al., 2023). Similarly, interview data from 244 respondents revealed that 37% had experienced suicidal thoughts over a lifetime, and 27% revealed having attempted suicide. This increased risk has been associated with a lack of family support, joblessness, and homelessness (Roy, 2010), ACES (Zatti et al., 2017), extreme negative affective states (Garland et al., 2017), more negative emotions (Wakaizumi et al., 2021), and comorbidity of disorders, especially mood and anxiety disorders (Cacciola et al., 2001).

Opioid overdose has become the primary cause of death during pregnancy and postpartum time, with rates rising by 80% between 2017 and 2020 (American Medical Association, 2024). The opioid crisis is also affecting neonates and children. The number of pregnant women with OUDs increased by 131% between 2010 and 2017 (Hirai et al., 2021). Women using opioids during pregnancy risk spontaneous abortion, fetal death, preeclampsia, premature rupture of membranes, and placental abruption (Qato & Gandhi, 2021). The increase in opioid-using women while pregnant has led to an increase in the number of children born with Neonatal Abstinence Syndrome (NAS). This condition can cause symptoms such as high-pitched/excessive cry, poor sleep, hypertonia, tremors, and gastrointestinal issues. Opioid use while pregnant can also lead to adverse effects including gastroschisis, sudden infant death, premature delivery, and low birth weight (Smith et al., 2015; Aliyu et al., 2014). The long-term effects of NAS may include potential vision, motor, and behavioral/cognitive problems in childhood and into adolescence (Maguire et al., 2016).

Simultaneous to the feelings of euphoria an opioid user feels are the "dysregulation of dopamine transmission, and a co-occurring impairment in the frontal brain regions," which negatively impacts cognition and function (Tolomeo et al., 2016). This can occur when opioids cross the blood-brain barrier to access the central nervous system (Schaefer et al., 2017). Impairments can include deficits in memory, attention, and executive functions such as inhibition control (Darke et al., 2012). These functions are used in gaining and maintaining a recovery lifestyle as they may be less likely to effectively problem solve, reason, and make good decisions (Tolomeo et al., 2016). Additionally, using images of the brain, it has been discovered that the brain loses mass and eventually, cognitive impairment is permanent and persists even without the drug being administered (Ersche et al., 2006).

Criminal Justice Approaches

According to the Congressional Research Services Report (2019), the DOJ has various grants that address the opioid epidemic. Some of these grants include:

- The Comprehensive Opioid Abuse Grant Program (COAP) for states, units of local government, and Indian tribes (34 U.S.C. 10701 et seq.). This grant supports projects primarily related to opioid abuse, including: (1) diversion and alternatives to incarceration projects; (2) collaboration between criminal justice, social service, and substance abuse agencies; (3) overdose outreach projects, including law enforcement training related to overdoses; (4) strategies to support those with a history of opioid misuse, including justice-involved individuals; (5) prescription drug monitoring programs; (6) development of interventions based on a public health and public safety understanding of opioid abuse; and (7) planning and implementation of comprehensive strategies in response to the growing opioid epidemic. This grant assists law enforcement officers in collecting and analyzing data whereby they can investigate physicians who prescribe controlled substances for drug dealers or abusers, pharmacists who falsify records to sell controlled substances, and people who forge prescriptions.
- The Community Oriented Policing Services (COPS) Office's Anti-Heroin Task Force (AHTF) Program provides funding assistance on a competitive basis to state law enforcement agencies to investigate illicit activities related to the trafficking or distribution of heroin or diverted prescription opioids. Funds are distributed to states with high rates of primary treatment admissions for heroin and other opioids. Furthermore, the program focuses its funding on state law enforcement agencies with multi-jurisdictional reach and interdisciplinary team structures such as task forces.
- The Drug Court Discretionary Grant program (Drug Courts Program) enhances drug court services, coordination, and SAT and recovery support services. It is a competitive grant program that provides resources to state, local, and tribal courts and governments to enhance drug court programs for non-violent substance-abusing offenders. Drug courts are designed to help reduce recidivism and substance abuse among participants and increase an offender's likelihood of successful rehabilitation through early, continuous, and intense judicially supervised treatment; mandatory periodic drug testing; community supervision; appropriate sanctions; and other rehabilitation services. In 2015, the Office of National Drug Control Policy placed the following restrictions on state drug courts receiving federal funding: (1) such courts cannot deny any appropriate and eligible client for the treatment drug court access to the program because of their use of FDA approved medications that are by an appropriately authorized prescription; or (2) mandate that a drug court client no longer use medications as part of the conditions of the drug court if such a mandate is inconsistent with a medical practitioner's recommendation or prescription (NIDA, 2018).
- The Veterans Treatment Court Program is offered through the Drug Courts Program to assist veterans with addiction and serious mental illnesses. These grants are awarded to state, local, and tribal governments to fund and establish treatment courts for veterans.
- The Opioid Affected Youth Initiative is a competitive grant program that funds state, local, and tribal government efforts in developing a data-driven response that identifies and addresses challenges of opioid abuse that impact the safety of youth and the

community. The program supports recipients in implementing strategies and programs to identify areas of concern, collect, and interpret data to help develop youth strategies and programming and implement services to assist children, youth, and families affected by opioid abuse.

- Residential SAT (RSAT) for State Prisoners Program is a formula grant program that supports state, local, and tribal governments in developing and implementing SAT programs in correctional and detention facilities. Funds may also be used to support reintegration services for offenders as they reenter the community after a period of incarceration.

These grants represent the paradigm shift that has taken place in the way the criminal justice system views those who suffer from OAs. Local, state, and tribal governments are now allowed the opportunity to apply for funding that will provide drug treatment; diversionary programs; community supervision; family counseling; and collaborations between criminal justice agencies, social services, and substance abuse agencies to assist, and hopefully, eliminate OA. However, more research needs to be done to ensure small towns and rural communities are aware of these funding opportunities.

Public Health Approaches

Public health approaches to OA are aimed at improving the health of populations as opposed to individuals. Populations can be geographical communities, ethnic or racial communities, populations of people with other shared variables or characteristics, and local, state, regional, national, and global impact. A public health framework to effectively address public health issues consists of *primary, secondary, and tertiary* strategies derived from an ecological model that emerges from interactions between individuals, institutions, communities, and policies (McLeroy et al., 1988). First, *primary* measures to address OA consist of actions aimed at preventing opioid misuse, abuse, and addiction from occurring. This may include decreasing opioid access, increasing protective factors, and reducing risk factors (Livingston et al., 2022). This can be building overdose tracking into existing sentinel surveillance systems, creating data dashboards that link information across service systems, and educating prescribers and patients better about the dangers of opioid misuse and addiction (Saloner et al., 2018). Improving prescribing guidelines, making nonpharmacological pain therapies more available, increasing prescription drug monitoring programs, improving access to mental health care (Livingston et al., 2022), pairing nonopioid alternatives with opioid prescriptions, and offering naloxone to all patients who are prescribed opioids (Mayo Clinic, 2024a), are other primary measures Next, *secondary* measures focus on the early identification of OUD and linkage to evidence-based treatment services (Livingston, 2022). This consists of improving the assessment of OUDs and the ability to find and connect individuals with appropriate treatment, including MAT as well as increasing mental health services and support. Expanding prearrest diversion programs, changing policing strategies to focus on increasing treatment options (Saloner et al., 2018), the initiation and continuation of treatment for incarcerated individuals, supporting primary care providers in providing OUD treatment, and leveraging extra support for pregnant women with OUD (Livingstone et al., 2022) are all secondary level measures. Third, *tertiary* measures consist of slowing the progression of addiction and/or reducing the negative consequences of OA

(Livingston et al., 2022). An example is the establishment of harm reduction programs in communities across the U.S. that provide safe consumption sites, access to clean syringes, fentanyl test strips, and naloxone would ease the disparity of available treatment (Saloner et al., 2018). In addition to these three levels of addressing OA, the ideal most effective measure for preventing OA and the wake of death it leaves behind is what is termed "primordial" prevention that addresses all social and environmental inequities that promote and perpetuate the problem such as poverty, ACES, socioeconomics, and systemic racism.

Public Health and Social Work Approaches

Many of the measures discussed in the section about methods that public health can use to address the opioid epidemic can be enhanced with the inclusion of social workers. For example, harm reduction strategies are effective in reducing opioid overdose deaths (Kennedy et al., 2017) in part because of the emphasis on the patient's decision-making capacity (Hawk et al., 2017). Social workers can join with public health to advocate for the expansion of harm-reduction programs and educate community members to reduce stigma and increase support for these services (Childs et al., 2021). Moreover, social workers can assist public health workers to engage patients in treatment compliance. When surveyed about attributes of treatment that were critical to their recovery, patients consistently responded with the importance of being made to feel human (Alves et al., 2021). Social workers are especially trained in the worth and dignity of every person (Council on Social Work Education, 2022). For this reason, they should share advisory roles with other healthcare professionals in OUD treatment programs and treatment overseeing bodies to ensure that humanistic practices and policies are in place and adhered to, to maximize patient engagement from the EM or primary care office through recovery. Social workers should also assist public health practitioners in developing, distributing, and implementing updated stigma-reducing education (Bascou et al., 2022).

Both public health and social work utilize community-based participatory approaches to research and engage communities in addressing public health issues such as the opioid crisis. An example of this is the National Institutes of Health HEAL Initiative designed to understand, manage, and treat pain and to improve prevention and treatment for opioid misuse and addiction (NIH, 2024). Public health, social work, and other professions from the scientific community, healthcare fields, advocacy groups, and community individuals have formed work groups and committees devoted to addressing the opioid epidemic. There are more than 1,800 projects, over 40 research programs, and nationwide initiatives in all 50 states.

Integrating Skills of Social Epidemiology to Address Disparities and Achieve Equity

An earlier chapter discussed the epidemiological triad model for addressing public health disease and events and explained its traditional three components: host, agent, and environment. The host component is composed of individual factors that determine the level of risk, the agent is an external causal factor, and the environment contains factors external to both that bring the host and agent together (Compton & Jones, 2019). In other words, "disease results from the interaction between the agent and the susceptible host in an

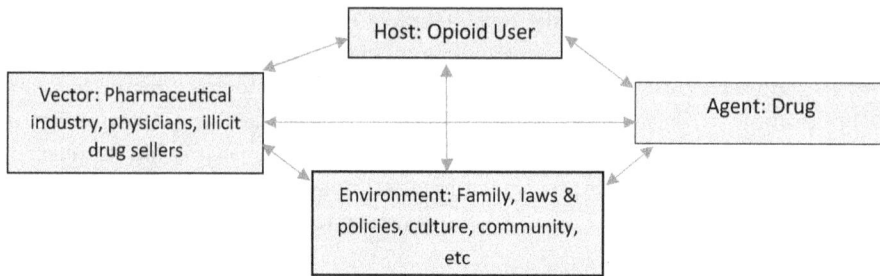

FIGURE 14.1   Epidemiological Triad Model + Vector.

environment that supports transmission of the agent from a source to that host" (National Center for State, Tribal, Local, and Territorial Public Health Infrastructure and Workforce, Division of Workforce Development, 2012). Due to the complexity of the opioid crisis and the significance of market structures and marketing techniques, the impetus behind illegal sellers and authorized providers of opioids and how they control drug use behaviors (Mars et al., 2015). Compton and Jones (2019) suggest that a new component representing market forces should be added to the triad and be referred to as *the vector*.

Figure 14.1 explains that the vector component forces those tackling the opioid crisis to consider the behaviors of illicit and licit drug manufacturers, drug dealers, and doctors to have a comprehensive understanding of how their behaviors have influenced and spread the crisis. This knowledge guides the creation and implementation of better-informed prevention and intervention measures. The use of the original triad, with the addition of the vector component, aids those in public health and other professions to isolate critical information about each component to effectuate positive change in both the opioid crisis and the health disparities linked to opioid misuse, abuse, and addiction. According to Compton and Jones (2019), evidence supports five significant strategies for intervention and prevention: healthcare provider education, primary prevention of all substance use, expanded treatment, access to naloxone, and increased harm reduction programs. Moreover, if disparities in evaluating and treating pain continue, persons of color will not receive the care they need and deserve. Therefore, it is imperative to address structural racism in the healthcare system since it would be a step toward dismantling disparities that push some people to seek pain relief in illicit forms (Compton & Jones, 2019). Attending to the social patterning of health—social inequality, social relationships, social capital, and work stress—motivates more in-depth inquiries into causation (Diez Roux, 2022). Working with police, legislators, and community leadership could lead to collaborations that seek to help, rather than, punish user that could reduce the number of mentally ill and addicted persons in the correctional system. Additional measures are discussed in the next section.

How Can Opioid Addiction Be Prevented?

While the public health epidemiological model assists in gathering data and other information needed for a thorough understanding of the opioid crisis, a social-ecological model of substance use and overdose prevention can help develop a comprehensive prevention strategy that works across multiple levels, using both *upstream* and *downstream* approaches (Jalali et al., 2020). When host, vector, environment, and agent information are strategically situated in the social-ecological model, prevention and intervention measures can be more accurately located and initiated.

Figure 14.2 presents the four levels that explain opioid use and prevention efforts. At the individual level, there are sociodemographic, health and mental health, biological, and psychosocial domain factors that influence opioid use, misuse, and overdose (Jalali et al., 2020). These factors include personal economics, race and ethnicity, health conditions, mental health diagnoses, and genetics, but there is also personal influences and conditions related to drug use such as chronic pain, in utero exposure, comorbid medical and mental health conditions, self-medication of untreated or undertreated pain, hopelessness and despair, stress, unhealthy coping, prescription misuse, lack of knowledge about OA and overdose risk, and using for the euphoria (Brady et al., 2023). Prevention strategies should include the reduction of unnecessary prescribing to youth and adults, better evaluations of pain levels to enhance culturally appropriate pain management for postpartum women and surgery patients of color, provide adequate access to opioid abuse and addiction treatment, including harm reduction, screen for and treat co-occurring disorders together, and assist in the proper management of opioid withdrawal (Jalali et al., 2020).

At the interpersonal level, factors that influence opioid misuse and addiction include marital stress and divorce, family conflicts, IPV, financial hardships, family substance abuse, social disconnection and isolation, drug use among peers, and trauma (experienced as a child or adult) (Brady et al., 2023). If there is a history of family substance use, vulnerability to initiating use may be heightened if a spouse uses and/or there is easy access to opioids from family, friends, and/or co-workers (Jalali et al., 2020). Prevention can begin in the home with parents disapproving of drug use explaining to youth about addiction risk linked to family history of abuse or addiction. School-based prevention programs to build protective factors that help to prevent or delay substance use have proven to be effective (Livingston et al., 2022). Interventions focusing on parenting skills have been shown to improve family functioning, reduce child problem behaviors, and prevent parental substance use relapse

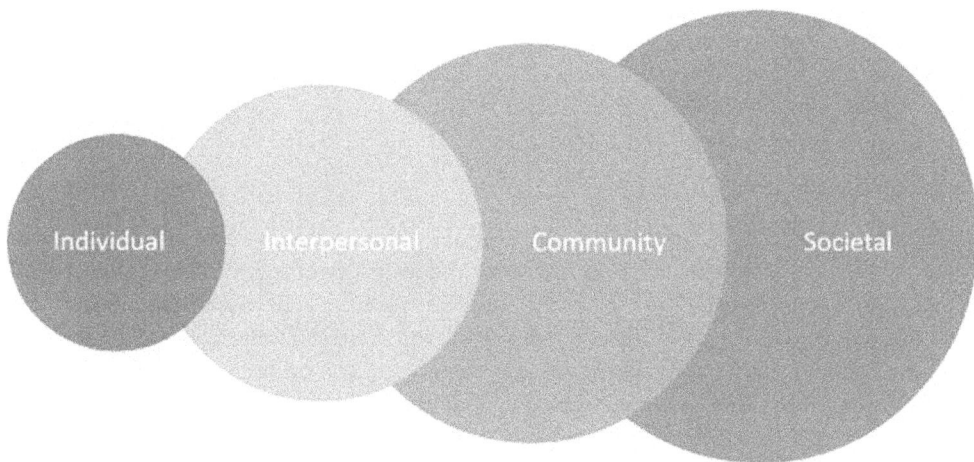

FIGURE 14.2 Social-Ecological Model.

(Dawe et al., 2003). Family therapy, IPV interventions, and assistance with job searching and home finances may help to lower stress. At the community level, impacting factors include unstable housing, unemployment, neighborhood crime, the criminalization of substance use, stigma, community economic inequality, food insecurity and accessibility, lack of harm reduction services, and poor access to health care and OUD treatment (Brady et al., 2023). The community level is also where care may or may not occur. Factors that can increase the risk for opioid misuse include "prescribers' perception of risk, over-prescription of opioids or under-treatment of pain, types of prescription opioid formulations available, community norms, and access to legal and illegal opioids" (Jalali et al., 2020, p. 4). Prevention measures may include access to culturally appropriate providers, supports, mental health services, drug disposal facilities, MAT, naloxone and naloxone training, and harm reduction programming (Minnesota Department of Health, 2024). Physicians should follow the CDC Guideline for Prescribing Opioids for Chronic Pain, practice opioid tapering, and use alternatives to opioid for pain management (Livingston et al., 2022). Community norms around drug use, as well as stigma around seeking treatment, can impact the likelihood of initiation of substance misuse, highlighting the need for both stigma reduction campaigns to encourage help-seeking behavior.

The societal level provides the larger social context, containing the opioid market forces of supply and demand, government regulations, economic conditions, and unemployment rates, discrimination, media and advertising, educational campaigns, and policing/law enforcement (Jalali et al., 2020). Influencing factors include the over or under-prescribing of opioids, provider stigma toward OUD, insufficient patient opioid use monitoring and education, patient-doctor and pharmacy shopping, limited access to opioid alternatives, no access to integrative chronic pain treatment, and the increased availability of both heroin and fentanyl (Brady et al., 2023). OA strategies can include a housing-first approach, changes in policing practices to reduce combative encounters with drug users, implementation of stigma-reduction campaigns to influence public opinion, use of destigmatizing language and imagery in news media, government communication, and medical practice, building overdose tracking into existing sentinel surveillance systems (Saloner et al., 2018) and training the healthcare workforce to address SUDs (USDHHS, 2018). Healthcare systems can assist by promoting integrated prevention, treatment, and recovery support services, "engage primary care providers as part of a comprehensive treatment solution," and "implement health information technologies to promote efficiency, actionable information, and high-quality care" (p. 29).

Policy Recommendations

Policy recommendations for addressing OA and the opioid crisis have been suggested for every level of possible intervention. They are many and interconnected, overlapping at critical points needing collaboration of ideas and funding. Below are a few recommendations.

Practitioners who treat pain should take a person-centered approach and establish hospital and clinic policies for tailored treatments that focus on recovery (Blanco et al., 2020), including post-overdose services (Massachusetts Health Officers Association, 2025). Health insurance plans can establish uniform policies that support the "use of opioid agonist and antagonist medication to treat opioid use disorders, offer incentives to prescribers to enhance access to buprenorphine treatment. . . and, most importantly, eliminate fail first requirements" before ordering best-practice treatments (Holton et al., 2018, p. 4).

Attention to the social determinants and contexts of OA is considered the first line of defense in this opioid crisis (Blanco et al., 2020). As pointed out previously, living in impoverished communities and circumstances, with little or no sufficient means for pain management, heightens one's probability of seeking out illicit substances. This puts an onus on local governments to establish spending policies and guidelines that provide adequate harm reduction and OUD treatment facilities in their communities. In tandem, cities and states can create policies and appropriate funding to support access to medication-assisted OUD treatment in jails and prisons (Saloner et al., 2018). State government can develop policies that increase accountability for agencies working on addiction issues, establish required minimum skill sets and competencies for those working in addiction treatment, and create drug policy advisory boards that include persons in recovery (National Association of Social Workers, 2025).

Due to the risk of overdose for recently released prisoners (CDC, 2022) and the large number of persons incarcerated diagnosed with an OUD (Bronson et al., 2020), detention policy should allow for the assessment, treatment, and recovery of those in custody. The policy should specifically indicate the availability of methadone or buprenorphine for the OUD treatment of pregnant women (Peeler et al., 2019). WHO's Guidelines for the Psychosocially Assisted Pharmacological Treatment of Opioid Dependence recommends that incarcerated persons have access to opioid "withdrawal, agonist maintenance, and naltrexone treatment should be available" (WHO, 2009, p. 12). The best evidenced-based treatment for pregnant women with OUD is MAT with either methadone or buprenorphine.

For greater, sustainable reform, local, state, and federal government divisions should take more responsibility. For example, legislatures should pass bills to develop overdose-tracking systems and support data surveillance and linkage (Saloner et al., 2018). Congress should appropriate funding and change laws that support county and city-wide safe consumption and harm reduction facilities. Congress should also amend regulations for controlled substances based on increased public input and public health best practices. Appropriations and support need to be continued for the Support for Patients and Communities Reauthorization Act (H.R. 4531) that funds OUD prevention, treatment, and recovery.

Summary

OA is a complex public health problem that requires multi-systemic approaches to prevention and intervention. While opioids can be effective pain relievers, they are highly addictive. When unable to obtain legal and sufficient pain management, some feel as though their only option is to seek illegal relief through street drugs such as heroin or illegal prescription pills. Unfortunately, this has led to an overdose epidemic primarily due to the rise in fentanyl availability and fentanyl-laced drugs. The misuse of opioid prescription drugs has also been a grave concern for all groups, including youth. Many have reported misusing opioids before trying heroin. The flow of fentanyl into the U.S. and the hands of drug traffickers is difficult to control. The Mexican Sinaloa Cartel and the Jalisco Cartel have sophisticated networks of smuggling drugs, people, weapons, and migrants, taking control of the U.S. drug market. Risk factors for OA include racial inequality, economic inequality, and several individual factors such as personal income, stressed personal relationships and IPV, genetics, residing in disadvantaged neighborhoods, identifying as LGBTQ+, justice system involvement, and having had or currently having under or untreated chronic pain. The risk of overdose increases with a history of substance abuse, increased opioid use, polysubstance use, high pain intensity levels, and the presence of comorbid mental health and/or physical conditions. The community where people reside may play a significant role in the rise of addiction and overdoses. If city or county governments cannot or will not fund treatment and harm reduction facilities, opioid abusers have nowhere to turn for help and medication-assisted relief. The answer they find is too often jail, overdose, or death. The war on drugs, beginning in 1971, intensified the criminalized substance-involved individuals, driving the prison population from 50,000 to over 400,000 within 17 years. This foreshowed what occurred during the crack cocaine years. However, by 2022, overdoses by any opioid had nearly doubled to 81,806. The toll on persons addicted to opioids can be tremendous, including possibly heart conditions, brain damage, overdose, and suicide. Public health officials, social workers, and government agencies have teamed up to find a better way forward, developing public education campaigns, advocating for more MAT access and harm reduction facilities, designing opioid education for healthcare providers, engaging in participatory research with those most affected, and trying new perspectives, such as the epidemiological triad model + vector, for gaining as much insight as possible. Scientific inquiry, systems analysis, and prevention programming occur at every level of the social-ecological model, spanning from individual intervention, family treatment, community campaigns, and policy advocacy. Though many programs and treatment protocols have been established, and while there are small victories, the opioid crisis continues. Until determinants of health, conditions fueling impoverishment, homelessness, and hopelessness are properly addressed, healthcare systems confront structural racism, law enforcement finds more effective mechanisms to slow drug cartels, and society puts aside its stigmatizing beliefs about persons suffering from pain, progressive change will continue to be delayed.

Discussion Questions

1 What are three determinants of health associated with the opioid crisis?
2 Which policy recommendation would be most effective in assisting to curb the opioid crisis and why?
3 Using the social-ecological model, in which level can intervention most impact the prevention of OUD? Why?
4 What are some lessons learned from the war on drugs?
5 What are some negative health consequences of opioid abuse?
6 How can the lack of legitimate access to prescribed pain medicine lead one to seek out street drugs?

References

Adler, N.E., & Newman, K. (2002). Socioeconomic disparities in health: Pathways and policies. *Health Affairs*, 21(2), 60–76. https://doi.org/10.1377/hlthaff.21.2.60

Aliyu, M.H., Cain, M.A., Mogos, M.F., Salemi, J.L., Whiteman, V., & Salihu, H.M. (2014). Maternal opioid drug use during pregnancy and its impact on perinatal morbidity, mortality, and the costs of medical care in the United States. *Journal of Pregnancy*, 2014(2014), 184–191. https://doi.org/ 10.1155/2014/906723

Altekruse, S.F., Cosgrove, C.M., Altekruse, W.C., Jenkins, R.A., & Blanco, C. (2020). Socioeconomic risk factors for fatal opioid overdoses in the United States: Findings from the mortality disparities in American communities study (MDAC). *PLoS One*, 15(1), e0227966. https://doi.org/10.1371/ journal.pone.0227966

Alves, P.C.G., Stevenson, F.A., Mylan, S., Pires, N., Winstock, A., & Ford, C. (2021). How do people who use drugs experience treatment? A qualitative analysis of views about opioid substitution treatment in primary care (iCARE study). *BMJ Open*, 11, Article e042865. https://doi.org/10.1136/ bmjopen-2020-042865

American Medical Association. (2024, February 29). *AMA report on overdose crisis in pregnant and postpartum people* [Press release]. American Medical Association. www.ama-assn.org/press-cen ter/ama-press-releases/ama-report-overdose-crisis-pregnant-and-postpartum-people

American Psychiatric Association (APA). (2025. Opioid use disorder.www.psychiatry.org/patients-families/opioid-use-disorder#:~:text=Opioid%20Use%20Disorder%20Symptoms&text=Tak ing%20larger%20amounts%20or%20taking,or%20recovering%20from%20its%20effects

Anderson, J.F., Reinsmith-Jones, K., Dyson, L., & Langsam, A. (2017). Nothing succeeds like failure: Lessons learned from combating crack cocaine and its impact on fighting the current opioid epidemic. *Journal of Law and Criminal Justice*, 5(2), 31–42. https://doi.org/10.15640/jlcj.v5n2a3

Anderson-Carpenter, K.D., Rutledge, J.D., & Mitchell, K. (2020). Prescription opioid misuse among heterosexual versus lesbian, gay, and bisexual military veterans: Evidence from the 2015–2017 National Survey of Drug Use and Health. *Drug Alcohol Depend*, 207. https://doi.org/10.1016/ j.drugalcdep.2019.107794

Austin, A., Favril, L., Craft, S., Thliveri, P., & Freeman, T.P. (2023). Factors associated with drug use in prison: A systematic review of quantitative and qualitative evidence. *The International Journal of Drug Policy*, 122, 104248. https://doi.org/10.1016/j.drugpo.2023.104248

Badreldin, N., Grobman, W.A., & Silver, R.K. (2019). Racial and ethnic disparities in opioid prescribing at hospital discharge after childbirth. *Obstetrics & Gynecology*, 133(5), 903–911. https://doi.org/10.1097/AOG.0000000000003248

Bascou, N.A., Haslund-Gourley, B., Amber Monta, K., Samson, K., Goss, N., Meredith, D., Friedman, A., Needleman, A., Kumar, V.K., & Fischer, B.D. (2022). Reducing the stigma surrounding opioid use disorder: Evaluating an opioid overdose prevention training program applied to a diverse population. *Harm Reduction Journal*, 19, Article 5. https://doi.org/10.1186/s12954-022-00589-6

Binswanger, I.A., Stern, M.F., Deyo, R.A., Heagerty, P.J., Cheadle, A., Elmore, J.G., & Koepsell, T.D. (2007). Release from prison—A high risk of death for former inmates. *The New England Journal of Medicine*, 356(2), 157–165. https://doi.org/10.1056/NEJMsa064115

Blanco, C., Wiley, T.R.A., Lloyd, J.J., Lopez, M.F., & Volkow, N.D. (2020). America's opioid crisis: The need for an integrated public health approach. *Translational Psychiatry*, 10(1), 167. https://doi.org/10.1038/s41398-020-0847-1

Bondurant, S.R., Lindo, J.M., & Swensen, I.D. (2018). Substance abuse treatment centers and local crime. *Journal of Urban Economics*, 104, 124–133. https://doi.org/10.1016/j.jue.2018.01.007

Brady, B.R., Taj, E.A, Cameron, E., Yoder, A.M., & De La Rosa, J.S.A. (2023). Diagram of the social-ecological conditions of opioid misuse and overdose. *International Journal of Environmental Research and Public Health*, 20(20), 6950. https://doi.org/10.3390/ijerph20206950

Brinkley-Rubinstein, L., Macmadu, A., Marshall, B.D.L., Heise, A., Ranapurwala, S.I., Rich, J.D., & Green, T.C. (2018a). Risk of fentanyl-involved overdose among those with past year incarceration: Findings from a recent outbreak in 2014 and 2015. *Drug and Alcohol Dependence*, 185, 189–191. https://doi.org/10.1016/j.drugalcdep.2017.12.014

Brinkley-Rubinstein, L., Zaller, N., Martino, S., Cloud, D.H., McCauley, E., Heise, A., & Seal, D. (2018b). Criminal justice continuum for opioid users at risk of overdose. *Addictive Behaviors*, 86, 104–110. https://doi.org/10.1016/j.addbeh.2018.02.024

Bronson, J., & Stroop, J. (2020, March). *Drug use, dependence, and abuse among state prisoners and jail inmates, 2007-2009*. Bureau of Justice Statistics. https://bjs.ojp.gov/content/pub/pdf/dudaspji0 709.pdf

Cacciola, J.S., Alterman, A.I., Rutherford, M.J., McKay, J.R., & Mulvaney, F.D. (2001). The relationship of psychiatric comorbidity to treatment outcomes in methadone maintained patients. *Drug and Alcohol Dependence*, 61(3), 271–280. https://doi.org/10.1016/S0376-8716(00)00148-4

Campbell, C.I., Weisner, C., LeResche, L., Ray, G.T., Saunders, K., Sullivan, M.D., Banta-Green, C.J., Merrill, J.O., Silverberg, M.J., Boudreau, D., Satre, D.D., & Von Korff, M. (2010). Age and gender trends in long-term opioid analgesic use for noncancer pain. *American Journal of Public Health*, 100(12), 2541–2547. https://doi.org/10.2105/AJPH.2009.180646

Capistrant, B.D., & Nakash, O. (2019). Lesbian, gay, and bisexual adults have higher prevalence of illicit opioid use than heterosexual adults: Evidence from the national survey on drug use and health, 2015–2017. *LGBT Health*, 6(6), 326–330. https://doi.org/10.1089/lgbt.2019.0060

Carlson, R.G., Nahhas, R.W., Martins, S.S., & Daniulaityte, R. (2015). Predictors of transition to heroin use among non-opioid dependent illicit pharmaceutical opioid users: A natural history study. *Drug and Alcohol Dependence*, 160, 127–134. https://doi.org/10.1016/j.drugalcdep.2015.12.026

Case, A., & Deaton, A. (2015). Rising morbidity and mortality in midlife among white non-Hispanic Americans in the 21st century. *Proceedings of the National Academy of Sciences – PNAS*, 112(49), 15078–15083. https://doi.org/10.1073/pnas.1518393112

Caulkins, J.P., Gould, A., Pardo, B., Reuter, P., & Stein, B.D. (2021). Opioids and the criminal justice system: New challenges posed by the modern opioid epidemic. *Annual Review of Criminology*, 4, 353–375. https://doi.org/10.1146/annurev-criminol-061020-125715

Centers for Disease Control and Prevention (CDC). (2014). Increases in heroin overdose deaths—28 states, 2010 to 2012. *Morbidity and Mortality Weekly Report*, 63(39), 849–854. mm6339.pdf

Centers for Disease Control and Prevention (CDC). (2022). *State unintentional drug overdose reporting system (SUDORS)*. Final data. US Department of Health and Human Services, CDC. www.cdc.gov/overdose-prevention/data-research/facts-stats/sudors-dashboard-fatal-overdose-data.html

Centers for Disease Control and Prevention (CDC). (2024a). Understanding the opioid overdose epidemic. Overdose Prevention | CDC.

Centers for Disease Control and Prevention (CDC). (2024b). Multiple cause of death 1999–2022. CDC WONDER online Database. 2022 Documentation Mortality Multiple Cause-of-Death Public Use Record Layout.

Centers for Disease Control and Prevention (CDC). (2024c). Opioid dispensing rate maps. www.cdc.gov/overdose-prevention/data-research/facts-stats/opioid-dispensing-rate-maps.html

Chatterjee, A., Larochelle, M.R., Xuan, Z., Wang, N., Bernson, D., Silverstein, M., Hadland, S.E., Land, T., Samet, J.H., Walley, A.Y., & Bagley, S.M. (2019). Non-fatal opioid-related overdoses among adolescents in Massachusetts 2012–2014. *Drug and Alcohol Dependence*, 194, 28–31. https://doi.org/10.1016/j.drugalcdep.2018.09.020

Childs, E., Biello, K, B., Valente, P. K., Salhaney, P., Biancarelli, D.L., Olson, J., Earlywine, J.J., Marshall, B.D., & Bazzi, A.R. (2021). Implementing harm reduction in non-urban communities affected by opioids and polysubstance use: A qualitative study exploring challenges and mitigating strategies. *International Journal of Drug Policy*, 90, Article 103080. https://doi.org/10.1016/j.drugpo.2020.103080

Cicero, T.J., Ellis, M.S., & Kasper, Z.A. (2017). Increased use of heroin as an initiating opioid of abuse. *Addictive Behaviors*, 74, 63–66. https://doi.org/10.1016/j.addbeh.2017.05.030

Compton, W.M., & Jones, C.M. (2019). Epidemiology of the U.S. opioid crisis: The importance of the vector. *Annals of the New York Academy of Sciences*, 1451(1), 130–143. https://doi.org/10.1111/nyas.14209

Congressional Research Service. (2019, June 28). *The opioid epidemic: Supply control and criminal justice policy—Frequently asked questions* (R45790). https://sgp.fas.org/crs/misc/R45790.pdf

Council on Social Work Education. (2022). EPAS 2022: Educational policy and accreditation standards for Baccalaureate and master's social work programs. www.cswe.org/getmedia/bb5d8 afe-7680-42dc-a332-a6e6103f4998/2022-EPAS.pdf

Curtin, M., & Goldstein, L. (2010). Cultural differences and pain management. *Practical Pain Management*, 10(5). www.practicalpainmanagement.com/resources/cultural

Darke, S., McDonald, S., Kaye, S., & Torok, M. (2012). Comparative patterns of cognitive performance amongst opioid maintenance patients, abstinent opioid used and non-opioid users. *Drug and Alcohol Dependence*, 126, 309–315. https://doi.org/10.1016/j.drugalcdep.2012.05.032

Darke, S., Ross, J., Marel, C., Mills, K.L., Slade, T., Burns, L., & Teesson, M. (2015). Patterns and correlates of attempted suicide amongst heroin users: 11-year follow-up of the Australian treatment outcome study cohort. *Psychiatry Research*, 227(2), 166–170. https://doi.org/10.1016/j.psychres.2015.04.010

Dasgupta, N., Beletsky, L., & Ciccarone, D. (2018). Opioid crisis: No easy fix to its social and economic determinants. *American Journal of Public Health*, 108(2), 182–186. https://doi.org/10.2105/AJPH.2017.304187

Dasgupta, N., Funk, M.J., Proescholdbell, S., Hirsch, A., Ribisl, K.M., & Marshall, S. (2016). Cohort study of the impact of high-dose opioid analgesics on overdose mortality. *Pain Medicine (Malden, MA)*, 17(1), 85–98. https://doi.org/10.1111/pme.12907

Dawe, S., Harnett, P., Rendalls, V., & Staiger, P. (2003). Improving family functioning and child outcome in methadone maintained families: the parents under pressure programme. *Drug and Alcohol Review*, 22, 299–307. https://doi.org/10.1080/0959523031000154445

Day, B.F., & Rosenthal, G.L. (2019). Social isolation proxy variables and prescription opioid and benzodiazepine misuse among older adults in the U.S.: A cross-sectional analysis of data from the national survey on drug use and health, 2015–2017. *Drug and Alcohol Dependence*, 204, 107518. https://doi.org/10.1016/j.drugalcdep.2019.06.020

Dhaliwal, A., & Gupta, M. (2023). *Physiology, Opioid Receptor*. StatPearls. Treasure Island (FL): StatPearls Publishing. www.ncbi.nlm.nih.gov/books/NBK546642/. www.ncbi.nlm.nih.gov/books/NBK546642/#:~:text=Opioid%20receptors%20are%20abundant%20in%20the%20resp iratory,slow%20breathing%2C%20eventually%20developing%20hypercapnia%20and%20 hypoxia

Diez Roux, A.V. (2022). Social epidemiology: Past, present, and future. *Annual Review of Public Health*, 43(1), 79–98. https://doi.org/10.1146/annurev-publhealth-060220-042648

Donziger, S.R. (1996). *The real war on crime: The report of the national criminal justice commission. The real war on crime: the report of the National Criminal Justice Commission: National Center on Institutions and Alternatives (U.S.)*. National Criminal Justice Commission: Free Download, Borrow, and Streaming: Internet Archive.

Drug Enforcement Agency (DEA). (n.d.). *Opium*. Drug Enforcement Agency.

Drug Enforcement Agency. (2021). *Sharp increase in fake prescription pills containing fentanyl and methamphetamine*. Public safety alert. Department of Justice, Drug Enforcement Agency. 2021 DEA Public Safety Alert.pdf.

Drug Enforcement Agency. (2023). *DEA operation last mile tracks down sinaloa and Jalisco Cartel associates operating within the United States*. Press Release. U.S. Department of Justice, Drug Enforcement Agency. DEA Operation Last Mile Tracks Down Sinaloa and Jalisco Cartel Associates Operating within the United States.

Drug Enforcement Administration (DEA). (2024a). Benzimidazole-opioids: Other name: Nitazenes. Diversion Control Division Drug & Chemical Evaluation Section. https://deadiversion.usdoj.gov/drug_chem_info/benzimidazole-opioids.pdf#:~:text=Mu-opioid%20receptor%20and%20%CE%B2-arrestin-2%20interaction%20has%20been%20implicated,and%20can%20prod uce%20dose-dependent%20respiratory%20depression%20and%20arrest

Drug Enforcement Administration (DEA). (2024b). *National drug threat assessment 2024*. U.S. Department of Justice, Drug Enforcement Agency. National Drug Threat Assessment 2024.

Duncan, D.T., Zweig, S., Hambrick, H.R., & Palamar, J.J. (2019). Sexual orientation disparities in prescription opioid misuse among U.S. adults. *American Journal of Preventive Medicine*, 56(1), 17–26. https://doi.org/10.1016/j.amepre.2018.07.032

Dwyer-Lindgren, L., Bertozzi-Villa, A., Stubbs, R.W., Morozoff, C., Kutz, M.J., Huynh, C., Barber, R.M., Shackelford, K.A., Mackenbach, J.P., van Lenthe, F.J., Flaxman, A.D., Naghavi, M., Mokdad, A.H., & Murray, C.J.L. (2016). US county-level trends in mortality rates for major causes of death, 1980–2014. *JAMA: The Journal of the American Medical Association*, 316(22), 2385–2401. https://doi.org/10.1001/jama.2016.13645

Ersche, K.D., Clark, L., London, M., Robbins, T.W., & Shahakian, B.J. (2006). Profile of executive and memory function associated with amphetamine and opiate dependence. *Neuropsychopharmacology*, 31(5), 1036–1047.

Federal Communications Commission (FCC). (n.d.). Connect2Health: Focus on broadband and opioids. www.fcc.gov/reports-research/maps/connect2health/focus-on-opioids.htmlFind-A-Code. (2025). 6C43 Disorders due to use of opioids: International classification of diseases for mortality and morbidity statistics, 11th Revision, v2024–01. www.findacode.com/icd-11/code-111507 461.html#:~:text=6C43%20Disorders%20due%20to%20use%20of%20opioids%20%2D%20 ICD%2D11%20MMS

Flanagan B.E., Ducharme, L., Taylor, B.G., & Johnson, A. (2024). factors associated with the availability of medications for opioid use disorder in US jails. *JAMA Network Open*, 7(9), e2434704. https://doi.org/10.1001/jamanetworkopen.2024.34704

Florence, C.S., Zhou, C., Luo, F., & Xu, L. (2016). The economic burden of prescription opioid overdose, abuse, and dependence in the United States, 2013. *Medical Care*, 54(10), 901–906. https://doi.org/10.1097/MLR.0000000000000625

Frankenfeld, C.L., & Leslie, T.F. (2019). County-level socioeconomic factors and residential racial, Hispanic, poverty, and unemployment segregation associated with drug overdose deaths in the United States, 2013–2017. *Annals of Epidemiology*, 35, 12–19. https://doi.org/10.1016/j.annepi dem.2019.04.009

Freeman, J., Lewis, T., Jones, R., Goldberg, S., & Snyder, T. (2025). 2024 LGBTQ+ youth substance abuse report. Human Rights Campaign Foundation. 3. LGBTQ+ Youth Substance Use

Friedman, J., Godvin, M., Shover, C.L., Gone, J.P., Hansen, H., & Schriger, D.L. (2022). Trends in drug overdose deaths among US adolescents, January 2010 to June 2021. *JAMA: The Journal of the American Medical Association*, 327(14), 1398–1400. https://doi.org/10.1001/jama.2022.2847

Friedman, J., & Hansen, H. (2024). Trends in deaths of despair by race and ethnicity from 1999 to 2022. *JAMA Psychiatry (Chicago, IL)*, 81(7), 731–732. https://doi.org/10.1001/jamapsychia try.2024.0303

Furr-Holden, D., Milam, A.J., Wang, L., & Sadler, R. (2021). African Americans now outpace whites in opioid-involved overdose deaths: A comparison of temporal trends from 1999 to 2018. *Addiction*, 116(3), 677–683. https://doi.org/10.1111/add.15233. Disparities in the overdose crisis? A comparison of Black and White communities in America – Recovery Research Institute.

Garland, E.L., Riquino, M.R., Priddy, S.E., & Bryan, C.J. (2017). Suicidal ideation is associated with individual differences in prescription opioid craving and cue-reactivity among chronic pain patients. *Journal of Addictive Diseases*, 36(1), 23–9. https://doi.org/10.1080/10550887.2016.1220800

Goldman-Hasbun, J., Kerr, T., Nosova, E., Shulha, H., Wood, E., & DeBeck, K. (2019). Initiation into heroin use among street-involved youth in a Canadian setting: A longitudinal cohort study. *Drug and Alcohol Dependence*, 205, 107579. https://doi.org/10.1016/j.drugalc dep.2019.107579

Gordon, M.S., Kinlock, T.W., & Schwartz, R.P. (2014). Medication-assisted treatment for opioid use disorders in correctional settings: An ethics review. *International Journal of Drug Policy*, 25(6), 1148–1154. https://doi.org/10.1016/j.drugpo.2014.07.009

Griffin, O.H., & Miller, B.L. (2011). OxyContin and a regulation deficiency of the pharmaceutical industry: Rethinking state-corporate crime. *Critical Criminology (Richmond, B.C.)*, 19(3), 213–226. https://doi.org/10.1007/s10612-010-9113-9

Han, B., Jones, C., Einstein, E., Dowell, D., & Compton, W. (2024). Prescription opioid use disorder among adults reporting prescription opioid use with or without misuse in the United States. *The Journal of Clinical Psychiatry*, https://doi.org/10.4088/jcp.24m15258

Harris, E., & Barraclough, B. (1997). Suicide as an outcome for mental disorders. A meta-analysis. *British Journal of Psychiatry*, 170(3), 205–228. https://doi.org/10.1192/bjp.170.3.205

Hatoum, A.S., Colbert, S.M.C., Johnson, E.C., Huggett, S.B., Deak, J.D., Pathak, G., Jennings, M.V., Paul, S.E., Karcher, N.R., Hansen, I., Baranger, D.A.A., Edwards, A., Grotzinger, A., Tucker-Drob, E.M., Kranzler, H.R., Davis, L.K., Sanchez-Roige, S., Polimanti, R., Gelernter, J., ..., Substance Use Disorder Working Group of the Psychiatric Genomics Consortium. (2023). Multivariate genome-wide association meta-analysis of over 1 million subjects identifies loci underlying multiple substance use disorders. *Nature Mental Health*, 1(3), 210–223. https://doi.org/10.1038/s44220-023-00034-y

Hawk, M., Coulter, R.W.S., Egan, J.E., Fisk, S., Friedman, M.R., Tula, M., & Kinsky, S. (2017). Harm reduction principles for healthcare settings. *Harm Reduction Journal*, 14, Article 70. https://doi.org/10.1186/s12954-017-0196-4

Hellman, J., & Raman, S. (2025, January 15). *DEA, HHS finalize rule allowing telehealth drug treatment*. Policy. DEA, HHS finalize rule allowing telehealth drug treatment – Roll Call.

Hirai, A.H., Ko, J.Y., & Patrick, S.W. (2021). US hospital data about neonatal abstinence syndrome and maternal opioid-related Diagnoses—Reply. *JAMA: The Journal of the American Medical Association*, 325(20), 2120–2120. https://doi.org/10.1001/jama.2021.4519

Holton, D., White, E., & McCarty, D. (2018). Public health policy strategies to address the opioid epidemic. *Clinical Pharmacology and Therapeutics*, 103(6), 959–962. https://doi.org/10.1002/cpt.992

Human Impact Partners & WISDOM. (2012, November). *Treatment alternatives to prison: A health impact assessment on diversion from incarceration in Wisconsin*. Human Impact Partners. Treatment Alternatives to Prison | Health Impact Assessment

Iheanacho, T., & Jordan, A., D. C. (2020). Underserved populations. In C. Marienfeld (Ed.), *Absolute addiction psychiatry review*. Springer. https://link.springer.com/chapter/10.1007/978-3-030-33404-8_18

Institute of Medicine. (2011). *Relieving pain in America: A blueprint for transforming prevention, care, education, and research*. National Academies Press.

Jackson, K.A., Bohm, M.K., Brooks, J.T., Asher, A., Nadle, J., Bamberg, W.M., Petit, S., Ray, S.M., Harrison, L.H., Lynfield, R., Dumyati, G., Schaffner, W., Townes, J.M., & See, I. (2018). Invasive methicillin-resistant *Staphylococcus aureus* infections among persons who inject drugs—Six sites, 2005–2016. *MMWR. Morbidity and Mortality Weekly Report*, 67(22), 625–628. https://doi.org/10.15585/mmwr.mm6722a2

Jalali, M.S., Botticelli, M., Hwang, R.C., Koh, H.K., & McHugh, R.K. (2020). The opioid crisis: A contextual, social-ecological framework. *Health Research Policy and Systems*, 18(1), 87. https://doi.org/10.1186/s12961-020-00596-8

Johnson, J.D., Asiodu, I.V., McKenzie, C.P., Tucker, C., Tully, K.P., Bryant, K., ... & Stuebe, A.M. (2019). Racial and ethnic inequities in postpartum pain evaluation and management. *Obstetrics & Gynecology*, 134(6), 1155–1162. doi:10.1097/AOG.0000000000003505

Joint Economic Committee Democrats. (2022, September 28). *The economic toll of the opioid crisis reached nearly $1.5 trillion in 2020*. United States Joint Economic Committee. www.jec.senate.gov/public/_cache/files/67bced7f-4232-40ea-9263-f033d280c567/jec-cost-of-opioids-issue-brief.pdf

Jones, C.M., Logan, J., Gladden, R.M., & Bohm, M.K. (2015). Vital signs: demographic and substance use trends among heroin users – United States, 2002–2013. *Morbidity and mortality weekly report (MMWR)*. Atlanta, GA: Centers for Disease Control and Prevention. www.cdc.gov/mmwr/preview/mmwrhtml/mm6426a3.htm

Jones, C.M., & McCance-Katz, E.F. (2019). Co-occurring substance use and mental disorders among adults with opioid use disorder. *Drug and Alcohol Dependence*, 197, 78–82. https://doi.org/10.1016/j.drugalcdep.2018.12.030

Kazour, F., Soufia, M., Rohayem, J., & Richa, S. (2016). Suicide risk of heroin dependent subjects in Lebanon. *Community Mental Health Journal, 52*(5), 589–596. https://doi.org/10.1007/s10 597-015-9952-7

Keen, C., Young, J.T., Borschmann, R., & Kinner, S.A. (2020). Non-fatal drug overdose after release from prison: A prospective data linkage study. *Drug and Alcohol Dependence, 206*, 107707. https://doi.org/10.1016/j.drugalcdep.2019.107707

Kennedy, M.C., Karamouzian, M., & Kerr, T. (2017). Public health and public order outcomes associated with supervised drug consumption facilities: A systematic review. *Current HIV/AIDS Reports, 14*, 161–183. https://doi.org/10.1007/s11904-017-0363-y

Krisberg, B., Marchionna, S., & Hartney, C. (2015). *American corrections: Concepts and controversies.* SAGE Publication.

Lent, M.R., Dugosh, K.L., Hurstak, E., Callahan, H.R., Mazur, K., Greater Philadelphia Opioid Use Disorder Research Group, & The Greater Philadelphia Opioid Use Disorder Research Group. (2023). Prevalence and predictors of suicidality among adults initiating office-based buprenorphine. *Addiction Science & Clinical Practice, 18*(1), 37–37. https://doi.org/10.1186/s13722-023-00393-y

Lindenfeld, Z., Mauri, A.I., & Chang, J.E. (2025). Examining the relationship between local governmental expenditures on the social determinants of health and county-level overdose deaths, 2017–2020. *Journal of Public Health Management and Practice, 31*(1), 20–28. https://doi.org/10.1097/PHH.0000000000001983

Livingston, C.J., Berenji, M., Titus, T.M., Caplan, L.S., Freeman, R.J., Sherin, K.M., Mohammad, A., & Salisbury-Afshar, E.M. (2022). American college of preventive medicine: Addressing the opioid epidemic through a prevention framework. *American Journal of Preventive Medicine, 63*(3), 454–465. https://doi.org/10.1016/j.amepre.2022.04.021

Maguire, D.J., Taylor, S., Armstrong, K., Shaffer-Hudkins, E., Germain, A.M., Brooks, S.S., Cline, G.J., & Clark, L. (2016). Long-term outcomes of infants with neonatal abstinence syndrome. *Neonatal Network, 35*(5), 277–286. https://doi.org/10.1891/0730-0832.35.5.277

Mars, S.G., Bourgois, P., Karandinos, G., Montero, F., & Ciccarone, D. (2014). "Every 'Never' I ever said came true": Transitions from opioid pills to heroin injecting. *The International Journal of Drug Policy, 25*(2), 257–266. https://doi.org/10.1016/j.drugpo.2013.10.004

Mars, S.G., Fessel, J.N., Bourgois, P., Montero, F., Karandinos, G., & Ciccarone, D. (2015). Heroin-related overdose: The unexplored influences of markets, marketing and source-types in the United States. *Social Science & Medicine (1982), 140*, 44–53. https://doi.org/10.1016/j.socsci med.2015.06.032

Massachusetts Health Officers Association. (2025). *Section II: Evidence-based opioid prevention interventions.* https://opioid-toolkit.mhoa.com/evidence-based-opioid-prevention-examples/

Mayo Clinic. (2024a). *The role of healthcare professionals in opioid addiction prevention.* Mayo Foundation for Medical Education and Research. www.mayoclinic.org/medical-professionals/tra uma/news/the-role-of-healthcare-professionals-in-opioid-addiction-prevention/mac-20561321

Mayo Clinic. (2024b). How opioid use disorder occurs. Mayo Foundation for Medical Education and Research. www.google.com/url?sa=t&source=web&rct=j&opi=89978449&url=https://www.may oclinic.org/diseases-conditions/prescription-drug-abuse/in-depth/how-opioid-addiction-occurs/ art-20360372&ved=2ahUKEwiYxs7955SMAxVWlYkEHb6uAI0QFnoECBQQAw&usg=AOvVa w0SH4WOPcUYKrqiuN9iHhEq

McLeroy, K.R., Bibeau, D., Steckler, A., & Glanz, K. (1988). An ecological perspective on health promotion programs. *Health Education Quarterly, 15*(4), 351–377. https://doi.org/10.1177/109 019818801500401

Memorial Sloan Kettering Cancer Center Library. (2025). *Public health: What is the Opioid epidemic?* https://libguides.mskcc.org/publichealth/opioids

Miech, R.A., Johnston, L.D., Patrick, M.E., & O'Malley, P.M. (2024). *Monitoring the Future national survey results on drug use, 1975–2024: Overview and key findings for secondary school students.* Monitoring the Future Monograph Series. Institute for Social Research, University of Michigan. https://monitoringthefuture.org/results/annual-reports/

Minnesota Department of Health. (2024, April 5). *Comprehensive Drug Overdose Prevention and Morbidity Act - Legislative Report*. www.health.state.mn.us/communities/opioids/documents/2024compaleg.pdf

Monnat, S.M. (2019). The contributions of socioeconomic and opioid supply factors to U.S. drug mortality rates: Urban-rural and within-rural differences. *Journal of Rural Studies*, 68, 319–335. https://doi.org/10.1016/j.jrurstud.2018.12.004

Moore, K.E., Roberts, W., Reid, H.H., Smith, K.M.Z., Oberleitner, L.M.S., & McKee, S.A. (2019). Effectiveness of medication assisted treatment for opioid use in prison and jail settings: A meta-analysis and systematic review. *Journal of Substance Abuse Treatment*, 106, 33–49. https://doi.org/10.1016/j.jsat.2019.07.014

Morgan, E., Feinstein, B.A., & Dyar, C. (2020). Disparities in prescription opioid misuse affecting sexual minority adults are attenuated by depression and suicidal ideation. *LGBT Health*, 7(8), 431–438. https://doi.org/10.1089/lgbt.2020.0220

Mossey, J.M. (2011). Defining racial and ethnic disparities in pain management. *Clinical Orthopaedics and Related Research®*, 469(7), 1859–1870. doi:10.1007/s11999-011-1770-9

Muhuri, P.K., Gfroerer, J.C., & Davies, M.C. (2013). Substance abuse and mental health services administration. Associations of nonmedical pain reliever use and initiation of heroin use in the United States. *CBHSQ Data Review*. Center for Behavioral Health Statistics and Quality, Substance Abuse and Mental Health Services Administration. www.samhsa.gov/data/sites/default/files/DR006/DR006/nonmedical-pain-reliever-use-2013.htm.

National Association of Addiction Treatment Providers. (2023). *Treatment methods & evidence-based practices*. www.naatp.org/addiction-treatment-resources/treatment-methods

National Association of County & City Health Officials. (2021). *Identifying the root causes of drug overdose health inequities and related social determinants of health: A literature review*. Identifying the Root Causes-of Drug Overdose Health Inequities pdf.

National Association of Social Workers. (2025). *Blueprint for the states: Policies to improve the ways states organize and deliver alcohol and drug prevention and treatment*. Policies to Improve Alcohol and Drug Prevention and Treatment.

National Center for State, Tribal, Local, and Territorial Public Health Infrastructure and Workforce, Division of Workforce Development. (2012). *Lesson 1: Introduction to epidemiology: section 8: Concepts of Disease Occurrence*. https://archive.cdc.gov/www_cdc_gov/csels/dsepd/ss1978/lesson1/section8.html#:~:text=A%20number%20of%20models%20of,the%20host%20and%20agent%20together

National Institute on Drug Abuse. (2018, June). *Medications to Treat Opioid Use Disorder* (NIH Publication No. 18-DA-8041). U.S. Department of Health and Human Services, National Institutes of Health. https://nida.nih.gov/sites/default/files/21349-medications-to-treat-opioid-use-disorder.pdf

National Institute on Drug Abuse (NIDA). (2021). *Prescription Opioids DrugFacts*. U.S. Department of Health and Human Services. National Institutes of Health. https://nida.nih.gov/publications/drugfacts/prescription-opioids

National Institute on Drug Abuse (NIDA). (2024). *Fewer than half of U.S. jails provide life-saving medications for opioid use disorder*. U.S. Department of Health and Human Services.

National Institutes of Health (NIH). (2018, May 22). *How opioid drugs activate receptors*. NIH Research Matters. National Institutes of Health. *U.S. Department of Health and Human Services*. www.nih.gov/news-events/nih-research-matters/how-opioid-drugs-activate-receptors

National Institutes of Health (NIH). (2020). Re-envisioning how the Criminal Justice System responds to the opioid crisis: Connecting justice-involved people with life saving medication treatment for opioid use disorder. https://heal.nih.gov>news>stories>about.JCOIN

National Institutes of Health (NIH). (2024). *What is the NIH HEAL Initiative?* https://heal.nih.gov/

National Library of Medicine. (2025). Health topics: *Prescription drug misuse*. National Library of Medicine, MedlinePlus. Prescription Drug Misuse: MedlinePlus

Netherland, J., & Hansen, H.B. (2016). The war on drugs that wasn't: Wasted whiteness, "dirty doctors," and race in media coverage of prescription opioid misuse. *Culture, Medicine, and Psychiatry*, 40(4), 664–686. https://doi.org/10.1007/s11013-016-9496-5

New York City Department of Health and Mental Hygiene. (2019). *Unintentional drug poisoning (overdose) deaths in New York City in 2018*. Epi Data Brief 116. databrief116.pdf.

Pan American Health Organization. (2021). *The burden of drug use disorders in the Region of the Americas, 2000–2019*. Noncommunicable Diseases and Mental Health Data Portal. Pan American Health Organization. www.paho.org/en/enlace/burden-drug-use-disorders

Paulozzi, L.J., Jones, C., Mack, K., & Rudd, R. (2011). Vital signs: Overdoses of prescription opioid pain relievers—United States, 1999–2008. *Morbidity and Mortality Weekly Report (MMWR)*, 60(43), 1487–1492.

Peeler, M., Fiscella, K., Terplan, M., & Sufrin, C. (2019). Best practices for pregnant incarcerated women with opioid use disorder. *Journal of Correctional Health Care*, 25(1), 4–14. https://doi.org/10.1177/1078345818819855

Peterson, T. (2025). *Complete list of opioids: Brand name, street name, strength*. Complete List of Opioids – Brand Name, Street Name, Strength | Healthy Place.

Pierce, M., Hayhurst, K., Bird, S.M., Hickman, M., Seddon, T., Dunn, G., & Millar, T. (2017). Insights into the link between drug use and criminality: Lifetime offending of criminally-active opiate users. *Drug Alcohol Depend*, 1(179), 309–316. https://doi.org/10.1016/j.drugalcdep.2017.07.024

Pitzer, L., Bennett, M., Simard, B., Schillo, B.A., Vallone, D.M., & Hair, E.C. (2020). Prescription opioid misuse: Examining the role of opioid-related attitudes among youth and young adults by sexual orientation. *Substance Use & Misuse*, 55(10), 1601–1609. https://doi.org/10.1080/10826084.2020.1753774

Qato, D.M., & Gandhi, A.B. (2021). Opioid and benzodiazepine dispensing and co-dispensing patterns among commercially insured pregnant women in the united states, 2007–2015. *BMC Pregnancy and Childbirth*, 21(1), 350. https://doi.org/10.1186/s12884-021-03787-5

Qeadan, F., Madden, E.F., Bern, R., Parsinejad, N., Porucznik, C.A., Venner, K.L., & English, K. (2021). Associations between opioid misuse and social relationship factors among American Indian, Alaska Native, and Native Hawaiian college students in the U.S. *Drug and Alcohol Dependence*, 222, 108667. https://doi.org/10.1016/j.drugalcdep.2021.108667

Raja, A.S., Miller, E.S., Flores, E.J., Wakeman, S.E., & Eng, G. (2017). Case 37-2017. A 36-year-old man with unintentional opioid overdose. *The New England Journal of Medicine*, 377(22), 2181–2188. https://doi.org/10.1056/NEJMcpc1710563. PMID: 29171813.

Ranapurwala, S.I., Shanahan, M.E., Alexandridis, A.A., Proescholdbell, S.K., Naumann, R.B., Edwards, D., & Marshall, S.W. (2018). Opioid overdose mortality among former North Carolina inmates: 2000–2015. *American Journal of Public Health*, 109(9), 1207–1213. https://doi.org/10.2105/AJPH.2018.304514

Richard Nixon Foundation. (2016. *Public enemy number one: A pragmatic approach to America's drug problem*. Public Enemy Number One: A Pragmatic Approach to America's Drug Problem » Richard Nixon Foundation.

Richesson, D., Magas, I., Brown, S., Linman, S., & Hoenig, J. (2024). *Key substance use and mental health indicators in the United States: Results from the 2023 National Survey on Drug Use and Health*. U.S. Department of Health and Human Services Substance Abuse and Mental Health Services Administration Center for Behavioral Health Statistics and Quality Office of Population Surveys. Publication Number PEP24-07-021. Key Substance Use and Mental Health Indicators in the United States: Results from the 2023 National Survey on Drug Use and Health.

Robinson, S. M., & Adinoff, B. (2016). The classification of substance use disorders: Historical, contextual, and conceptual considerations. *Behavioral Sciences*, 6(3), 18. https://doi.org/10.3390/bs6030018

Rollston, R., Clear, B., & Clark, K. J. (2021, February 11). *Treating the Opioid Crisis: Current Trends and What's Next*. The Medical Care Blog, Harvard Medical School. www.themedicalcareblog.com/treating-opioid-crisis-part1/

Ropero-Miller, J.D., & Speaker, P.J. (2019). The hidden costs of the opioid crisis and the implications for financial management in the public sector. *Forensic Science International: Synergy*, 1, 227–238. https://doi.org/10.1016/j.fsisyn.2019.09.003

Roy, A. (2010). Risk factors for attempting suicide in heroin addicts. *Suicide & Life-Threatening Behavior*, 40(4), 416–420. https://doi.org/10.1521/suli.2010.40.4.416

Royall, M. 2024. *Social workers can help with the substance use crisis*. National Association of Social Workers. www.socialworkers.org/Practice/Tips-and-Tools-for-Social-Workers/Social-Workers-Can-Help-with-The-Substance-Use-Crisis

Rushovich, T., Arwady, M.A., Salisbury-Afshar, E., Arunkumar, P., Aks, S., & Prachand, N. (2020). Opioid-related overdose deaths by race and neighborhood economic hardship in Chicago. *Journal of Ethnicity in Substance Abuse*, 21(1), 22–35. https://doi.org/10.1080/15332640.2019.1704335

Saloner, B., McGinty, E.E., Beletsky, L., Bluthenthal, R., Beyrer, C., Botticelli, M., & Sherman, S.G. (2018). A public health strategy for the opioid crisis. *Public Health Reports (1974)*, 133(1S), 24S–34S. https://doi.org/10.1177/0033354918793627

Schaeffer, C.P., Tome, M.E. & Davis, T.P. (2017). The opioid epidemic: A central role for the blood brain barrier in opioid analgesia and abuse. *Fluids and Barriers of the CNS*, 14(32), 1–11.

Schnoll, S. (1982). Pain. In S. Cohen, D. Katz, C. Buchwalk, & J. Solomon (Eds.), *Frequently prescribed and abused drugs: Their indications, efficacy and rational prescribing* (pp. 41–55). National Institute on Drug Abuse.

Schuler, M.S., Dick, A.W., & Stein, B.D. (2019). Sexual minority disparities in opioid misuse, perceived heroin risk and heroin access among a national sample of US adults. *Drug Alcohol Depend*, 201, 78–84. https://doi.org/10.1016/j.drugalcdep.2019.04.014

Siddiqui, N., & Urman, R.D. (2022). Opioid use disorder and racial/ethnic health disparities: Prevention and management. *Current Pain and Headache Reports*, 26, 129–137. https://doi.org/10.1007/s11916-022-01010-4

Smith, M.V., Costello, D., & Yonkers, K.A. (2015). Clinical correlates of prescription opioid analgesic use in pregnancy. *Maternal and Child Health Journal*, 19(3), 548–556. https://doi.org/10.1007/s10995-014-1536-6

Spencer, M.R., Warner, M., Cisewski, J.A., Miniño, A.M., Dodds, D., Perera, J., & Ahmad, F.B. (2023, April). *Vital statistics rapid release. Estimates of drug overdose deaths involving fentanyl, methamphetamine, cocaine, heroin, and oxycodone: United States, 2021* (Report No. 27). Centers for Disease Control and Prevention. www.cdc.gov/nchs/data/vsrr/vsrr027.pdf

Stoeber, M., Jullié, D., Lobingier, B.T., Laeremans, T., Steyaert, J., Schiller, P.W., Manglik, A., & von Zastrow, M.A. (2018). Genetically encoded biosensor reveals location bias of opioid drug action. *Neuron*, 98(5), 963–976.e5. https://doi.org/10.1016/j.neuron.2018.04.021

Substance Abuse and Mental Health Services Administration (SAMHSA). (2017). *National survey on Drug Use and Health, 2016*. Key Substance Use and Mental Health Indicators in the United States: Results from the 2016 National Survey on Drug Use and Health | CBHSQ Data

Substance Abuse and Mental Health Services Administration (SAMHSA). (2024a). *Behavioral health by race and ethnicity: Results from the 2021–2023 national surveys on drug use and health* (SAMHSA Publication No. PEP24-07-022). Center for Behavioral Health Statistics and Quality, Substance Abuse and Mental Health Services Administration. Behavioral Health by Race and Ethnicity: Results from the 2021-2023 National Surveys on Drug Use and Health

Substance Abuse and Mental Health Services Administration (SAMHSA). (2024b). *Key substance use and mental health indicators in the United States: Results from the 2023 national survey on drug use and health* (HHS Publication No. PEP24-07-021, NSDUH Series H-59). Center for Behavioral Health Statistics and Quality, Substance Abuse and Mental Health Services Administration. www.samhsa.gov/data/report/2023-nsduh-annual-national-report

Tadros, A., Layman, S. M., Davis, S.M., Davidov, D.M., & Cimino, S. (2015). Emergency visits for prescription opioid poisonings. *The Journal of Emergency Medicine*, 49(6), 871–877. https://doi.org/10.1016/j.jemermed.2015.06.035

Tanz, L.J., Dinwiddie, A.T., Mattson, C.L., O'Donnell, J., & Davis, N.L. (2022). Drug overdose deaths among persons aged 10–19 years—United States, July 2019–December 2021. *Morbidity and Mortality Weekly Report*, 71, 1576–1582. http://dx.doi.org/10.15585/mmwr.mm7150a2

Tanz, L.J., Stewart, A., Gladden, R.M., Ko, J.Y., Owens, L., & O'Donnell, J. (2024). Detection of illegally manufactured fentanyls and carfentanil in drug overdose deaths – United States, 2021–2024. *MMWR. Morbidity and Mortality Weekly Report*, 73(48), 1099–1105. https://doi.org/10.15585/mmwr.mm7348a2

Tolomeo, S., Gray, K., Steele, J.D. & Baldacchino, A. (2016). Multifaceted impairments in impulsivity and brain structure abnormalities in opioid dependence and abstinence. *Psychological Medicine*, 46(13), 2841–2853. https://doi.org/10.1017/S0033291716001513

Tracy, N. (2025). *What is Heroin? Information about Heroin.* HealthyPlace. www.google.com/search?q=https://www.healthyplace.com/addiction/heroin/what-is-heroin-information-about-heroin

United Nations Office on Drugs and Crime. (2023a). *World Drug Report 2023.* www.unodc.org/unodc/en/data-and-analysis/world-drug-report-2023.html

United Nations Office on Drugs and Crime (UNODC). (2023b). *Online world drug report 2023 – Latest data and trend analysis.* www.unodc.org/unodc/en/data-and-analysis/wdr-2023-online-segment.html

United States Department of Health and Human Services (USDHHS), Office of the Surgeon General. (2018). *Facing addiction in America: The surgeon general's spotlight on opioids.* HHS. Facing Addiction in America: The Surgeon General's Spotlight on Opioids.

United States Department of Health & Human Services. (2022). National opioids crisis: health and resources- *What are opioids?* www.hhs.gov/opioids/prevention/index.html

United States Department of Justice. (2008, September 29). *Biopharmaceutical company, Cephalon, to pay $425 million & enter plea to resolve allegations of off-label marketing* [Press release No. 08-860]. www.justice.gov/archive/opa/pr/2008/September/08-civ-860.html

United States (U.S.) Department of Justice (DOJ). (2023). Practitioners' Manual: An informational outline of the Controlled Substances Act. Drug Enforcement Administration. Practitioner's Manual

United States Department of Labor Statistics. (2023). *Occupational Employment and Wages.* Division of Occupational Employment and Wage Statistics. www.bls.gov/oes/2023/may/oes211023.htm#nat

United States Food and Drug Administration. (n.d.). *Timeline of selected FDA activities and significant events addressing substance use and overdose prevention.* Retrieved July 15, 2025, from www.fda.gov/drugs/food-and-drug-administration-overdose-prevention-framework/timeline-selected-fda-activities-and-significant-events-addressing-substance-use-and-overdose

Vanderplasschen, W., Wolf, J., Rapp, R.C., & Broekaert, E. (2007). Effectiveness of different models of case management for substance-abusing populations. *Journal of Psychoactive Drugs*, 39(1), 81–95. https://doi.org/10.1080/02791072.2007.10399867

Venner, K.L., Donovan, D.M., Campbell, A.N.C., Wendt, D.C., Rieckmann, T., Radin, S.M., Momper, S.L., & Rosa, C.L. (2018). Future directions for medication assisted treatment for opioid use disorder with American Indian/Alaska Natives. *Addictive Behaviors*, 86, 111–117. https://doi.org/10.1016/j.addbeh.2018.05.017

Villarosa, L. (2019, August 14). Myths about physical racial differences were used to justify slavery—And are still believed by doctors today. *The New York Times.* www.proquest.com/newspapers/myths-about-physical-racial-differences-were-used/docview/2851364998/se-2?accountid=10639

Visconti, A.J., Santos, G.M., Lemos, N.P., Burke, C., & Coffin, P.O. (2015). Opioid overdose deaths in the city and county of San Francisco: Prevalence, distribution, and disparities. *Journal of Urban Health*, 92(4), 758–772. https://doi.org/10.1007/s11524-015-9967-y

Wakaizumi, K., Vigotsky, A.D., Jabakhanji, R., Abdallah, M., Barroso, J., Schnitzer, T.J., Apkarian, A.V., & Baliki, M.N. (2021). Psychosocial, functional, and emotional correlates of long-term opioid use in patients with chronic back pain: A cross-sectional Case–Control study. *Pain and Therapy*, 10(1), 691–709. https://doi.org/10.1007/s40122-021-00257-w

Weerasinghe, I., Jimenez, Y., & Wilson, B. (2020). *Between the lines: Understanding our country's racialized response to the opioid overdose Epidemic.* The Center for Law and Social Policy.

Between the Lines: Understanding Our Country's Racialized Response to the Opioid Overdose Epidemic | CLASP.

Wilcox, H.C., Conner, K.R., & Caine, E.D. (2004). Association of alcohol and drug use disorders and completed suicide: An empirical review of cohort studies. *Drug and Alcohol Dependence*, 76, S11–S19. https://doi.org/10.1016/j.drugalcdep.2004.08.003

Williams, J.R., Cole, V., Girdler, S., & Cromeens, M.G. (2020) Exploring stress, cognitive, and affective mechanisms of the relationship between interpersonal trauma and opioid misuse. *PLoS One*, 15(5), e0233185. https://doi.org/10.1371/journal.pone.0233185

Wilson, J.D., Sumetsky, N.M., Coulter, R.W.S., Liebschutz, J., Miller, E., & Mair, C.F. (2020). Opioid-related disparities in sexual minority youth, 2017. *Journal of Addiction Medicine*, 14(6), 475–479. https://doi.org/10.1097/ADM.0000000000000628

Winkelman, T., Chang, V.W., & Binswanger, I.A. (2018). Health, polysubstance use, and criminal justice involvement among adults with varying levels of opioid use. *JAMA Network Open*, 1(3), e180558. https://doi.org/10.1001/jamanetworkopen.2018.0558

World Health Organization (WHO). (2009). Guidelines for the psychosocially assisted Pharmacological Treatment of Opioid Dependence. 9789241547543_eng.pdf

World Health Organization (WHO). (2025). *Importance of ICD*. www.who.int/standards/classificati ons/frequently-asked-questions/importance-of-icd

Zaller, N., McKenzie, M., Friedmann, P.D., Green, T.C., McGowan, S., & Rich, J.D. (2013). Initiation of buprenorphine during incarceration and retention in treatment upon release. *Journal of Substance Abuse Treatment*, 45(2), 222–226. https://doi.org/10.1016/j.jsat.2013.02.005

Zatti, C., Rosa, V., Barros, A., Valdivia, L., Calegaro, V.C., Freitas, L.H., Ceresér, K.M.M., Rocha, N.S.d., Bastos, A.G., & Schuch, F.B. (2017). Childhood trauma and suicide attempt: A meta-analysis of longitudinal studies from the last decade. *Psychiatry Research*, 256, 353–358. https://doi.org/10.1016/j.psychres.2017.06.082

Zedler, B.K., Saunders, W.B., Joyce, A.R., Vick, C.C., & Murrelle, E.L. (2018). Validation of a screening risk index for serious prescription opioid-induced respiratory depression or overdose in a US commercial health plan claims database. *Pain Medicine (Malden, MA)*, 19(1), 68–78. https://doi.org/10.1093/pm/pnx009

15
TOWARD AN EPIDEMIOLOGICAL APPROACH TO STUDY VIOLENCE AND CRIME

Introduction

Violence and crime are aspects of the human experience that are unlikely to go away since they have existed since the beginning of time. They are global behaviors that directly and indirectly impact the lives of millions of people each year. Criminal justice experts, criminologists, and public health researchers contend that these behaviors are matters of national as well as global importance since they often have a "rippling" effect when they spread from individuals, families, communities, and societies. It is incumbent on the entire society to properly address violence and crime as quickly as possible lest the number of victims and offenders will increase (Akers & Sellers, 2005). Research reveals that in the aftermath of assaultive violence when offenders are apprehended and processed by the justice system, victims often experience a host of physical, emotional, as well as psychological injuries that are concerning given it implicates the public health system. While the justice system is responsible for capturing, arresting, and processing offenders, the public health system must treat the physical and psychological injuries sustained by victims that can either endure for the short or long term (Rosenberg & Fenley, 1991). Studies show that when victims of violence and crime are not properly treated, they can easily become the byproducts of the "cycle of violence" and engage in similar predatory behavior against others. Because of its prevalence, devastation, and economic toll on the global level, researchers in the social sciences, as well as natural sciences, are committed to engaging in research investigations to find viable solutions regarding the etiology of violence and crime, and more specifically, what can be done to prevent such threatening behaviors from reoccurring and causing serious health consequences to the population. This concern has sparked the need for studies that focus on why people commit crime and violence, the effect of the law on criminal behavior, prevention, and the punishment offenders receive for their law violations. Violence and crime experts argue that the study of these and other areas has led to the development of academic disciplines such as criminal justice, criminology, and public health (Dantzker, 1998; Schneider, 2020).

DOI: 10.4324/9781003373001-15

Criminal Justice

Because of increasing crime problems that emerged in the late 1960s, the *American Bar Foundation* and other research projects engaged in collaborative efforts that led to developments that were designed to acquire a better understanding of the role and operations of police, courts, and corrections in society. This resulted in the creation of academic programs designed to study the criminal justice system (Remington, 1990). Criminal justice historians cite the *Law Enforcement Assistance Administration (LEAA)* funding by *the Omnibus Crime Control Act of 1968* as a primary reason why criminal justice was able to create its separate identity from its roots in sociology and public administration (Lanier, 2010). Some scholars contend that criminal justice as an academic discipline is an interdisciplinary science that uses the scientific method to focus on the operations of police, courts, corrections, and the application of the law and how they work to dispense justice (Champion, 1997). Others argue that "criminal justice examines crime control policies and the criminal justice system and its components" (Kraska & Neuman, 2012, p. 6). Perhaps a better definition is provided by Rush (2003, p. 95) where he provided criminal justice pertains to crime prevention, control, reduction, or the enforcement of criminal law that includes police efforts (to prevent, control, or reduce crime by apprehending offenders), court activities with jurisdiction over criminals and other agencies (such as prosecutorial authority and defender services); along with correctional activities (such as institutional, probation and parole) designed to prevent, control, or reduce crime, but also programs related to preventing and reducing juvenile delinquency, and drug addiction. Criminal justice research disproportionately asks applied questions. It is often focused on the agencies of social control that are in place to ensure that citizens confirm their behaviors to the requirements of the law and maintain social order. Justice experts are also concerned with whether agencies (e.g., police, court, corrections) are dispensing justice as required by the law and its consequences on society (Siegel, 1998).

Criminology

Criminology dates back to the 18th century. Experts contend that positivistic criminology emerged in the 19th century and quickly overshadowed classical criminology (after 100 years of dominance) largely because of advances in science. Positivism advanced the notion that crime was caused by biological, psychological, and environmental factors that could be measured and rigorously studied (Williams & McShane, 1999). It is important to note that classical criminology never disappeared, it remained in the backdrop. However, because of social, political, and economic changes that occurred in the U.S., it experienced a resurgence in the 1970s, but was called, choice theory (Williams & McShane, 1999). Criminology is a multidisciplinary approach that focuses on the study of crime causation, how crime is defined, patterns, and trends as well as how society reacts and responds to crime (Kraska & Neuman, 2012). Criminology is used as a framework to inform policies designed to reduce and prevent violence and crime (Schram & Tibbetts, 2014). Criminology relies on the scientific method to study the nature, extent, and control of criminal behavior. While some contend that criminal justice and criminology have stark differences, others contend that their commonalities and overlaps outweigh their differences. Kraska (2006) reported the criminal justice and criminological literature is replete with studies conducted by criminologists that are focused on practical and not abstract crime control matters. Comparatively, there is a large body of theoretical research conducted on crime control and other criminal justice topics (Kraska & Neuman, 2012).

Public Health

Public health is primarily concerned with the health status of a population by addressing diseases and other emerging problems (e.g., violence and crime) that present negative health consequences. Experts contend that public health is focused on preventing and eradicating diseases that impact communities (Lanier, 2010). Unlike medical care that is individualized to patients, public health is utilitarian, in that, it concentrates on providing the maximum benefit to the greatest number of people in each population, but its goal of prevention is pivotal to its mission (Krug et al., 2002). Public health is also interdisciplinary and relies on the scientific method to perform research that investigates why disease, violence, and crime occur and what are the best ways to prevent them. Public health officials are also challenged with addressing social norms and attitudes of people who have normalized violence and crime as acceptable aspects of life. Consequently, they must also educate the public to reject such contentions (Rosenberg & Mercy, 1991). Public health approaches enlist and draw on knowledge from disciplines that include professionals in medicine, epidemiology, criminal justice, criminology, psychology, social work, sociology, economics, education, and others to work together to understand causes and solutions (Rosenberg & Fenley, 1991). Through effective collaborations, these disciplines have had to agree on definitions and build compatible datasets (Rosenberg & Fenley, 1991, p. 11). As a result, public health has been able to successfully respond to challenges such as diseases, violence, crime, illnesses, and injuries with devastating consequences for millions of people worldwide (Krug et al., 2002). Health experts attribute public health effectiveness to its commitment to join forces with other disciplines and professionals by forming collaborative partnerships that reach beyond public health exclusively and rely on other sectors (e.g., social services, justice and policy, community-based services, education, and other stakeholders who are better able to address issues and areas that are not medical) to address the many social determinants that influence and impact diseases, violence, and crime. Particularly, those experts in the areas of social services, justice and policy, and education. In fact, those who advocate the public health approach, contend that each stakeholder in disease, violence, and crime prevention must be aware that they have an equally important role to play since each contribution has the potential to reduce disease, violence, and crime. Public health's main contribution has been getting society to recognize that disease, violence, and crime are problems that transcend criminal justice and enter the realm of public health (Rosenberg & Fenley, 1991).

Epidemiology and Epidemiological Techniques

Epidemiology is one of the five branches of public health that studies the determinants of disease frequency and distribution in human populations (Schneider, 2020). Some contend that epidemiology is focused on methodology with particular emphasis on the study of variables, vectors, and factors that influence the spread of disease and violence. Epidemiologists approach violence and crime as though they are diseases which requires that they first define the behavior to ensure that it can be counted as a disease (Schneider, 2020). The logic of using epidemiological approaches to combat violence is that epidemiologists use public health strategies as part of their interventions on violence and crime, the same way it would treat diseases that threaten public health. When it comes to defining a disease (or violence/crime) to study, epidemiologists often refer to the matter as a health outcome. Like criminal justice experts and criminologists who focus on the nature and extent of crime, epidemiologists study the *frequency* and *distribution* of acts of assaultive violence or injuries related to violence with the expectation that they will develop interventions to prevent negative health outcomes associated with the behavior by merging epidemiological and criminal justice theory, methodologies, and practices (Schneider, 2020; Lanier, 2010). When they measure the *frequency* of violence and crime, they count the number of known cases in relation to the size of the population under investigation which yields a rate. When determining the rate, the denominator is the population or community at risk. For example, what is the impact of a new deadly illegal drug that has infected an impoverished community? An epidemiologist could calculate it by dividing the number of cases by the number of drug users in the neighborhood, but not the total population of the city (Schneider, 2020).

Health experts contend that epidemiologists are concerned with two types of frequency measures: *incidence rates* and *prevalence rates*. First, *incidence rates* include the number of new cases of violence in a particular or defined population over a specified timeframe. This can be acquired from the number of cases that are reported to police. Health experts also postulate that these rates help identify causes of violence. Second, the other frequency measure is *prevalence rates* which is defined as the total number of cases that exist in a defined population at one point in time (Schneider, 2020). This information can be measured by using a survey instrument. Scholars report that there is an overlap between *incidence* and *prevalence*, but it is contingent on how long people are affected by violence. For example, if a certain form of assaultive violence kills victims, or if they recover, the incidence can be high, but its prevalence can be low (Schneider, 2020).

Epidemiological techniques and methods are designed and used to study health problems at the population level (Dufort & Infante-Rivard, 1998; Rothman, 1986). These methods are used to address injury etiology which allows for an understanding of causal, as well as risk factors associated with diseases, violence, and crime. Experts contend that some of the most frequently used designs in population-based studies include *experimental studies, quasi-experimental designs, observational studies, analytical studies, and descriptive studies.* As a rule, the question that the researcher seeks to address always determines the methodology to use in the investigation (Dufort & Infante-Rivard, 1998; Maxfield & Babbie, 2008; Anderson, 2022). Epidemiologists use *experiments* to determine cause and effect, but before this can occur, a researcher must randomly select a population of victims or offenders (some assigned to a treatment group and others to a control group). The treatment group receives a treatment or independent variable, also known as the intervention, while the other group receives a placebo (lacking any known medicinal or curative value) for comparison purposes. *Quasi-experimental designs* are often used when *randomization* of selection to either the experimental or control group is not available. When this occurs, researchers typically select one group and based on the characteristics it contains, use matching to select a comparison group. If this is not achieved, the experiment is considered *contaminated* before the study begins. *Observational studies* are used when the researcher goes into the social environment where the study is being conducted and makes observations of the setting, people, behavior, lifestyles, and culture to gain a better understanding of the behavior from the perspective of the subjects. While there, they often interview subjects of their investigation by getting the information directly from the words of subjects. *Analytical studies* are those designed to measure the association between exposure and a disease, violence, or crime by gathering data collected from people (e.g., *victims/offenders*). In these investigations, the instrument is a survey or questionnaire that provides primary data collected in official statistics or aggregated data compilations. However, some other types of analytical epidemiology research designs include *cross-sectional studies*, *case–control studies*, *cohort studies*, and *controlled clinical trials*. It also relies on hypothesis testing of independent variables (e.g., causal factors) and dependent variables (e.g., violence, crime, diseases) to determine causation. *Descriptive studies* can be taken from observations made to describe or characterize the distribution of a disease or violence/ crime that is experienced by a group of people in a population. These studies provide significant data that reveal which people are impacted, the social setting or place where the incidents occurred, the time that these actions were reported to have occurred, and what consequences these behaviors have on the population (Schneider, 2020).

Epidemiological Data and Other Types of Epidemiological Research Designs

Epidemiologists use *primary* and *secondary* data when conducting their studies. *Primary data* do not exist until they are collected by a researcher who has a specific purpose (Schneider, 2020). These data are often gathered using an instrument such as a survey or interview which requires a researcher to rely on a respondent to provide information after asking questions that are designed to measure a particular area. For example, an epidemiologist could use a survey to ask residents if illegal drugs are a problem in their neighborhood. The information that they provide is considered primary data that did not exist prior to the epidemiologist asking the question. Research experts contend that collecting primary data can be time-consuming depending on the number of respondents surveyed or interviewed (Maxfield & Babbie, 2011). If an epidemiologist surveyed ten people in an investigation, this would not be considered challenging. However, if she engaged in a more ambitious study designed to survey 500 subjects in the investigation, this would place a greater demand on the researcher's time compared with the first example. If the former is conducted, the researcher could be at the mercy of respondents if data are collected using a mail survey. If the latter occurs, there may be logistical problems that have to be sorted between the researcher and the interviewees such as meeting times and locations that correspond with everyone's schedule (Maxfield & Babbie, 2011). Conversely, *secondary data* are existing information that was collected by someone else, an organization, or an agency to answer research questions. These data are typically statistics, books, articles, manuscripts, or any material gathered by others. However, they are used by other researchers and cited as part of the literature (Maxfield & Babbie, 2011). *Secondary data* are used to address a different set of research questions. Returning to the example of the epidemiologist who collected primary data by asking residents questions related to illegal drugs in their neighborhood, she can also use secondary data about the same neighborhood by reviewing police crime statistics, especially drug-related arrests, birth and death certificates, mortality rates for the areas as well as several other official records such as population census reports. Some other types of analytical epidemiology research designs include *cross-sectional studies, case–control studies, cohort studies, and controlled clinical trials.*

Cross-Sectional Studies

Epidemiologists use *cross-sectional* or nonexperimental research studies to measure the association of disease, injuries, or assaultive violence with variables of interest. Experts often use these designs to isolate the attitudes, behaviors, and characteristics of subjects or respondents at a single point in time (Bachman & Schutt, 2020). When these studies are used, the method allows for a singular measurement in time without knowing if changes will occur in the future. Some refer to this method as offering a snapshot in time. Stated differently, epidemiological cross-sectional research measures the prevalence of health outcomes or determinants of health, or both, in a population at one point in time or over a short period. Cross-sectional studies are interesting since they can be conducted by surveying a group of community residents about the prevalence of diseases, injuries, violence, and community factors that they believe influence health outcomes (Wang & Cheng, 2020; Rennison & Hart, 2019).

Case–Control Studies

Case–control studies are observational studies that examine factors associated with diseases or outcomes. These studies compare two groups of interest (or patients) to determine if there is a connection between a health outcome and exposure (Tenny et al., 2023). They also require looking back retrospectively to measure how frequently the exposure to a risk factor is present in both groups to measure the relationship between risk factors and the disease (Tenny et al., 2023). Epidemiologists use the *case–control* method to determine if being exposed to a determinant is associated with an outcome such as a disease, injury, or violence. The approach requires that the researcher identifies the cases such as a group known to have the variable of interests which for the epidemiologist is the disease, injury, or violence and the controls (a group known to be free of the outcome). After the two groups are selected, the researcher engages in a retrospective act of looking back in time to investigate which subjects in each group were exposed and compare the frequency of the exposure in the case group to the control group. If the exposure is observed more often in the cases, rather than the control, one can hypothesize that the exposure is linked to the outcome of interest (Tenny et al., 2023; Lewallen & Courtright, 1998).

Cohort Studies

In *cohort studies* or longitudinal designs, epidemiologists observe a group of people who share similar characteristics who have been exposed to a variable or condition such as disease, injury, or assaultive violence for an extended period of time to measure changes in their health outcome. The logic of the cohort study is that it is representative of a defined subpopulation which provides several advantages (Dantzker et al., 2018). According to Szklo (1998), its advantages include allowing the estimation of distribution and prevalence rates of relevant variables to the targeted population, an examination of risk factor outcomes that are distributed at different periods in a longitudinal examination of the group that can be used for comparative purposes, and other variables are often revealed that go beyond what was believed in the stated research hypothesis.

Controlled Clinical Trials

Controlled clinical trials are also referred to as *randomized controlled trials* used by epidemiologists to determine if treatment or an intervention has a causal effect on health outcomes. Health experts view them as the most rigorous methods to determine whether a causal relationship exists between treatment and outcome since they use *randomized* selection to intervention groups, patients should not know what intervention was given to them until the study is finished, and all intervention groups are treated the same except for the intervention, patients are analyzed within the group to which they are placed, and the analysis must be focused on estimating the size of the difference in predefined outcomes between the intervention groups (Sibbald & Roland, 1998). Studies show that epidemiologists consider them as the gold standard of clinical and epidemiological studies because they are rigorous, well-designed, and effective (Sibbald & Roland, 1998). They rely on the use of randomized selection to obtain equivalence among groups in a study. There can be no differences since it would contaminate the results. Controlled clinical trials also provide great control since people (e.g., patients) are randomly selected to either two or more treatment groups, followed over a predetermined amount of time. The technique is effective at producing evidence-based results to improve health outcomes and safety. Clinical trials can be used to investigate many questions such as whether a new treatment works, or what effect health education has on a targeted population (Sibbald & Roland, 1998).

Emergence of Criminal Justice, Criminology, and Public Health

Experts in criminal justice, criminology, and public health observe similarities in their areas of research (e.g., high-risk people, people with drug abuse histories), problem behavior (e.g., crime, violence, incarceration, health problems, prevention) as well as root causes of problems (i.e., poverty/unequal distribution of resources) they address. They are also aware that they are driven to promote and protect public safety. Because they overlap, researchers in criminal justice, criminology, and public health are beginning to see that their academic differences are becoming blurred, yet their theoretical and methodological connections remain elusive since research reveals that they lack integrative approaches (Akers & Lanier, 2009). Experts contend that to effectively study violence and crime, what is needed are the combined strategies that encompass those methods and statistics used by researchers in criminal justice, criminology, and public health. Scholars contend that when transdisciplinary thinking and approaches are conjoined, they provide a shared understanding of the problem under investigation. Thus, moving away from ideas and approaches that are discipline-specific to advancing the creation of new knowledge and a deeper understanding of real-life experiences (Ellington et al., 2022; Reingle et al., 2017; Lawlor et al., 2015; Miner-Romanoff & King, 2013). Those approaches that provide connections between epidemiological theories and models integrated with criminal justice and criminological tools tend to present a holistic strategy that better addresses violence and crime (Akers & Lanier, 2009).

Research reveals that criminal justice and criminology have played a dominant role for decades in providing scientific explanations for what causes violence and crime in the U.S., and what was thought at the time to be the most appropriate ways to address it. Studies on violence and crime are replete with theoretical arguments as well as methodological and statistical approaches used to isolate factors that cause violence and crime, and yearly efforts to measure their nature and extent and offer recommendations that guide public policy to control, deter, as well as prevent these behaviors from occurring. Despite criminal justice and criminology's best efforts, critics argue they tend to be more reactionary, rather than proactive or preventative, which serves to perpetuate more violence and crime (Rosenberg & Mercy, 1991). Consequently, they failed to attack many of the essential root sources. These same critics contend that what is noticeably missing from these efforts is the addition of epidemiology since the current criminal justice and criminological literature ignores and neglects its full inclusion in its analysis of the study of criminal behavior and preventative approaches (Akers & Lanier, 2009).

Crime and Public Health

Given the extent of violence and crime that occurs worldwide, they are known as both public health as well as global problems that bring negative health consequences to millions of people each year (Barcy, 2023). Experts at the *Centers for Disease Control and Prevention (CDC)* and *World Health Organization (WHO)* report that globally, crime impacts the quality of health found in communities, but it especially takes a greater toll on the physical and mental well-being of people who are disproportionately impacted by economic disparities and various forms of neighborhood deprivation, namely poverty (Matz et al., 2012). Research also supports the notion that one's mental health can invariably affect crime. For example, the criminal justice and criminological literature is saturated with studies that find people who suffer from mental health illnesses face a greater risk of being incarcerated since they are disproportionately stopped, arrested, taken into custody, and processed in the criminal justice system. These studies also find that many people with mental health problems who experience legal processing also have substance abuse issues (Hall et al., 2019). However, some public health researchers view this matter as not being caused by a singular explanation, but rather they conclude that this results from multiple determinant factors such as structural poverty, racism, substandard housing, stigma, history of trauma, co-occurring substance abuse, and mental health problems (Nishar et al., 2023). They further contend that mental illness is symptomatic of larger problems that proliferate in many communities, and it drives behaviors that often get a criminal justice, rather than public health response. Therefore, the lack of access to mental health services and resources often contributes to people with mental health issues becoming criminalized since they face a greater likelihood of engaging in behavior that often requires police attention (Hartford et al., 2007; Hall et al., 2019; Nishar et al., 2023).

The Intersection between Public Health and Criminology

Potter and Rosky (2013, p. 276), postulated that the intersection of public health and criminology is premised on preventing negative health outcomes. For example, public health's primary goals are to prevent and treat diseases and injuries caused by violence, while the primary goals in criminal justice/criminology are prevention and treatment where possible. This suggests that there is an overlap in their functions and purposes. Furthermore, they intersect because both fields have subdisciplines that are involved in the nuances of processes, structures, treatments, and outcomes (Potter & Rosky, 2013). A good example of their similarities can be demonstrated using a public health response. Since public health responses are concerned about disease prevention, at the *primary level*, it uses a combination of vaccination to immune the population from infectious diseases, but it takes other prevention measures such as engaging in educational campaigns on the need for healthy lifestyles and behavioral choices such as abstaining from alcohol, smoking, and drug use. Similar prevention approaches have been directed at all forms of assaultive violence. At the *secondary level*, public health prevention efforts have relied on epidemiological approaches to identify the root causes or sources of diseases as well as assaultive violence. Public health initiatives also use *tertiary-level* intervention when medical care is needed for chronic, acute, and infectious diseases and even for mental health treatment among people who have contracted communicable diseases (Potter & Rosky, 2013).

Where criminal justice is concerned, law enforcement has a public health duty of care to prevent crime by engaging in a host of prevention strategies aimed at crime problems. They also enforce safety regulations such as speed limits, seat belt regulations, drive under the influence (DUI) enforcement, and proper adherence to vehicle operations. These are efforts to prevent injuries. Another justice function that concerns public health occurs in adult incarcerations and juvenile justice since they overlap at the *primary, secondary, and tertiary* levels of public health. At the *primary* level, the need exists to control and prevent diseases from occurring in institutional corrections (e.g., jails, prisons, inpatient treatment facilities) since a showing of deliberate indifference to the health of inmates infringes on the *Eighth Amendment* prohibition against cruel and unusual punishment (Kosiak, 2022). Furthermore, because of health and safety concerns, correctional institutions prohibit the use of alcohol, smoking, and drugs. They have also passed the *Prison Rape Elimination Act of 2003* to prevent violence including sexual assaults against the inmate population, especially those who identify as members of the *LGBTQ+* community (Kosiak, 2022). At the *secondary* level, the criminal justice system has been remiss in adult as well as juvenile corrections since after offenders are incarcerated, they only provide supervision. However, at the *tertiary* level, the system is responsible for making sure that offenders, especially juveniles get the medical and psychological services they need given the state acts as guardians (Potter & Rosky, 2013).

Experts also contend that public health and criminology share common links to promoting environmentally sustainable societies. As such, they can use their similarities to enhance the safety and well-being of communities throughout society. When this occurs, it increases overall well-being and quality of life for everyone (Blaustein et al., 2018; Redo, 2017). Some feel that criminologists, unlike others, who have been called on for their crime expertise, must provide a framework for addressing issues of violence and crime and their control in a coordinated as well as systematic manner to impact the public with the results of their research. These efforts are needed to assist with creating research design, implementation, and evaluation of all projects devoted to local, community, societal, and global safety (Blaustein et al., 2018). Similarly, Macassa and McGrath (2024) report that there are five areas of intersection between public health and criminology that include social determinants, epidemiological criminology (EpiCrim), intervention and experimentation, prevention approaches, and sustainable development and safety.

Social Determinants of Health and Criminal Behavior

Criminal justice, criminology, and public health share commonalities in their focus, especially where research is concerned. Though they are interdisciplinary, they remain predominantly singular (Akers & Lanier, 2009). Scholars suggest that as more challenges emerge in society or globally regarding what causes violence and crime and how to better respond with prevention efforts to reduce the number of victims and offenders, and the overall toll they take on society, more collaborations are needed. Specifically, when it comes to addressing common problems, these disciplines should consider combining research efforts with other academic disciplines such as social work, psychology, psychiatry, and law (Potter & Akers, 2010; Akers et al., 2013). Moreover, some criminal justice experts, criminologists, and other social scientists have long pointed to social determinants such as race and ethnicity, classes differences, gender, and political as well as economic factors as having an impact on violence, crime, and health disparities (Oliver & Hilgenberg, 2006). Therefore, health experts contend that collaboration is necessary given that violence and crime tend to morph by touching the lives of many people in a community (e.g., victims, offenders, witnesses, neighbors), and those in the broader society since they can be vicariously impacted. It is also important to note that violence and crime also impact other social determinants that affect the health status of people in a community (Akers et al., 2013).

Health researchers posit that social determinants of health conditions cannot be ignored since they include factors that people often have no control over such as where they are born, grow up, live, and more broadly, the economic systems, structures, social situations, settings, social norms, and political systems that shape the conditions of their lives. As such, some health experts argue that they are the root causes of violence and crime (Newburn, 2016; Caruso, 2017; Armstead et al., 2021). To that extent, they identify health inequities and disparities as social determinants that also contribute to violence and crime. They recommend that researchers consider factors such as poverty, socioeconomic status, abuse and domestic violence, housing, mental illnesses, education, the environment, access to health care as social determinants when making efforts to prevent violence and crime and improve public safety (Caruso, 2017). Where research is concerned, this requires that criminal justice, criminology, and public health studies incorporate a social determinant perspective to better understand violence and crime. This requires that collaborative efforts examine social inequalities and how unequal distributions of resources and access to healthcare impact crime (Newburn, 2016). An understanding of inequalities must also be used when considering prevention and intervention programs that address violence, crime, and health disparities (Caruso, 2017).

Epidemiological Criminology (EpiCrim)

Experts define EpiCrim as an emerging field of study that combines epidemiology and criminology to better understand the root causes of crime. According to Lanier (2010), EpiCrim emerged because of factors such as globalization, the increased number of crime- and health-related concerns that have crossed boarders, and the need for academic disciplines to engage in theoretical integration to seek viable solutions (Barak, 1998). It also considers health inequities as a major contributing factor to violence and criminal behavior (Akers & Lanier, 2009; Akers et al., 2013; Potter & Akers, 2013). To that end, EpiCrim relies on the use of public health approaches, along with traditional criminal justice, criminological approaches, and theories to examine causes of violence and crime and other behaviors that are addressed by the criminal justice system. To many scholars, EpiCrim highlights the need for formulating a theoretical basis for interventions that blend academic disciplines (Lanier, 2010). Potter and Akers (2013), provide that EpiCrim must be viewed as an integration of theories, methods, and technologies taken from public health, criminal justice, and criminology and infused into an interdisciplinary framework of epidemiology and criminology.

By moving toward an EpiCrim, researchers can form and facilitate interdisciplinary research teams with criminal justice/criminology and public health officials (e.g., criminologists and epidemiologists) that can better understand crime and health and its intersectionality by using their theories, methods, and approaches (Macassa & McGrath, 2024). Experts citing the commonalities between epidemiology and criminology contend that prevention efforts can easily be combined since they are not dissimilar. They argue that the former uses public health strategies aimed at *primary*, *secondary*, and *tertiary prevention*, while the latter engages in *primary* and *secondary* prevention efforts often referred to as opportunity reduction theories of crime (Akers & Lanier, 2009). In moving beyond criminal justice/criminology, or public health alone, researchers can join forces and collaborate when studying violence and crime. In doing so, they come to rely on transdisciplinary efforts that are more robust since they will offer more information and understanding about determinant factors that contribute to both criminal and health risks (e.g., *social, economic, legal, geospatial, and environmental*) (Potter & Akers, 2013). Researchers who advocate for an EpiCrim framework (*e.g., biological, psychological, economic, and social factors*) argue that crime, health, and disease often converge since they have similar root sources. Regarding crime prevention, EpiCrim allows researchers to develop evidence-based interventions to reduce and prevent violence and crime by combining shared theories, methods, and approaches. The approach also reveals that health determinants of violence and crime are like those that produce poor health outcomes (Akers & Lanier, 2009).

Intervention and Experimentation

Scholars such as Akers et al. (2013) and others argue that the use of interventions and experiments is important to the link between criminology and public health since they both focus on investigating the etiology of violence and crime through understanding its determinants including health inequities, as well as identifying interventions, to use in efforts to reduce violence and crime (Macassa & McGrath, 2024). While many public health studies are complex and need preventative actions on several levels (such as environmental, biological, socioeconomic) to have a positive effect on research including violence and health, studies show that they often lack multilevel population-level intervention evidence from experimental designs. Ridgeway (2019), contended that to improve our understanding of violence, crime, and the criminal justice system, criminologists are expanding their research efforts to incorporate statistical methods that include the use of experiments. More specifically, he discussed studies where criminologists used daylight saving time to measure racial bias and natural disasters to measure the effect of displacement and relocation on desistance from violence and crime. Similarly, Andersen and Hyatt (2020), argued to develop more robust findings regarding what is more effective at reducing violence and crime, criminal justice experts, criminologists, and public health researchers must include interventions and experiments in their methodologies. Moreover, by integrating approaches from EpiCrim, they may strengthen their theoretical accuracy and advancement in understanding the etiology that leads to violence and crime, along with prevention measures to reduce the negative health consequences, including death (Akers & Lanier, 2009; Akers et al., 2013; Macassa & McGrath, 2024).

The Public Health Approach to Crime Prevention

Because criminological and public health researchers have identified similar determinants in the etiology of violence and crime as well as ill health, many experts suggest that they can be complementary in efforts toward prevention (Cereda et al., 2018). For decades, criminal justice approaches faced criticisms for being too reactive, punitive, and contributing to increases in the number of victims and offenders given its historically high recidivism rates. Consequently, experts are calling for public health approaches that focus on treating victims and offenders to prevent the continuation of behaviors that affect the overall health of a community. Public health strategies use multilayered approaches that rely on *primary prevention* (strategies designed to stop violence, crime, and disease before they occur); *secondary prevention* (strategies that focus on immediate interventions on violence, crime, or disease before they manifest); and *tertiary prevention* (strategies that focus on long-term care, and treatment such as rehabilitation and reintegration to reduce the long-term effect of trauma and violence before injuries or diseases become more severe) given the status of violence and crime (Battams et al., 2021; Krug et al., 2002; Schneider, 2020). While these efforts address social determinants of violence and crime, they also focus on disparities of health which are linked to environmental, social, and economic factors. They examine the physical and psychological well-being of populations throughout the U.S. and offer the best approaches to use to promote health outcomes for everyone in the social structure given the issues it presents to many living in poverty such as discrimination, racism, and income inequality that challenges access to adequate and proper healthcare. By employing its ecological model, public health officials assert that there is no single factor that explains why people act in a violent manner, but rather violence is caused by the interplay of many determinant factors. Therefore, public health approaches consider the individual, relationship, community, cultural, and societal factors and the role they play in contributing to violence, crime, and health disparities (Krug et al., 2002; Rotter & Compton, 2022). Public health officials also contend that this approach helps address health disparities among people by identifying the need to engage in intersectional collaboration with community organizations, social service groups, residents, as well as criminal justice officials. In fact, some experts suggest that criminal justice approaches can be used in conjunction with public health-specific prevention strategies (Gebo, 2016).

Sustainable Development and Safety

Since criminologists, epidemiologists, public authorities, and civil society are concerned about community safety, its overall health well-being, and inequities in health and quality of life, experts argue that they should join forces to transform the world by creating sustainable development goals and safety for each community and the boarder society (Fortune et al., 2018; Macassa & McGrath, 2024). They warn that sustainable development is threatened when people's safety and health are challenged by acts such as violence, crime, disease, and other adverse conditions that impact a community or population's health. Some experts argue that because of its large scope, health promotion designs can offer benefits to health and sustainable development, but they caution the work is considerable given that multisectoral tools are needed locally, nationally, and globally to address the vast problems including those that are health-related (Fortune et al., 2018, p. 622). These conditions must be removed and replaced with operational conditions (Nilson, 2018). Some studies report that sustainable development brings safety and provides for health promotion that empowers people with the control that is necessary to improve their health status since it alters the economic, environmental, institutional, and social contexts where health decisions are made (Fortune et al., 2018, p. 621; Nilson, 2018). Literature reveals that in the past decades, several efforts have been made to advance health promotion that has relied on strategies such as bringing together multilevel interventions to promote healthy environments, reorienting health services, and making healthy choices by enlisting community residents, influencing public policy initiatives, and helping at-risk people control social determinants that impact their behavior (Edington et al., 2016; Whitelaw et al., 2001).

A recent example by the *United Nations* is instructive in this regard since it created an agenda that has sustainable goals designed to promote global peace among nations by providing access to justice, building effective, accountable, and inclusive institutions at every level. It is also committed to working toward reducing all forms of violence, death rates, trafficking in people and firearms, and other types of devastation that challenge human well-being, health, and safety (VanderWeele, 2019). Health researchers contend that the goals of sustainable development and safety should be embraced by criminologists, epidemiologists, and others in public health given their intersectionality, mutual interests, goals, methods, and priorities on matters such as violence, crime, health disparities, and its impact on society. Additionally, more data are needed on the impact of multisectoral collaborations focused on providing health services designed to promote equity, especially when generating current data on violence-related deaths, conflict-related deaths, and data that measure other forms of collective violence (Holfler et al., 2022; Fortune et al., 2018).

Epidemiological Surveillance

Epidemiological surveillance is the ongoing systematic collection, analysis, and interpretation of data that are disseminated in a timely fashion to those who are responsible for preventing and controlling disease and injuries linked to violence. To be effective, surveillance must provide quick access to valid data so that problems can be quickly identified and given an appropriate response with an effective intervention (Krug et al., 2002, p. 229). As such, surveillance systems are extremely important to officials in disease and violence prevention because they are tools that enable health officials and scholars concerned about the health of the population to quickly and routinely monitor what is occurring and know when interventions are needed and the effect of those interventions on the overall health status of the population or a particular segment that is affected by disease or assaultive violence. Chief among its uses are surveillance systems that collect valid data and empower policymakers by providing evidence-based results that allow timely and effective managerial decisions aimed at targeting resources and evaluating programs designed to promote healthy public health (Thacker & Stroup, 1998; Krug et al., 2002). Experts even contend that the success of fighting the battle against diseases and violence is contingent on the strength of good epidemiological surveillance systems (e.g., from public health, criminal justice, and criminology) that rely on scientific and factual databases that inform policymakers on how to use more effective intervention programs that provide instructions on the appropriate designs to implement. They also suggest that the results from interventions must be properly analyzed and disseminated when they prove effective (Krug et al., 2002). These efforts are most effective when surveillance systems draw on the combined efforts of multiple disciplinary approaches of criminal justice, criminological, and public health resources.

EpiCrim Surveillance: Combining the Best of Both Worlds

EpiCrim surveillance should be used to prevent violence and crime since it combines the best of both worlds: epidemiology and criminological approaches. Public health data from the WHO, *National Institutes of Health (NIH)*, and the *National Centers for Health Statistics (NCHS)* allow researchers to document the health status of the *population* and of important subgroups by identifying health disparities and health and healthcare services by race/ethnicity, socioeconomic status, region, and other population characteristics; describing experiences with the healthcare system; monitoring trends in health status and healthcare delivery; identifying health problems; supporting biomedical and health services research; providing data for making change in public policies and programs; and evaluating the impact of health policies and program. The *NCHS* plays a critical role in the nation's public health infrastructure and provides key surveillance information that helps to identify and address critical health problems (Anderson, 2022). Since EpiCrim surveillance relies on data from public health and criminal justice/criminology to monitor crime trends, it can also track geographic locations, examining crime patterns that are distributed unequally throughout the population regarding socioeconomic status and the demographical characteristics of offenders and victims of crime and violence since the U.S. *Census Bureau* is also involved in collecting victimization data. These data are collected by the *Federal Bureau of Investigation*s' Uniform Crime Reports (UCR), and the *National Incident-Based Reporting System* (NIBRS) which relies on annual police data that are collected from over 19,000 participating agencies nationwide and provided to the federal government.

Other criminal justice and criminological surveillance data come from the *National Crime Victimization Survey (NCVS)*. This data compilation also examines environmental factors and reveals where violence occurs which helps to determine crime patterns. Yet, another data surveillance comes from the *U.S. Bureau of Justice Statistics*. These data lend themselves to examining and analyzing crime "hotspots" by using spatial data and identifying risk or determinant factors (e.g., social and environmental including poverty, unemployment, lack of education, or gang presence) that are linked to crime and violence since they focus on individual and neighborhood characteristics (Chainey et al., 2008). These data reveal that crime is not random, nor organized in space and time, but rather, it is affected by social, political, economic, and lifestyle characteristics that leave patterns of action that increase one's likelihood of experiencing victimization (Ratcliffe, 2010). Moreover, EpiCrim surveillance and crime surveillance data lend themselves to "crime mapping" which allows researchers to identify incidences of violence and crime (e.g., gang-related homicides, intimate personal violence, child abuse, substance abuse, elder abuse), hotspots and areas of concentrated high crime from location information reported about criminal activity to detect spatial patterns. Crime mapping allows for an examination of spatial patterns and the role that geography (as a determinant) contributes to violence and crime. Some experts contend that crime mapping enables researchers to create specific violence-preventative programs for certain places (Ratcliffe, 2010). These data can be used to evaluate the effectiveness of crime and violence prevention efforts and interventions by tracking crime patterns to determine whether targeted areas are experiencing more reported cases of violence which can be measured by a time series analysis, or surveys that monitor before and after implementing an intervention (Macassa & McGrath, 2024). Some experts contend that EpiCrim surveillance data allow for spatial and temporal analysis, and risk factor identification (Macassa & McGrath, 2024).

Need for EpiCrim Studies

Assaultive Violence and EpiCrim

According to *WHO, NIH, Amnesty International, UCR, NCVS*, and other surveillance data, assaultive violence is a local, state, regional, national, and global problem that impacts millions of people worldwide. While it disproportionately occurs among people from impoverished backgrounds (even cross-culturally), it does not exclude people based on race/ethnicity, nor gender since its negative health consequences extend beyond those who are immediately involved in impacting others at the individual, relational, community, and societal levels (Krug et al., 2002). Assaultive violence is rooted in common determinant factors such as poverty, lack of education, culture, and societal norms to name a few. When assaultive violence occurs, it becomes obvious to those directly and vicariously involved that a criminal justice response is immediately needed to protect its victims. However, what is not always understood at the local, state, regional, or even international level is that assaultive violence transcends the justice system and also requires a public health response (Schweig, 2014; Gebo, 2022). Most people do not give thought to what happens in the aftermath of crime to address the negative health consequences that are a byproduct of assaultive violence, namely the need for hospitalization, medication, and treatment (e.g., gunshot wounds, debilitating injuries, and others). Moreover, the traumatic aspects that many victims experience after certain acts of violence (e.g., rape/sexual assault), often require psychological treatment and counseling post victimization for anxiety, depression, post-traumatic stress disorders (PTSDs), and others. Unfortunately, treatment may be required either for the short or long term. Because of this, studies on assaultive violence require researchers to partner with other scholars who can fuse their areas of expertise to engage in more effective and robust research that treats assaultive violence as a criminal justice/ criminological as well as a public health issue (Schweig, 2014; Gebo, 2022). Experts contend that EpiCrim approaches combine criminological and epidemiological strategies to study assaultive violence as both a crime and disease. In doing so, it uses mixed methodologies, theories, and prevention efforts that focus on creating better interventions for prevention since, the combined effort views violence as preventable.

Child Abuse and EpiCrim

Child abuse is a global problem (Krug et al., 2002) that is defined differently based on culture. Experts at *WHO* contend that any approach to measure or understand child abuse must consider the different standards and expectations of parenting used globally and how they extend beyond boarders and cultures which often makes it more challenging for researchers to find global consensus on which parental practices are abusive or neglectful (*National Research Council*, 1993; Krug et al., 2002). Moreover, the type of child abuse varies, but it often includes behavior that can be characterized as either fatal or non-fatal abuse. With the former, it ends in death, while the latter inflicts injuries. Health experts relying on the ecological model to examine global child abuse data report that within the context of the family, child abuse stems from several determinant factors including the characteristics of the abused child (e.g., *female or male*), his or her family (e.g., *violence in the home*), traits of the caregiver or perpetrator (e.g., *young, single, poor, unemployed, less educated*) status of the local community, as well as the social economics and cultural environments (e.g., *high levels of unemployment, concentrated or chronic poverty*) where the abuse occurs (Crouter, 1978; Belsky, 1980). As such, a lack of information regarding the magnitude of child abuse distorts studies and renders research in this area tentative at best. Researchers suggest that little is being done to investigate or properly evaluate the effectiveness of child abuse prevention intervention programs (MacMillian, 2000). Emphasis must be placed on *primary prevention approaches* that are designed to prevent child abuse from occurring by determining what causes the behavior. *Secondary prevention* strategies must be used to reduce the number of children at risk or those who have already been abused from being revictimized. *Tertiary prevention* efforts are also required to prevent offenders from engaging in additional abuse. Experts contend that the latter approach can address child abuse on the local, state, regional, and societal levels since the use of punishment should send a deterrence message (Quadara et al., 2015). Some approaches for improving parenting and family support interventions include engaging in massive education programs to inform parents about proper child development and providing parental skills with management skills needed to improve their children's behavior (Wolfe et al., 1988). Another vital intervention is to receive screening by healthcare professionals which often identifies, treats, and refers cases of abuse and neglect to the appropriate health authority. EpiCrim can be most effective given that this collaborative effort will allow for both sectors to bring a balance of prevention and reaction to behavioral changes in communities where child abuse is reported (Swensen et al., 2020).

Child Sexual Abuse and EpiCrim

Child sexual abuse for boys and girls is a global problem (Krug et al., 2002). Data from *Unicef* (2024), revealed an estimated one in every five women, and one in every ten men reported being sexually abused as a child. While the actual extent of this problem cannot be truly known, researchers postulate that the number of cases is always underreported given the nature of this crime, shame, guilt, and stigma that attaches, especially considering the gender dynamics: boys compared with girls (Choudhary et al., 2012). Despite this, health experts contend that child sexual abuse comes with serious short- and long-term negative health consequences. Recently, professionals in the social and biomedical sciences have started to reconceptualize child sexual abuse and other forms of violence as both a criminal justice as well as a public health issue (Mccartan & Prescott, 2020; Skvortsova, 2013). This integrative approach highlights the need to better understand determinant factors such as developmental, psychological, social, and behavioral histories that often influence one's decision to engage in serious violence. EpiCrim can be used to inform research, theory, and practice by allowing health officials, practitioners, researchers, and justice officials to work together by forming partnerships that rely on the use of *primary, secondary, and tertiary* prevention efforts when responding either before or in the aftermath of and preventing child sexual abuse and other forms of violence (Wattermaurer & Akers, 2014). Researchers in the *U.K.* revealed that collaborative efforts are emerging in the use of EpiCrim that addresses the theoretical gap in the field of child sexual abuse that existing theories fail to consider, especially with respect to the intersect between behavioral, individual, and societal factors and how they affect the health of society. By relying on EpiCrim and its combined methods in criminal justice and public health, researchers in the *U.K.* contend that it fills the theoretical gap and has directly isolated adverse childhood experiences that have resulted in the implementation of trauma-informed care, strengths-based approaches, desistance, and rehabilitation programs to be used by offenders and victims. These researchers also contend that EpiCrim uses a framework that is well suited to study the complexities of child sexual abuse, and it allows criminal justice officials to adequately communicate and educate the public about child sexual abuse which has contributed to the international growth in sexual prevention research and practices that have been ongoing for a decade (Mccartan & Prescott, 2020; Skortsova, 2013).

Sexual Assault and EpiCrim

Sexual assault is also a global issue that is under and unreported because of its personal nature. Of the many sources of data that are used to measure this crime, researchers contend that official statistics, especially police reports may be the most reliable data when determining the extent of the problem. Researchers who study sexual assaults are impaired by victims' willingness to report this information to the police. Experts argue the lack of trust people have toward police officials extends beyond boarders (Jewkes & Abrahams, 2002). As such, public health officials recommend and encourage the use of health data since sexual assault is also a public health issue. These data can lend themselves to comparative analysis over periods and can be used to compare incident rates of other countries. The example of researchers in *Africa* who used sexual assault data collected by police to examine the epidemiology of rape is instructive in this regard. Police data from *Africa* were compared with rape statistics in the *U.S.* Jewks and Abrahams (2002), examined sexual assault crime statistics and compared incidents of rape in the *U.S.* with incidents of rape in *Botswana*. The study revealed that in 1990, there were 102,255 reported cases of rape in the *U.S.*, or an annual rate of 80 per 100,000 females, while there were 132 incidents of rape per 100,000 women in *Botswana* in 1993. Beyond the use of police data, the *Department of Health* (1998), reported that rape data revealed the age of the victims, the rate of rape and attempted rapes, the age of victims as proportioned in the population, the gender distribution of rape victims (e.g., mostly girls over age 9). These data showed that teenagers face a higher risk of rape than others in the population.

   Martin (1999), research examined the epidemiology of rape in central and southern *Johannesburg, South Africa* using surveillance, but relied on medico-legal clinic data that revealed the characteristics of women who were rape survivors. Seventy-five percent were between the ages 17 to 34 years, 12.4% were over 35 years old. Most women were raped by a man of the same racial group. Moreover, 80% of the attacks were committed by a stranger. Rapes committed on girls 16 and younger were more common among men known to the victim. However, this was not true of rapes committed against older women. Gang rapes were also common. Research by Swart and colleagues (1999), which relied on rape surveillance data from district surgeons' offices from 1996 to 1998 reported that in *Johannesburg*, rapes were more likely to occur over weekends with an estimated 25% occurring on Saturdays. A third of them occurred between 6 p.m. and 10 p.m. A common method used by attackers was to engage in rapes in open spaces such as fields (31%) in the rapist's home (29%) and in the victim's home (44%). These data showed that a weapon was used 55% of the time. More specifically, a knife was used in 51% of all cases, and firearms were used 35% of the time. Many rapes occurred as women traveled to and from work.

Data collected by EpiCrim can be used globally to define and monitor acts of sexual assault. Since these data are gathered from several research sources (e.g., police records, UCR, NCVS, WHO, *Amnesty International*, hospital charts, medical examiners, population-based surveys, and others), they will reveal the who, what, when, where, and how these victimizations occur. This can be used in *primary prevention*. Researchers will be able to identify risk and protective factors that will lead them to where interventions are most needed. This is instrumental in providing *secondary prevention* to people in families and communities who are already identified as victims. After analyzing data and findings conducted after a needs assessment, community surveys, stakeholders' interviews, and others, researchers will work to design effective intervention programs so that the behavior will not reoccur or by offering support to victims and holding offenders accountable for their behavior. Those using the public health approach are hopeful that *secondary* and *tertiary* prevention efforts will reduce the behavior. After the programs are implemented and evaluated, they can be widely disseminated to help victims and offenders on the family, community, societal, and global levels (Schweig, 2014).

Intimate Partner Violence and EpiCrim

Intimate partner violence is a global issue that affects millions of people each year. In fact, forth eight population-based surveys conducted globally revealed that between 10% and 69% of women reported that they have been physically assaulted by an intimate male partner during some point in their lives. These numbers are even higher when considering abuse statistics reported by members of the *LGBTQ+* community (Chen et al., 2013). Intimate partner violence is rarely singular behavior, but rather it is linked to other forms of abuse. Accordingly, research reports that in intimate relationships, physical violence is often followed by psychological abuse and is present in one-third to over half of sexual abuse cases (Leibrich et al., 1995; Yoshihama & Sorenson, 1994). In a study conducted in *Japan* on the abuse women suffer at the hands of their partners, research found that among 613 women who had experienced abuse, 57% suffered physical, psychological, and sexual abuse. The study revealed that less than 10% only experienced physical abuse (Yoshihama & Sorenson, 1994). Some experts contend that various types of abuse tend to coexist in these relationships that transcend culture (Krug et al., 2002). In a similar investigation that occurred in *Monterrey, Mexico*, researchers reported that 52% of women who experienced physical assault were also sexually abused by their partner (Granados-Shiroma, 1996). In another study that examined intimate partner violence in *Leon, Nicaragua*, Ellsberg and colleagues (2000), found that 60% of women who were abused during the previous

12 months had also experienced an attack several times, and 20% had experienced other severe violence an estimated six or more times. Specifically, 70% of the women in the study reported experiencing severe abuse (Ellsberg et al., 1999). In *London, England,* and the *U.S.*, surveys conducted in 1996 reported that women revealed the average number of physical assaults during the previous year who were still suffering abuse was seven and three, respectively (Mooney, 1993; Tjaden & Thoennes, 2000).

EpiCrim uses its framework to focus on preventing injuries while relying on public health approaches. The framework examines structural and organizational determinants that influence the behavior. Research suggests intimate partner violence is a learned behavior that is acquired throughout the socialization process and is used by abusers to achieve a certain aim. While this form of violence is global, it is more pronounced in areas characterized by poverty, low educational attainment, and among men who assert dominance over their female counterparts. Socialization toward an acceptance of this behavior mostly occurs among boys and men within intimate groups (e.g., *friends, cliques, fraternities*), family, community, and society. Violence is easily transmitted within the context of those interactions that people have with each other and in important institutions that either directly or indirectly reinforce sexist and stereotypical behaviors related to traditional roles in relationships. Notwithstanding, when violence is internalized, it encourages and leads to poor decision-making and risk-taking behavior that have negative health consequences. The task for epidemiological criminologists is to understand what causes the behavior and the poor health outcomes that it presents to the population and use integrative approaches to apply *primary*, *secondary*, and *tertiary* prevention strategies to educate the public, treat both offenders and victims, and minimize the degree of harm as soon as possible (Potter & Akers, 2013).

Elderly Abuse and EpiCrim

Elderly abuse is a global problem with serious negative health consequences since it often manifests in physical, sexual, psychological, and financial forms (Krug et al., 2002). It is composed of actions that are either committed intentionally or unintentionally by an abuser which in many cases is a family member. Some experts also argue that neglect is a form of elderly abuse (Acierno, 2003; Hudson, 1991). Despite the type of abuse, elderly victims typically experience unnecessary and preventable suffering, injury, pain, or loss of human rights as well as a diminished quality of life (Hudson, 1991). Epidemiological data on elderly abuse is often obtained from criminal justice as well as public health data sources such as (1) agency record review; (2) criminal justice statistics translated to focus on age and perpetrator; (3) interviews of elderly victims; (4) interviews of caregivers/family members; and (5) sentinel reports from trained observers employed by agencies that serve older adults (Acierno, 2003).

Elderly abuse is concerning for several reasons and chief among them is the fact that by 2025, it is estimated that the global population of elderly people between the ages of 60 and older will have increased from 542 million in 1995 to about 1.2 billion. Statistics also show that among the elderly living in developing countries, the population will more than double by 2025. They will also make up 12% of the population in the developing world. However, in countries such as *Kenya, Thailand, Columbia,* and *Indonesia*, the elderly population is expected to increase fourfold (Randal & German, 1999). Regarding the nature and extent of elderly abuse, researchers often rely on data that are collected in advanced nations since they are collected more consistently and are considered robust. As a result, there have been five surveys conducted in the past decade in five advanced nations (Pillemer & Finkelhor, 1988; Podnieks, 1992; Ogg & Bennett, 1992; Comijs, 1998). These data reveal that when considering physical, psychological, financial, and neglect, the abuse rate is estimated at between 4% and 6% among the elderly. Among the five surveys on elderly abuse, *Canada*, *the Netherlands*, and the *U.S.* focused on abuse that occurred during the preceding year. The *Finland* study examined abuse that the elderly experienced since the age of retirement, while *Great Britain* investigated cases that occurred in the past few years. The results from the first study composed of *Canada, the Netherlands,* and the *U.S.*, reported no significant differences in the rate of abuse by age or sex. Results from the second study in *Finland* revealed that more females were victimized compared with their male counterparts at 7% and 2.5%, respectively. In the third study, *Britain* did not make any designations in its survey regarding age or sex (Pillemer & Finkelhor, 1988; Podnieks, 1992; Ogg & Bennett, 1992; Comijs, 1998). Research literature shows that in a recent family violence study conducted in *Canada*, an estimated 7% of older people reported experiencing emotional abuse, 1% financial abuse, and 1% physical, or sexual abuse from either their children, caregivers, or partner during the past five years. Among those reporting abuse, men were 9% more likely than women (6%) to report emotional or financial abuse (Podnieks, 1992).

The epidemiological approach to studying and preventing elderly abuse uses an integrative model that delineates risk factors for this abuse. It contends that instead of relying on studies that disproportionately focus on interpersonal and family violence, elderly abuse is better understood by examining individual, relationship, community, and societal factors as major determinants. Individual factors include family members or caregivers with mental health and substance abuse problems (Wolf & Pillemer, 1989). Gender is also a factor that especially affects older men who are more at risk of being victims of spousal abuse or victimized by their children and other relatives (Pillemer & Finkelhor, 1988). Relationship stress is a factor that contributes to elderly abuse. Research reveals that it alone does not cause abuse. In cases where elder patients have dementia, those working with them may be triggered to act with violence owing to stress, the relationship between the caregiver and recipient, the disruptive and aggressive behavior of the elder, and whether the caregiver suffers from depression (O'Loughlin & Duggan, 1998). Regarding community and societal factors, research reveals that social isolation and a lack of interaction and integration with others can be a cause and consequence of elderly abuse (Podnieks, 1992; Wolf & Pillemer, 1989). This finding transcends culture in both developing and advanced societies given cultural norms and traditions such as global views shared regarding ageism, sexism, and cultures of violence that impact the treatment of elders (e.g., not worthy of respect, weak, dependent, frail, less worthy of government investments) (Gorman & Petersen, 1999; Kwan, 1995).

Suicidal Violence and EpiCrim

Suicide death is a global criminal justice and public health problem since it is the 13th leading cause of death worldwide (Favril, 2021). However, self-inflicted injuries are the fourth leading cause of death among people between the ages of 15 and 44. Suicide attempts are also the sixth leading cause of ill health for people in this age group (Favril, 2021; Krug et al., 2002). Literature reveals that when comparing adults in the free community with incarcerated persons in jails and prisons, the latter groups are at a greater risk of considering, attempting, and carrying out successful suicides which creates increasing concerns for penal institutions worldwide (Favril, 2021). Global statistics indicate that there are an estimated 10 million prisoners with additional inmates transitioning through prison systems (Fair & Walmsley, 2021). In these prisons, suicide is the leading cause of death accounting for an estimated 30% each year (Favril et al., 2019; Kaur et al., 2019; Rabe, 2012). Cross-cultural studies show that suicides among inmates in ten countries in *South America* have consistently found that they far exceed successful and attempted suicides of people in the free society with a rate that ranges from 3 to 9 (Fritz et al., 2021). In a recent investigation, Fazel and colleagues (2017) reported that in a cross-national study that included 24 high-income countries, the number of suicide rates among male prisoners were four times higher than their age-equivalent community counterparts (Fazel et al., 2017). The study also revealed that the highest rate of prison suicides was reported in *Nordic* countries, followed by *France* and *Belgium* where the rates were 100 suicides per 100,000 prisoners (Fazel et al., 2017). The study cautioned that because deaths in jails and prisons are often misclassified (e.g., suicides by self-poisoning recorded as unintentional overdoses), the actual number of cases may be underestimated (Duthé et al., 2014; Favril et al., 2019; Fazel et al., 2017; Kaur et al., 2019; Morthorst et al., 2021; Opitz-Welke et al., 2013).

Other prison studies find similar rates of suicides. In a recent meta-analysis that examined the results of 77 studies, Zhong and colleagues (2021), reported that factors that were associated with inmate suicides included the quality of the inmates' mental health which influenced suicidal ideation, history of suicide attempts, history of self-harm, and current psychiatric diagnosis. The study also found that penal institutional factors often increased the likelihood of inmate suicides. It identified factors that include single cell occupancy, not receiving visitors from outside, serving a life sentence, being remanded before trial, and having been sentenced for committing a violent crime (Zhong et al., 2021). In research by Vanhaesebrouck and colleagues (2024), that examined every incarceration in *France* from 2017 to 2020 to determine factors that influenced suicide risk, researchers relied on official data from the *National Prison Service*. Data revealed an estimated 350,000 incarcerations with 450 reported suicides. The study analyzed socio-demographics, criminal, and prison characteristics and found that nationality of a *European* country, older age, being separated, and having a high school diploma were suicidal risk factors. Moreover, the investigation revealed early stages of incarceration (first weeks), being incarcerated for a violent crime, especially homicide, prison overcrowding, being confined in personal housing, and having children were associated with suicide, but this measure was inconsistent. Results from the Vanhaesebrouck and colleagues (2024), the study revealed that during 2017–2020, *France* prison suicide rate was 173 per 100,000 inmates. The act also has a rippling effect on others since surviving family members and friends report experiencing a range of emotions, grief, along with suffering socially as well as economically. Researchers and economists in the U.S., estimate that suicides and attempts at self-inflicted injuries cost taxpayers billions of dollars annually (Stoudemire et al., 1986).

When considering risk factors associated with suicides, the public health view examines the vulnerabilities of people in the free society as well as inmates by focusing specifically on the status and quality of their mental health and whether their health needs are addressed. When people commit crimes and are taken into the justice system, public health officials and those responsible for their custody (e.g., correctional officers), must render a duty of care since prisoners with mental health issues import them into the penal setting. In contrast, the criminal justice view focuses on the impact of being institutionalized and how the penal environment and isolation affect prisoner's behavior, especially efforts to self-harm and suicide attempts (Favril et al., 2017; Liebling & Ludlow, 2016). Consequently, criminal justice experts and criminologists (e.g., penologists) advocate changing the custodial environment of jails and prisons and those experiences that often precipitate the decision to self-harm (Favril, 2021). Because of this, officials at *WHO* recommend evidence-based prevention efforts that are designed to make *primary and secondary prevention efforts* or early identification of high-risk people who would benefit from targeted intervention. Prison officials must recognize how vulnerable inmates are in the correctional environment given that with its many deprivations, it can be challenging to navigate. Therefore, health experts advise prison officials to develop a comprehensive suicide prevention program that includes targeted strategies directed at prisoners who exhibit high-risk behavior within the context of environmental stressors (e.g., victimization [*physical and sexual assault*], boredom, mental health, and isolation [Marzano et al., 2016; Rivlin et al., 2010]). Klonsky and colleagues (2021), argue that the process of preventing inmate suicide is not always easy since thinking about committing self-harm does not necessarily manifest into the behavior. They suggest that prison officials must recognize when suicidal thoughts can transition into suicidal behavior which is a process with distinct predictors. As a result, prison officials should create interventions that target suicidal ideation that are meant to impede the progression to suicidal behavior among inmates already thinking about self-harm. According to Marzano and colleagues (2016), programs that are designed to prevent inmate suicide must not be limited to merely monitoring newly arrived inmates, but rather, they must provide a process that continuously monitors inmates at regular intervals throughout the duration of an inmate's incarceration.

Police Violence and EpiCrim

Police violence is a form of policing that uses the amount of force or coercion that exceeds what is reasonably necessary to accomplish a legitimate policing objective (del Carmen, 1991). While police violence has always been viewed as a criminal justice problem in the U.S., it has recently been named a public health problem given its prevalence in some communities and people compared with others as well as its adverse physical, mental, and emotional impact on the health of the population (DeVylder et al., 2022; Cooper, 2004). Other scholars report that police violence also spills over into other groups who are punished and criminalized for having mental health disorders, being homeless, or simply living in poverty. Some health experts contend that police interactions often exacerbate health inequities. As previously stated, police violence, despite its short- and long-term effects on people in the U.S., has not been considered a public health issue for long (DeVylder et al., 2022). In a study conducted by Cooper and colleagues (2004), that examined 65 black adults in New York City and their violent encounters with police and the impact those experiences had on their health, the idea became accepted in mainstream society after the study's findings emphasized that police violence is a threat to public health in the U.S. This, and other studies have recorded many negative health consequences associated with police violence and found that they typically lead to chronic health conditions such as acute injuries, fatal injuries, high mortality rates, and symptoms such as PTSD, depression, distress, suicidal behavior, and symptoms of psychosis (Coulter et al., 1999; Hirschtick, et al., 2020). Other negative consequences of police brutality include excessive arrests, incarceration, poor school performance, medical and funeral bills, incomplete high school education, and systematic disempowerment of minorities and members of the *LGBTQ+* community (Bor et al., 2018).

Police violence is also a global problem, as revealed in state-sponsored universal responses to global protests of police violence, racism, and white supremacy in 2020. For example, *Amnesty International* (2020), reported that in *Nigeria*, at least 56 people were killed by *Nigerian* police forces as citizens protested police repression. Furthermore, data from the *U.K.* show that police often target and criminalize Blacks and other minorities. A 2018 survey revealed that blacks were nine times more likely to be stopped by police compared to other groups with only one in ten of those stops resulting in arrest (Shiner et al., 2020). In another study, research showed that while Blacks in the *U.K.* represent 3% of the population, they were the victims of police use of force (e.g., electric shock), 20% of the time compared to the rest of the population at 16% (*UK Home Office*, 2019). Axleby and Waight (2020) reported that in *Australia*, *Aboriginal* and *Torres Strait Islanders* make up 28% of adults confined in prison, but represent only 2% of the population. Other studies also highlight the racism that minority populations experience at the hands of police. According to *Human Rights Watch* (2016), at least 8,000 people have been killed by *Brazil's Rio de Janeiro* police force in the past decades in what has been declared unlawful killings. The demographics reveal that most victims have been young Black men. Moreover, a 2019 study estimated that 1,731 people were killed in police custody in *India*. The victims were disproportionately *Muslims* and *Hindus* from *Scheduled Caste* and *Tribes* (Gettleman & Yasir, 2020). Notwithstanding, comparative policing experts on violence report that though fatal police violence is not as common as nonfatal acts of violence police perpetrate on minorities, statistics show that when it comes to fatal acts of police violence, the U.S. accounts for more fatal acts of homicides (e.g., an approximately 8%) annually compared with any other advanced nation (Edwards et al., 2018). Despite this, some scholars report that this public health concern (police-inflicted homicides) receives scant attention in the literature. This is concerning to many scholars and researchers given that there are no national standards in the U.S. that require police to report the mortalities that they are involved (Feldman et al., 2019).

Preventing police violence is concerning on a global level, but experts contend it is to EpiCrim because of the harm and devastation it causes to victims and other people in society, namely members of marginalized communities globally. Researchers who study police violence rely on data collected by criminal justice experts, criminologists, public health officials (*WHO*), *Amnesty International*, and others to show how the behavior impacts the justice and public health systems. Because of this, some experts suggest using a social determinant and health framework approach. Where justice is concerned, police violence must be addressed to restore public trust and confidence in policing efforts to make society safe. This includes holding police accountable when they engage in misconduct or state crimes by either arresting, convicting, and sentencing police for the use of excessive or deadly force which may include filing a civil action against the officer, department, and municipality holding them responsible for injuries inflicted or wrongful death suits brought by surviving family members (del Carmen, 1991). Regarding public health, people and their respective families are impacted by police violence in several ways that include the immediate effects of physical injuries, untimely deaths, and subsequent links to mental health and the short- and long-term effects of chronic physical pain. Through collaborative efforts, EpiCrim relies on combined data collections, methodologies, and theories to reveal the disparities in police violence that are often delineated by race/ethnicity, gender and sexual minority status, housing status, presence of mental illness, disability, and others (DeVylder et al., 2022). Some scholars contend that while we have improved our understanding of the prevalence, disparities, and physical and psychological effects of police violence, we have failed to uncover the mechanisms that link police violence exposure to public health outcomes. Other scholars state that we have limited published studies on the structural factors that influence the rates of exposure and disparities in the rate of exposure. Because of the gaps in the literature as well as our understanding of police violence, EpiCrim holds promise that these and other salient matters can be addressed in future policy directions to shift from relying solely on punitive measures to educational and training programs that emphasize the need to address structural and systemic racism to reeducate police and engage in proactive and preventive social services (DeVylder et al., 2022).

Teenage Violence and EpiCrim

Teenage violence is a global problem that impacts millions of lives annually. Research on violence reveals that it holds the distinction of being the most visible form of violence in society (Krug et al., 2002). When it occurs, it often harms victims, friends, families, health workers treating firearm-related injuries, and others in the community (Hureau et al., 2022). Juvenile experts contend that youth violence also has a global presence since it leaves behind deaths, injuries, disabilities, and illnesses that often impact one's psychological and social functioning, along with a diminished quality of life for perpetrators and victims (Krug et al., 2002). Research reveals that both nationally and globally, the victims and perpetrators of youth violence are disproportionately juveniles who either encounter each other on the streets, schools, or via gangs (Reza et al., 2001). Young people account for a significant number of premature deaths, injuries, and disabilities because of their involvement in homicides as well as non-fatal assaults. Therefore, youth violence is considered a criminal justice and public health issue. It's a criminal justice problem because it is directly related to law violations and harming people in society. Conversely, it is also a public health issue given the number of youths who engage in violence along with the negative health consequences it causes teenagers and others. Research shows that globally, an estimated 193,000 homicides are committed by young (mostly male on male) between the ages of 15 and 29 each year making it the leading cause of death among youths in this age group (WHO, 2024). Experts contend that this represents an average of 565 children, adolescents, and young adults who die because of an act of interpersonal violence each day. Moreover, statistics reveal variation by regions in international comparative homicide rates (Krug et al., 2002). WHO data provides that homicide rates for youth are highest in *Latin America* (84.4 per 100,000 in *Columbia*), (50.2 per 100,000 in *El Salvador*), the *Caribbean* (41.8 per 100,000 in *Puerto Rico*), the *Russian Federation* (18 per 100,000), and some countries in south-eastern *Europe* (28.2 per 100,000 in *Albania*). In the *U.S.*, the rate is 11 per 100,000. However, most countries with a youth homicide rate above 10 per 100,000 are either developing countries or experiencing social and economic changes. In contrast, countries with low rates of youth homicides are often from *Western European* countries such as *France (0.6 per 100,000), Germany (0.8 per 100,000)*, and the *U.K. (0.9 per 100,000)* or in *Asia* such as *Japan (0.4 per 100,000)* (Krug et al., 2002). A recent report revealed that from 2000 to 2019, in most nations, the number of youth homicides experienced a decline. However, this occurred mostly in high-income nations.

The rate of fatal violence incidents is concerning given the high prevalence of youth involvement, especially in cases where firearm violence is acted out in schools. According to a nationwide survey conducted in the U.S., an estimated 51% of students revealed that they worry about either being killed or seriously injured in a school shooting (Southern Poverty Law Center, 2023). Health experts contend that students and teenagers who survive school shootings and other nonfatal acts of violence often experience declines in health and well-being, engage in risky behaviors, display increased absenteeism, perform poorly academically, and increased antidepressant use (Louis-Phillippe & Kim, 2016). When teenagers survive acts of firearm-related violence, they often require hospitalization that far exceeds the number of persons killed by violence. Acts of sexual violence are also common in youth violence. Studies report that one in five girls and one in seven boys report being sexually abused. Moreover, bullying and physical fighting are pervasive among the youth (WHO, 2024). In a comparative study, researchers reported that in 40 developing countries, 42% of boys and 37% of girls revealed that they were victims of bullying (WHO, 2024). Health experts suggest an increased focus on *primary prevention* efforts that rely on a comprehensive public health approach as a conceptual framework to prevent teenage violence. The use of *secondary prevention* strategies that actively target groups at risk of engaging in violence and being the victim of violence, and *tertiary prevention* efforts in response to violence so that the behavior will not occur again (Cant et al., 2022). Experts contend that troubled youths need treatment and counseling, instead of punishment. They also suggest victims of violence require treatment, counseling, and hospitalization which exceeds the reach and resources of the criminal justice system. Youth violence also impacts the economy since it contributes to the expensive costs of health and welfare services, reduced productivity, decline in property values, and can invariably undermine the fabric of society (Krug et al., 2002).

Workplace Violence and EpiCrim

Workplace violence is a national as well as global problem with far-reaching consequences (Krug et al., 2002). Experts at the *Occupational Safety and Health Administration* (OSHA), argue that it is pervasive in society impacting an estimated 2 million American workers and another 3 million workers in the *European Union* who have reported experiencing physical violence (Krug et al., 2002). A global survey conducted revealed some workplaces and occupations are more suspectable of experiencing violence. They include taxi drivers, healthcare workers, people working alone, teachers, social workers, domestics in foreign nations, employees working at night, and people working in the retail industry who report significant amounts of workplace violence (International Labor Organization, 2022). Workplace violence is not only physical, but rather, it has a broad scope that includes any act where an employee is abused, threatened, intimidated, or physically assaulted in the work environment. OSHA reported that some other forms of workplace violence include being subjected to bullying, sexual harassment, rumors, swearing, verbal abuse, pranks, arguments, property damage, vandalism, sabotage, pushing, theft, psychological trauma, anger-related incidents, rape, arson, and murder, especially deaths linked to love triangles or retaliation (Occupational Safety and Health Administration [OSHA], 2015).

Workplace violence is a criminal justice and public health issue because it contributes to many injuries, premature and untimely deaths, as well as other physical injuries (e.g., gunshot wounds, stabbings) and psychological injuries (e.g., PTSD, high levels of stress, anxiety) inflicted on co-workers by other employees. Regarding deaths in the U.S., Chappell and DiMartin (1998), reported that an estimated 1,000 killings occur in the workplace yearly. It is a public health problem because it causes negative health outcomes within the population such as short- and long-term injuries and disruptions to interpersonal relationships in the work environment that can have devastating consequences on the individual, family, and community (Krug et al., 2002). Economists contend workplace violence creates direct and indirect costs to the rest of society. Some economists site direct costs such as disabilities, deaths, high levels of absenteeism in the labor force that results in the loss of billions of dollars in revenues annually and high employee turnover. The indirect costs typically include low productivity owing to the level of morale, diminished quality products and services, along an environment that is not conducive to work. While OSHA estimates that workplace violence costs $120 billion in loss, the *National Safety Council* (2024) reports it costs society $171 billion annually.

Workplace violence is a serious global problem as evidenced by official statistics that indicate it is the second leading cause of death in the workplace for men and women next to traffic accidents. Cross-cultural comparative studies reveal that female migrant workers from the *Philippines*, especially those working in domestic service, or the entertainment industry are disproportionately the victims of violence within the context of engaging in work (Krug et al., 2002). Studies from the *U.K.* show that 53% of employees suffered from bullying at work, while 78% of employees reported witnessing violence in the workplace. In another comparative study, research conducted on workplace violence in *South Africa* found that hostile work environments are not rear but rather are the rule with rates that are abnormally high given an estimated 78% of employees who were surveyed, reported they experienced bullying at work by a coworker. A comparative study conducted in *Sweden* reported that acts of violence in the workplace, especially bullying, sexual harassment, and threats were linked to between an estimated 10% and 15% of suicides (Krug et al., 2002). More recently, the combined efforts from the *UN's International Labor Organization* and *Lloyd's Register Foundation*, along with a global study that used a Gallup self-reported survey that included 121 countries and over 74,000 workers, showed that one in five workers, or 23% of all workers worldwide experienced violence (e.g., physical and psychological) along with sexual harassment at work during some point in their lifetime (Crabtree, 2022). The study revealed that psychological violence and harassment were the most common types of violence and those most vulnerable were young women between the ages of 15 and 24. The survey concluded that workplace violence does not occur in isolated incidents given that more than three in five victims reported experiencing violence on several occasions with the most recent incident occurring within the past five years (Crabtree, 2022).

Experts contend that workplace violence is preventable since efforts can be taken to address this form of assaultive violence. Prevention is possible through collaborative efforts of EpiCrim and employers who can identify risk factors and determine who is at a greater risk of being the victims and perpetrators of workplace violence. Researchers report that in most workplaces, employers have a legal obligation to provide workers with a safe environment and can easily assess the worksites and identify risk factors so that violent assaults can be prevented. California has passed State Bill 553 which includes *Labor Code section 6401.9* outlining the elements that are required in a workplace violence prevention plan. It makes every employer responsible for creating, implementing, and maintaining an effective prevention plan that must contain aspects such as training on workplace safety, workplace violence recordkeeping, and the responsibility of immediately reporting any serious incidents such as deaths, injuries, or illnesses that occur in the workplace to OSHA (Rodriguez & Tynan, 2024). Additionally, workplace violence can also be prevented by using data collected by EpiCrim on employees and places where workplace violence occurs that contains information on employee's history of violence, threatening behavior, intimidating behavior, increase in personal stress, negative personality characteristics, and observed changes in mood or behavior to create safe working spaces. The efforts of EpiCrim can create typologies based on the demographical data of victims and offenders and the types of assaultive violence that employers are likely to commit. These data will contain the physical warning signs (e.g., bizarre behavior, irrational ideas, depressed appearance, social isolation, and others) that precipitate workplace violence. OSHA (2015), suggests that workplace violence can be prevented if businesses and occupations implement a workplace violence prevention plan that requires all employees to undergo training on how to reduce workplace violence. Within these programs, businesses are responsible for informing employees and providing them with information on risk factors and the extent of violence that exists in the workplace to increase awareness of workplace violence. The plan should include an emergency response protocol, training provisions, and procedures to identify and evaluate workplace violence inspections (Rodriguez & Tynan, 2024).

Firearm Injuries and EpiCrim

Firearm violence is a national as well as global problem that factors prominently in the U.S. and throughout the world. Health officials argue that the morbidity and mortality caused by firearm violence continue to rise and have profound negative health consequences on individuals, families, communities, and adverse impacts on the broader society. It is also the leading cause of death for U.S. children and adolescents between the ages of 1 and 19 (Goldstick et al., 2022). Because of its pervasiveness, it is a public health and global problem (Fontanarosa et al., 2022). According to Kegler and colleagues (2022), data from the *CDC* reveal that an estimated 45,000 firearm-related deaths and 71,000 nonfatal injuries occurred in the U.S. in 2020. In a recent national survey, Schumacher and colleagues (2023), reported that firearm violence is so pervasive in the U.S. that an estimated 54% of adults revealed that either they or a family member have experienced a firearm-related incident. Kegler and colleagues' study revealed that more than half of the deaths were acts of suicide, while more than 40% were due to homicide. They also show firearm mortality demonstrates racial inequities since data from 2020 show that the firearm homicide rate was substantially greater for Blacks compared with Whites at 22.6 per 100,000 and 2.2 per 100,000, respectively (Kegler et al., 2023).

In the U.S., gun-related killings are common occurrences in places such as schools, churches, workplaces, shopping malls, night clubs, and recreational activities. Experts report that there is variation in rates of firearm deaths cross cultures. Some global statistics find that firearm mortality was highly concentrated among six countries in *the Americas-Brazil, the U.S., Mexico, Columbia, Venezuela, and Guatemala.* In 2016, these areas accounted for 50.5% of all deaths. Experts estimate that percentage, 32% of the deaths occurred in *Brazil* and the *U.S.* with 25% of all firearm deaths attributed to *Brazil*, while the *U.S.* accounted for 35% of all suicides (Rivera et al., 2018). Statistics reveal that the lowest firearm suicide rate was 0.1 per 100,000 in *Singapore*, and the rate was 6.4 per 100,000 persons in the *U.S.* However, the firearm homicide rate was close to zero in *Singapore* to 38.9 per 100,000 in *El Salvador.* Homicide data in countries such as *Brazil, Columbia, Mexico, the Philippines,* and *South Africa* show that most firearm-related deaths were homicides and suicides accounted for a small number (Rivara et al., 2018). Research reveals the opposite was true in affluent countries such as *Australia, Canada, France, Germany,* and *Sweden* where the number of suicides dwarfed the reported number of homicides. According to statistics, the firearm-related suicide rate was 6.6 times higher compared with the firearm-related homicide rate in *France* and 7.5 times higher in *Germany.* However, in a small number of countries such as *China* and *Saudi Arabia,* the most common types of firearm-related deaths were reported as unintentional (Rivara et al., 2018). Furthermore, global comparisons of firearm-related deaths show the U.S. has significantly higher rates than other high-income countries. Specifically, data collected by the *CDC* and *WHO* in 2015, revealed all firearm-related deaths in the U.S. were 11.4 times higher than in 28 other higher-income nations (Grinshteyn & Hemenway, 2019). What is more concerning about the statistics is that during this time, the *U.S.* accounted for about 31% of the combined population of the 29 countries but was responsible for 83.7% of all firearms-related deaths (Grinshteyn & Hemenway, 2019).

Another consistency that emerges in cross-cultural comparative studies on homicide data is that the U.S. has the dubious distinction of having the highest firearm-related mortality rate among peer nations. For data from 2015 revealed that among 29 countries, an estimated 97% of children from the U.S., or 9 in 10 between the ages of 0 and 14, and 92% of children between the ages of 5 and 14 who died from firearms-related injuries, lived in the U.S. (Grinshteyn & Hemenway, 2019). In a recent study, data from the *Institute for Health Metrics and Evaluation* found that in 2019, a comparison of firearm mortality among children and adolescents in the *U.S., Canada,* and *Sweden* showed that the U.S. remains the leader among deaths of children linked to firearms-related injuries within the U.S., having 36.4 per 1 million or 5 times the rate of firearms mortality compared with *Canada* at 6.2 per 1 million, about 18 times the rate of firearm mortality in *Sweden* with 2.0 per 1 million, and exceeds *Australia* by more than 22 times with a rate of 1.6 per 1 million firearm mortality for children and adolescents between the ages of 1 and 19 (McGough et al., 2023). While the number of fatal injuries is alarming, VanDyke and colleagues (2022) reported that firearm-related injuries far exceed the number of fatal injuries and contribute substantially to victimizations. They reported that from 2018 to 2021, an estimated 100,000 persons experienced either fatal or nonfatal firearms injuries each year that required an emergency room or hospital visit.

Firearm violence is also preventable and can be achieved with multisectoral collaborative efforts of EpiCrim, policing, public health officials, and other stakeholders since it will bring experts together across multiple disciplines and occupations such as criminal justice, criminology, public health, and politics working to define and monitor the problem of firearm violence; identify risk and protective factors; develop and test prevention strategies; and ensure widespread adoption of effective strategies. Experts advise that *primary prevention* efforts are highly effective when conducted early, especially among people, groups, and places that are discovered to be at a high risk for victimization. These efforts typically include using measures such as media and educational campaigns to reduce firearm injuries and improve firearm-related safety by changing attitudes, behavior, and social norms about the danger of firearms (Krug et al., 2002). Some efforts are made by defraying the cost of airtime on radio and television to educate the public on the pervasiveness of intentional and unintentional firearm violence and the toll it takes on human life in certain communities. This strategy of educating the public can reach large numbers of listeners and viewers within minutes. Experts are quick to suggest that these efforts can have both a specific and general deterrence effect in the targeted as well as the general population. Another effective educational tool is the use of billboards in high-risk communities that present the harsh reality of gun violence. Other areas that need to be addressed are poor infrastructures in some communities such as environmental factors in certain locations, namely high-risk places (e.g., impoverished areas) that are dimly lit, isolated, and where people congregate and consume alcohol. Because a disproportionate amount of firearm violence occurs in economically challenged areas nationally as well as globally, experts recommend that improvements must be made to the infrastructure in impoverished areas to offer community residents better alternatives such as educational and economic opportunities. Health experts and EpiCrim contend that local and national interventions can be directed at preventing firearms violence by passing legislation on gun sales and ownership and efforts to get illegal guns off the streets such as buyback programs (Krug et al., 2002). In the U.S., media critics have argued that *Hollywood* has constructed a culture of violence that has normalized nearly all types of assaultive violence. Some experts argue that violent media presentations have desensitized American viewers and arguably the world community to extreme levels of violence (Barak, 1994). However, the same experts argue that the media can be used to help change violence-related attitudes and behavior as well as social norms that perpetuate the behavior by presenting anti-violence themes and messages via movies and other television productions (Barak, 1994).

Problems and Limitations of Epidemiological Studies

Public health researchers argue that the goal of epidemiological studies is to determine cause and effect by using a threefold approach. First, observing an association between exposure to a disease or violence. Second, developing a hypothesis about the cause-and-effect relationship. Third, testing the hypothesis by using a formal epidemiological design. The researchers also warn that though such studies may find strong support for conclusions that isolate certain exposures that cause a particular disease or violence, there are many potential mistakes in drawing such conclusions, especially given that some diseases and types of violence have several determinants and develop over extended periods of time that are subject to mistakes (Schneider, 2020). Despite this, some researchers believe that since all epidemiological studies use samples of people, this increases the likelihood that mistakes or errors are inevitable. This view has led researchers to suggest that no matter how well-designed epidemiological studies are, mistakes are often unavoidable. Thus, rendering researchers unable to establish cause-and-effect. According to Farmer (2007) and Lilienfeld (1983), epidemiological studies rarely prove causality on their own owing to the need for other data and the likelihood that there are often flaws in their designs or execution. Consequently, epidemiologists often use language such as risk factors associated with diseases and violence, rather than, causes (Schneider, 2020). Given the gravity of this statement, a few examples are instructive in this regard. If a researcher engages in a rigorous scientific study using a *randomized controlled trial* to monitor two groups for interpersonal violence intervention: one receiving treatment and the other group does not, it is virtually impossible to control the behavior of people who are not kept in a secured environment with specific conditions to adhere to. As such, the results derived from this investigation may not be what the researcher hypothesized since subjects in a control group or experimental group may not adhere to a research protocol (e.g., treatment and control approaches), and adjust their behavior accordingly.

Because a *randomized controlled trial* may fail to achieve adequate results, a researcher may opt to use a group of people similarly situated (e.g., victims of interpersonal violence) to test the same hypothesis by placing them in a *cohort study* and monitoring them for three years. The study could be made into a time-series longitudinal design whereby the same group will be contacted twice a year for a total of six interventions to measure whether their health status improved since the start of the *cohort study*. Research reveals that the use of this design can also be problematic because subjects who volunteer to participate in a study are often different from non-volunteers in that they are more likely to desire and seek help to change. They may be less representative of others or inclined to repeat victims or engage in the type of violence against others that were committed against them. This suggests that these subjects were at a low or reduced risk of interpersonal violence.

After experiencing failure with a *case study* design, a researcher may engage in an *observational study*. However, these studies are also problematic since the investigator lacks control over nearly every aspect of the study, namely who gets exposed to a disease or act of violence under observation. The investigator cannot predict when subjects are exposed or any determinant factors that may impact a disease or violence that affects the subjects under observation or pinpoint with accuracy, exactly when a disease or violence initially occurred. Farmer (2007) contends that this design is also limited by the fact that in *observational studies*, the data that are collected are always incomplete. Another type of study a researcher could use is the *case–control design* which requires the selection of a group of people who already have a disease or experienced violence (e.g., interpersonal). The researcher could visit and interview victims at a domestic violence recovery center to collect data. As a comparison, the researcher could select a similar group of people with respect to demographics (e.g., race, ethnicity, age, gender, and others) to serve as a control group. The researcher could interview both groups and ask questions regarding their current and past relationships with partners about violence to measure if the hypothesis is correct regarding the cause-and-effect of interpersonal violence. Unfortunately, research reveals that this design is also problematic given that people are often embarrassed about sharing their personal experiences, unwilling to report to strangers about private matters, have problems recalling events, exaggerate their partner's role in the matter, and downplay the seriousness of their injuries and the research questions. While not intended to be an exhaustive list, experts argue that these and other shortcomings, conspire to make findings from epidemiological studies unreliable. Lilienfeld (1983), suggested that despite such challenges, epidemiological studies have increased our understanding of how environmental factors impact human populations. Therefore, these challenges do not necessarily mean that no valid conclusions can be derived from epidemiological studies, but rather, they represent that mistakes are very common in research. Lilienfeld (1983) and others suggest that investigators who engage in epidemiological studies must be vigilant in selecting and improving study designs as well as managing their execution. They must be cautious about the interpretations of research findings (Farmer, 2007).

As stated in Chapter 3, epidemiologists, criminal justice experts, and criminologists rely on several data sources when conducting research investigations. Some methodologies include tools such as *official agency data (e.g., statistics), experiments, surveys, questionnaires, case studies, observational studies, case–control desig*ns, and others. It is important to note that the instrument and research design have serious implications for the findings of the investigation (Thygesen & Ersboll, 2014). Scholars report that studies that rely on data collected from surveys or questionnaires are designed only to capture information that appears as one of the items in the instrument. Consequently, research questions are crafted by the investigator's prior knowledge, attempt to test the hypothesis that is being investigated, and to some extent, the researchers' bias (Farmer, 2007). To the latter point, Smith (2001) reported that a major limitation of epidemiological research in recent years has been that its failure to be a value-free approach, but instead, is used as a research tool to support predetermined goals. Another concerning aspect of epidemiological studies that has received considerable attention is its use of small samples to derive meaningful findings. Farmer (2007) contends that this is not meant to diminish the value of using small samples in research, but rather some scholars argue that the design of epidemiological studies can only be improved when more rigorous measurements are added to exposed small samples instead of being content with findings that often use poorly exposed measurements in larger samples. These, alone, make the findings of epidemiological investigations limited (Farmer, 2007). Because of this, experts argue that consumers of research must always consider the amount of selectivity placed on the questions and limitations found in a study's design when evaluating its results (Farmer, 2007).

Researchers point out that recent studies have uncovered mistakes in many questionnaires used to conduct epidemiological studies that reveal questionable results. An investigation that attempted to collect exposure data to determine the risk of breast cancer is instructive in this regard. The instrument used asked the mothers (of women in a study who were diagnosed with breast cancer) about the dietary habits of their daughters when they were between the ages of 3 and 5 years old. The findings were deemed suspicious at best given that the mothers were asked to complete the questions by reflecting on what they fed their daughters 40 years ago (Michels et al., 2006). Similarly, problems were discovered by Nielsen and colleagues (2005) who reported in a study on the effects of stress and the risk of breast cancer, researchers gave a group of women a questionnaire designed to measure how often and what degree of intensity they experienced stress. The researchers used the findings to determine the risk of breast cancer for the next 18 years after estimating the reported stress levels. The study was criticized because the researchers hypothesized that self-reported stress levels could affect the risk of breast cancer without considering any other evidence to validate data collected from the questionnaire. Moreover, the presentation of the results of a study is crucial. Scholars contend that if we overinterpret the results of *randomized control trials, cohort studies, observational studies, case–control designs,* or any other, it can lead to erroneous information or a misunderstanding about disease and violence causation that may be better explained by other determinants not found in the study where data are collected and inferences drawn (Farmer, 2007). With that said, Smith (2001) reports that all epidemiological investigations should be designed to test the hypothesis by using several types of data sources that are designed to rigorously measure many social determinants (e.g., social, economic, historical, and others) instead of relying solely on one method or determinants. This requires improving the study design (Smith, 2001). If a significant result emerges, it indicates that the association is not due to chance. However, experts advise that a non-significant finding does not necessarily mean that there is no association between an exposure and the outcome. It means that the hypothesis was supported. Early evaluation of epidemiological research is important and should be reported with prudence (Farmer, 2007).

Summary

Researchers and other professionals who study and examine assaultive violence argue that greater efforts must be made to advance the use of epidemiological approaches that combine the collaborative efforts of criminal justice, criminology, and public health officials since they sure similar concerns and interests about violence and crime that can be used to strengthen their theoretical as well as methodological rigors that can make findings more robust. The wisdom is that the use of mixed instruments, tools, and methods from several academic disciplines instead of continuing the historical practice of using separate academic disciplines' own theories, methods, and statistics to examine violence and crime, will likely yield better results if research investigators integrate the efforts of other professionals and stakeholders when working to prevent violence and crime. Many experts are beginning to embrace the idea that violence and crime (given their pervasiveness and the negative health consequences they present nationally as well as globally), transcend criminal justice and should be viewed as an epidemic similar to other diseases that have spread and negatively impacted the overall health of a population and how public health officials have responded to diseases with success using epidemiological approaches. The professionals who embrace this idea believe that effectively preventing violence and crime from occurring or repeating, requires the use of criminal justice as well as epidemiological surveillance and prevention approaches, namely *primary, secondary, and tertiary* responses. They contend that to successfully prevent violence and crime, requires that those working together toward prevention must rely on using multiple forms of data sources in criminal justice, criminology, and public health to better address and understand assaultive violence. This can invariably lead to the emergence of EpiCrim. More specifically, when seeking the causes of assaultive violence, researchers in their respective disciplines must examine determinant factors, risk factors, and preventative factors from those areas. These data must come from local, state, regional, national, as well as global efforts to address violence given it is a preventable issue that affects nearly everyone either directly or indirectly starting at the individual, family, community, and societal levels. Each data source allows for a more complete picture of the nature, extent, and magnitude of assaultive violence on a national as well as global level. While there are many types of methods that are used in studying violence, some of the more popular approaches include *cross-sectional studies, case–control studies, cohort studies, and controlled clinical studies.* Because of the harm that violence and crime do to society, more studies need to be conducted in the areas of child abuse, child sexual abuse, sexual assaults, intimate partner violence, elderly abuse, suicidal violence, police violence, teenage violence, workplace violence, and firearm injuries. While experts contend that EpiCrim holds much promise in explaining crime and helping to move toward prevention, they also report that there are problems and limitations in the epidemiological approach.

Discussion Questions

1 What are some benefits of using EpiCrim to address assaultive violence?
2 List and explain two types of epidemiological research designs.
3 How is epidemiological surveillance used to study violence and crime?
4 How does criminal justice, criminology, and public health intersect?
5 How are controlled clinical studies used in epidemiological investigations?
6 Discuss two limitations of epidemiological studies.

References

Acierno, R. (2003). Elder mistreatment: Epidemiological assessment methodology. In R.J. Bonnie & R.B. Wallace (Eds.), *Elder mistreatment: Abuse, neglect, and exploitation in an aging America* (pp. 261–302). The National Academies Press.

Akers, R.L., & Sellers, C. (2005). *Criminological theories: Introduction, evaluation, and application* (4th ed.). Roxbury.

Akers, T.A., & Lanier, M.M. (2009). Epidemiological criminology: Coming full circle. *American Journal of Public Health*, 99(3), 397–402.

Akers, T.A., Potter, R.H., & Hill, C.L. (2013). *Epidemiological criminology: A public health approach to crime and violence*. John Wiley.

Andersen, S.N., & Hyatt, J. (2020). Randomized experiments in Scandinavian criminal justice: Reviewing the past and looking to the future. *European Journal of Criminology*, 17(2), 224–244.

Anderson, J.F. (2022). *Criminal Justice Research Methods* (1st ed.). Cognella Publishing.

Armstead, T.L., Wilkins, N., & Nation, M. (2021). Structural and social determinants of inequities in violence risk: A review of indicators. *Journal of Community Psychology*, 49(4), 878–906.

Axleby, C., & Waight, N. (2020). We need to go beyond empty gestures if we're going to end Aboriginal deaths in custody. *The Guardian*. www.theguardian.com/commentisfree/2020/jun/29/we-need-to-go-beyond-empty-gestures-if-were-going-to-end-aboriginal-deaths-in-custody

Bachman, R.D., & Schutt, R.K. (2020). *The practice of research in criminology and criminal justice* (7th ed.). Sage.

Barak, G. (1994). *Media, process, and the social construction of crime: Studies in newsmaking criminology*. Garland Publishing.

Barak, G. (1998). *Integrating criminologies*. Allyn and Bacon.

Barcy, A. (2023). *Seeing crime and violence as public health issues*. MI Blues Perspectives. www.mibluesperspetives.com/stories/social-determinants-of-health/seeing-crime-and-violence-as-public-health-issues

Battams, S., Delaney-Crowe, T., Fisher, M., Wright, L., McGreevy, M., McDermott, D., & Baum, F. (2021). Reducing incarceration rates in Australia through primary, secondary, and tertiary crime prevention. *Criminal Justice Policy Review*, 32(6), 618–645.

Belsky, J. (1980). Child maltreatment: An ecological integration. *American Psychologist*, 35, 320–335.

Blaustein, J., Pino, N.W., Fitz-Gibbon, K., & White, R. (2018). Criminology and the UN sustainable development goals: The need for support and critique. *The British Journal of Criminology*, 58(4), 767–786.

Bor, J., Venkataramani, A.S., Williams, D.R., et al. (2018). Police killings and their spillover effects on the mental health of black Americans: A population-based, quasi-experimental study. *Lancet*, 392, 302–310.

Cant, R.L., Harries, M., & Chamarette, C. (2022). Using a public health approach to prevent child sexual abuse by targeting those at risk of harming children. *International Journal on Child Maltreatment: Research, Policy and Practice*. https://doi.org/10.1007/s42448-022-00128-7

Caruso, G.D. (2017). *Public health and safety: The social determinants of health and criminal behavior*. ResearchersLinks Books.

Cereda, M., Tracy, M., & Keyes, K.M. (2018). Reducing urban violence: A contrast of public health and criminal justice approaches. *Epidemiology*, 29, 142–150.

Chainey, S., Tompson, L., & Uhling, S. (2008). The utility of hotspot mapping for predicting spatial patterns of crime. *Security Journal*, 21(1–2), 4–28.

Champion, D.J. (1997). *The Roxbury dictionary of criminal justice: Key terms and major court cases*. Roxbury Publishing Company.

Chappell, D., & DiMartino, V. (1998). *Violence at work*. International Labor Office.

Chen, P.H., Jacobs, A., & Rovi, S.C.D. (2013). Intimate partner violence: IPV in the LGBT community. *FP Essentials*, 412, 28–35.

Choudhary, E., Gunzler, D., Tu, X., & Bossarte, R.M. (2012). Epidemiological characteristics of male sexual assault in a criminological database. *Journal of Interpersonal Violence*, 27(3), 523–546.

Comijs, H.C. et al. (1998). Elder abuse in the community: Prevalence and consequences. *Journal of the American Geriatrics Society*, 46, 885–888.

Cooper, H., Moore, L., Gruskin, S., & Krieger, N. (2004). Characterizing perceived police violence: implications for public health. *American Journal of Public Health*, 94(7), 1109–1118.

Coulter, M.L., Kuehnle, K., Byers, R., & Alfonso, M. (1999). Police-reporting behavior and victim – Police interactions as described by women in a domestic violence shelter. *Journal of Interpersonal Violence*, 14(12), 1290–1298.

Crabtree, S. (2022). Global study: 23% of workers experience violence/harassment. news.gallup.com/opinion/gallup/406793/global-study-workers-expereince-violence-harassment-aspx

Dantzker, M.L. (1998). *Criminology and criminal justice comparing, contrasting and intertwining disciplines*. Butterworth-Heinemann.

Dantzker, M.L., Hunter, R.D., & Quinn, S.T. (2018). *Research methods for criminology and criminal justice* (4th ed.). Jones & Bartlett Learning.

del Camen, R.V. (1991). *Civil liabilities in American policing: A text for law enforcement personnel*. A Prentice Hall Division.

Department of Health. (1998). South Africa. Demographic and Health Survey: Final report. Pretoria: Department of Health. www.dhsprogram.com/pubs/pdf/FR131/FR131.pd

DeVylder, J.E., Anglin, D.M., Bowleg, L., Fedina, L., & Link, B.G. (2022). Police violence and public health. *Annual Review of Clinical Psychology*, 18, 527–552.

Dufort, V.M., & Infante-Rivard, C. (1998). Housekeeping and safety: An epidemiological review. *Safety Science*, 28(2), 127–138.

Duthé, G., Hazard, A., & Kensey, A. (2014). Trends and risk factors for prisoner suicide in France. *Population*, 69(4), 463–494.

Edington, D.W., Schultz, A.B., Pitts, J.S., & Camilleri, A. (2016). The future of health promotion in the 21st century: A focus on the working population. *American Journal of Lifestyle Medicine*, 10(4), 242–252.

Edwards, F., Esposito, M.H., & Lee, H. (2018). Risk of police-involved death by race/ethnicity and place, United States, 2012–2018. *American Journal of Public Health*, 108(9), 1241–1248.

Ellington, R., Barajas, C.B., Drahota, A., Meghea, C., Uphold, H., Jamil, S., Lewis, E.Y., & Furr-Holden, D. (2022). An evaluation framework of a transdisciplinary collaborative center for health equity research. *American Journal of Evaluation*, 43(3), 357–377.

Ellsberg, M.C. et al. (1999). Wife abuse among women of childbearing age in Nicaragua. *American Journal of Public Health*, 89 241–244.

Ellsberg, M.C. et al. (2000). Candies in hell: Women's experience of violence in Nicaragua. *Social Science and Medicine*, 51, 1595–1610.

Fair, H., & Walmsley, R. (2021). *World prison population list* (13th ed.). World Prison Brief, Birkbeck.

Farmer, R. (2007). The problems with some epidemiological studies. *Maturitas*, 57, 11–15.

Favril, L. (2021). Epidemiology, risk factors, and prevention of suicidal thoughts and behavior in Prisons: A literature review. *Psychologica Belgica*, 61(1), 341–355.

Favril, L., Vander Laenen, F., Vandeviver, C., & Audenaert, K. (2017). Suicidal ideation while incarcerated: prevalence and correlates in a large sample of male prisoners in Flanders, Belgium. *International Journal of Law and Psychiatry*, 55, 19–28.

Favril, L., Wittouck, C., Audenaert, K., & Vander Laenen, F. (2019). A 17-year national study of prison suicides in Belgium. *Crisis*, 40(1), 42–53.

Fazel, S., Ramesh, T., & Hawton, K. (2017). Suicide in prisons: An international study of prevalence and contributory factors. *Lancet Psychiatry*, 4(12), 946–952. doi:10.1016/S2215-0366(17)30430-3. www.pubmed.ncbi.nlm.nih.gov/29179937/

Feldman, J.M., Gruskin, S., Coull, B.A., & Krieger, N. (2019). Police-related deaths and neighborhood economic and racial/ethnic polarization, United States, 2015–2016. *American Journal of Public Health*, 109(3), 458–464.

Fontanarosa, P.B., & Bibbons-Domingo, K. (2022). The unrelenting epidemic of firearm violence. *JAMA*, 328(12), 1201–1203.

Fortune, K. et al. (2018). Health promotion and the agenda for sustainable development, WHO region of the Americas. *Bulletin of the World Health Organization*, 96, 621–626.

Fritz, F.D., Fazel, S., Benavides, S. et al. (2021). 1324 prison suicides in 10 countries in South America: Incidence, relative risks, and ecological factors. *Social Psychiatry and Psychiatric Epidemiology*, 56(2), 315–323.

Garbarino, J., & Crouter, A. (1978). Defining the community context for parent-child relations: The correlates of child maltreatment. *Child Development*, 49, 604–616.

Gebo, E. (2016). An integrate public health and criminal justice approach to gangs: What can research tell us? *Preventive Medicine Reports*, 4, 376–380.

Gebo, E. (2022). Intersectoral violence prevention: The potential of public health-criminal justice partnerships. *Health Promotion International*, 37(3), 1–11.

Gettleman, J., & Yasir, S. (2020). Hundreds of police Killings in India, but no mass protests. *The New York Times*. Available: www.nytimes.com/2020/08/world/asia/india-police-brutality.html

Goldstick, J.E., Cunningham, R.M., & Carter, P.M. (2022). Current causes of death in children and adolescents in the United States. *The New England Journal of Medicine*, 386(2), 1955–1956.

Gorman, M., & Petersen, T. (1999). *Violence against older people and its health consequences: Experience from Africa and Asia*. HelpAge International.

Granados-Shiroma, M. (1996). *Salud reproductive y violencia contra la mujuer: un analisis desde la perspectiva de genero* [*Reproductive health and violence against women: A gender perspective.*] Nuevo Leon, Asociacion Mexicana de población, Consejo Estatal de Poblacion.

Grinshteyn, E., & Hemenway, D. (2019). Violent death rates in the US compared to those of the other high-income countries, 2015. *Preventive Medicine*, 123, 20–26.

Hall, D., Lee, L.W., Manseau, M.W., Watson, A.C., & Compton, M.T. (2019). Major mental illness as a risk factor for incarceration. *Psychiatric Services*, 70(12), 1088–1093.

Hartford, K., Carey, R., & Mendonca, J. (2007). Pretrial court diversion of people with mental illness. *Journal of Behavioral Health Services & Research*, 34(2), 198–205.

Hirschtick, J.L., Homan, S.M., Rauscher. G., Rubin, L.H., Johnson, T.P., et al. (2020). Persistent and aggressive inter- actions with the police: potential mental health implications. *Epidemiology and Psychiatric Sciences*, 29, e19.

Hoeffler, A., Kaiser, F., Pfeifle, B., & Risse, F. (2022). Tracking the SDGs: A methodological note on measuring deaths caused by collective violence. *The Economics of Peace and Security Journal*, 17(2), 32–46.

Hudson, M.F. (1991). Elder mistreatment: A taxonomy with definitions by Delphi. *Journal of Elder Abuse and Neglect*, 3, 1–20.

Human Rights Watch (2016). Brazil: Extrajudicial executions Undercut Rio security: Police killings persist as summer Olympics approach. Available: www.hrw.org/news/2016/07/07/brazil-extraj udicial-executions-undercut-rio-security

Hureau, D.M., Wilson, T., Rivera-Cuadrado, W., & Papachristos A.V. (2022). The experience of secondary traumatic stress among community violence interventionists in Chicago. *Preventive Medicine*, 165(Part A), 107186. https://doi.org/10.1016/j.ypmed.2022.107186

International Labor Organization (2022). Experience of violence and harassment at work. A global first survey.

Jewkes, R., & Abrahams, N. (2002). The epidemiology of rape and sexual coercion in South Africa: An overview. *Social Science and Medicine*, 55(7), 1231–1244. www.doi:10.1016/s0277-9536(01)00242-8. www.pubmed.ncbi.nlm.nih.gov/12365533/

Kaur, J., Manders, B., & Windsor-Shellard, B. (2019). *Drug-related deaths and suicide in prison custody in England and Wales: 2008 to 2016*. Office for National Statistics.

Kegler, S.R., Simon, T.R., & Sumner, S.A. (2023). Notes from the field: Firearm homicide rates, by race and ethnicity-United states, 2019-2022. *The Morbidity and Mortality Weekly Report*, 72(41), 1149–1150. doi:10.15585/mmwr.mm7242a4. www.pubmed.ncbi.nlm.nih.gov/37856328/

Kegler, S.R., Simon, T.R., Zwald, M.L. et al (2022). Changes in firearm homicide and suicide rates-United States, 2019-2020. *Morbidity and Mortality Weekly Report*, 71, 656–663.

Klonsky, E.D., Dixon-Luinenburg, T., & May, A.M. (2021). The critical distinction between suicidal ideation and suicide attempts. *World Psychiatry*, 20(3), 439–441.

Kosiack, D. (2022). *Legal aspects of corrections management* (4th ed.). Jones & Bartlett Learning.

Kraska, P.B. (2006). Criminal justice theory: Towards an infrastructure. *Justice Quarterly*, 23, 167–185.

Kraska, P.B., & Neuman, W.L. (2012). *Criminal justice and criminology research methods* (2nd ed.). Pearson.

Krug, E.G., Dahlberg, L.L., Mercy, J.A., Zwi, A.B., & Lozano, R. (2002). *World report on violence and health*. World Health Organization.

Kwan, A.Y. (1995). Elder abuse in Hong Kong: A new family problem from the east? In J.I. Kosberg & J.L. Garcia (Eds.), *Elder abuse: International and cross cultural perspectives* (pp. 65–80). Haworth Press.

Lanier, M.M. (2010). Epidemiological criminology (EpiCrim): Definition and application. *Journal of Theoretical and Philosophical Criminology*, 2(1), 63–103.

Lawlor, E.F., Kreuter, M.W., Sebert-Kuhlmann, A.K., & McBride, T.D. (2015). Methodological innovations in public health education: Transdisciplinary problem solving. *American Journal of Public Health*, 105(suppl 1), S99–S103.

Leibrich, J., Paulin, J., & Ransom, R. (1995). *Hitting home: Men speak out about domestic violence abuse of women partners*. Department of Justice and AGB McNair.

Lewallen, S., & Courtright, P. (1998). Epidemiology in practice: Case-control studies. *Community Eye Health*, 11(28), 57–58.

Liebling, A., & Ludlow, A. (2016). Suicide, distress and the quality of prison life. In Y. Jewkes, B. Crewe, & J. Bennett (Eds.), *Handbook on prisons* (pp. 224–245). Routledge.

Lilienfeld, A.M. (1983). Practical limitations of epidemiologic methods. *Environmental Health Perspectives*, 52, 3–8.

Louis-Philippe, B., & Kim, D. (2016). The effect of high school shootings on schools and student performance. *Educational Evaluation and Policy Analysis*, 38(1), 113–126.

Macassa, G., & McGrath, C. (2024). Common problems! and common solutions?- Teaching at the intersection between public health and criminology: A public health perspective. *Annals of Global Health*, 90(1), 12, 1–11. https://doi.org/10.5334/aogh.4375

MacMillian, H.L. (2000). Preventive health care, 2000 update: prevention of child maltreatment. *Canadian Medical Association Journal*, 163, 1451–1458.

Martin, L. (1999). Violence against women: An analysis of the epidemiology and patterns of injury in rape homicide in Cape Town and in rape in Johannesburg. Unpublished M.Med. Forensic Pathology Thesis, University of Cape Town.

Marzano, L., Hawton, K., Rivlin, A., Smith, E.N., Piper, M., & Fazel, S. (2016). Prevention of suicidal behavior in prisons. *Crisis*, 37(5), 323–334.

Matz, A.K., Wicklund, C., Douglas, J., & May, B. (2012). Justice-health collaboration: Improving information exchange between corrections and health/human service organizations. www.search.org/files/pdf/Justice-HealthCollaBusinessCase.pdf

Maxfield, M.G., & Babbie, E. (2008). *Research methods for criminal justice and criminology* (5th ed.). Thomson/Wadsworth.

Maxfield, M.G., & Babbie, E. (2011). *Research methods for criminal justice and criminology* (6th ed.). Wadsworth Cengage Learning.

Mccartan, K., & Prescott, D. (2020). Epidemiological criminology as a means to understanding sexual offending. Association for the Treatment & Prevention of Sexual Abuse (ATSA). Blog. https://blog.atsa.com/2020/03/epidemioloigcal-criminology-as-means-html

McGough, M., Amin, K., Panchel, N., & Cox, C. (2023). Child and teen-firearm mortality in the U.S. and peer countries KFF. www.kff.org/mental-health/issue-brief/child-and-teen-firearm-mortality-in-the-us-and-peer-countries/

Michels, K.B., Rosner, B.A., Chumlea, W.C., Colditz, G.A., & Willett, W.C. (2006). Preschool diet and adult risk of breast cancer. *International Journal of Cancer*, 118(3), 749–754.

Miner-Romanoff, K., & King, L. (2013). Crime and public health: Interdisciplinary approach to education. Presented as part of scholarship forum. Columbus, OH. https://fuse.franklin.edu/forum-2013/12

Mooney, J. (1993). *The hidden figure: Domestic violence in north London*. Middlesex University.

Morthorst, B.R., Mehlum, L., Palsson, S.P., Muhlmann, C., Hammerlin, Y., Madsen, T., et al. (2021). Suicide rates in Nordic prisons 2000–2016. *Archives of Suicide Research*, 25(3), 704–714.

National Research Council (1993). *Understanding child abuse and neglect*. National Academy of Sciences Press.

National Safety Council (2024). Assault at work. NSC: Injury facts. www.injuryfacts.nsc.org/work/safety-topics/assault/

Newburn, T. (2016). Social disadvantage, crime, and punishment. In D. H. Platt (Ed.), *Social advantage and disadvantage* (pp. 322–340). Oxford University Press.

Nielsen, N.R., Zhang, Z.F., Kristensen, T.S., Netterstrom, B., Schnohr, P., & Gronback, M. (2005). Self-reported stress and risk of breast cancer: Prospective cohort study. *BMJ*, 331(7516), 548.

Nilson, C. (2018). Community safety and well-being: Concept, practice, and alignment. *Journal of Community Safety and Well-Being*, 3(3), 96–104.

Nishar, S., Brumfield, E., & Mandal, S. et al. (2023). "It's a revolving door": Understanding the social determinants of mental health as experienced by formerly incarcerated people. *Health Justice*, 11(26). https://doi.org/10.1186/s40352-023-00227-8

Occupational Safety and Health Administration (OSHA) (2015). Preventing workplace violence: A road map for healthcare facilities. Department of Labor. www.osha.gov/sites/default/files/OSHA3827.pdf

Ogg, J., & Bennett, G.C.J. (1992). Elder abuse in Britain. *British Medical Journal*, 305, 998–999.

Oliver, W.M., & Hilgenberg, J.F. (2006). *A history of crime and criminal justice in America*. Pearson/Allyn and Bacon.

O'Loughlin, A., & Duggan, J. (1998). Abuse, neglect, and mistreatment of older people: An exploratory study. National Council on Ageing and Older People. (Report No. 52).

Opitz-Welke, A., Bennefeld-Kersten, K., Konrad, N., & Welke, J. (2013). Prison suicides in Germany from 2000 to 2011. *International Journal of Law and Psychiatry*, 36(5–6), 386–389.

Pillemer, K., & Finkelhor, D. (1988). Prevalence of elder abuse: A random sample survey. *The Gerontologist*, 28, 51–57.

Podnieks, E. (1992). National survey on abuse of the elderly in Canada. *Journal of Elderly Abuse and Neglect*, 4, 5–58.

Potter, R.H., & Akers, T.A. (2010). Improving the health of minority communities through probation-public health collaborations: An application of the epidemiological criminology framework. *Journal of Offender Rehabilitation*, 49(8), 595–609.

Potter, R.H., & Akers, T.A. (2013). Epidemiological criminology and violence prevention: Addressing the co-occurrence of criminal violence and poor health outcomes. In A.M. Viens, J. Coggon, & A.L. Kessel (Eds.), *Criminal law, philosophy, and public health practice* (pp. 171–191). Cambridge University Press.

Potter, R.H., & Rosky, J.W. (2013). The iron fist in the latex glove: The intersection of public health and criminal justice. *American Journal of Criminal Justice*, 38, 276–288.

Quadara, A., Nagy, V., Higgins, D., & Siegel, N. (2015). Conceptualising the prevention of child sexual abuse: Final report (Report No. 33). Australian Institute of Family Studies. https://aifs.gov.au/publications/family-relationships-and-disclosure-institutional-child-sexual-abuse

Rabe, K. (2012). Prison structure, inmate mortality and suicide risk in Europe. *International Journal of Law and Psychiatry*, 35(3), 222–230.

Randal, J., & German, T. (1999). *The ageing and development report: Poverty, independence, and the world's people*. HelpAge International.

Ratcliffe, J. (2010). Crime mapping: Spatial and temporal challenges. In A.R., Piquero & D. Weisburd (Eds.), *Handbook of Quantitative Criminology*. https://doi.org/10.1007/978-0-387-77650-7_2

Redo, S. (2017). The 2030 United Nations sustainable development agenda and academic criminology. *International Annals of Criminology*, 55(1), 132–146.

Reingle, J.M., & Akers, T.A. (2017). Transdisciplinary research perspective: Epidemiological criminology as an emerging framework for substance abuse research. In J.B. VanGeest et al., (Eds.), *Research methods in the study of substance abuse* (pp. 27–40). Springer International Publishing. https://doi.org/10.1007/978-3-319-55980-3_2

Remington, F. (1990). Development of criminal justice as an academic field. *Journal of Criminal Justice Education*, 1, 9–20.

Rennison, C.M., & Hart, T.C. (2019). *Research methods in criminal justice and criminology*. Sage.

Reza, A., Mercy, J.A., & Krug, E. (2001). Epidemiology of violent deaths in the world. *Injury Prevention*, 7, 104–111.

Ridgeway, G. (2019). Experiments in criminology: Improving our understanding of crime and the criminal justice system. *Annual Review of Statistics and Its Application*, 6(1), 37–61.

Rivara, F.P., Studdert, D.M., & Wintermute, G.P. (2018). Firearm-related mortality: A global public health problem. *JAMA*, 320(8), 764–765.

Rivlin, A., Hawton, K., Marzano, L., & Fazel, S. (2010). Psychiatric disorders in male prisoners who made near- lethal suicide attempts: case-control study. *British Journal of Psychiatry*, 197(4), 313–319.

Rodriguez, R.C., & Tynan, K.F., (2024). California's workplace violence prevention plan law, SB 553, takes effect on July 1, 2024: Three weeks until required compliance. Ogletree Deakins.

Rosenberg, M.L., & Fenley, M.A. (1991). *Violence in America: A public health approach*. Oxford University Press.

Rothman, K.J. (1986). *Modern epidemiology*. Little Brown & Co.

Rotter, M., & Compton, M. (2022). Criminal legal involvement: A cause and consequence of social determinants of health. *Psychiatric Services*, 73(1), 108–111.

Rush, G.E. (2003). *The dictionary of criminal justice: With summaries of Supreme Court cases affecting criminal justice* (6th ed.). Dushkin/McGraw-Hill.

Schneider, M.J. (2020). *Introduction to public health* (6th ed.). Jones and Bartlett Learning.

Schram, P.J., & Tibbetts, S.G. (2014). *Introduction to criminology*. Sage.

Schumacher, S., Kirzinger, A., Presiado, M., Valdes, I., & Brodie, M. (2023). *Americans experience with gun-related violence, injuries, and deaths.* KFF. www.kff.org/other/poll-finding/americans-experiences-with-gun-related-vioelnce-injuries-and-deaths/

Schweig, S. (2014). Healthy communities may make safe communities: Public health approaches to violence prevention. *National Institute of Justice Journal.* https://nij.ojp.gov

Shiner, M., Carre, Z., Delsol, R., & Eastwood, N. (2020). The colour of injustice: 'Race', drugs and law enforcement in England and Wales. The London School of Economics and Political Science. Available: www.lse.ac.uk/united-states/Assets/Documents/the-Colour-of-Injustice.pdf

Sibbald, B., & Roland, M. (1998). Understanding controlled trials: Why are randomized controlled trials important? *The* BMJ, 316(7126), 201. https://doi.org/10.1136/bmj.316.7126.201

Siegel, L.J. (1998). *Criminology* (6th ed.). West/Wadsworth Publishing.

Skvortsova, T. (2013). Epicrim and child sexual abuse: A public health theory for a criminal justice epidemic. Unpublished Thesis: University of Alabama. Tuscaloosa, Alabama.

Smith, G.D. (2001). Reflections on the limitations to epidemiology. *Journal of Clinical Epidemiology,* 54, 325–331.

Southern Poverty Law Center (2023). Everytown for gun safety support fund, & polarization and extremism research and innovation lab. U.S. Youth Attitudes on Guns Report. www.splcenter.org/peril-youth-attitudes-guns-report

Stoudemire, A. et al. (1986). The economic burden of depression. *General Hospital Psychiatry,* 8, 387–394.

Swart, L., Gilchrist, A., Butchard, A., Seedat, M., & Martin, L. (1999). Rape surveillance trough district surgeons' offices in Johannesburg, 1996–1998: Evaluation and prevention implications. Institute of Social and Health Sciences. University of South Africa.

Swensen, K., Murza, G., Sulzer, S.H., & Voss, M.W. (2020). Public health violence prevention: Supporting law enforcement (2020). *All Current Publications.* Paper 2123.https://digitalcommons.usu.edu/extension_curall/2123

Szklo, M. (1998). Population-based cohort studies. *Epidemiologic Review,* 20(1), 81–90.

Tenny, S., Kerndt, C.C., & Hoffman, M.R. (2023). Case control studies. In: StatPearls Treasure Island: StatPearls Publishing: 2024. PMID: 28846237.

Thacker, S.B., & Stroup, D.F. (1998). Public health surveillance and health services research. In H.K. Armenian & S. Shapiro (Eds.), *Epidemiology and Health Services* (pp. 61–82). Oxford University Press.

Thygesen, L.C., & Ersboll, A.K. (2014). When the entire population is the sample: Strengths and limitations in register-based epidemiology. *European Journal of Epidemiology,* 29, 551–558. doi: 10.1007/s10654-013-9873-0

Tjaden, P., & Thoennes, N. (2000). Full report of the prevalence, incidence, and consequences of violence against women: Findings from the National Violence Against Women Survey. Washington, DC, National Institute of Justice, Office of Justice programs, United States Department of Justice and Centers for Disease Control and Prevention (NCJ 183781).

UK Home Office (2019). Police use of force statistics, England and Wales. April 2018 to March 2019. Available: www.gov.uk/government/statistics/police-use-of-force-statistics-england-and-wales-april-2018-to-march-2019

Unicef (2024). Sexual violence. https://data.unicef.org/topic/child-protection/violence/sexual-violence/

VanderWeele, T.J. (2019). Measures of community-well-being: A template. *International Journal of Community Well-Being,* 2, 253–275.

VanDyke, M.E., Chen, M.S., Sheppard, M. et al. (2022). Country-level social vulnerability and emergency department visits for firearm injuries-10 U.S. jurisdictions. *Morbidity and Mortality Weekly Report,* 11(27), 873–877.

Vanhaesebrouck, A., Fovet, T., Melchior, M., & Lefevre, T. (2024). Risk factors of suicide in prisons: A comprehensive retrospective cohort study in France, 2017-2020. *Social Psychiatry and Psychiatric Epidemiology,* 59, 1931–1941.

Wang, X, & Cheg, Z. (2020). Cross-sectional studies: Strengths, weaknesses, and recommendations. *Chest*, 158(1S), S65–S71.

Wattermaurer, E., & Akers, T. (2014). *Epidemiological criminology* (1st ed.). Routledge.

Whitelaw, S., Baxendale, A., Bryce, C., MacHardy, L., Young, I., & Witney, E. (2001). Setting based health promotion: A review. *Health Promotion International*, 16(4), 339–354.

WHO (2024). Youth violence. www.who.int/news-room/fact-sheets/detail/youth-violence

Williams, F.P., & McShane, M.D. (1999). *Criminological theory* (3rd ed.). Prentice-Hall.

Wolf, R.S., & Pillemer, K.A. (1989). *Helping elderly victims: The reality of elder abuse*. Columbia University Press.

Wolfe, D.A. et al. (1988). Early intervention for parents at risk of child abuse and neglect. *Journal of Consulting and Clinical Psychology*, 56, 40–47.

Yoshihama, M., & Sorenson, S.B. (1994). Physical, sexual, and emotional abuse by male intimates: Experiences of women in Japan. *Violence and Victims*, 9, 63–77.

Zhong, S., Senior, M. et al. (2021). Risk factors for suicide in prisons: A systematic review and meta-analysis. *Lancet Public Health*, 6(3), e164–e174.

INDEX

Note: Figures are shown in *italics* and tables in **bold** type. "EpiCrim" refers to epidemiological criminology

abandonment, of elderly 266, 273
abuse: elderly 117–118, 264–285; emotional *see* emotional abuse; financial *see* financial abuse; online 228, 232, 250; physical *see* physical abuse; psychological *see* psychological abuse; sexual *see* sexual abuse; *see also* neglect; stalking
access to healthcare *see* healthcare
accidental deaths 93, 438, 439, 449, 452
acculturative stress 307, 318
ACEs (adverse childhood experiences) 112, 116, 298, 495, 504; and suicide 304–305, 306
acquaintance/date rape 192
acquired immune deficiency syndrome (AIDS) 15, 77, 204, 239, 243; and blood-borne disease risk 503–504
active surveillance 10, 21
adult interpersonal violence 118–119
adverse childhood experiences (ACEs) 112, 116, 298, 495, 504; and suicide 304–305, 306
affluence 4, 40, 41, 99, 361, 497, 551
aggressive behavior 57, 110, 198, 235; in children 34; children witnessing 86–87; in elderly 469, 543; learning of 44, 195; *see also* bullying
AHTF (Anti-Heroin Task Force) Program 505
AIDS *see* acquired immune deficiency syndrome (AIDS)
alcohol use 29, 32, 88, 105, *149*, 204, 234, 306, 312, 384
American Public Health Association (APHA) 55, 112, 116, 121, 309, 314–315, 349, 350, 358, 359, 364, 412, 428, 463

Amnesty International 201–202, 342, 351, 538, 541, 546
anti-bullying campaigns and policies 124, 384, 391, 392, 393
anticipatory guidance and firearm-retirement counseling 469
Anti-Heroin Task Force (AHTF) Program 505
anti-LGBTQIA hate crimes 103–104
APHA *see* American Public Health Association (APHA)
apprehending offenders 6–7, 111, 200, 205, 525
Asians: crimes against 102–103; and teenage bullying 378
assaultive violence (AS) 99–100, 126–127; as criminal justice issue 111–112, 119–120; definition of 100; and EpiCrim 538; international comparative statistics for 113–115; nature and extent of 100–101; negative health consequences of 116–119; policy recommendations for 125–126; prevention of 123–125; as public health issue 112–113, 115–117, 120–121; risk factors for 105–107; roots of 104–105; and social epidemiology 122–123; as social work issue 115–117, 121; and social-ecological model 107–111; types of 102–104; *see also* intimate partner violence (IPV)
assisted dying 308
asthma 27, 101, 116, 117, 161, 204, 244, 353
ATF (Bureau of Alcohol, Tobacco, Firearms, and Explosives) 450, 460, 462, 497, 498
attachment element of social bonds 48–49, *148*, *149*, 196, 312
auto-accidents, public health approaches to 16–18

behavior: aggressive *see* aggressive behavior; changes in 18–19, 247, 539; criminal *see* criminal behavior; problem 31, 172, 343–344, 381, 509–510, 530
behavioral parent training programs 172
beliefs element of social bonds 48, 49
biological causes, of violence 33–34, 235, 277
bipolar disorder 161, 300, 305, 306, 486
Black males 5, 28, 29, 31, 55, 343, 365; and firearm violence 440, 456; police violence against 337–338; protesters 336–337, 365; suicide of 302–303, 316, 318
Black youth 298–299, 302–303, 309, 343, 457
Blacks: crimes against 102; and teenage bullying 378
blood-borne disease risk 503–504
body cameras 356
bourgeoisie 52–53
broken windows 57–58, 236
bullying 118; *see also* cyberbullying; teenage bullying (TB)
burdensomeness 278, 302, 318
Bureau of Alcohol, Tobacco, Firearms, and Explosives (ATF) 450, 460, 462, 497, 498

CA *see* child abuse (CA)
CAC (Children's Advocacy Center) 157
campus rape 192–193
CAP (Child Access Prevention) laws 470, 472
capitalism 52–53, 54–55, 194
CAPTA (Child Abuse and Prevention and Treatment Act) 136, 147
cardiovascular disease (CVD) 28, 158, 277, 354
caregiver disability 143
caregiver mental illness 285
caregiver relationships 271
case–control studies 528, 529, 553, 554–555
census data 77–78, 93
child abuse (CA) 135, 175–176; as criminal justice issue 157–158, 162–164; definition of 135–137; and EpiCrim 538–539; global statistics on 114–115, 159–160; nature and extent of 137–138; negative health consequences of 161–162; policy recommendations for 173–175; prevention of 170–173; as public health issue 158–159, 164–166; risk factors for 142–147, *148–151*; roots of 141–142; and social epidemiology 166–170; as social work issue 166; types of 138–141, **139–140**; *see also* child sexual abuse; child sexual exploitation and abuse (CSEA)
Child Abuse and Prevention and Treatment Act (CAPTA) 136, 147
Child Access Prevention (CAP) laws 470, 472
Child Maltreatment Report Rates 143–144
child protection 136, 157, 164, 165–166, 168–169

Child Protective Services (CPS) 137
child sexual abuse (CSA) 152–156; definitions of 147, 151–152; and EpiCrim 539–540
child sexual exploitation and abuse (CSEA) 153–154, 155
childcare 167, 170, 171, 174, *150*
Children's Advocacy Center (CAC) 157
child-to-parent family violence 59–60
choice theory 36–37, 525; rational (RCT) 36–37, 38
class: dominant 53, 60–61, 344; inequality of 31; lower *see* lower class; middle 41–42, 43, 110; upper 41, 43, 44, 53–54, 110; working 53
COAP (Comprehensive Opioid Abuse Grant Program) 505
cognitive causes, of violence 33, 34, 56, 87, 380
cognitive processing therapy (CPT) 203, 242, 311
cohort studies 105, 553, 528, 529, 554–555
commitment element of social bonds 47, 48, *48*, 49
community education 203, 281, 386
community health 275–276, 279, 280, 285, 358, 364, 465
Community Oriented Policing Services (COPS) 462, 505
community overdose response inequity 495–497
community partnerships 280
community policing 7, 8, 21, 282
community risk factors 529; for assaultive violence 109–110, 116, 124; for elder abuse 271–273; for firearm injuries 440, 448–449; for intimate partner violence 236, 251; for opioid addiction 495–497; for police violence 344, 346; for sexual violence 198, 215; for suicide 307–308; for teenage bullying 382–383; for workplace violence (WPV) 408, 410
community support networks 167
Community Violence Intervention (CVI) 462, 467, 468, 472
community-based proactive law enforcement 460
community/societal risk factors, for child abuse 147, *148–151*
Comprehensive Opioid Abuse Grant Program (COAP) 505
conflict theory 51
consent: and cyberbullying 377; and disclosure of employee information 420; relationships based on 249; for sexual activity 141, 147, 151, 173, 188, 192, 203, 205, 228
constitutional rights 111, 201, 348, 355, 357, 450
containment theory 47–48, *48*
contextual stressors, for violence 55–60
control theory 47–49, *48*; self- 194, 195–196; social 48, 49

controlled clinical trials 528, 530
COPS (Community Oriented Policing Services) 462, 505
coronary heart disease 17, 116
COVID-19: elder abuse during 265; and firearms 227, 438, 442, 443, 449; and health data 74–75; and health inequalities 91; and health spending 90; and intimate partner violence 231; and race 30; as social stressor 59, 438; and suicide 438; and violence against healthcare workers 412; and violent crime 1; and youth drug use 487
CPS (Child Protective Services) 137
CPT (cognitive processing therapy) 203, 242, 311
crack cocaine epidemic 16, 117, 347, 499–500
crime, definition of 2–3
crime rates 1, 40, 83, 84, 101, 346, 349, 365, 490
crime reduction 8, 50, 58, 62, 106, 120, 459–461, 525
criminal behavior, social determinants of 532–533
criminal justice: as academic discipline 525; and assaultive violence 111–112, 119–120; emergence of 530–531; approaches to violence and crime 19–20
criminogenic health disparities 30–32
criminological explanations, of violence 35–44
criminology: as academic discipline 525–526; emergence of 530–531; and public health 531–532; of violence 26–63, *33, 48, 61*
cross-sectional studies 83, 346, 443, 467, 528, 529, 555
CSA (child sexual abuse) 152–156; definitions of 147, 151–152; and EpiCrim 539–540
CSEA (child sexual exploitation and abuse) 153–154, 155
cultural context, effect on violence of 56
Cultural Deviance Theory 39, 43–44
cultural stereotypes 43–44, 344, 378
culture, effect on violence of 56
culture of violence theory 196–197
CVD (cardiovascular disease) 28, 158, 277, 354
CVI (Community Violence Intervention) 462, 467, 468, 472
cyberbullying 118, 126, 298, 303; teenage 375, 376, 377–378, 383, 385, 391, 392, 393
cyberstalking 232
cycle of violence 61, 195, 207, 208, 228–229, 236, 239, 342, 524

dash cameras 356
data dissemination 15, 21
date/acquaintance rape 192
date-related physical violence 241
death rates 30, 334, 536; firearm 437, 441–442, 454; high 29–30; overdose 496

delinquency 39–40, 43, 45, 47, 158, 236; juvenile 32, 62, 171, 172, 525; violent 233
Department of Health and Human Services 17, 18, 57, 81, 137, 138, 140–141, 142, 158, 190, 192, 274, 304, 313, 390, 496–497, 503–504
deprivation 2, 26, 100, 106, 233, 303, 409–410, 413, 531, 545
deviance 49, 419; cultural 39, 43–44; primary 50; secondary 50
diabetes 3, 37, 78, 81, 88, 239, 242, 301, 353, 354, 361, 442, 459; Type 2 28, 29, 161
Diagnostic and Statistical Manual of Mental Disorders, Fifth Edition, Text Revision (DSM-5-TR) 486–487
differential association theory 44–46
differential reinforcement theory 44, 45–46
disability 27, 28, 74, 78, 102; and bullying 376, 377, 381, 384, 392; caregiver 143; children with 146, *149,* 155–156; and gun violence 463, 467; inequalities due to 146, 155–156; mental 29, 266, 300; physical 266, 270, 272, 300
disgruntled employee/coworker 405, 406
domestic violence 143, 405, *411,* 447; *see also* intimate partner violence
dominant class 53, 60–61, 344
Drug Court Discretionary Grant program 505
drug use *see* opioid addiction
DSM-5-TR (*Diagnostic and Statistical Manual of Mental Disorders, Fifth Edition, Text Revision*) 486–487

EA *see* elderly abuse (EA)
early education 167, 170, 171
economic abuse 231; elder 266
economic burden 29, 30, 85, 152, 284
economic inequality 493, 510, 511–512
economic insecurity 144, *150,* 199, 241
economic support, for families 166–167, 170–171
ECV (exposure to community violence) 116
educational campaigns 18–19, 21, 126, 213, 214, 510, 532, 552
Educational Fund to Stop Gun Violence (EFSGV) 440, 448, 463
EJA (Elder Justice Act) 268, 273, 276
EJI (Elder Justice Initiative) 268, 273–274, 278, 279
elder abandonment 266, 273
elder abuse *see* elderly abuse
elder economic abuse 266
elder financial exploitation 266
Elder Justice Act (EJA) 268, 273, 276
Elder Justice Initiative (EJI) 268, 273–274, 278, 279
elder neglect 266
elder physical abuse 265

elder psychological abuse 266
elder sexual abuse 265–266
elderly abuse (EA) 117–118, 264, 284–285;
    as criminal justice issue 273–274, 278–279;
    definition of 264; and EpiCrim 542–543;
    international comparative statistics for
    275; nature and extent of 265; negative
    health consequences of 277–278; policy
    recommendations for 283–284; prevention
    of 282–283; as public health issue 274,
    279–281; risk factors for 268–273; roots of
    267–268; and social epidemiology 281–282;
    as social work issue 275–277, 281; types of
    265–267
EMDR (eye movement desensitization and
    reprocessing) 203, 242
emotional abuse 114, 405; of children 136, 138,
    140, *148*, 155, 158, 162, 173; of elderly 266,
    267, 275, 283, 543; of intimate partners 226,
    228, 229–230, 235, 239
environment, effect on violence of 57–58
EpiCrim (epidemiological criminology)
    533–534; and assaultive violence 538; and
    child abuse 538–539; and child sexual abuse
    539–540; and elderly abuse 542–543; and
    firearm injuries 550–552; and intimate
    partner violence 541–542; and police violence
    545–547; and sexual assault 540–541; and
    suicidal violence 543–545; surveillance
    537–538; and teenage violence 547–548; and
    workplace violence 548–550
epidemics, violence and crime as 5, 10, 14,
    15–16, 21
epidemiological approach, to study violence and
    crime 19–20, 26–27, 524–556
epidemiological criminology *see* EpiCrim
    (epidemiological criminology)
epidemiological studies 530; problems and
    limitations of 552–555
epidemiological triangle 33, *33*
epidemiology: as academic discipline 526–527;
    and criminology of violence 26–63, *33*, *48*,
    61; data of 528; how it works 32; research
    designs of 528–530; social *see* social
    epidemiology; techniques of 527–528
ethnic inequality 335
evolutionary theory 194, 196, 215
exposure to community violence (ECV) 116
eye movement desensitization and reprocessing
    (EMDR) 203, 242

families, economic support for 166–167,
    170–171
family court 163, 164
family violence: child-to-parent 59–60; parent-
    to-child 59, 60
Fatal Force Database 462
feminist theory 215; Marxist 54–55; radical 194

financial abuse 228, 231, 265, 266, 267, 270,
    272, 274, 275, 285, 405, 543
firearm death rates 437, 441–442, 454; *see also*
    firearm mortality
firearm homicides 105, 437, 438, 453, 467;
    rates of 105, 438, 441–442, 468, 550, 551
firearm injuries 436–474, *444*, *445*, *447*, **451**,
    455, *456*, *465*; as criminal justice issue
    449–452, **451**, 459–462; definition of
    436–437; and EpiCrim 550–552;
    international comparative statistics for
    453–454; negative health consequences of
    458–459; policy recommendations for
    471–474; prevention of 468–470; as public
    health issue 463–466, *465*; risk factors for
    440–449, *444*, *445*, *447*; as social work issue
    465–466
firearm mortality 31, 454–455; global statistics
    on 550–551; *see also* firearm death rates
firearm violence 31–32
firearm-retirement counseling 469
Floyd, George 336, 341, 449

gang activity 8, 42, 43
gang violence 115, 116, 120
gangs 41–42, 44, 47, 56, 110, 346, 376, 440,
    547; and opioid addiction 490, 497, 499
gender: and child abuse 144–145; effect on
    violence of 56; and elder abuse 270
gender identity 102, 295, 297, 299, 341, 376,
    378, 379, 392
gender inequality 144–145, 155, 199, 209, 213,
    245, 379
gender stereotypes 249
general strain 42
Germ Theory of Disease 34
global statistics: on assaultive violence (AV)
    113–115, 127; on child abuse 114–115; on
    child sexual exploitation and abuse (CSEA)
    153–154; on firearm mortality 550–551; on
    homicides 114; on prison population 544
grand juries 6, 111, 349, 356
guns: homicide rate 105, 438, 441–442, 468,
    550, 551; laws on 81, 439, 440, 448, 449,
    450, **451**, 459, 465, 466; restrictions on use
    of 449; smart technology for 469; violence
    involving 104, 119, 127, 349, 552; *see also*
    firearm injuries

hate crimes 52, 102, 273, 340, 377, 388, 408,
    412, 423; anti-LGBTQIA 103–104
health, social determinants of 532–533
health data 12, 537, 540, 542; on injuries
    85–86; for victimization 35, 73–94
health disparities: consequences of 29–30;
    criminogenic 30–32; definition of 27; and
    health equities 116, 161, 203–204, 242–243,
    276–277, 311–312, 353, 386, 414; notable

28–29; *see also* cancer; cardiovascular disease (CVD); diabetes; infant mortality; mental health; stroke
health equities, and health disparities 116, 161, 203–204, 242–243, 276–277, 311–312, 353, 386, 414
health inequality 62, 91, 122, 168, 233
health insurance 77–78, 89–90, 91, 458
healthcare: access 4, 27, 62, 90–91, 110, 122, 166, 208, 210, 307, 350, 359, 361, 510, 533; systems 1, 2, 17, 88, 89–90, 94, 122, 203, 227, 413, 472, 508, 510, 512, 537; workforce 274, 280, 284, 510
high death rates, and lack of insurance 29–30
HIV/AIDS *see* acquired immune deficiency syndrome (AIDS)
homicide rates 16, 452; firearm 105, 438, 441–442, 468 550, 551; and impoverished Black males 5; and income inequality 106; and younger Americans 4; youth 547–548
homicides: firearm 105, 437, 438, 453, 467; global statistics on 114
hot spots 8, 119–120, 388, 459
humiliation 34, 195, 266, 351

ICD (International Classification of Diseases) *444, 445,* 487
illegal drugs 109, 125, 235, 491, 528; *see also* street drugs
income inequality 122, 213, 440, 466, 467, 473, 535; effect on violence of 58–59
individual parent/child relationship risk factors, for child abuse 146
individual risk factors 37, 543; for assaultive violence 107–108; for child abuse 146; for elder abuse 270–271; for firearm injuries 440, 442–446, *444, 445*; for intimate partner violence (IPV) 233, 235, 251; for opioid addiction 493–495, 507, 512; for police violence 344, 345; for rape 197, 198, 215; for sexual assault 197, 198, 215; for sexual violence 197; for suicide 304–306; for teenage bullying (TB) 381–382; for workplace violence (WPV) 408, 409
INEP (International Network for Epidemiology in Policy) 471, 473–474
inequalities 4, 39; in assaultive violence (AS) 106–107; and Black youth 448; in bullying 381; and capitalism 53; in child abuse (CA) 143–146; in child sexual abuse (CSA) 154–156; class 31; disability 146, 155–156; economic 493, 510, 511–512; in elder abuse 268–270; ethnic 335; and firearm injuries 440–442; gender 144–145, 155, 199, 209, 213, 245, 379; health 62, 91, 122, 168, 233; income 58–59, 122, 213, 440, 466, 467, 473, 535; and intimate partner violence (IPV)

234–235; and Latinx youth 448; in mortality 282; in opioid addiction 492–493; in police violence 344–345; racial 31, 122, 145–146, 155, 213, 335, 441, 442, 511–512; and sexual violence 199, 213; social 35, 122, 147, 209–210, 248, 440, 508, 533; socioeconomic 147, 199, 214, 492; in status in society 34; structural 247, 249, 346, 347, 361, 440–441, 448; and suicide 302–304; in teenage bullying 380–381; and women 54, 245; in workplace violence (WPV) 408–409; *see also* poverty
inequity *see* inequality
infant mortality 28, 40, 77
injuries, health data on 85–86
inmates: deliberate indifference to health of 532; opioid addiction of 498–499, 500; suicide of 312–313, 544–545; *see also* jail/prison rape
Institute of Medicine and National Research Council 55
institutions, and elder abuse 271–272
insurance 27, 29; health 77–78, 89–90, 91, 458; lack of 29–30, 467; and opioid addiction 510–511
inter-adult violence 87
International Classification of Diseases (ICD) *444, 445,* 487
international comparative statistics: for assaultive violence 113–115; for elderly abuse 275; for firearm injuries 453–454; for intimate partner violence 240–241; for opioid addiction 501; for police violence 350–352; for rape 201–203; for sexual assault 201–203; for suicide 310; for teenage bullying 385–386; for workplace violence 414
International Network for Epidemiology in Policy (INEP) 471, 473–474
interpersonal theory of suicide 302, 306
interpersonal violence 241–242, 247, 437, 547, 553; adult 118–119; and suicide 306; *see also* elderly abuse (EA)
intervention 5–6; evaluation of 11, 21
intimate partner domestic violence *see* intimate partner violence (IPV)
Intimate Partner Resource for Action 249
intimate partner violence (IPV) 117, 224–251, 405–406; as criminal justice issue 237–238, 244–245; definition of 225–226; and EpiCrim 541–542; international comparative statistics for 240–241; negative health consequences for men of 243–244; policy recommendations for 250; prevention of 249; as public health issue 238–240, 245–248; risk factors for 233–237; as social work issue 247–248
involvement element of social bonds 48, 49
IPDV *see* intimate partner violence (IPV)
IPV *see* intimate partner violence (IPV)

isolation 140, *149*, 166, 168, 235, 359, 410, 438, 443; and elderly abuse 264, 269, 270, 271, 272, 276, 278, 284; and epidemiology 543, 545, 550; and opioid addiction 494, 495, 509; and suicide 301, 302, 306, 318

jail/prison rape 193
job training 167, 389
Johns Hopkins Center for Gun Violence 473–474
justice system-involved opioid addiction 494
juvenile court 39–40, 142, 164
juvenile delinquency 32, 62, 171, 172, 525

labeling theory 49–51
law enforcement 19–20, 79, 82, 83, 164, 174–175, 278–279; and bullying 387–388; and crime reduction 459–461; and firearm violence 442; and LGBTQ+ community 339–340; militarized 338; and officer suicide 308–309, 313, 314; and opioid addiction 505; proactive 459–460
lead poisoning 3, 31
learning theories 44–47
lethal means restrictive counseling 468–469
lethal violence 78–80, 93, 343
LGBTQIA community: crimes against 103–104; intimate partner violence within 232–233; and opioid addiction 494; police violence against 339–341; and suicide 297–298
life skills 172
life-course approach 62–63
loneliness *149*, 278, 301, 318, 442, 458, 469
longitudinal designs 105, 553, 528, 529, 554–555
love triangle 405–406, 549
lower class 39, 41–42, 43–44, 53–54, 194, 234, 362; and assaultive violence 101, 106, 108, 109–110
Lower-Class Status Frustration and Gang Formation 41–42

made to penetrate (MTP) 204
mandatory federal database, of police shootings 356–357
Mapping Police Violence 334, 338, 346, 347, 357
Marxist feminist theory 54–55
Marxist theory 52–55
mass shootings 1, 100, 436, 438, 439, 450, 452, 453, 463
mental disability 29, 266, 300
mental health 29; disorders of 27, 161, 205, 242, 306, 311, 353, 437, 455, 457, 503, 545; services for 166, 167, 168, 272, 298, 299, 303, 309, 317, 473, 506, 510, 531
mental illness 27, 29, 57, 271; caregiver 285; history of 304; and suicide 305, 307, 311, 495

middle class 41–42, 43, 110
militarized law enforcement 338
military personnel 193, 208, 301
military rape 193
minority populations 28, 52, 91, 277, 546
minority women 105–106, 226–227
MTP (made to penetrate) 204
multidisciplinary issue, violence as 60–61

National Center for Education Statistics (NCES) 383
National Center for Injury Prevention and Control (NCIPC) 61, 101, 105, 239, 240, 458, 492
National Centers for Health Statistics (NCHS) 74, 76, 77, 80, 537
National Child Abuse and Neglect Data System (NCANDS) 135–136, 142–143
National Children's Alliance (NCA) 137–138
National Coalition of Anti-Violence Programs 227, 340
National Crime Victimization Survey (NCVS) 75, 82–83, 84–85, 91–92, 93–94, 102, 103, 152, 189, 383, 403, 537
National Crimes against Children Investigators Association (NCACIA): public health model of 167–168; strategies of 166–167, 168–169, 170
National Incident-Based Reporting System (NIBRS) 75, 82, 84, 91, 93–94, 201, 537
National Intimate Partner and Sexual Violence Survey (NISVS) 78, 190, 227, 304
National Policy Summit on Elder Abuse 279
National Violent Death Reporting System (NVDRS) 79, 93, 297, 303–304, 305–306, 409
NCA (National Children's Alliance) 137–138
NCACIA *see* National Crimes against Children Investigators Association (NCACIA)
NCANDS (National Child Abuse and Neglect Data System) 135–136, 142–143
NCES (National Center for Education Statistics) 383
NCHS (National Centers for Health Statistics) 74, 76, 77, 80, 537
NCIPC (National Center for Injury Prevention and Control) 61, 101, 105, 239, 240, 458, 492
NCVS *see* National Crime Victimization Survey (NCVS)
negative health consequences: 1, 3, 17, 21; of assaultive violence 116–119; of child abuse 161–162; of elderly abuse 277–278; of firearm injuries 458–459l; of intimate partner violence for men 243–244; of opioid addiction 504; of police violence 354; of rape 204–205; of sexual assault 204–205; of suicide 312; of

teen bullying 387; of workplace violence 418–419
negative punishment 46
negative reinforcement 45, 46, 124
negative social control 405
neglect: of children 140–141; elder 266
Neoclassical School of Criminology 37–38
neutralization theory 44, 46
NIBRS (National Incident-Based Reporting System) 75, 82, 84, 91, 93–94, 201, 537
NISVS (*National Intimate Partner and Sexual Violence Survey*) 78, 190, 304
non-intimate partner abusers 271
NVDRS (National Violent Death Reporting System) 79, 93, 297, 303–304, 305–306, 409

obesity 28, 88, 117, 158, 175, 491; and police violence 353, 354, 361, 365
observational studies 412, 527–528, 529, 553, 554–555
OC (Operation Ceasefire) 119–120
offenders: apprehending of 6–7, 111, 200, 205, 525; prosecuting of 6–7, 20, 459, 460, 498; punishing of 6–7, 112, 119, 205, 208
Office of Juvenile Justice and Delinquency Prevention (OJJDP) 157, 388
online abuse 228, 232, 250
operant conditioning 45, 46
Operation Ceasefire (OC) 119–120
opioid addiction 485–486, 511–512; as criminal justice issue 497–499, 505–506; definition of 486–487; international comparative statistics for 501; nature and extent of 487–488; negative health consequences of 504; paradigm shift in 499–500; policy recommendations for 510–511; prevention of 508–510, 509; as public health issue 500–501, 502–504, 506–507; risk factors for 492–497; roots of 491–492; and social epidemiology 507–508, 508; as social work issue 502–504, 507; types of 488–491
Opioid Affected Youth Initiative 505–506
oppression 52, 55; and LGBTQI+ status 155; racial 58, 155, 354; of women 54, 55
overdose death rate 496
overdose prevention 497; social-ecological model of 508–509, 509

parental physical violence (PPV) 382, 390, 393
parental rights, termination of 163, 164
parenting skills 167, 170, 171, 172, 250, 509–510
parent-to-child family violence 59, 60
partner/spousal rape 191
passive surveillance 10
Patient Protection and Affordable Care Act 273
personal economics 493–494, 509

person-focused proactive law enforcement 460
physical abuse 8788; of children 138–140, 144–145, 161; of elderly 265, 267, 270, 273, 275
physical disability 266, 270, 272, 300
physical violence 60, 104; date-related 241; and intimate partners 228, 243; parental (PPV) 382, 390, 393
place, effect on violence of 55–56
place-based proactive law enforcement 459
police officer recruitment 355
police officer training 355–356
police shootings 81, 441, 442, 459, 463; mandatory federal database of 356–357; and police violence 332, 334, 335, 343, 344, 346, 348, 349, 356
police violence 332–333, 365; against Black male protesters 336–337; against Black males 336–338; as criminal justice issue 348–349, 354–358; definition of 333; and EpiCrim 545–547; international comparative statistics for 350–352; against LGBTQIA 339–341; against media 341; against medics 341; nature and extent of 333–336; negative health consequences of 354; policy recommendations for 364; prevention of 362–363; as public health issue 349–350, 352–353, 358–361; risk factors for 343–348; roots of 341–343; and social epidemiology 361–362; as social work issue 352–353, 360–361; types of 336–341; against women 338–339
poly-victimization, of elders 267
poor neighborhoods 125, 493, 496
pornography 147, 151, 152, 195, 265
positive parenting 150, 167, 170, 171
positive punishment 46
positive reinforcement 45, 46, 124, 150
post-traumatic stress disorder (PTSD) 5, 29, 57, 82, 158; and assaultive violence 101, 105, 108, 112, 118; and firearm injuries 457, 458; and intimate partner violence 230, 239, 242, 244; and police violence 342–343, 345, 354; and rape 203, 204, 207; and sexual assault 203, 204, 207; and suicide 298, 306, 307; and workplace violence 418, 419
poverty 39, 40, 53, 58, 106; and child abuse 143–144, 167; and child sexual abuse 154; and rape 199; and sexual assault 199
power threat theory (PTT) 51–52
PPV (parental physical violence) 382, 390, 393
prescription medications 488–489
prevention 5–6; of assaultive violence (AV) 123–125; of child abuse (CA) 170–173; of crime 8–9; of elderly abuse 282–283; of firearm injuries 468–470; of intimate partner violence (IPV) 249; of opioid addiction 508–510, 509; of overdoses 508–509, 509; of

police violence 362–363; of rape 210–212; of sexual assault 210–212; of suicide 316–317; of teenage bullying (TB) 390–391; of violence 9–11; of workplace violence 424–426

primary care 171, 247, 274, 506, 507, 510

primary deviance 50

prison/jail rape 193

proactive law enforcement 459–460

problem behavior 31, 172, 343–344, 381, 509–510, 530

Problem-Solving Policing (PSP) 8, 21, 359, 460

problem-solving proactive law enforcement 460

proletariat 52–53

prosecution: of offenders 6–7, 20, 459, 460, 498; of parents 163, 164

protective factors 10–11, 12–13, 32, 165; caregiver 283; and violence prevention 421, 463

PSP (Problem-Solving Policing) 8, 21, 359, 460

psychological abuse 228, 406; of children 140; of elderly 265, 266, 267, 268, 271, 273, 275, 285; of intimate partners 228, 230, 240, 244, 250, 541

PTSD *see* post-traumatic stress disorder (PTSD)

PTT (power threat theory) 51–52

public health 5, 9–11, 55; as academic discipline 526; action on 14, 15; and assaultive violence 112–113; and crime 531; and criminology 531–532; definition of 3–4; emergence of 530–531; NCACIA model 167–168; perspectives on violence of 55; for prevention of violence and crime 9–11; and social work 115–116, 160, 203–204, 241–243, 275–277, 310–312, 352–353, 414–418; surveillance 10, 11–15, 21, 75, 165; and violence prevention 120–121

punishment 35; negative 46; of offenders 6–7, 112, 119, 205, 208; positive 46

race, and child abuse 145–146

racial inequality 31, 122, 145–146, 155, 213, 335, 511–512; and firearm injuries 441, 442; and opioid addiction 492–493

racial oppression 58, 155, 354

racial profiling 49, 339, 342, 345, 362

racial stereotypes 345, 347, 348, 355, 356, 359, 362

radical feminist theory 194

RAINN (Rape, Abuse and Incest National Network) 190

random shootings 5, 438

rape 187, 214–215; campus 192–193; as criminal justice issue 200, 205–207; date/acquaintance 192; definition of 188; international comparative statistics for 201–203; jail/prison 193; military 193; nature and extent of 188–190; negative

health consequences of 204–205; policy recommendations for 212–214; prevention of 210–212; as public health issue 200–201, 203–204, 207–209; risk factors for 197–199; roots of 193–197; and social epidemiology 209–210; as social work issue 203–204, 209; spousal/partner 191; statutory 192; stranger 191–192, 540–541; typologies of 191–193

Rape, Abuse and Incest National Network (RAINN) 190

Rape Prevention and Education (RPE) programs 210–211

RAT (routine activity theory) 37, 38–39

rational choice theory (RCT) 36–37, 38

reinforcement: negative 45, 46, 124; positive 45, 46, 124, *150*

relationship risk factors: and assaultive violence 108–109; for elderly abuse 270–271; for firearm injuries 446–448, *447*; for intimate partner violence 235–236; for opioid addiction 495; for police violence 345–346; for rape 198; for sexual assault 198; for sexual violence 198; and suicide 306; for teenage bullying 382; for workplace violence (WPV) 409–410

relationship violence (RV) 306, 405, 409, 414, **417**

Residential SAT (RSAT) for State Prisoners Program 506

RESPECT women 212, 249

rippling effects 126, 240, 524, 544

risk factors 10–11; for assaultive violence (AV) 105–106; for child abuse (CA) 142–147, *148–151*; for elderly abuse 268–273; for firearm injuries 440–449, *444, 445, 447*; for intimate partner violence (IPV) 233–237; for opioid addiction 492–497; for police violence 343–348; for rape 197–199; for sexual assault 197–199; for sexual violence 197–199; for suicide 302–308; for teenage bullying (TB) 380–383; for workplace violence 408–410

risk reduction, and firearm injuries 472–473

routine activity theory (RAT) 37, 38–39

RPE (Rape Prevention and Education) programs 210–211

RSAT (Residential SAT) for State Prisoners Program 506

ruralness 272–273

RV (relationship violence) 306, 405, 409, 414, **417**

safe storage 468, 469, 470

safety planning 203, 311, 315, 420, 469

schizophrenia 37, 300, 305, 486

school shootings 80, 438–439, 450, 453, 457, 548

SDI (sociodemographic index) profiles 455

SDI (suicide and death ideation) 302–303
secondary deviance 50
Section 1983 litigation 355, 357
self-control theory 194, 195–196
sentinel surveillance 10, 506, 510
SES *see* socioeconomic status (SES)
sexist social norms 199
sexual abuse: of children 141; elder 265–266
sexual aggression 194, 197, 198
sexual assault 187, 214–215; as criminal justice
     issue 200, 205–207; definition of 188; and
     EpiCrim 540–541; international comparative
     statistics for 201–203; nature and extent
     of 188–190; negative health consequences
     of 204–205; policy recommendations for
     212–214; prevention of 210–212; as public
     health issue 200–201, 203–204, 207–209; risk
     factors for 197–199; roots of 193–197; and
     social epidemiology 209–210; as social work
     issue 203–204, 209; typologies of 191–193
sexual orientation 102, 190, 297, 299, 341,
     376, 377, 378–379
sexual violence, and intimate partners 228–229
sexually transmitted infections (STIs), public
     health approaches to 16–18
shame 34–35, 49, 140, 145, 188–189, 200,
     212–213, 285, 299, 312, 539
situational causes, of violence 33, 34, 37
smart gun technology 469
smoking, public health approaches to 16–18
social bonds 48–49
social conflict theories 35, 51–55, 60–61
social control 40, 52, 55; informal mechanisms
     of 198, 236; negative 405; theory of 48, 49
social disorganization theory 39–40
social epidemiology: of assaultive violence (AV)
     122–123; of child abuse (CA) 166–170; of
     elderly abuse 281–282; of firearm injuries
     466–468; of intimate partner violence (IPV)
     248; of opioid addiction 507–508; of police
     violence 361–362; of rape 209–210; of
     sexual assault 209–210; of suicide 315–316;
     of teenage bullying (TB) 390; of workplace
     violence 422–424
social inequality 35, 122, 147, 209–210, 248,
     440, 508, 533
social isolation *see* isolation
social learning theory 195
social norms 49, 110, 211, 247, 249, 250, 526,
     533, 552; sexist 199; for parental support
     170–171, 173; and teenage bullying 377, 379
social problems, caused by violence 61–63, *61*
social process theories 44–51, *48*
social stressors 59, 60
social structure theories 39–44
social work: and public health 115–116, 160,
     203–204, 241–243, 275–277, 310–312,

352–353, 386–387, 414–418; and violence
     prevention 121
social-ecological model 61–62, *61*, 107–111,
     246, 423; and assaultive violence 107–111; of
     substance use and overdose prevention
     508–509, *509*
socialization causes, of violence 33, 34, 44, 108,
     124, 542
societal risk factors: for assaultive violence
     110–111; for child abuse 147; for intimate
     partner violence 236–237; for police violence
     346–348; for rape 198–199; for sexual assault
     198–199; for sexual violence 198–199
sociodemographic index (SDI) profiles 455
socioeconomic inequality 147, 199, 214, 492
socioeconomic status (SES) 4, 28, 29, 199, 233,
     268–269, 440, 533; and access to healthcare
     90, 94; and bullying 381–382; and child
     abuse *148*, 154, 166, 170, 174
sociological model, of violence 35
spousal/partner rape 191
SPRC (Suicide Prevention Resource Center) 309,
     312–313, 316, 469
stalking 304, 377, *411*, 419, 420; cyber- 232;
     and intimate partner violence 230–231,
     238–239, 241, 244
statutory rape 192
stereotypes 174, 175, 189, 191, 205, 206, 212,
     213; cultural 43–44, 344, 378; gender 249;
     racial 345, 347, 348, 355, 356, 359, 362
stigma 77, 155, 162, 189, 241, 297, 299, 302,
     308, 315, 318, 507, 510, 531, 539
STIs (sexually transmitted infections), public
     health approaches to 16–18
strain theories 40–43
stranger rape 191–192, 540–541
street drugs 491, 496, 497, 511; *see also* illegal
     drugs
stressors, for violence 55–60
stroke 28, 101, 112, 116, 161, 242, 419
structural inequality 247, 249, 346, 347, 361,
     440–441, 448
substance use: social-ecological model of
     508–509, *509*; and suicide 305–306; *see also*
     alcohol use; opioid addiction
suicidal violence, and EpiCrim 543–545, *556*
suicide 295–318; of adolescents 298; of
     American Indians and Alaskan natives (AI/
     AN) 303–304; of Black adults 302–303; of
     Black youth 298–299, 302–303; as criminal
     justice issue 308–309, 312–314; definition
     of 295–296; and elder abuse 277–278;
     of Hispanic youth 299; international
     comparative statistics for 310; interpersonal
     theory of 302, 306; of LGBTQ youth
     299; of LGBTQIA adults 297–298; of
     military personnel 299–301; negative health

consequences of 312; policy recommendations for 317; prevention of 316–317; as public health issue 309–310, 314–315; risk factors for 302–308; as social work issue 315
suicide and death ideation (SDI) 302–303
suicide attempts 117, 235, 265, 278, 353, 381, 387, 443, 495, 543–544, 545; and suicide 295, 296, 297, 298, 299, 301, 303, 304, 306, 312, 314, 316, 317, 318
suicide clusters 307
suicide ideation 230, 244, 278, 353, 443; and suicide 295, 296, 297, 298, 299, 302, 311, 312, 316; and teenage bullying 381, 384, 385, 393
suicide plans 299, 318, 443–444
Suicide Prevention Resource Center (SPRC) 309, 312–313, 316, 469
Surgeon General 19, 101, 388, 389, 438, 453, 471–472, 474, 503–504
surveillance 9–10; active 10, 21; of child abuse 165; passive 10; public health 10, 11–15, 21, 75, 165; sentinel 10, 506, 510; syndromic 10
syndromic surveillance 10
systemic factors, of violence 58

teenage bullying (TB) 375–376, 392–393; against Asians 378; against Blacks 378; as criminal justice issue 383–384, 387–388; definition of 376; international comparative statistics for 385–386; against LGBTQIA 378–379; nature and extent of 376–378; negative health consequences of 387; policy recommendations for 391–392; prevention of 390–391; as public health issue 384–385, 386–387, 388–390; risk factors for 380–383; roots of 379–380; and social epidemiology 390; as social work issue 386–387, 389–390; types of 378–379
teenage violence 246, 556; and EpiCrim 547–548
theoretical causes, of violence 26–27, 33–35
tool in commission of crime 438
transgender population 104, 193, 232, 233, 297, 299, 332, 339, 340, 379, 392
trauma and violence-informed care (TVIC) 121
trauma-informed interventions 167
TVIC (trauma and violence-informed care) 121
Type 2 diabetes 28, 29, 161

unemployment 8, 35, 40, 109, 116, 147, 199, 315, 409–410, 510, 537, 539

United Nations Office on Drugs (UNODC) 114, 496, 501
U.S. Centers for Medical & Mediciad Services 90
upper class 41, 43, 44, 53–54, 110

Veterans Treatment Court Program 505
vicarious trauma 119
victimization 35, 73–94; violent 101, 102, 118, 189, 191, 194
violence, definition of 2
Violence Against Women Act 209, 210–211, 238
violence prevention: public health approaches to 120–121; social work approaches to 121
violent crime 101; etiological causes of 26–27; rates of 1–2, 113
violent delinquency 233
violent victimization 101, 102, 118, 189, 191, 194
vital statistics 12, 76–77, 79, 80, 93, 170

water contamination 3
weapons: and intimate partner violence 227; *see also* firearm injuries; guns
White privilege 52
women: inequalities 54, 245; minority 105–106, 226–227; oppression of 54, 55
working class 53
workplace violence (WPV) 402, 428; as criminal justice issue 410–412, *411*, 419–420; definition of 402–403; and EpiCrim 548–550; international comparative statistics for 413–414; nature and extent of 403–404; negative health consequences of 418–419; policy recommendations for 426–428; prevention of 424–426; as public health issue 412–413, 414–418, 420–422; risk factors for 408–410; roots of 406–407; and social epidemiology 422–424; as social work issue 414–418, 421–422; types of 404–406
World Report on Violence and Health 27
WPV *see* workplace violence (WPV)
wrongful death lawsuits 357–358

youth homicide rate 547–548
youth violence 80, 117, 118, 384, 390, 391, 392, 465, 547, 548

zone of transition 40

For Product Safety Concerns and Information please contact our EU
representative GPSR@taylorandfrancis.com
Taylor & Francis Verlag GmbH, Kaufingerstraße 24, 80331 München, Germany

www.ingramcontent.com/pod-product-compliance
Lightning Source LLC
Chambersburg PA
CBHW080127270326
41926CB00021B/4386